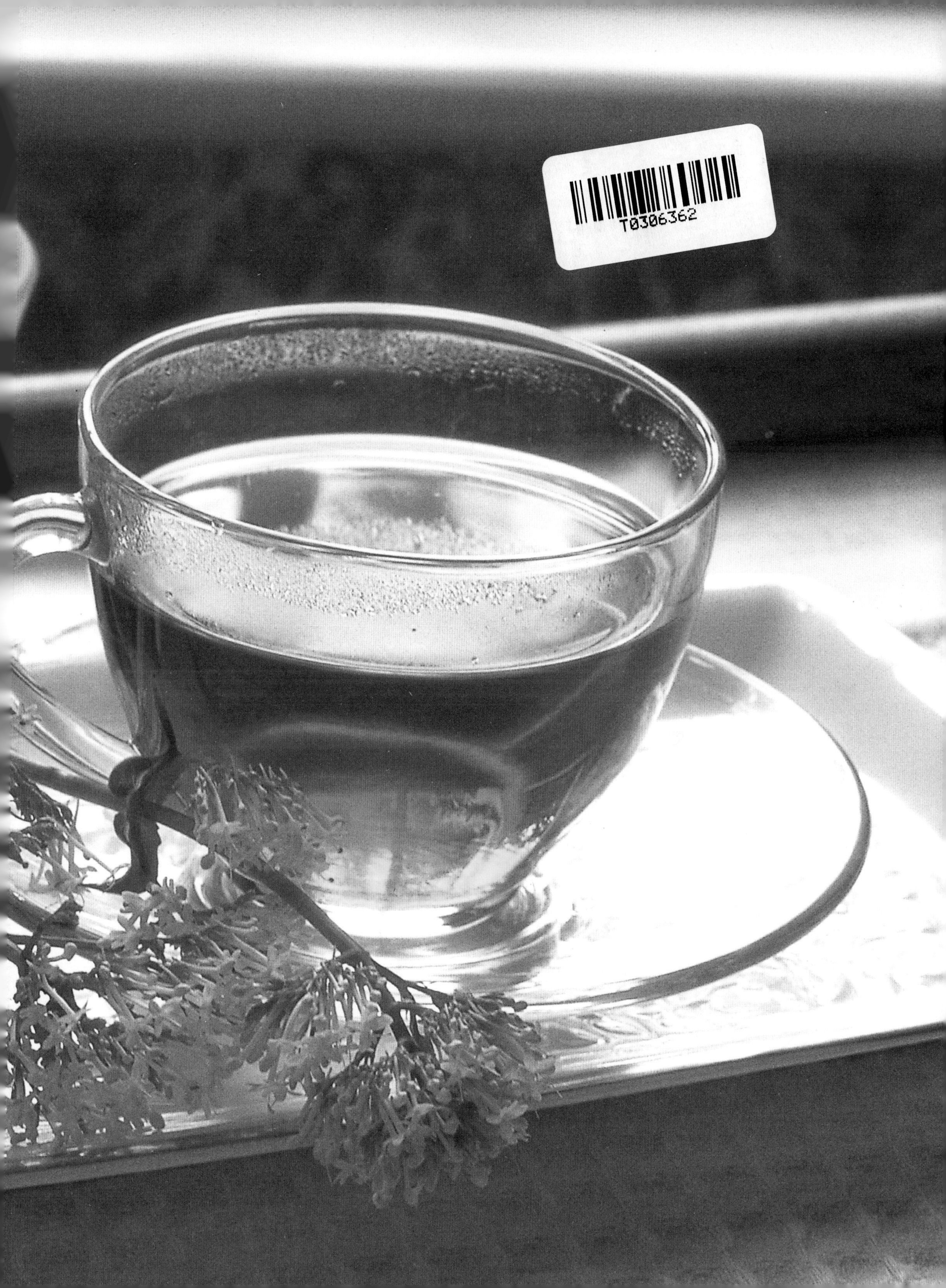

HERBAL
HOME REMEDIES

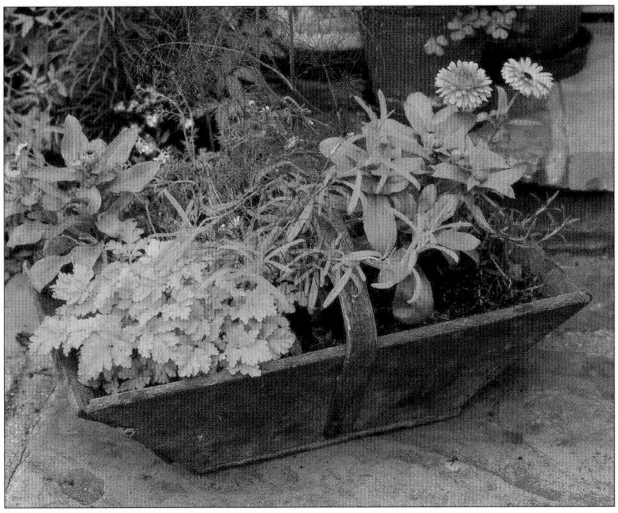

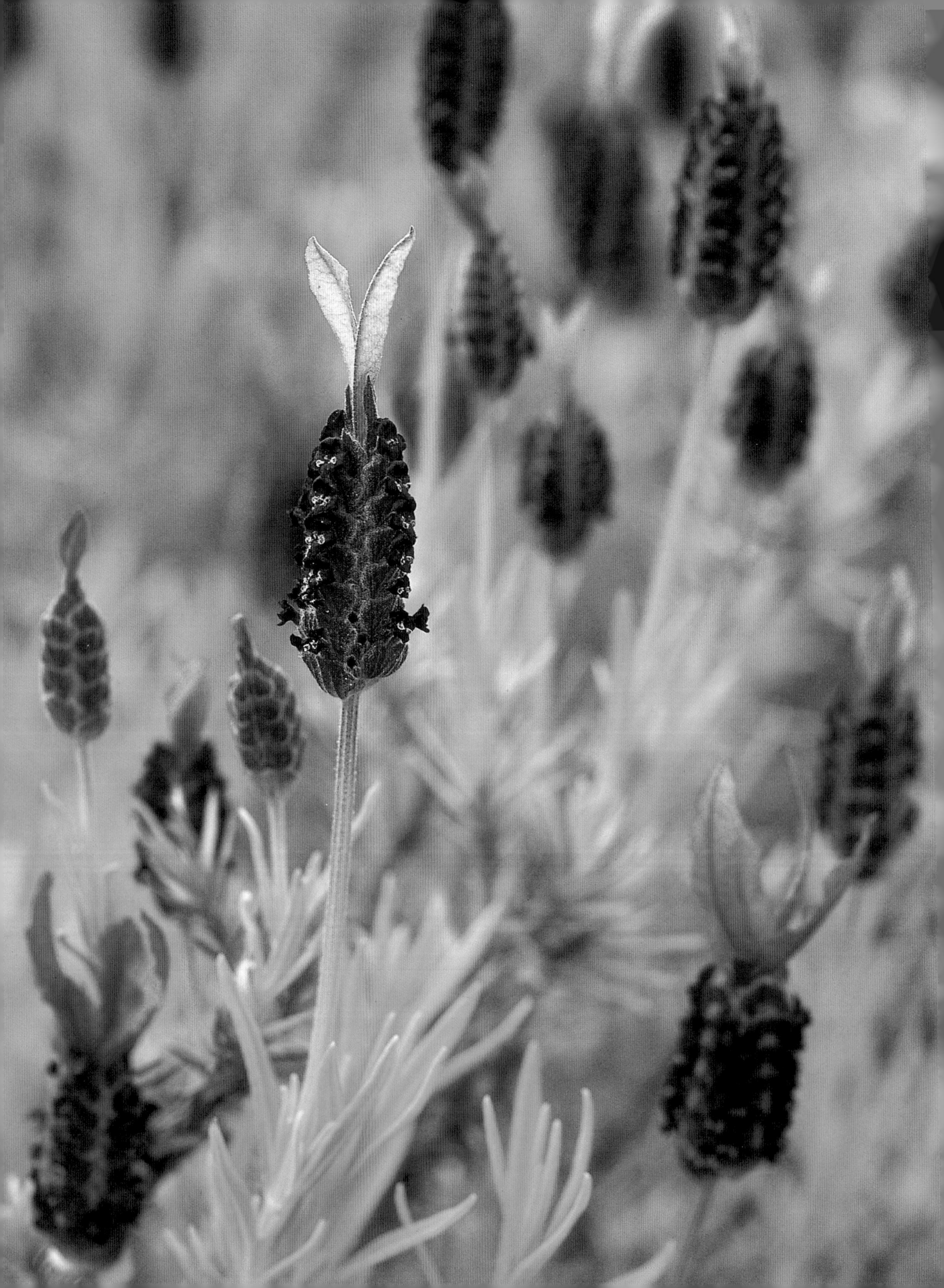

HERBAL HOME REMEDIES

Simple instructions for mixing and preparing herbs for traditional remedies that can help relieve common ailments, shown in more than 750 photographs

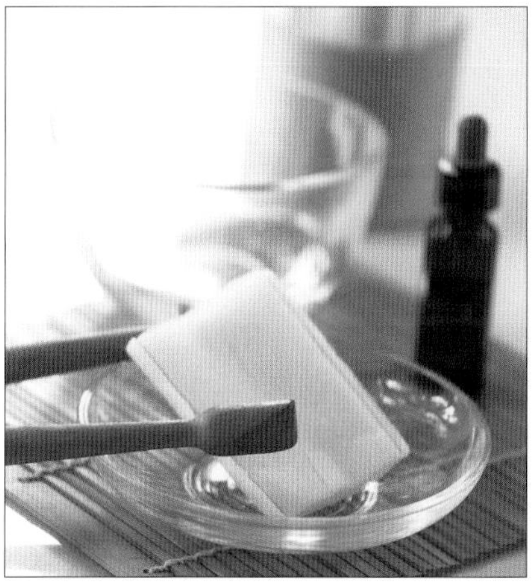

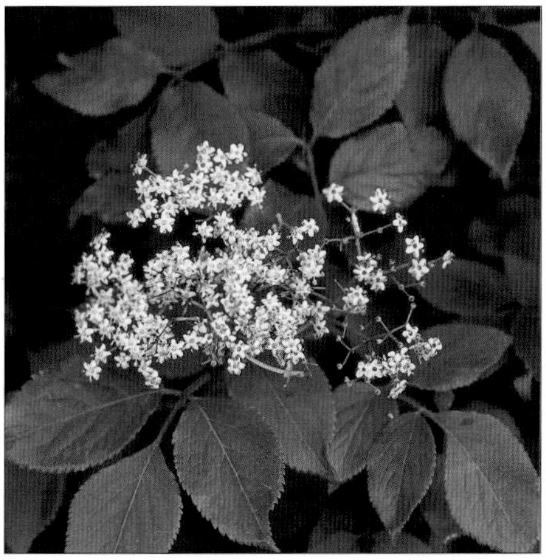

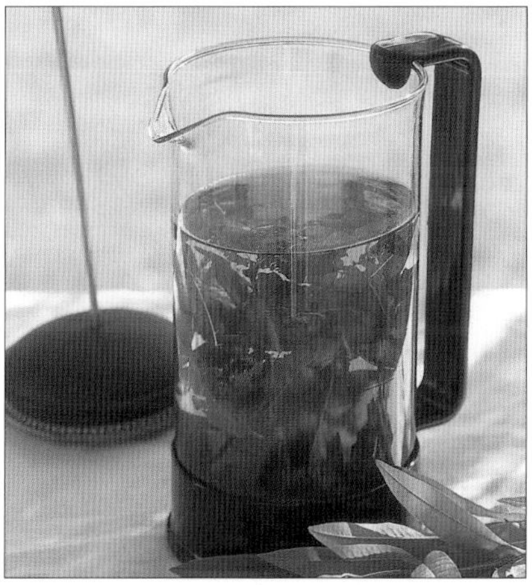

Includes a comprehensive botanical A–Z encyclopedia of 235 herbs, with clear descriptions of the general and medicinal uses of each one

JESSICA HOUDRET

LORENZ BOOKS

CONTENTS

This edition is published by Lorenz Books
an imprint of Anness Publishing Ltd
info@anness.com
www.lorenzbooks.com
www.annesspublishing.com

Publisher: Joanna Lorenz
Editorial director: Helen Sudell
Editor: Simona Hill
Text updates: Clare Goulding
Designer: Nigel Partridge
Production controller: Ben Worley

A CIP catalogue record for this book is available from the British Library.

PUBLISHER'S NOTE

This book is intended as a source of information on herbs and their uses, and does not provide recommendations as a replacement for professional medical advice and treatment. The publishers and the author cannot accept responsibility for any specific individual's reactions, nor for any harmful or ill effects or damage, arising from the use of the general data and suggestions this book contains, whether in remedy form or otherwise. Nor is any responsibility taken for mistaken identity or inappropriate use of any of the plants. It is always advisable to consult a medical practitioner or qualified medical herbalist before using herbal treatments or remedies, particularly if you are pregnant, suffering from an ongoing medical condition or taking any other medication.

ABOUT THE AUTHORS

Jessica Houdret was a long-standing member and past Chairman of the Herb Society and for many years was on the council of the British Herb Trade Association. Jessica wrote articles on herbs for national publications and wrote many books on herbs and herb gardening, including *The Home Apothecary* and the *Ultimate Book of Herbs and Herb Gardening*.

Claire Goulding, MNIMH is a Medical Herbalist, Facilitator and Aromatherapist based in the southwest of England, with over 15 years of experience working in education, environmental conservation and the complementary therapy sector. Claire holds a BSc (Hons) in Clinical Herbalism and runs a specialist Women's Health Clinic in Bristol and online for Napiers. www.learnbotanics.co.uk

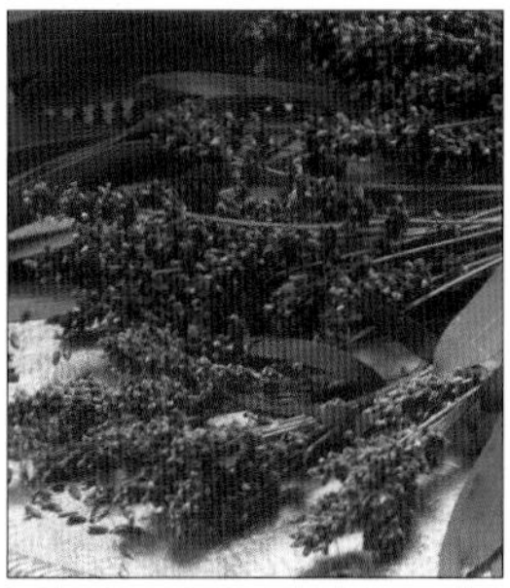

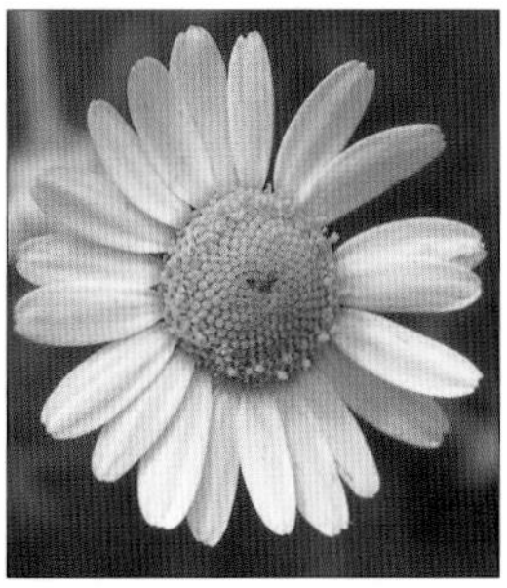

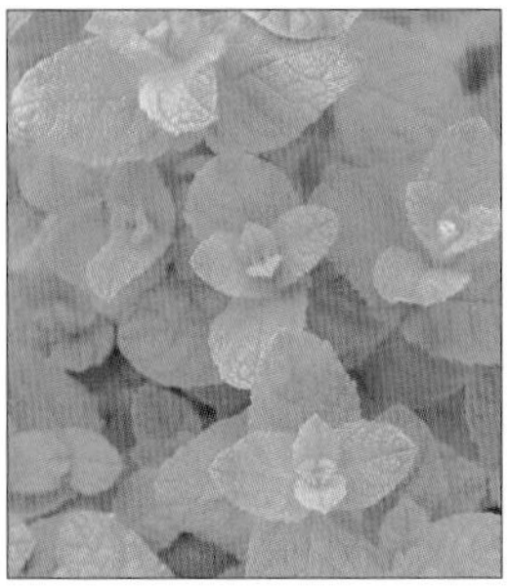

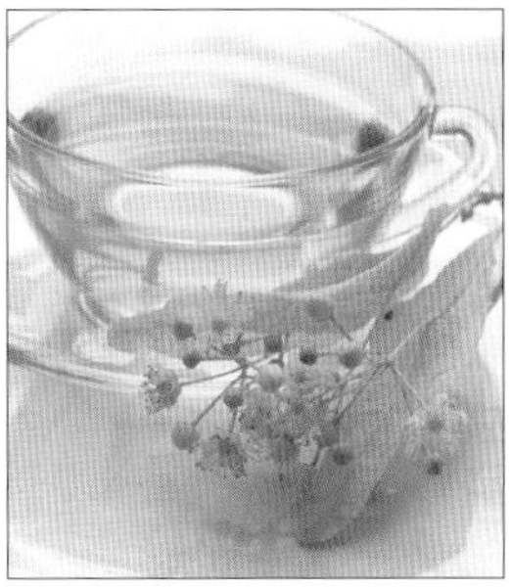

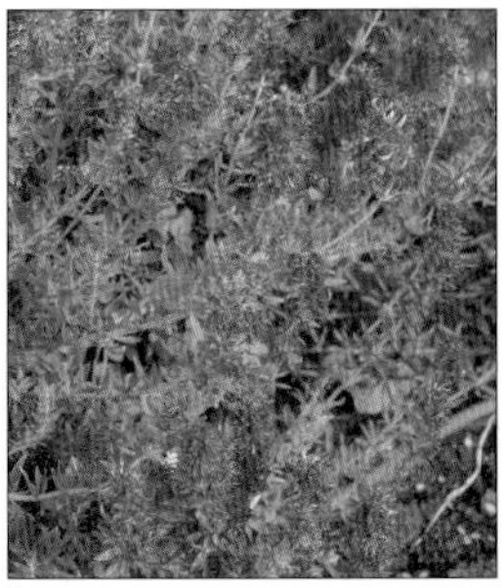

Introduction

Herbs and home remedies can play a major role in promoting health and well-being. They are often effective in alleviating the symptoms of everyday illnesses, such as coughs and colds or aches and pains, and are useful as first aid for a range of minor accidents, from cuts and grazes to insect bites and stings.

This book is intended as a practical guide to using herbs in the home as part of a healthy way of living. In order to do so to best advantage, it helps to understand how herbal remedies work and why.

Self-treatment is sensible and appropriate for everyday ailments, or for relieving the discomfort of ongoing conditions that are not critical. However, for more serious problems it should never take the place of professional medical advice. If you stub your toe, a comfrey poultice is a good way to take away the pain, but if you develop bronchitis or pneumonia, you must consult your doctor.

Herbal medicine may also be appropriate where a specific condition is not responding to orthodox medical treatment. But in such a case self-treatment is again unwise, and you should consult a qualified herbal practitioner for proper advice on which herbal treatments would be best for your individual requirements.

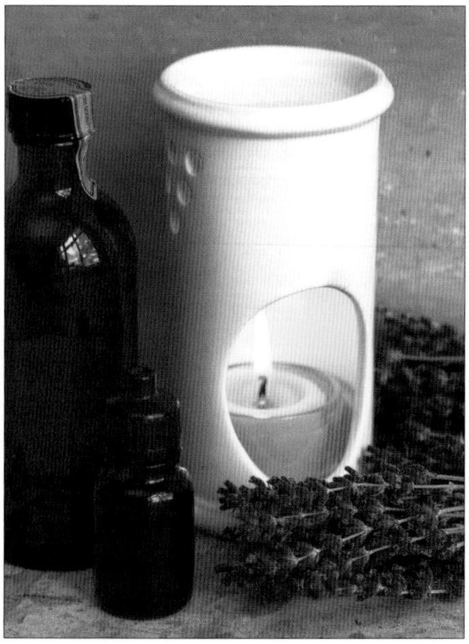

Left *Essential oils, such as lavender, can be used in aromatherapy to lift the mood and aid relaxation.*

How herbal remedies work

Plants have been used as medicine for centuries, and modern research has confirmed the therapeutic properties of many. Some contain potent alkaloids and other constituents, which is why they work effectively and why many of them form the basis of modern pharmaceutical drugs. It is also why some of them may interact with pharmaceutical drugs. But there is a difference between using the most powerful constituent of a herb, isolated and extracted in a laboratory and usually synthesized (as in pharmaceutical drugs), and using a home preparation made from the whole plant. Herbs should always be used with care in home remedies, and warnings respected.

The constituents of herbs cause them to act on the body in a variety of ways. Some have a sedative action; others are stimulants. There are those that enhance the circulation of blood, and those with an astringent action, which means that they constrict bodily tissues and are useful in healing cuts and wounds. Some herbs have a detoxifying effect, helping to eliminate toxins and waste from the system, and some stimulate digestion and aid the absorption of nutrients. Many more fight infections, due to their antiseptic, antibacterial or antifungal properties, and a few have more complex actions, such as regulating hormonal activity.

Herbal remedies remain a valuable resource for many minor ills, but it would be foolish to ignore scientific advances and not to take advantage of modern medical knowledge when dealing with more serious health conditions.

Herbs for general well-being

No alternative therapy should be seen as a quick cure-all to be taken in isolation. For herbal remedies to have any impact they must be part of a healthy lifestyle. It's a question of "rounding up all the usual suspects": paying attention to diet, not smoking, not drinking too much, taking exercise and regulating stress by finding time for relaxation techniques.

This is where herbs also play an important role. They are vital as agents for maintaining general well-being. Incorporating them in food adds flavour and interest, making it easier to keep to a healthy diet, as well as providing an opportunity to benefit from their intrinsic properties. In beauty products they provide the ingredients for a range of simple preparations to make at home, which may be used to supplement or replace commercially manufactured beauty products, many of which can contain potentially harmful chemicals. These may be present in only small amounts in each individual product, but the effect can be cumulative, and changing to a herbal beauty regime is all part of a healthy lifestyle based on holistic principles.

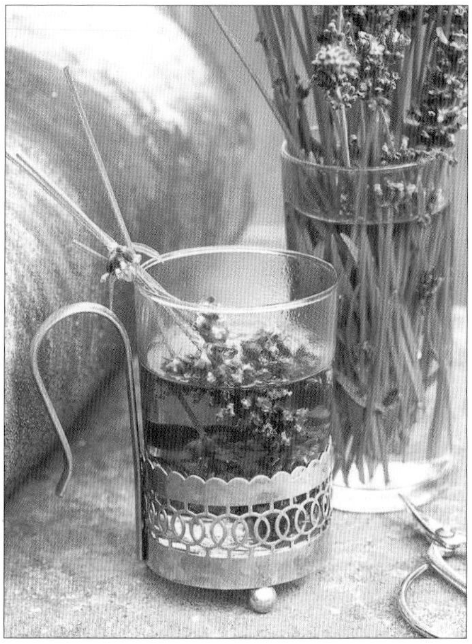

Above *Infusions are a simple way to enjoy the benefits of herbs.*

Right *Dried leafy herbs and flowers have plenty of uses around the home as well as having a therapeutic use in many herbal remedies. Growing herbs, harvesting, drying and then using them is rewarding and can be life-enhancing.*

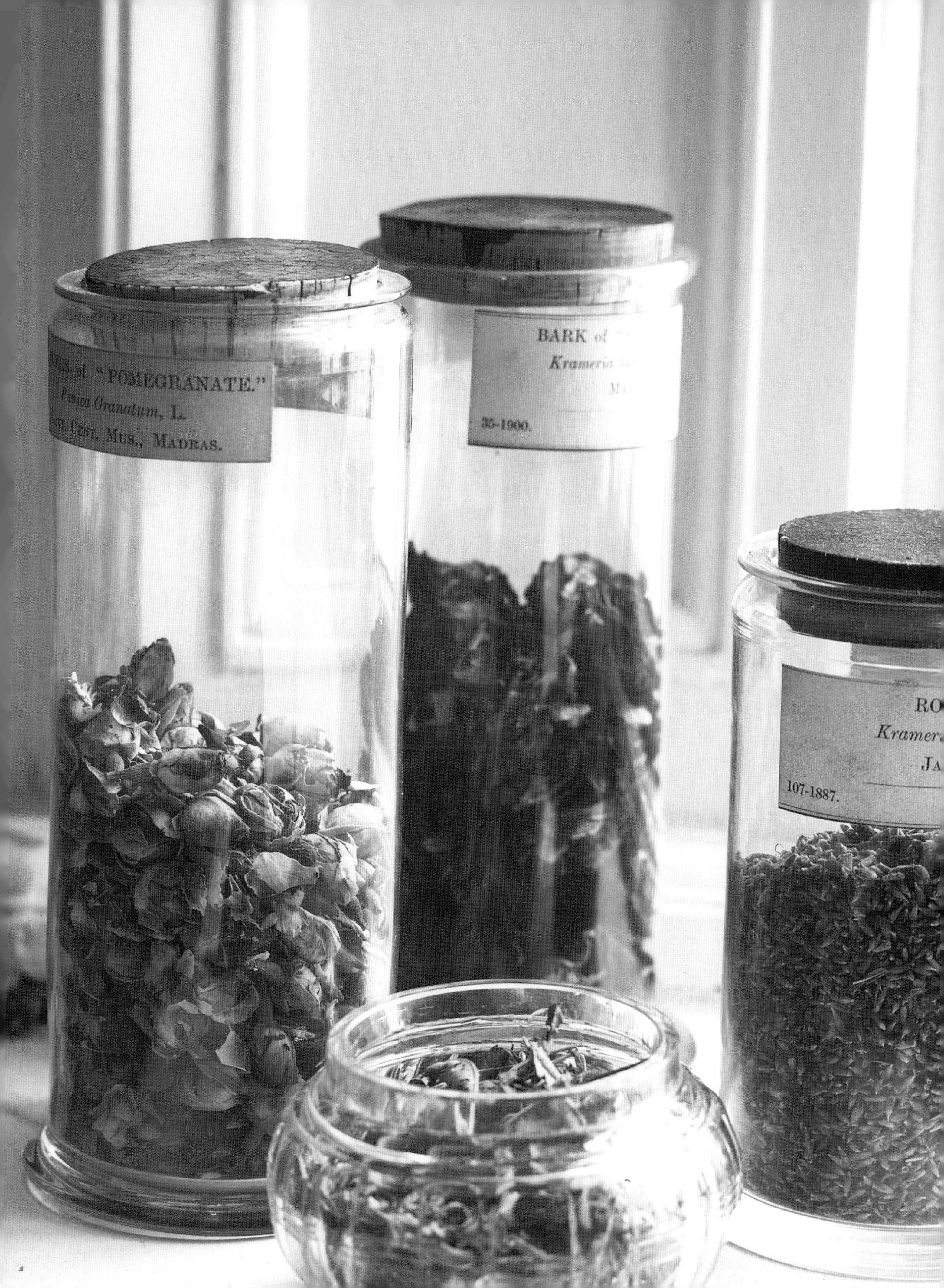

of "POMEGRANATE."
Punica Granatum, L.
CENT. MUS., MADRAS.
BARK of
Krameria
35-1900.
107-1887.

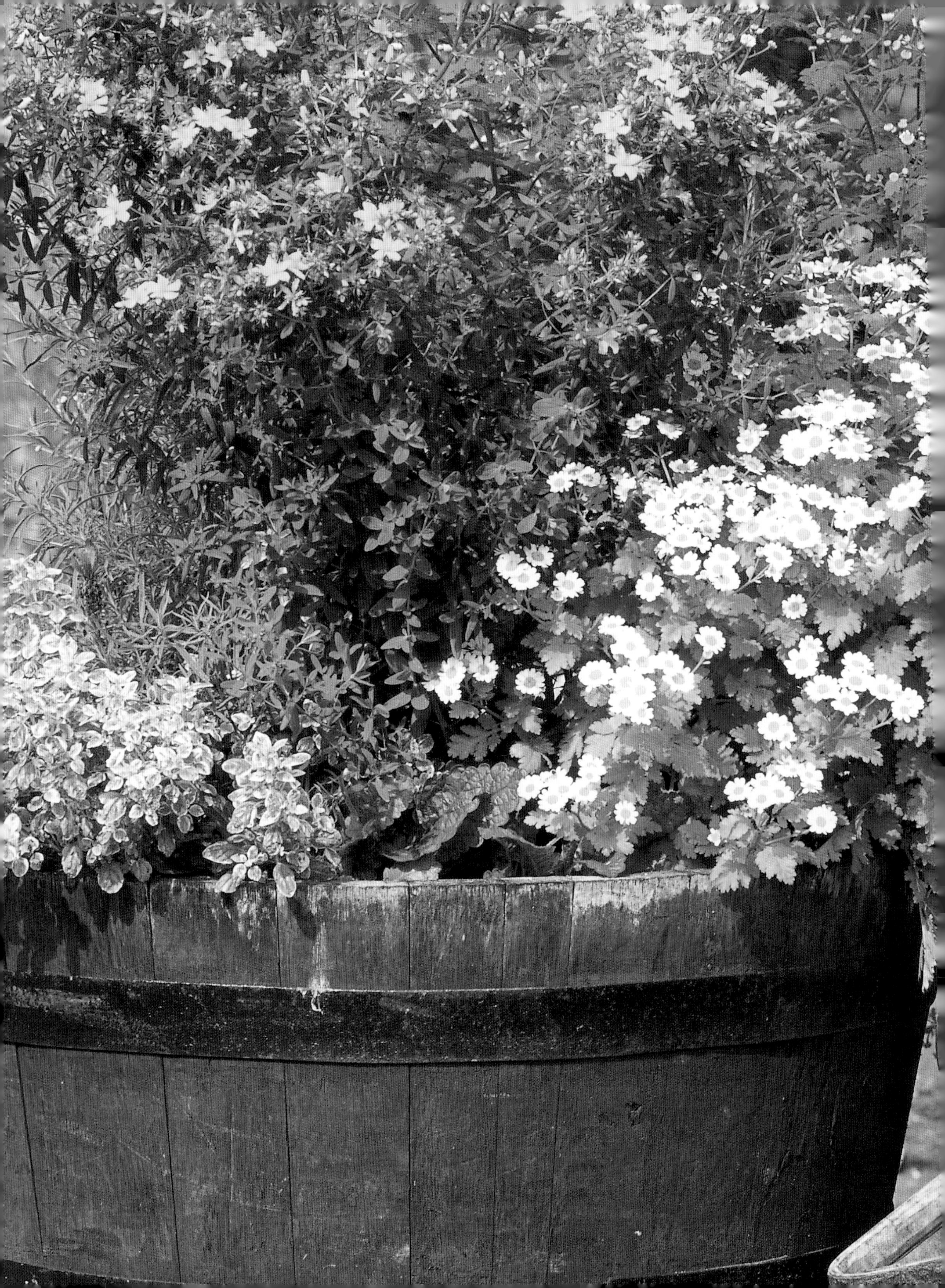

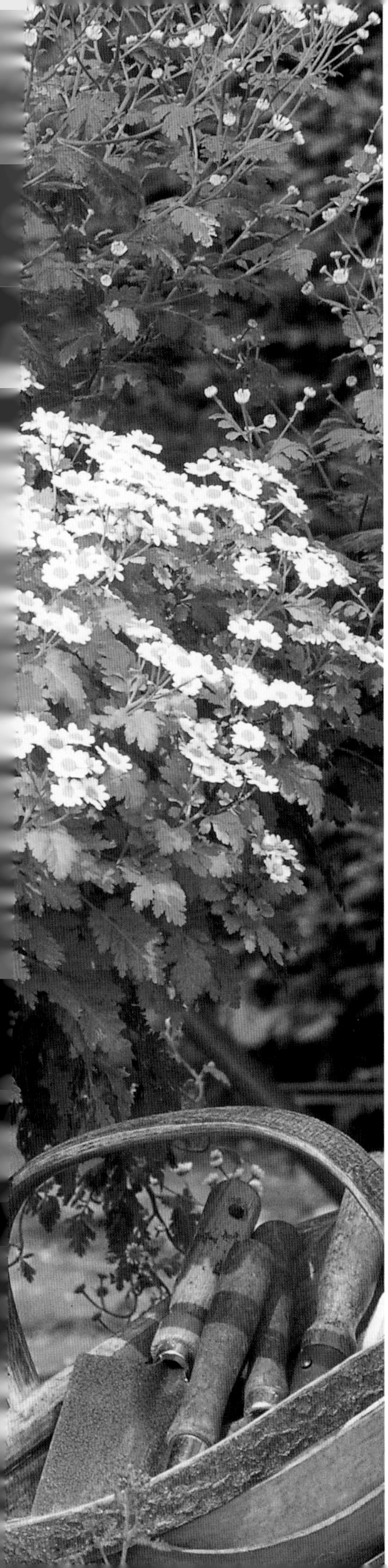

Using Medicinal Herbs

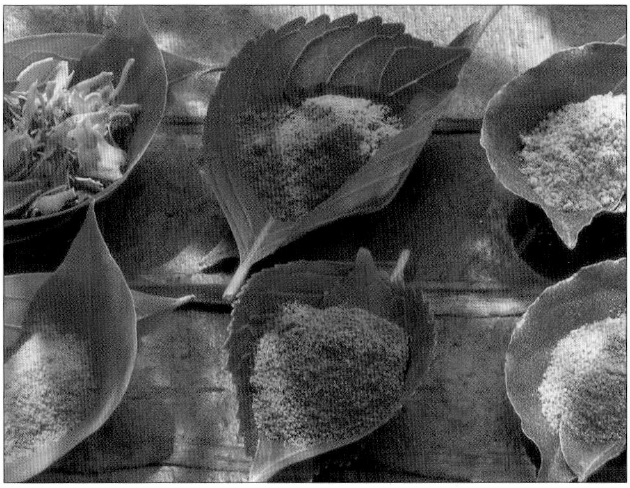

Medicinal herbs have been used throughout history to cure ills and promote well-being. Despite huge advances in modern medical science, they remain popular today, with 80 per cent of the world's population relying on herbal medicine for primary healthcare. Safety is an important issue, however, and it should be stressed that these plants are effective because they contain potent constituents. Dosages, diagnosis and quality of product are crucial and it is vital to remember that herbs can interact with pharmaceutical drugs. If in doubt as to what to take and when, professional guidance should be sought. Used sensibly and with care, medicinal herbs can greatly add to the quality of life.

Above *Many herbs and spices have antibacterial properties.*

Left *Growing herbs can be an attractive talking point in the garden, as well as providing fresh material for your medicinal requirements.*

A History of Herbal Medicine

Plants are the basis of life. They supply us with oxygen and are the primary source of food for the animal kingdom. They have also been used as medicines, probably since humans first roamed the earth and certainly since civilizations began.

There is ample evidence of the medicinal use of herbs in antiquity by the Egyptians, from papyri and inscriptions in tombs and temples, dating back as far as 2800BC. The oldest complete herbal comes from China, written around 200BC and credited to the legendary Yellow Emperor, Huang Ti; Ayurvedic medicine, from India, is another long-standing system based on herbs.

In ancient Greece, herbal medicine was widely practised and recorded; and in Rome, Dioscorides, a Greek physician living there in the first century AD, produced *De Materia Medica*, a herbal describing 600 plants and their healing properties. It became the standard work on the subject and influenced European herbalism for the next 1,500 years. After the fall of the Roman Empire, herbal knowledge persisted and prospered in Christian monasteries. In Britain during this period, Anglo-Saxon writings show a wide knowledge of herbs and evidence of correspondence with centres in Europe.

During the 10th century, Avicenna, an Arab polymath, was the first to produce attar of roses by distillation and was instrumental in the discovery of plant essential oils. In the medieval period, European crusaders trying to seize the Holy Land from Muslim control brought home new herbs and spices from the Middle East that became part of the herbal canon.

The 16th and 17th centuries saw further advances in the study of the healing properties of plants. This was the age of the great herbalists (including Gerard, Parkinson, Clusius and Dodoens) in Britain and throughout Europe. It was also the era of the New World explorations, when many plants that had long been used by Native Americans in their traditional medicine were brought to Europe. Seeds and plants, including such familiar plants as parsley, savory and thyme, were taken the opposite way, too, by the early American colonists.

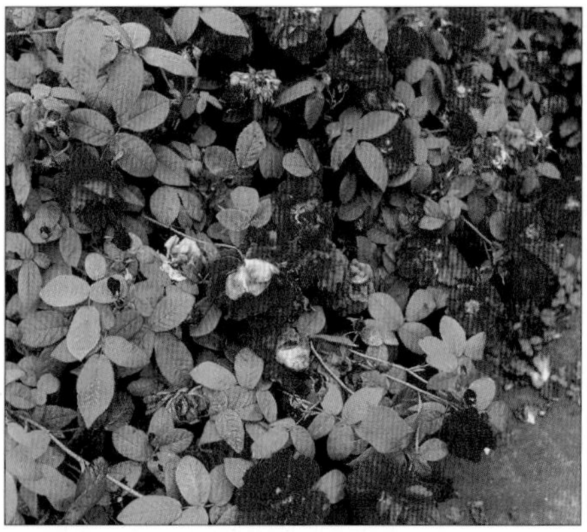

Left *The apothecary's rose (*R. gallica officinalis*) was used in the Middle Ages to relieve indigestion, rashes and sore throats.*

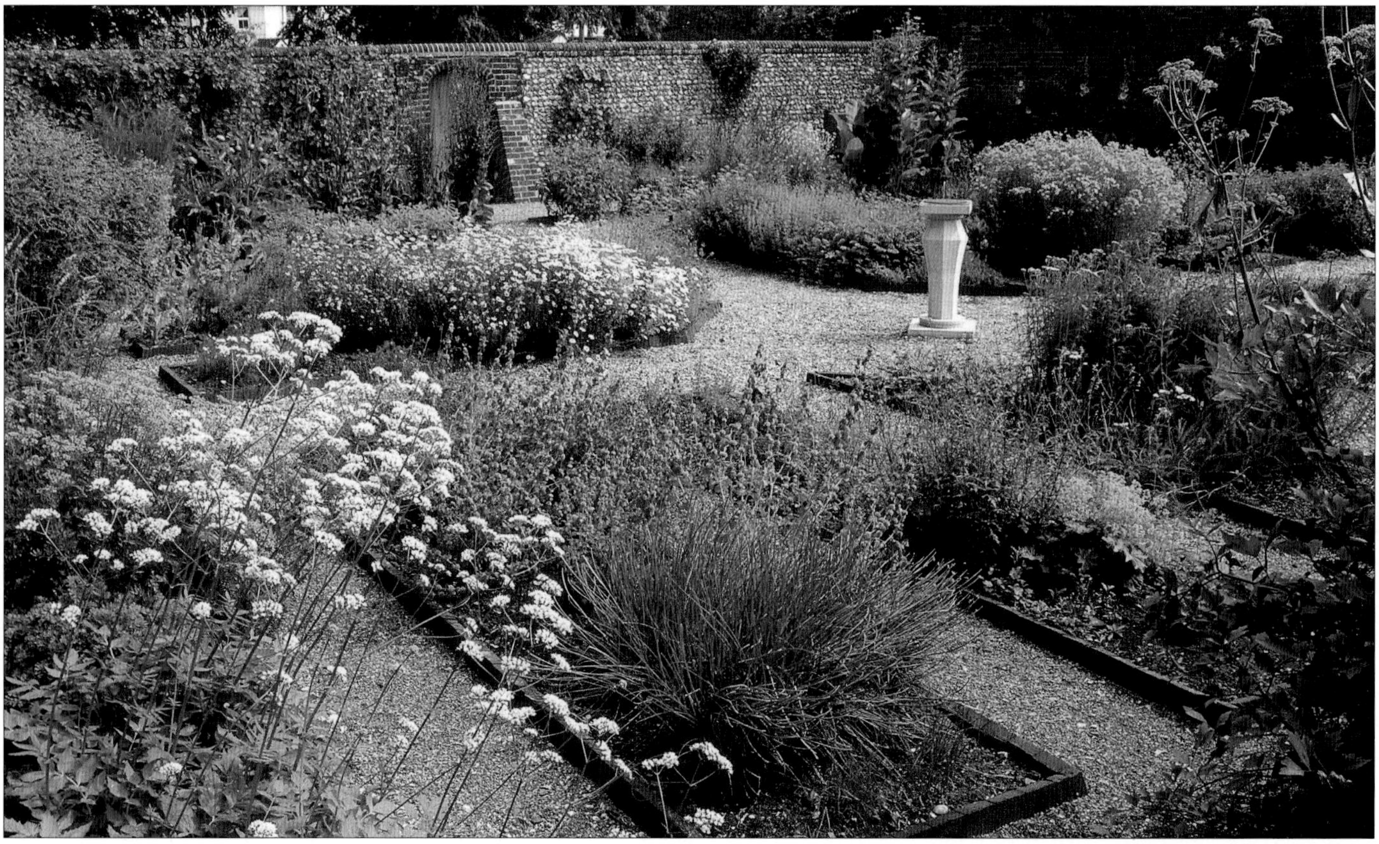

Below *In medieval gardens, herbs were grown in small rectangular beds for ease of harvesting.*

Until the 18th century, botany and medicine were closely allied, but with the rise of modern scientific enquiry they drew apart as separate disciplines. During the 19th century the medical establishment turned away from plant-based remedies, and synthetic drugs, produced in the laboratory, began their ascendancy. This is not to say that the old herbal remedies entirely disappeared: traditions were kept alive, especially in rural areas, and in much of Europe they never fell completely out of use. The history of herbs adds up to a long tradition of use and a large body of accumulated knowledge.

Herbal medicine today

New research has endorsed much of the traditional knowledge, in that many herbs have been found to possess therapeutic properties and to have a powerful effect on the way the body functions. Some previously accepted ideas and theories have lost credibility, and some old recipes and ingredients seem quaint or far-fetched by modern standards, but much remains valid.

World Health Organization figures reveal that 80 per cent of the world's population currently relies on herbal medicine for primary health care. In some poorer countries it is the only option for many people, but in the more affluent nations an interest in herbal medicine is steadily increasing. In the UK up to 40 per cent of people are said to use herbal remedies on a regular basis; in Australia the proportion is thought to be even higher, and in the USA it is claimed that one in five Americans now uses some form of alternative therapy, compared with one in fifty in 1990. Germany is a world centre for phyto-medicine (or plant-based medicine) and much research is carried out there.

Many herbs work well as remedies because they contain potent substances. Plants are, after all, the basis of many modern pharmaceutical drugs. Aspirin, originally derived from meadowsweet following the isolation of salicylic acid (also present in willow bark), is one of the best known. Key anti-cancer agents have been derived from plants, with more than 50 per cent of cancer drugs based at least to some extent on natural plant sources: taxol, from yew, is a well-known example.

Herbs and pharmaceutical drugs

Pharmaceutical drugs that are derived from plants are made by extracting a single active constituent from the plant source, which is then synthesized in the laboratory for mass manufacture.

Herbal remedies are different in that they use the whole plant (or the whole of a part of it, such as the leaves or the roots) in extracts containing hundreds or thousands of constituents, which all work together to produce a balanced effect.

For example, pharmaceutical diuretic drugs reduce the potassium level in the body, which then has to be restored with potassium supplements. A herbal preparation for the same purpose might be made with dandelion leaves, which have a diuretic action but also contain potassium to replace any that is lost.

As home treatments, herbs and herbal products are most appropriate when taken to relieve the symptoms of conditions which will heal by themselves over time.

Plants as sources of pharmaceutical drugs

Plant	Constituent	Drug
• *Mentha* spp (Mint)	Menthol	Used in throat lozenges and respiratory medicaments
• *Gaultheria procumbens* (Wintergreen)	Methylsalicylate	Used in ointments for rheumatic conditions
• *Digitalis purpurea* (Foxglove)	Digitoxin	Heart condition medication
• *Cinchona* spp	Quinine	First anti-malarial drug
• *Catharanthus roseus* (Madagascan periwinkle)	Vinblastine, vincristine	Anti-cancer drugs for leukaemia and Hodgkin's disease
• *Taxus brevifolia* (Yew)	Taxol	Anti-cancer drug
• *Rauwolfia serpentina*	Reserpine	Anti-hypertensive drug and sedative
• *Curarea* spp (Curare)	Tubocurarine	Muscle relaxant

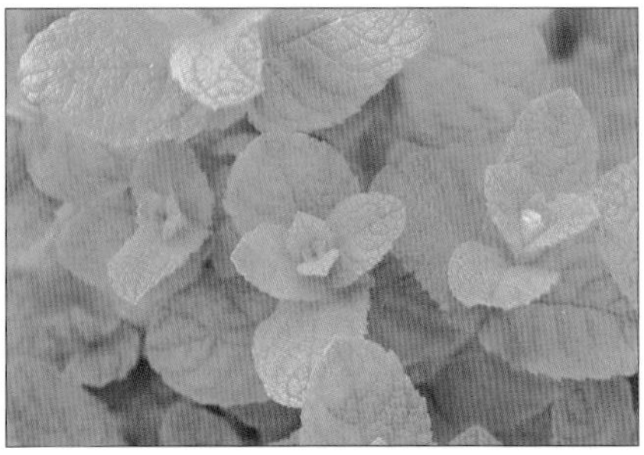

Above *Menthol is a major constituent of mint.*

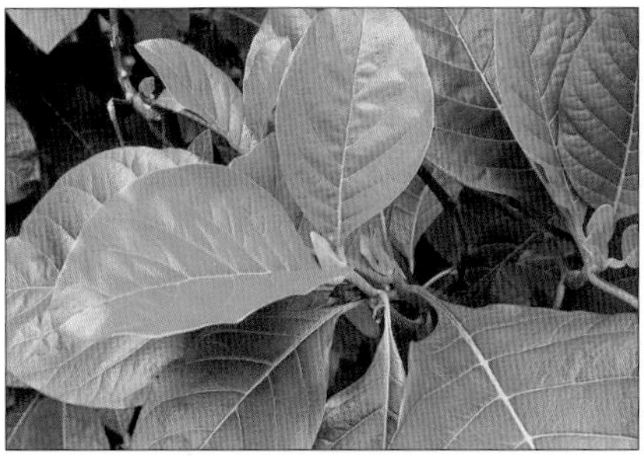

Above *Quinine is derived from* Cinchona *spp.*

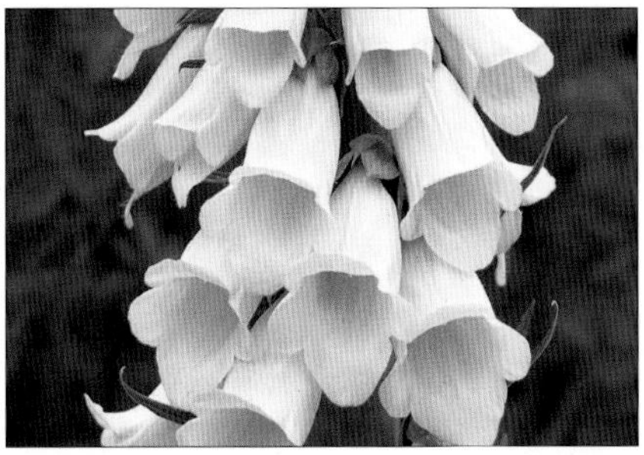

Above *Foxglove is the source of digitoxin.*

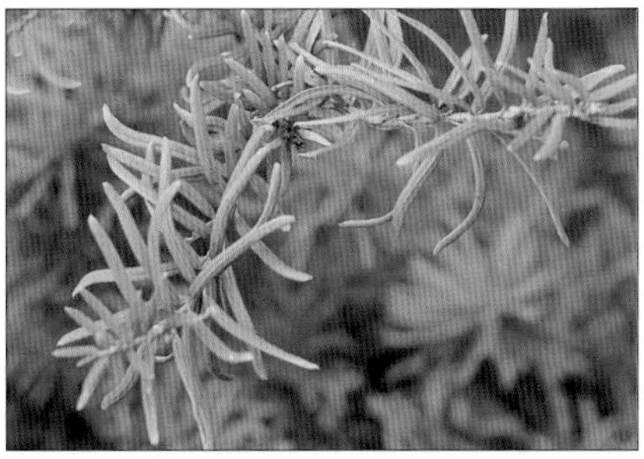

Above *Yew provides the cancer drug taxol.*

How Safe are Herbal Remedies?

There is a lot of controversy over the safety of herbal remedies, with new research constantly highlighting potential risks and previously unsuspected side effects. It is as well to remember that this also applies to medical drugs, food and drink, and many of the products we use in our everyday lives. Reports appear, almost daily, on newly discovered health risks in these areas.

If taken with due care and in the correct dosage, herbal remedies have a good safety record. Self-diagnosis and self-treatment can be hazardous however, and there are a number of factors to take into account before taking any herbal remedies. None of the remedies suggested in this book are intended to replace professional medical treatment or advice, and it is always best to speak to your doctor before embarking on any alternative therapy.

Toxic plants

Just because something is "natural" does not mean it is good for you. Some natural substances, including plants, are highly toxic to humans. Correct identification is crucial when picking herbs to use in herbal preparations. Some toxic plants resemble others that are harmless. For example, cow parsley and hemlock, which are poisonous, bear a strong resemblance to sweet cicely (*Myrrhis odorata*), a delightful herb that can be used to add sweetness to food.

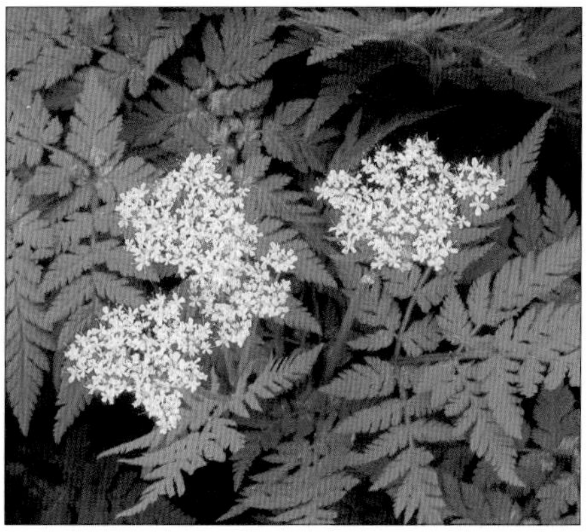

Above *The leaves of sweet cicely (*Myrrhis odorata*) are edible.*

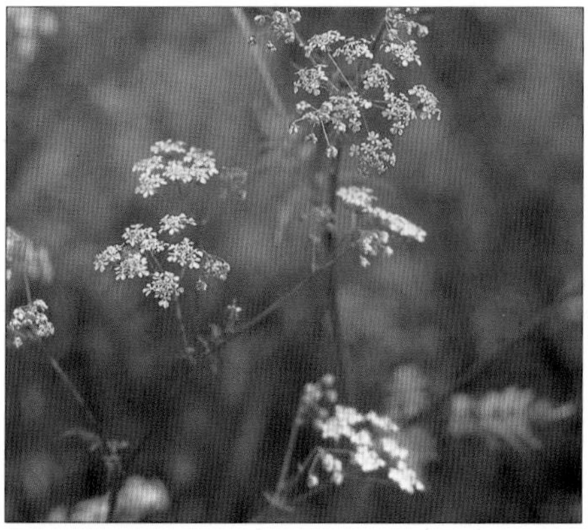

Above *Cow parsley (*Anthriscus sylvestris*) should not be confused with sweet cicely.*

Side effects

Some herbs may cause side effects, such as gastro-intestinal upsets, headaches or rashes. A few may have more serious adverse effects, including liver damage, usually in rare cases or when taken in large amounts. At the first sign of any adverse reaction, stop taking the herb immediately and consult a qualified herbalist or medical practitioner.

Others, including seemingly innocuous plants such as pot marigold (*Calendula officinalis*), may cause allergic reactions in certain people. For anyone prone to allergies, it is sensible to start with a small amount of any herbal product, and then step up the dose if all seems well.

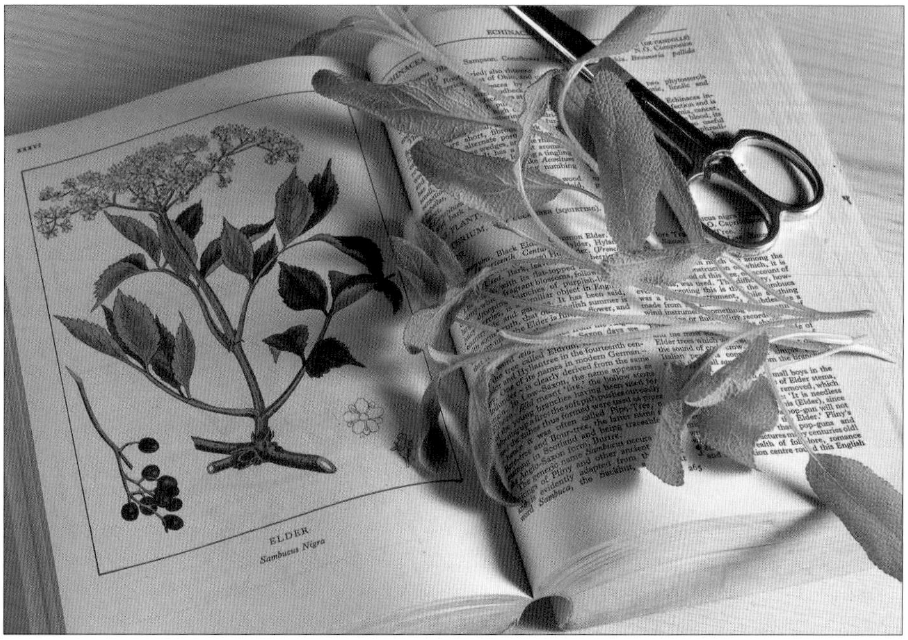

Below *Before you use any medicinal plant you have gathered yourself, make sure that you have identified it correctly.*

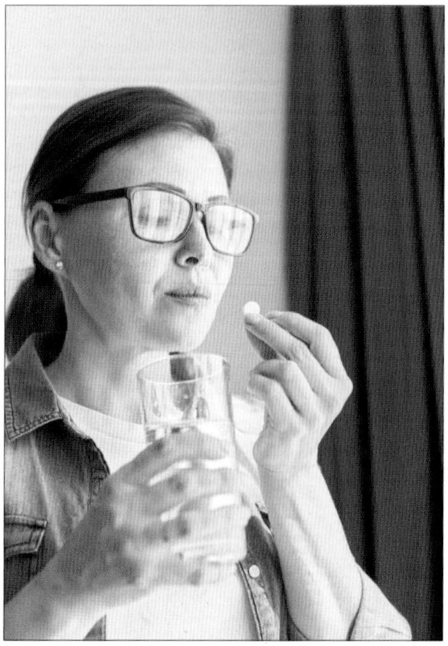

Below *Some herbs may interfere with certain pharmaceutical drugs, so seek medical advice before taking herbal remedies*

Contra-indications

Some illnesses and pre-existing health conditions can be made worse by a specific herb, so if herbs are to be taken medicinally, try each first to ensure there are no adverse reactions. Liquorice (*Glycyrrhiza glabra*), for example, can increase high blood pressure through its action on the adrenal glands. As some people may be unaware that their blood pressure is raised when they are taking a remedy for a different condition, it is generally unwise to use liquorice in herbal preparations. For this reason it does not feature in any recipes in this book, despite its otherwise beneficial properties.

Safety checklist

- Remember that "natural" does not necessarily mean "safe".
- Check that you have correctly identified herbs for use in remedies.
- Buy dried herbs and herbal products from a reliable source.
- Do not exceed recommended doses.
- Remember that some herbs are safe in low doses but toxic in large doses.
- Do not take any herbal remedy continuously for more than 2–3 weeks.
- Do not use poultices or compresses continuously for more than 1–2 days.
- If prone to allergies, start by taking a low dose, gradually increasing it if no adverse reaction is experienced.
- Do not take essential oils internally.
- If you experience any adverse reaction to a herbal remedy, seek professional advice immediately.
- Herbal remedies should not be taken if elderly, or pregnant, or by young children without professional advice.
- If you have a pre-existing health condition, including high blood pressure, seek medical advice before taking herbal remedies.
- If you are taking pharmaceutical drugs or prescribed medication, seek medical advice before taking herbal remedies.

CAUTION Pharmaceutical drugs include many common over-the-counter products, such as aspirin, as well as prescribed medicines.

So many herbs are contra-indicated during pregnancy or when breastfeeding that it is wisest not to take any at such times, especially in larger, medicinal doses, without first seeking professional advice.

Interactions

Some herbs may interact with certain pharmaceutical drugs, usually by increasing or decreasing their effect, although this is rare in practice. Some interactions may be minor, but others can be life-threatening. St John's wort (*Hypericum perforatum*), hailed until fairly recently as the natural way to treat depression without the side effects of many medical antidepressant drugs, has since been found to interact with vital medically prescribed drugs for other conditions, and can therefore no longer be recommended for internal use in home remedies or for self-treatment.

Herbal remedies and pharmaceutical drugs are not necessarily mutually exclusive, but decisions on taking both at the same time should be left to professionals. The rule is simple: never take herbal remedies at the same time as prescribed medication without telling your doctor. Equally, a professional herbal consultant should always be informed during a consultation of any pharmaceutical drugs you are taking. The main categories of pharmaceutical drugs that may be affected by herbal preparations are: anticoagulants (blood-thinning drugs, including aspirin and warfarin); antidepressants; drugs for epilepsy; medication for diabetes; drugs used to treat heart disorders; immuno-suppressants; the contraceptive pill; HRT and fertility treatment.

Below *Liquorice may raise blood pressure if taken in large, medicinal doses.*

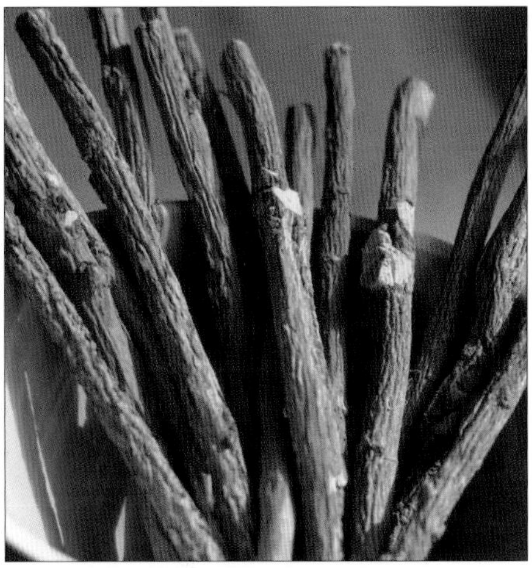

Herb–drug interactions

This list includes some herbs commonly used as remedies, and the main categories of pharmaceutical medicines with which they may interact:

Herb	Drugs that may be affected
• Angelica (*Angelica archangelica*)	anticoagulants
• Chaste tree (*Vitex agnus-castus*)	contraceptive pill, fertility treatment, HRT
• Devil's claw (*Harpagophytum procumbens*)	various
• Echinacea (*Echinacea angustifolia, E. purpurea*)	various
• Evening primrose (*Oenothera biennis*)	epilepsy drugs
• Feverfew (*Tanacetum parthenium*)	anticoagulants
• Fenugreek (*Trigonella foenum-graecum*)	anticoagulants, diabetic medicine
• Garlic (*Allium sativum*)	anticoagulants
• Ginger (*Zingiber officinalis*)	anticoagulants
• Ginseng (*Panax ginseng*)	high blood pressure, diabetes medication
• Hawthorn (*Crataegus* spp)	high blood pressure, heart medication
• Liquorice (*Glycyrrhiza glabra*)	antibiotics, PPIs (proton pump inhibitors)
• St John's wort (*Hypericum perforatum*)	contraceptive pill, immuno-suppressants anti--depressants
• Turmeric (*Curcuma longa*)	anticoagulants
• Valerian (*Valeriana officinalis*)	epilepsy drugs

Quality Control and Dosage

Using herbs safely is not just about finding the correct remedy. It's vital to be confident about the quality of the ingredients and to observe the guidelines on dosage.

Home-grown herbs and remedies

There are many advantages to using herbs you have grown yourself, not least that you will know the plant material is clean, and has not been mixed with soil or other species or sprayed with pesticides. If you dry your own herbs, you will know how old they are and that they have not been adulterated with suspect material. All these things can be enormously reassuring.

Buying herbs for use in remedies

Quality is more of an issue when it comes to buying dried herbs to make your own preparations. Herb crops are subject to natural variation, due to changing weather and growing conditions, and some batches will be of higher quality than others. More seriously, one of the problems of buying dried herbs is that they are easy to adulterate, and there have been instances when toxic plant material has been accidentally mixed in with beneficial herbs.

Always buy from a reputable source, preferably one where products have been standardized or there is some guarantee of quality control. Remember that this will not apply to all internet sources.

Chinese herbs

There have been some reports of batches of imported Chinese herbs being severely contaminated. At the time of writing there is no reliable way of being sure of their safety, and quality issues on this score remain a health concern.

Below *Growing your own herbs for use in home remedies ensures a safe supply.*

Legislation on herbal products

In the USA, herbal remedies are mostly classified as food supplements and come under regulations for retailing food, rather than medicines. In the European Union and Australia, legislation on quality standards and labelling requirements for herbal medicinal products has been put in place. In Europe, the Traditional Herbal Medicinal Products Directive now requires anything sold as a herbal remedy to be licensed, an extremely costly procedure that will inevitably result in fewer products being available. At present only the components of the remedy may be stated on the label, but by 2011, provided the product is licensed, the manufacturer will be allowed to include information on the ill-health condition it is intended to treat. The legislation is applied to dried herbs only if they are sold as medicines, and of course it does not prevent you growing and using your own herbs.

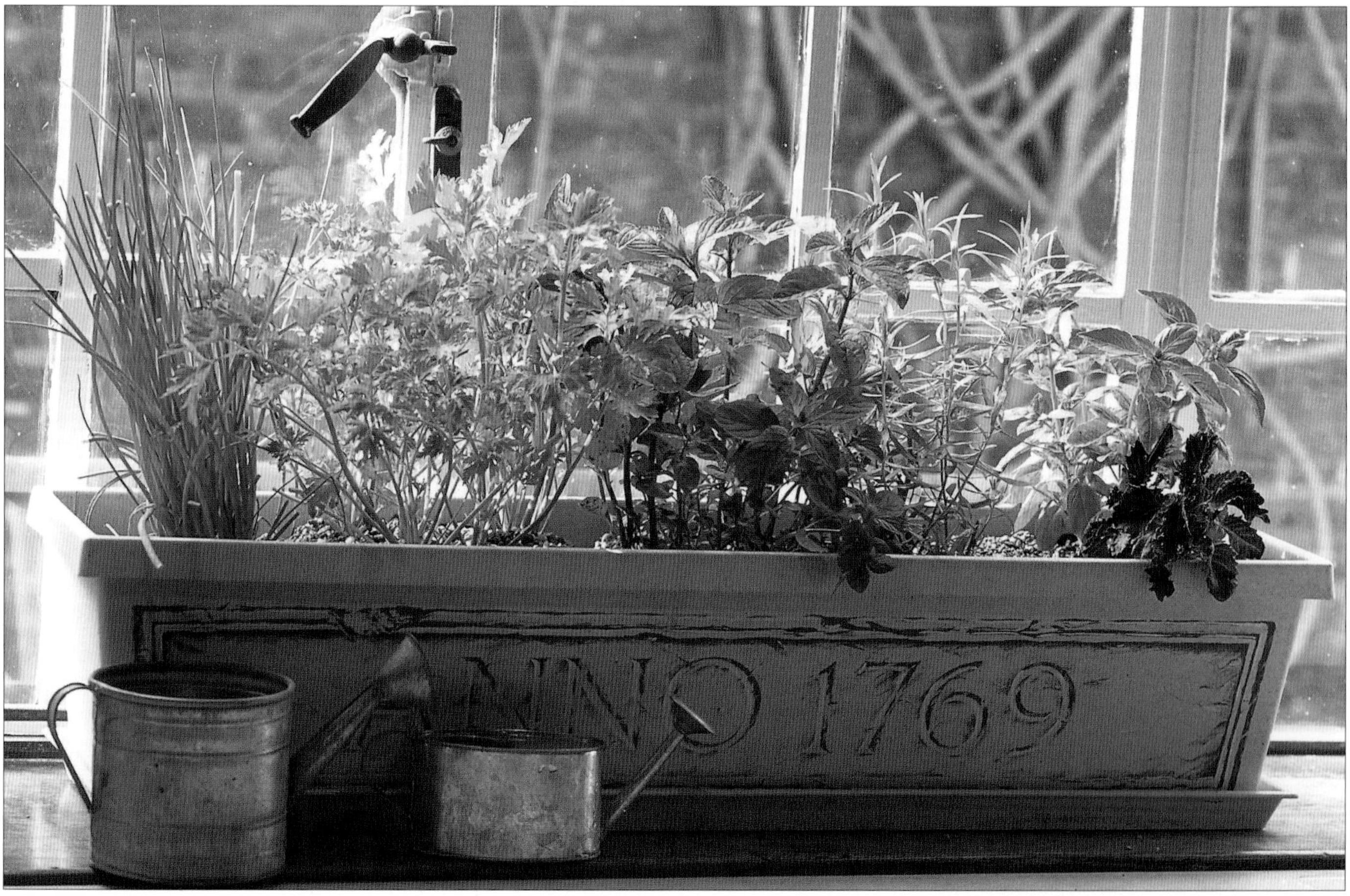

Right *You can dry home-grown herbs to make your own herbal preparations. Choose a warm morning to harvest them, before the essential oils have evaporated.*

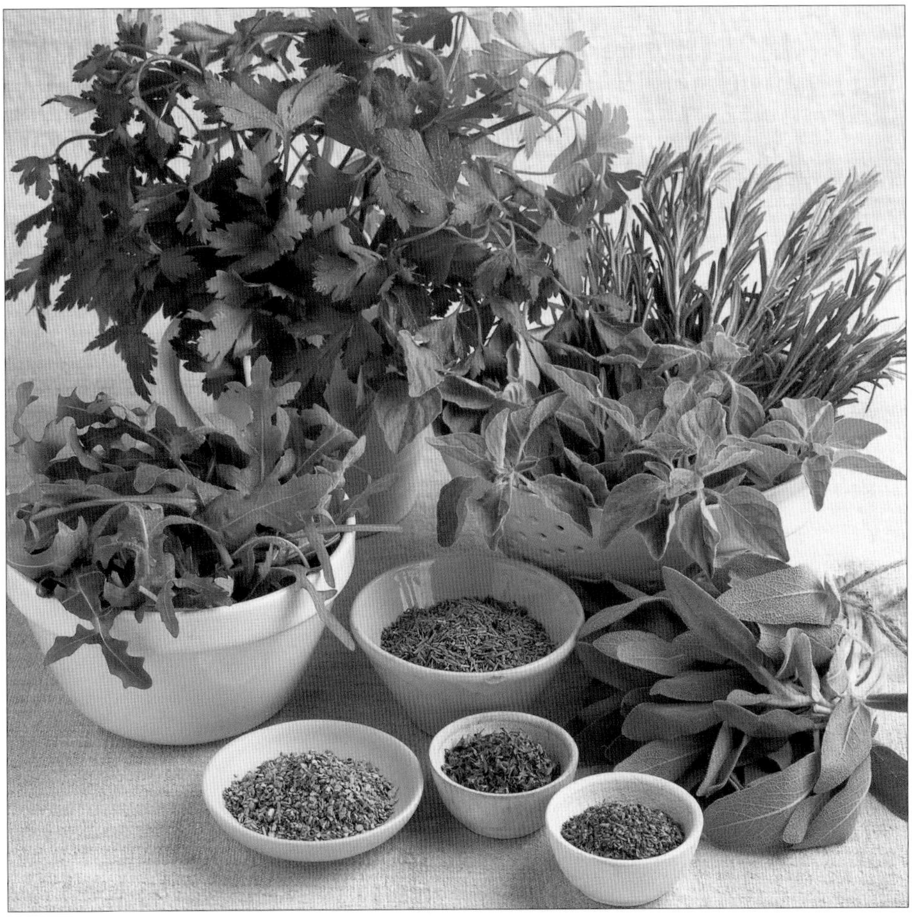

Changes and updates are ongoing, and the Medicine Control Agency (dedicated to safety issues associated with herbal medicines) reviews the current situation on its website.

Sensible dosages

Anything, including water and carrot juice, can be harmful if taken in vast quantities. How much you take of any herb, and in what form or concentration, is crucial to safety. Taking more of a herbal product to remedy a particular problem, far from making it better more quickly, is likely to make things worse. Some herbs, even culinary herbs such as sage, are perfectly safe in normal, recommended quantities, but toxic in large amounts. Herbal preparations work gently on the system, and results may not be felt immediately. It is important that herbs should be taken only in the quantities recommended and, for maximum effect, in conjunction with a healthy lifestyle. Doses need to be carefully monitored when taking herbs as extracts or in manufactured medicinal preparations, and essential oils should not be taken internally without professional advice. (See the guidelines for standard adult doses.) Always follow guidelines carefully and use common sense when taking herbal remedies. It is no good expecting herbal remedies to work if you take no exercise and eat badly.

Below *Consult a healthcare professional for advice before taking herbal remedies.*

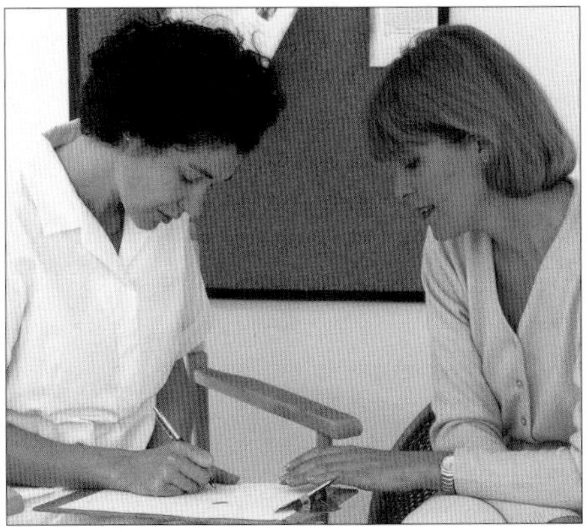

Guidelines for standard adult doses

For children under 12 and the elderly, seek the advice of a professional herbalist before using herbal remedies.

- Infusions (teas): 1 cup 3 times daily.
- Decoctions: 1 cup 3 times daily.
- Syrups: 5–10ml/1–2 tsp 3 times daily.
- Tinctures (home-made): 5ml/1 tsp diluted in a little water or fruit juice, 3 times daily.
- Tinctures (bought): These vary in strength, and should be taken according to the manufacturer's directions, or following professional advice.
- Capsules (bought): According to manufacturer's directions.
- Compresses: Apply as often as required, for 10–15 minutes at a time (for no longer than 1–2 days).
- Poultices: Apply 2–3 times a day for 2–3 hours at a time (for no longer than 1–2 days).
- Steam inhalations: 2–3 times a day, for up to 10 minutes at a time.
- Essential oils in bath: 5–6 drops.
- Essential oils for massage: 1–2 drops essential oil in 5ml/1 tsp base oil (10–12 drops in 30ml/2 tbsp).
- Essential oils in a vaporizer: 5–8 drops initially, topping up as necessary.

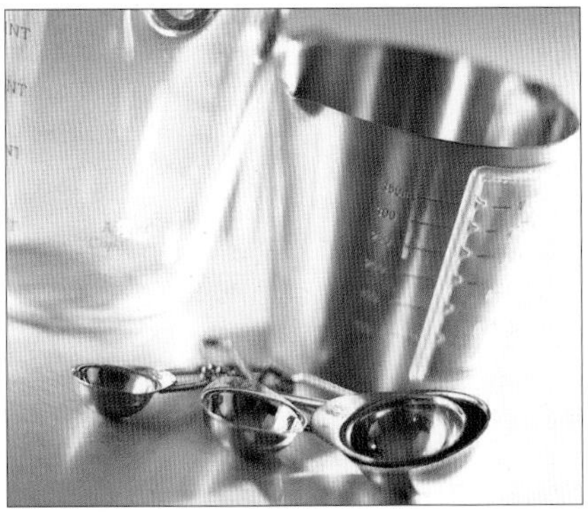

Left *Measuring jugs (cups) and spoons are essential for accurately measuring any remedies that are taken orally. Taking too much may be harmful.*

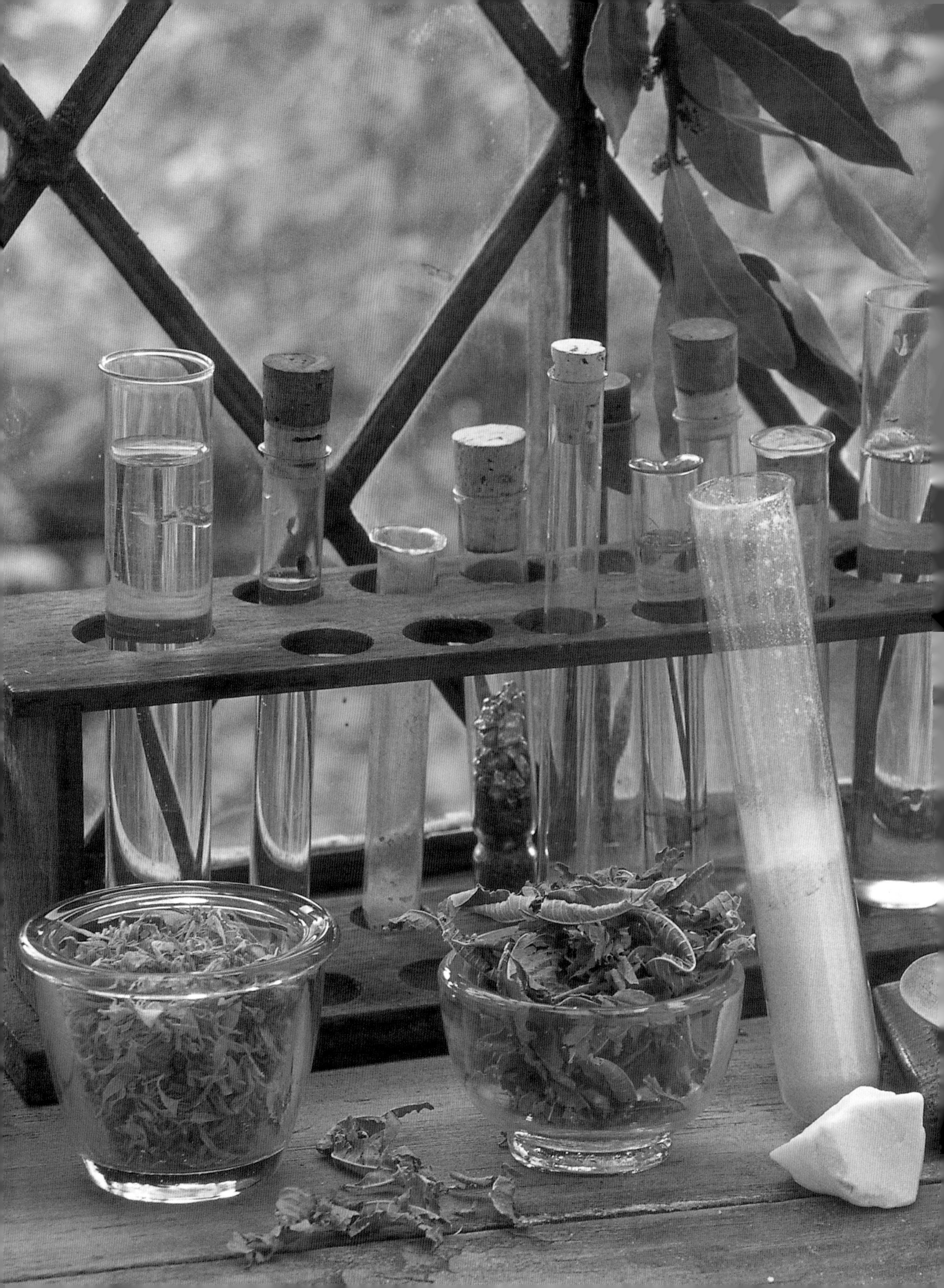

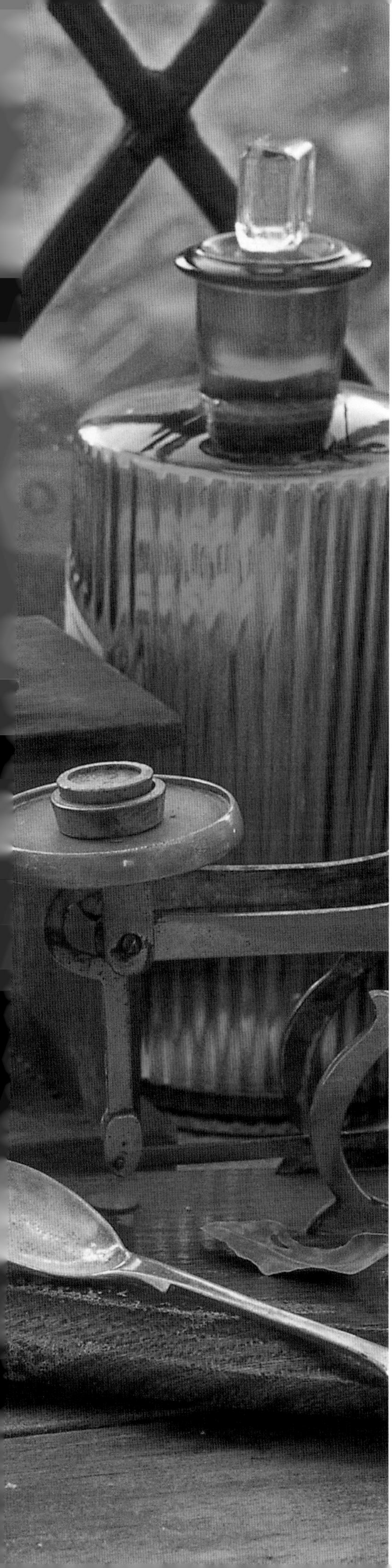

Herbal Preparations

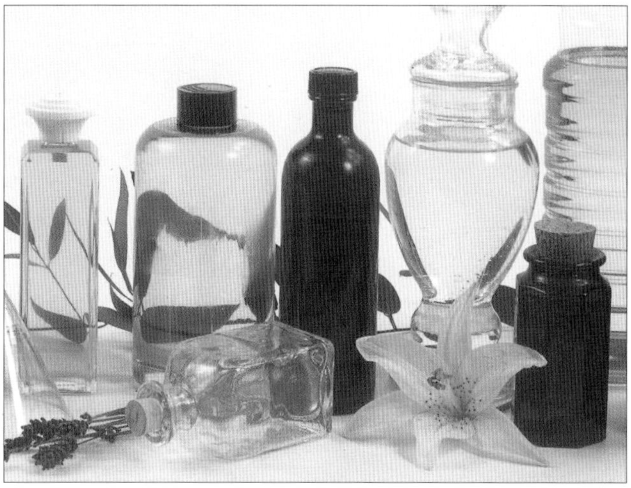

Growing your own herbs for use in herbal preparations provides a steady source of fresh material that you can guarantee has not been sprayed or contaminated in any way. Wild plants are also a valuable resource. Drying and storing the leaves, flowers, roots or seeds, as appropriate, will ensure a year-round supply. Some components, including essential oils, you will need to buy, and ready-made remedies also have their uses. Making your own infusions, decoctions, tinctures, syrups, creams and lotions is not difficult: follow the step-by-step sequences given here, and you will have the reward of knowing you are using natural ingredients, simply prepared.

Above *A collection of jars and bottles is useful for storing your home-made herbal products.*

Left *Dried herbs and other ingredients for use in home preparations.*

Wild Herbs

Many medicinal herbs are wild plants, and if you are tempted to pick them for use in home preparations you should be careful to follow the code of conduct for harvesting plants from the wild. Remember that some species are protected by law.

Commercial wild harvesting

Plants for use in commercial herbal medicines and products are still gathered from the wild in parts of Europe and in the developing world. This practice has brought many species to the point of extinction, such as golden seal (*Hydrastis canadensis*) and *Echinacea* in North America. To counteract this trend, some countries have instituted large-scale cultivation of medicinal herb crops, such as German chamomile (*Matricaria chamomilla*) and *Ginkgo biloba*.

Other useful herbs are familiar as common 'weeds' and as such can be encouraged to grow in the untended areas of your garden, or even cultivated.

Wild herbs to harvest

- Chickweed (*Stellaria media*) – A creeping ground-cover plant, rich in vitamins, which comes up in cleared ground in spring.
- Cleavers (*Galium aparine*) – It is tempting to pull out this prolific, sticky creeper as soon as you see it, but leave a patch to grow over a wall or fence for use as a spring tonic.
- Dandelion (*Taraxacum officinale*) – An easy plant to cultivate, its cheery yellow flowers feature in spring and summer. It self-seeds freely and even if the whole plant is dug up it will regenerate from a tiny portion of root left in the soil. The leaves are packed with vitamins and minerals.
- Stinging nettles (*Urtica dioica*) – For maximum medicinal potency these should not be grown in rich soil. Allow clumps to flourish where they come up, in a wild corner of the garden.
- Yarrow (*Achillea millefolium*) – A common grassland weed with astringent properties, traditionally used to staunch bleeding, it will be improved if you dig it up and re-plant in cultivated soil. There are many ornamental *Achillea* varieties but they do not have the same medicinal properties as the species.
- Elder (*Sambucus nigra*) – If you do not have room in the garden for an elder tree ("the poor man's medicine chest"), this is one that can be harvested from the wild, provided the wild harvesting code of conduct is followed.

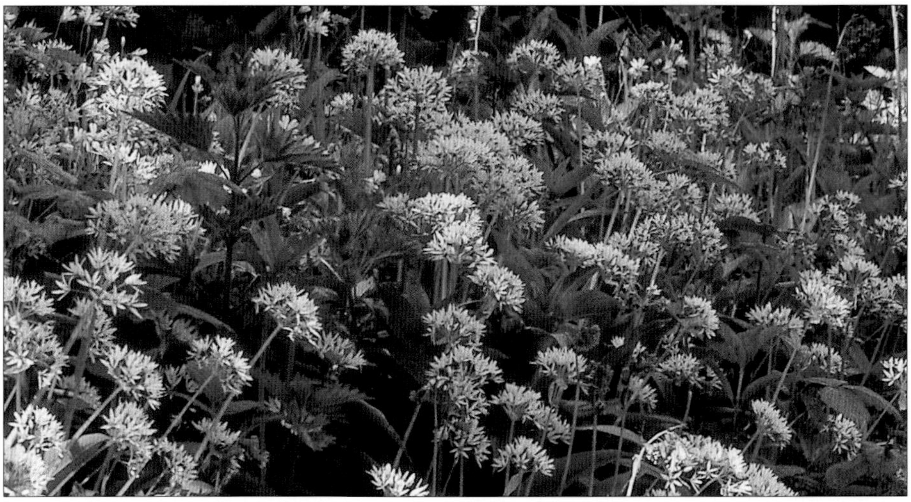

Above *Herbs with medicinal properties can be found growing wild in many different plant habitats.*

Below *Dandelions have many uses in herbal remedies.*

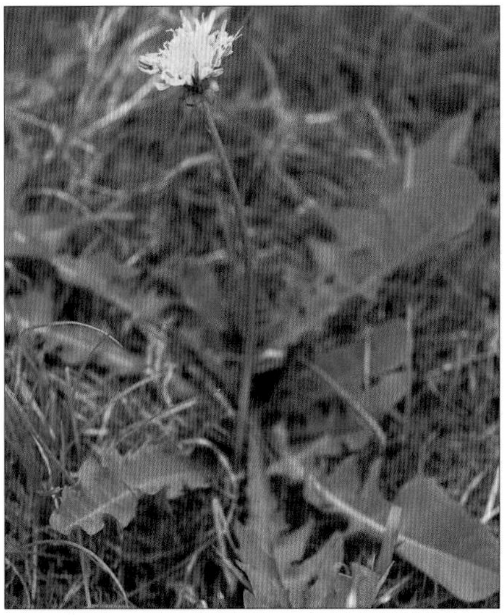

Below *Elderflowers can be made into soothing teas and lotions.*

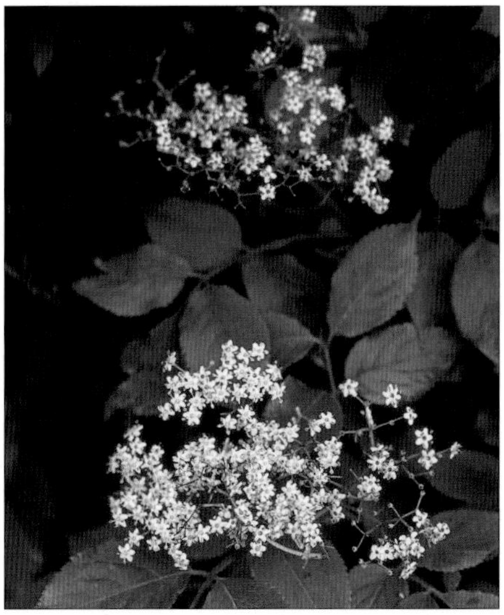

Code of conduct for harvesting from the wild

- Always be sure you have identified the plant correctly.
- Do not pick near roadsides, or at field edges where crops may have been sprayed with pesticides.
- Make sure the plant you pick is not legally protected.
- Never uproot a wild plant.
- Do not always pick from the same area, or where the species is scarce.
- Avoid plants that are stunted or do not look healthy.

Garden Herbs

There are many advantages to growing your own plants for use in herbal preparations:

- You can be sure that they have not been contaminated or sprayed with pesticides.
- Identification is secure (provided you have grown the right variety and labelled it correctly).
- You will have fresh material to hand just when you need it.
- If you are using dried material from herbs you have grown, you can ensure it has not been kept too long.
- You can pick material for drying at the optimum time of day.
- There is a wide range of seeds and plants from which to choose.

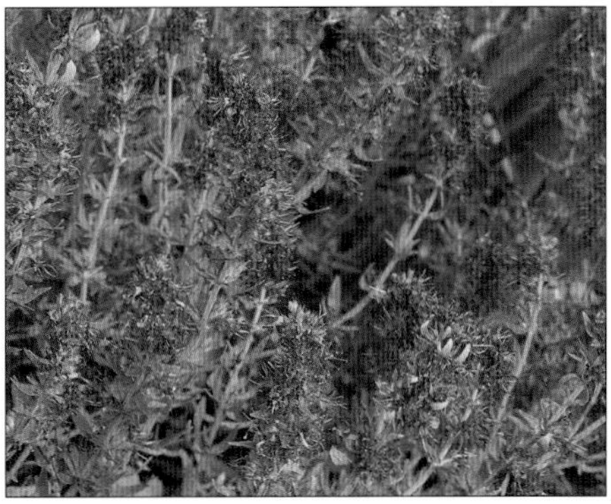

Above *Hyssop (*Hyssopus officinalis*) has colourful flowers and is easy to grow in the garden for use in home remedies. It needs a sunny spot in well-drained soil.*

Herbs to grow in the garden

Plants that can be used in herbal home preparations come from all over the world. Some flourish in tropical climates, but there are a large number that originate from temperate regions and can withstand frost. Tender plants, such as *Aloe vera*, can be successfully grown as houseplants.

The lists below are not exhaustive but will form the basis of a useful collection as the source of fresh ingredients for home-made herbal preparations.

Remember that many herbs fulfil more than one purpose and cannot necessarily be categorized as exclusively medicinal or culinary.

Annuals and biennials

These are best grown from seed.

- Angelica (*Angelica archangelica*)
- Basil (*Ocimum basilicum*)
- Borage (*Borago officinalis*)
- Calendula (*Calendula officinalis*)
- Chervil (*Anthriscus cerefolium*)
- Coriander (*Coriandrum sativum*)
- Wild (German) chamomile (*Matricaria chamomilla*)
- Parsley (*Petroselinum crispum*)
- Garlic (*Allium sativum*) – grow from a "clove" or small bulblet.

Below *Buy seed from a reputable supplier to be sure of good quality.*

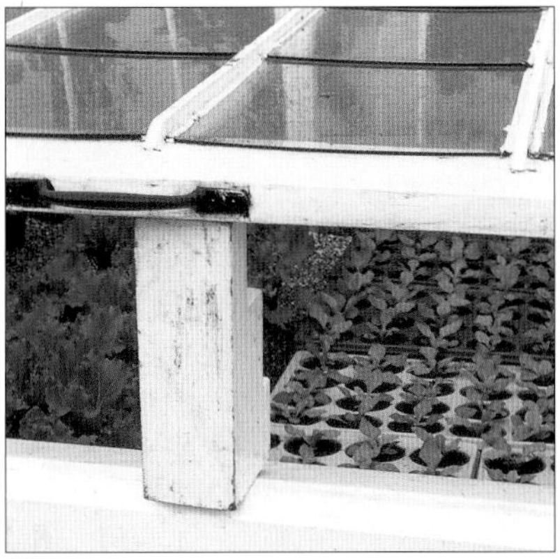

Perennials

It is easier to buy most of these as little plants, or to obtain them as root divisions or offsets from existing plants. Some may also be grown successfully from seed.

- Anise hyssop (*Agastache foeniculum*)
- Boneset (*Eupatorium perfoliatum*)
- Chamomile (*Chamaemelum nobile*)
- Comfrey (*Symphytum officinalis*)
- Cotton lavender (*Santolina chamaecyparissus*)
- Echinacea (*Echinacea purpurea*)
- Elecampane (*Inula helenium*)
- Fennel (*Foeniculum vulgare*)
- Feverfew (*Tanacetum parthenium*)
- Globe artichoke (*Cynara scolymus*)
- Houseleek (*Sempervivum tectorum*)
- Hyssop (*Hyssopus officinalis*)
- St John's wort (*Hypericum perforatum*)
- Lavender (*Lavandula* spp)
- Lemon balm (*Melissa officinalis*)
- Lemon verbena (*Aloysia triphylla*)
- Marjoram (*Origanum* spp)
- Marshmallow (*Althaea officinalis*)
- Mint (*Mentha* spp)
- Rose (*Rosa* spp)
- Rosemary (*Rosmarinus officinalis*)
- Sage (*Salvia officinalis*)
- Soapwort (*Saponaria officinalis*)

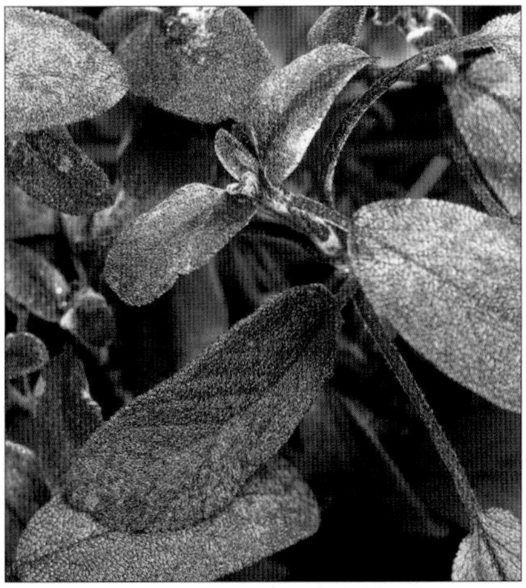

Above *Purple sage (*Salvia officinalis purpurea*) is an attractive sub-shrub.*

- Southernwood (*Artemisia abrotanum*)
- Thyme (*Thymus* spp)
- Valerian (*Valeriana officinalis*)

Climbers

- Hops (*Humulus lupulus*)
- Passion flower (*Passiflora incarnata*)

Shrubs

- Elder (*Sambucus nigra*)
- Witch hazel (*Hamamelis virginiana*)

Growing Herbs in the Garden

A carefully designed and stocked herb garden will provide all the fresh plant material you need for making your own herbal preparations. Herbs are not fussy or difficult plants to grow, but giving them the right soil and situation will ensure that you get the best from them.

Site and soil

A sunny sheltered position and light, dryish soil suits most herbs best. For many of them, the sunnier and hotter the site is, the more fragrance and flavour they will have and the higher will be the proportion of active constituents. The smell and taste of herbs is largely due to the production of essential oils within the plants. If they are grown in hot conditions, the concentrations of essential oils will be greater. Dull, damp conditions and a very moist rich soil will produce lush, leafy plants with a milder flavour and little scent. To cater for moisture lovers, such as angelica *(Angelica archangelica)*, add extra organic matter in the area where they grow.

Layout and design

Although herbs can be grown throughout the garden, it is more convenient when using them as ingredients for preparations to plant them together in a designated herb garden. A formal, symmetrical design of small rectangular beds, divided by gravel or paved paths, is a traditional layout that makes tending and harvesting easy. Some beds could be devoted to a single species, in the style of a medieval apothecary's garden, or collections of principally medicinal, culinary or fragrant herbs could be grouped together in larger beds. An informal cottage-garden style provides plenty of scope for imaginative planting and requires a little less maintenance than the more formal designs.

Watering and maintenance

Most herbs will withstand dry summers, but some, such as parsley (*Petroselinum crispum*) and chervil (*Anthriscus cerefolium)*, are apt to bolt in dry conditions and may need watering. Herbs with a root system of vigorous runners, such as mint (*Mentha* spp), can become invasive unless you restrict the roots by growing them in a bucket with the bottom removed, sunk in the soil. Remove heads of rampant seeders, such as lemon balm (*Melissa officinalis*), promptly to prevent unwanted seedlings germinating all over the garden.

Stocking the herb garden

For a good range of plants you will need to start by buying some in pots from a specialist outlet. For economy, choose small pots, though larger specimens will provide material to cut more quickly. Other herbs are best grown from seed, especially annuals. If you have access to established plants, digging up and dividing clumps of fibrous-rooted herbs, such as marjoram or chives, is a good way to increase stocks as well as rejuvenate existing plants. Some herbs, including houseleek (*Sempervivum tectorum*) and chamomile (*Chamaemelum nobile*) conveniently provide offsets or runners for planting out.

SOWING SEEDS

To give plants an early start and maximize germination, sow seeds in trays, in the spring, under glass. Label the tray with the seed name (all seedlings look very similar when they have just germinated).

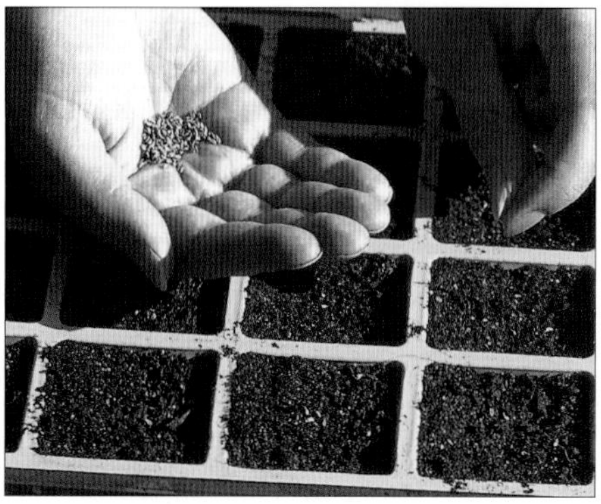

1 Fill a seed tray with soilless compost (growing medium). A tray divided into cells makes it easier to sow the seeds thinly and to pot up seedlings later on. Water the compost first, then scatter two or three seeds in each compartment.

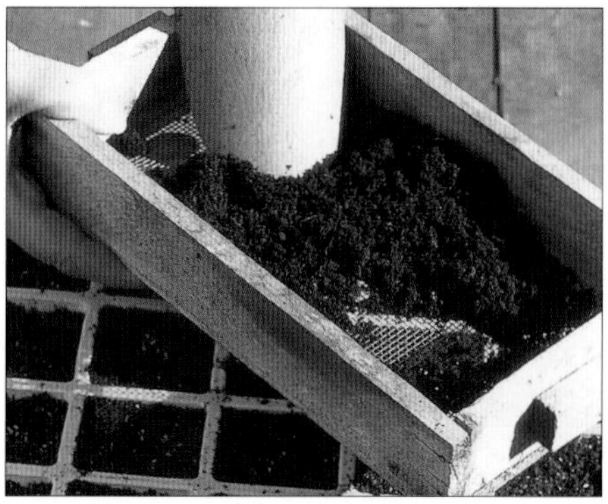

2 Cover the tray with a thin layer of sieved compost. Water again very lightly.

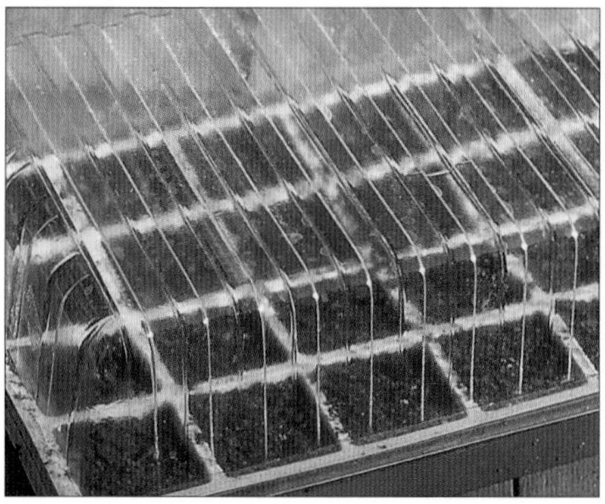

3 Put a polythene (plastic) dome over the tray, or enclose it in a clear plastic bag. Put the tray on a windowsill or in the greenhouse and cover with black polythene until the seedlings begin to show.

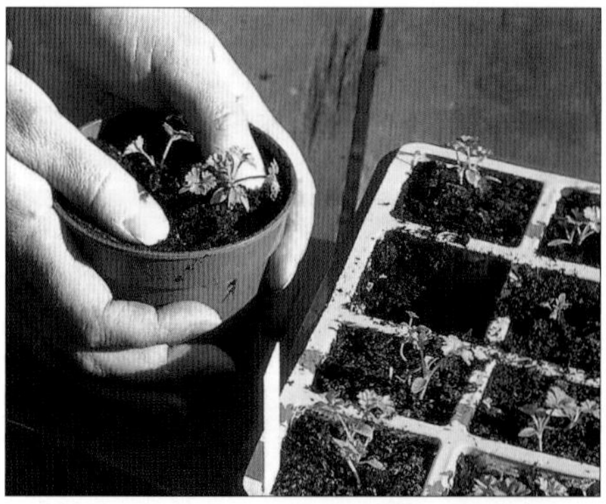

4 When the seedlings come through, remove the cover and keep them moist. As soon as they are large enough to handle, pot them up individually and harden off before planting outside.

PLANTING OFFSETS

Plants such as chamomile (*Chamaemelum nobile)* and houseleek (*Sempervivum tectorum)* send out little satellite plants, or offsets (offshoots), which can be separated and replanted, either directly in the garden or in pots. Replant them in spring.

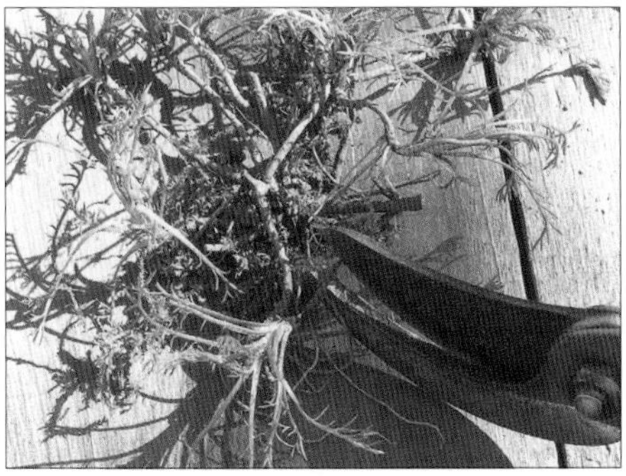

1 Lift a plant (in this case, chamomile) and separate the offsets, making sure each piece has some root attached.

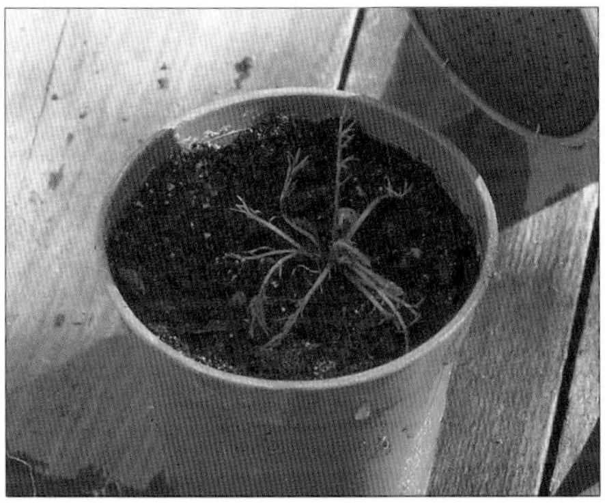

2 Press each new plantlet into a pot of compost (growing medium). Water and leave in a shady place until new roots develop.

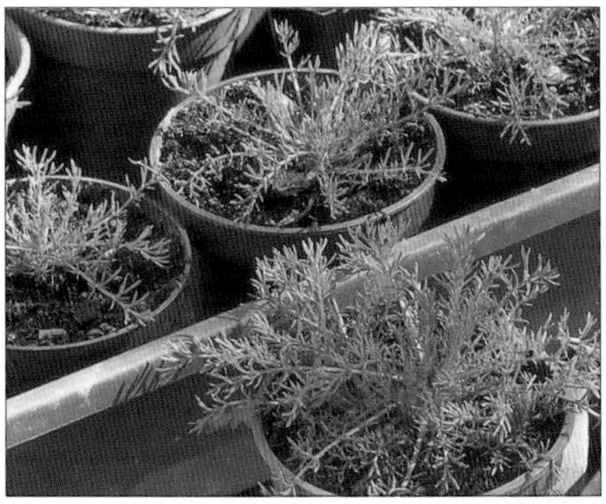

3 The cuttings will grow into bushy plants in 2–3 weeks, when they can be potted on into larger pots or planted out in the garden.

PLANTING A HERB GARDEN

Spring is a good time for planting a herb garden. The ground starts to warm up and the days lengthen, providing optimum growing conditions. Annuals, such as chervil (*Anthriscus cerefolium)* and coriander (*Coriandrum sativum)* (cilantro) are best sown directly where they are to grow. Others, including parsley (*Petroselinum crispum)* and basil (*Ocimum basilicum)*, are successful when raised in trays for growing on and setting out later. Half-hardy herbs, such as basil and nasturtium (*Tropaeolum majus)*, should not be planted outside until all danger of frost is past.

Shrubby plants like lavender (*Lavandula* spp*)*, and trees, such as elder (*Sambucus nigra)* or bay (*Laurus nobilis)*, can also be planted out in autumn. Prepare the ground well first.

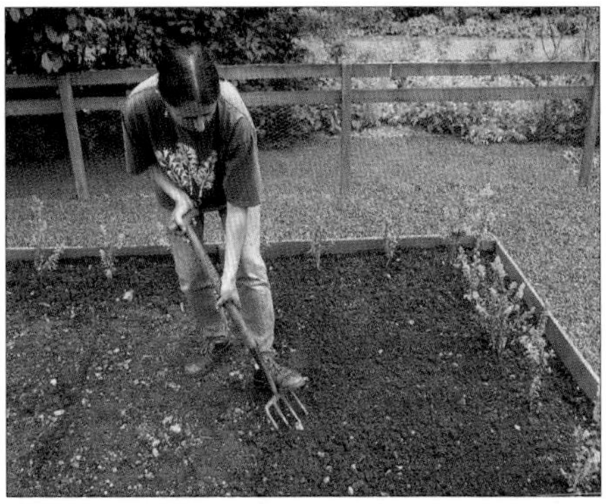

1 Fork over the planting area, removing weeds and breaking up and turning over the soil. Improve very heavy soils by digging in grit and compost to improve drainage. Work the soil to a fine tilth.

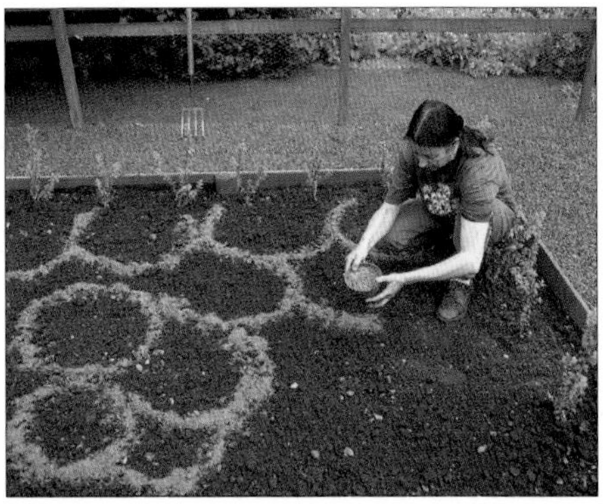

2 Using sand, divide the area into planting bays, allowing sufficient room in each for a plant to spread and grow.

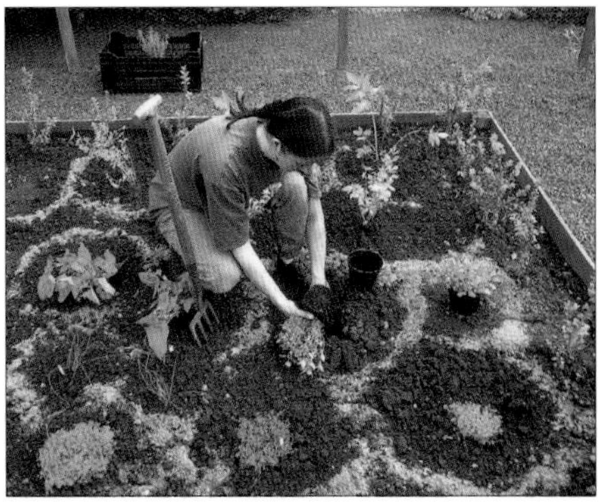

3 Dig a hole in the centre of each area deep enough to plant the herb. Tap the plant out of its container, position it and backfill with soil. Adding compost or organic matter at the planting stage gives plants a good start.

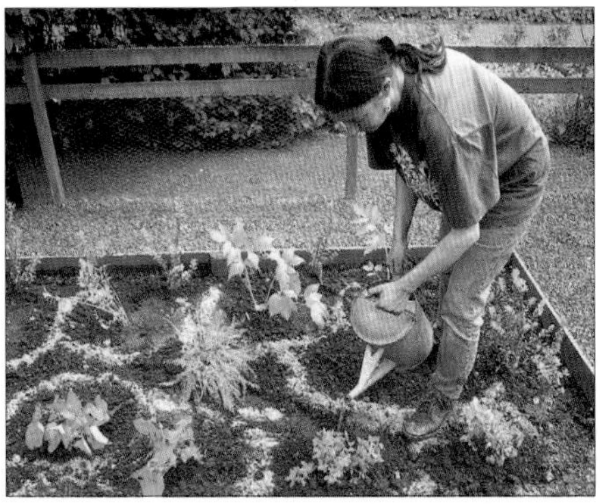

4 Soak plants well in their pots for an hour before setting them out in the garden. Water them again immediately after planting. Keep them well watered until the roots are fully established in the surrounding soil.

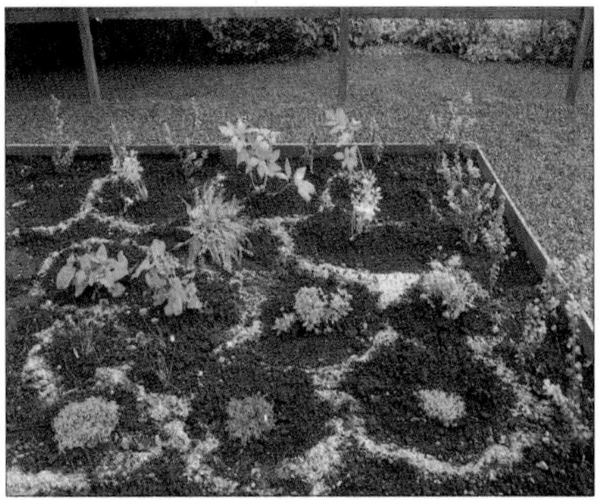

5 Keep the whole area weed free to give the plants a chance to become well established. As they spread and outgrow their space, some of the herbs can be dug up and replanted elsewhere.

Growing Herbs in Containers

There are many advantages to growing herbs in containers. Even in the smallest of gardens there is always room for a few pots. Sited near the house, they provide the added convenience of being handy for harvesting. As part of a garden scheme, containers can be placed in a bed to fill a temporary bare patch, used as focal points or arranged symmetrically to link different elements of a design.

Planting

Growing a single species in a container gives plants room to develop and to provide plenty of leafy growth. For larger specimens, such as bay (*Laurus nobilis*), sage (*Salvia officinalis*) and lemon verbena (*Aloysia triphylla*), it is essential that they do not have to share a pot if they are to be left undisturbed for several years. The pot should be large enough to allow roots to spread. Mixed herb pots make very attractive features and are a good way of growing a variety of plants in a small space, but the plants are inevitably cramped and the roots become congested. Annual repotting is usually necessary for a mixed planting.

Plants that are kept in the same container for several years should have the top layer of compost, about 5cm/2in, scraped off and replaced with a fresh layer every year. They will need re-potting in a larger container as roots become congested – try not to leave this until the plant is suffering, with roots bursting out of the pot, yellowing leaves and poor, straggly growth.

Growing medium

Most herbs flourish in a free-draining environment and, as a general rule, a 3:1 mixture of soilless compost (planting medium) and loam-based compost (soil mix) gives the best results. For shrubby herbs, such as bay, sage and rosemary (*Rosmarinus officinalis*), and for scented pelargoniums, add a few handfuls of grit (gravel) to the mix to improve drainage. Do not be tempted to use ordinary garden soil to fill containers; it will not provide enough nutrients and is likely to harbour weeds and pests.

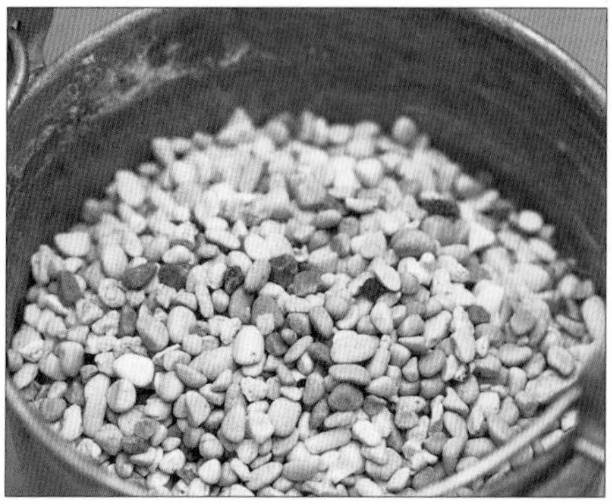

Above *Good drainage is one of the keys to success. Check that there is a large hole in the base of the pot. Put in a layer of broken terracotta pots, then cover with a layer of sand or grit (gravel) before filling the pot with potting compost (soil mix).*

Maintenance

Extra fertilizer must be added to the containers after about four weeks, with subsequent weekly feeds throughout the growing season. An organic plant food based on seaweed extract is preferable, but slow-release fertilizer granules save time as they are added when potting up.

Pot-grown plants need frequent watering during the growing season. As a general rule, it is better to let the plants almost dry out and then give them a good soaking, rather than to keep dribbling in small amounts of water. Water-retaining gel mixed into the growing medium at the time of planting makes watering less of a chore. During the winter months pot-grown perennials should be given the minimum amount of water possible, to allow them a period of dormancy.

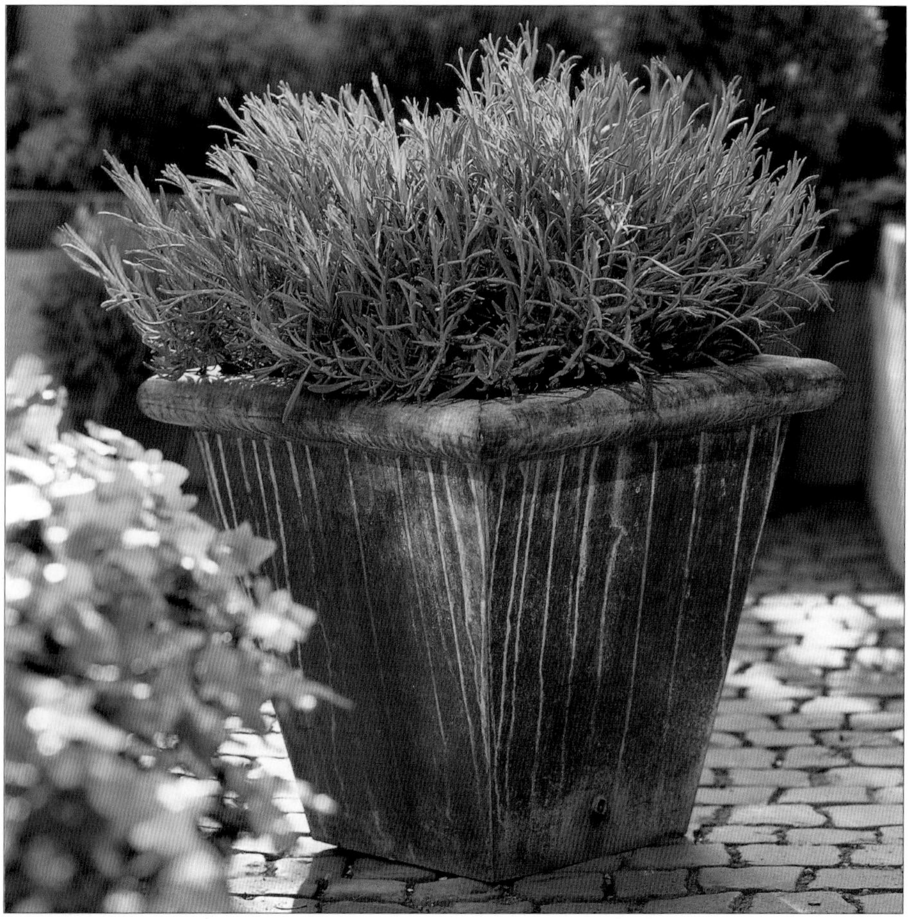

Left *Grow herbs in containers if you are short of space. This lavender plant will thrive if well watered.*

A CONTAINER FOR COLD REMEDIES

Herbs for use in teas and other cold remedies make a useful collection. Most of them keep their leaves through the winter, when they can still be picked on a daily basis in small quantities. However, they do not have the same potency while dormant, so it is advisable to harvest them while they are growing vigorously and dry them for later use.

Ingredients

Thyme (*Thymus* spp)
Sage (*Salvia* spp)
Horehound (*Marrubium vulgare)*
Hyssop (*Hyssopus officinalis)*
Peppermint (*Mentha spicata*)

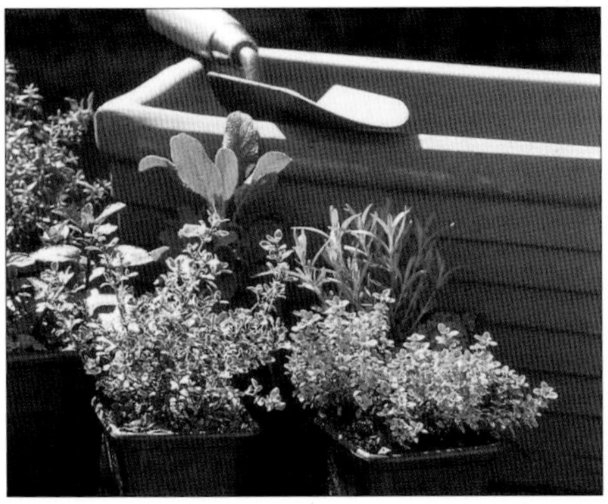

1 Put a layer of broken terracotta pots over the drainage holes in the bottom of the container. Top with a layer of horticultural grit (gravel), and fill with a potting compost (soil mix). Leave room for the plants.

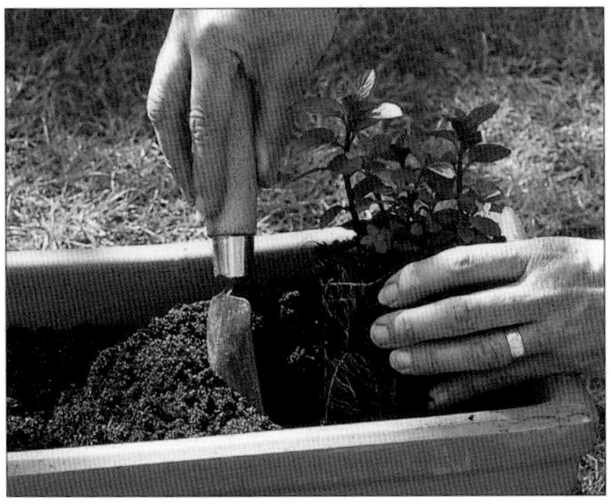

2 Position the plants while they are still in their pots, then take them out and plant them, firming around each one with extra compost. Put the tallest plants (horehound, hyssop, sage and peppermint) at the back and the thymes in front.

MAINTENANCE Do not let the trough dry out. Feed every 2–3 weeks with a liquid fertilizer during the growing season. Replant annually, using fresh compost (soil mix).

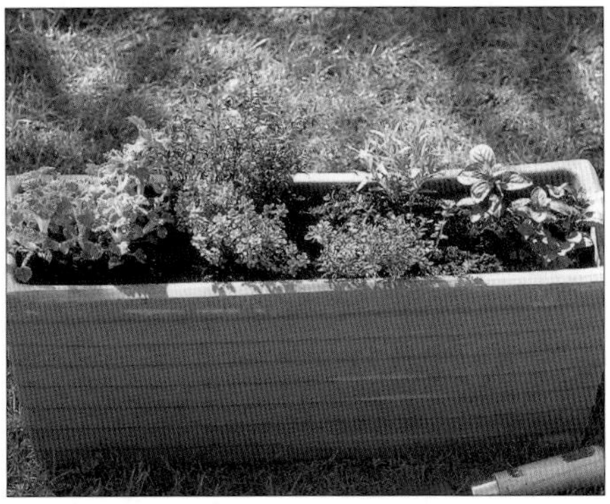

3 Top up with extra compost as necessary and water the plants in well. It is best to replant a mixed container like this annually to prevent the plants becoming overgrown. For best results do not include large shrubby herbs in a small mixed container.

A THYME POT

The antiseptic properties of thyme make it the first choice of herb for treating sore throats, coughs and colds. The essential oil contains a high level of antioxidants. Recent research has also established a link between thyme and slowing the ageing process.

Fortunately, thyme is easy to grow in pots so you can always have a ready supply. *Thymus vulgaris* is best for medicinal use. You could also include lemon thyme (*T.* x *citriodorus)*. Ornamental thymes do not have the same medicinal properties. Choose a planter with generously sized pockets so that the plants are not squashed. The same method can be used for planting pots with a selection of mixed herbs – thyme, lavender (*Lavandula* spp), peppermint (*Mentha spicata)*, chamomile (*Chamaemelum nobile*) and feverfew (*Tanacetum parthenium)* for a medicinal collection, or scented pelargoniums for fragrance.

Water regularly, but allow to dry out between waterings. The same planting should last for several years if you keep it in a sheltered place during winter. Trim in spring and feed with liquid fertilizer.

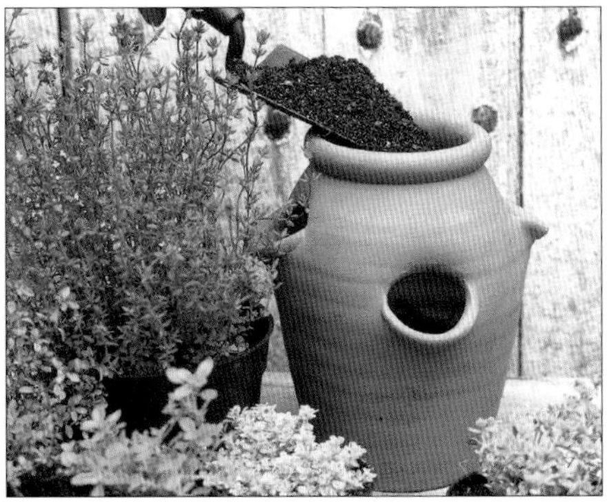

1 Put a layer of crocks in the bottom of the pot. Mix slow-release fertilizer and water-retaining gel, following the manufacturer's instructions, into a potting medium made up of equal parts of soilless compost (growing medium) and loam-based compost (soil mix). Fill to the first hole.

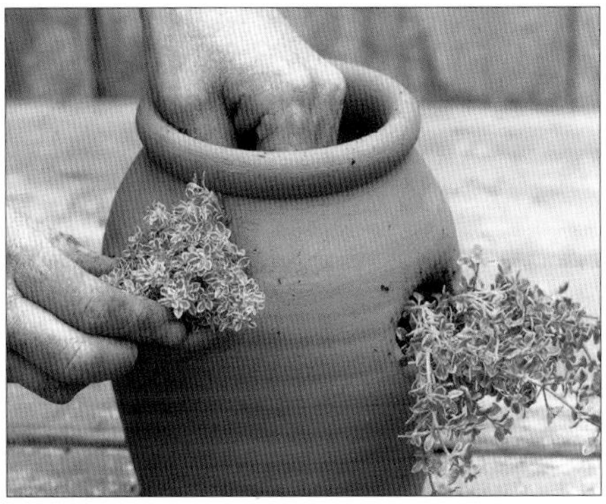

2 Tap a thyme plant out of its pot and feed it gently into place through a hole, working from the inside outwards. Cover the roots with more compost and firm it down before adding a further layer. Put in more plants until all the holes are filled.

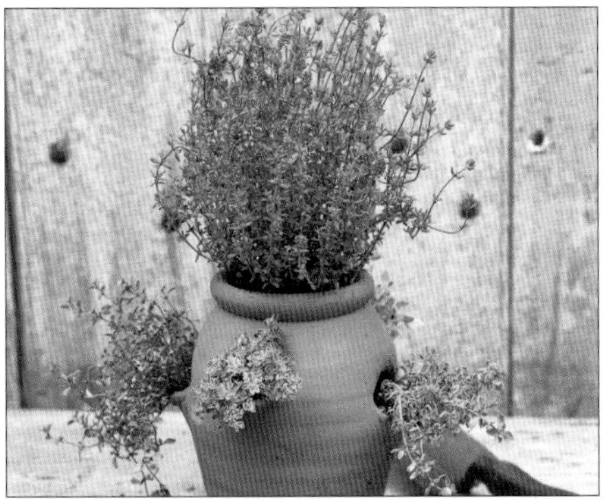

3 Plant the top of the container with one or more good, bushy specimens of thyme and water the plants thoroughly.

Harvesting, Drying and Storing

Growing your own herbs means you can preserve them for later use. This is particularly beneficial during the winter when plants are dormant. Harvesting plants at the right time and drying and storing them carefully will ensure they retain maximum fragrance and medicinal properties for as long as possible.

Harvesting herbs

The various parts of a herb, including the leaves, flowers, fruits and seeds, may be gathered at different times, depending upon the plant and the part that provides the desirable properties. Annual leafy herbs such as basil (*Ocimum basilicum*) and parsley (*Petroselinum crispum*) should be carefully picked, never taking more than about 10 per cent of the growth in a single picking.

The same is true of perennials such as sage (*Salvia officinalis*), thyme (*Thymus vulgaris*) and rosemary (*Rosmarinus officinalis*), because severe pruning or overstripping of the leaves will weaken the plant. It is important that you do not remove more than one-third of the growth at any one time. If you harvest carefully you will get a more vigorous leaf growth that will result in healthier plants.

As a general rule, pick herbs just before the plant is about to flower, which is when the leaves have the strongest flavour. Pick leaves when they are fresh and at their sweetest, selecting blemish-free upper leaves. Collect the leaves in the early morning or evening, provided they are dry, rather than in bright afternoon sun when the plant's sap is rising. The aroma of herbs is at its strongest at this time of day and it is easily lost if picked then. Flowers such as borage (*Borago officinalis*) and lavender (*Lavandula* spp), however, are best picked just before they reach full bloom and once they begin to open in the heat of the day.

Roots and rhizomes, such as black cohosh (*Actaea racemosa*) and echinacea (*E. purpurea*), are collected in autumn, when the maximum amount of nutrition has been stored. Use a fork to tease the roots from the soil; avoid "hand-pulling" them. Choose

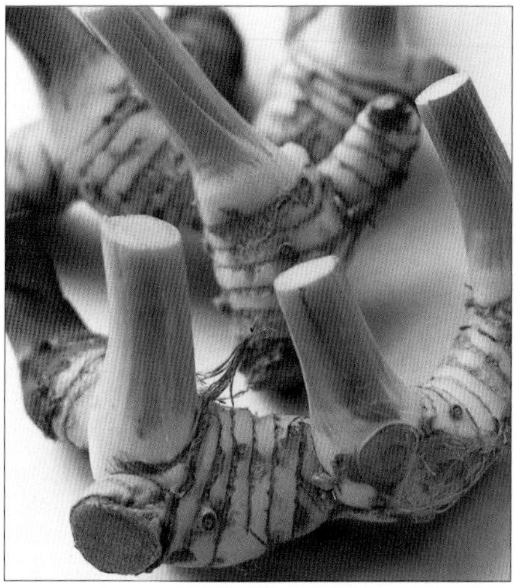

Above *Galangal* (Alpinia officinarum) *root is harvested for use in culinary and herbal preparations.*

the best and use a brush to loosen any dirt. If you need to wash them, avoid soaking as this can leach out active constituents.

Harvesting seeds tends to vary from plant to plant. Some seeds, like those of borage (*Borago officinalis*), fall to the ground as soon as they are ripe. Thyme (*Thymus* spp) seeds are very small and hard to see. Parsley (*Petroselinum crispum*) and coriander (*Coriandrum sativum*) seeds shake off easily, and frequently the plants will have sown next year's crop for you before you realize they have gone to seed. One method of harvesting any seed that is difficult to collect is to tie a small paper bag over the flower head when the seeds start to form, ensuring that you can collect the seed without losing any. Use this method for collecting from plants with small seeds, as they can drop off when ripe or may spring from the plant.

Drying herbs

One of the most popular methods of preserving herbs for use during the winter months is drying. This method may actually improve the flavour of bay leaves (*Laurus nobilis*).

When drying herbs, the temperature of the area should not exceed 30°C/86°F because the plants' essential oils will evaporate at or above this temperature. Do not dry your herbs in the kitchen where they will be spoiled by steam.

Spread leaves, flowers or petals on newspaper or put small bunches of herbs into brown paper bags. Store them in a dry, dark, warm place until the herbs inside are crumbly, shaking the bags occasionally so that the plants dry evenly. The process should take up to a week. Roots are best chopped into small pieces and dried in a very low oven.

Drying seeds

Collect the seeds just as they are ripening. Remove any chaff or plant debris and spread the seeds out on a tray or in a paper or muslin bag. Leave in a cool, dark place for a few days until the seed is completely dry. Once the seeds have been dried they can be stored in airtight containers, such as dark-coloured glass jars with well-fitting lids. Label the jars with the name of each herb and the date of picking for future reference, and store them in a cool, dry place, protected from light.

Below *Set a space aside for preparing herbs, and keep it clean so that the dried herbs do not become contaminated.*

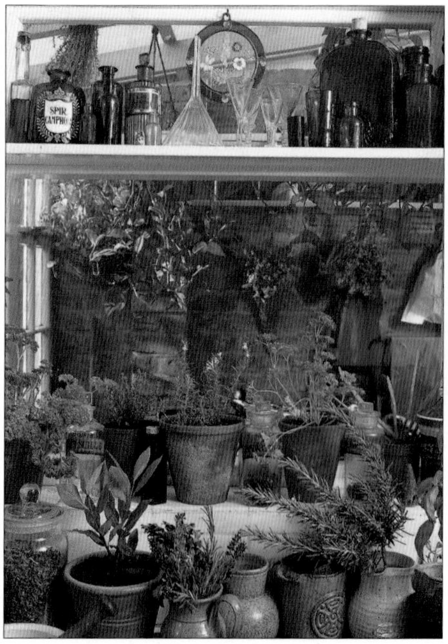

Storing herbs

Rub leafy herbs off their stems once they are dry. The job is easier if you wear light cotton gloves. Dried herbs deteriorate quickly if left out in the light and air, so store them in a cool, dark place in airtight, dark glass or pottery jars. Herbs also keep well in sealed brown paper bags. Cellophane bags are fine for short periods, but do not use polythene (plastic) bags or containers as they draw out residual moisture in the material. Dried herbs should not be exposed to any dampness. If left in unsealed containers, they will take in moisture from the surrounding air.

Although many herbs retain an aromatic scent for several years after drying, it is best to replace stocks every year since their potency declines with age. Drying your own herbs allows you to know exactly how old your stock is.

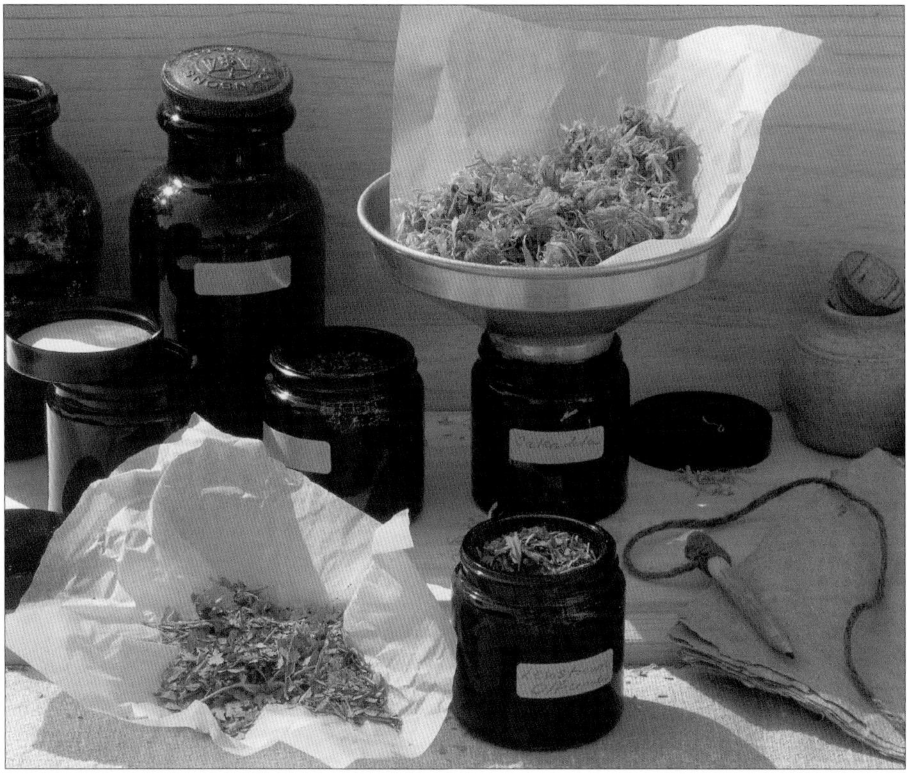

Above *Store home-dried herbs in dark glass jars to prevent deterioration. Ensure the stock is thoroughly dried and that it is not contaminated with dust. Label the jars with the date and name of the herb.*

Other ways of preserving and storing herbs

Although drying is the most common way to preserve leafy herbs for use when fresh are not in season, it is not the only possibility. Other traditional ways of preserving herbs include steeping them in oil or vinegar, or in sugar syrups, all of which take on their flavours. The methods described below are also effective ways of retaining the properties and fragrance of herbs for later use.

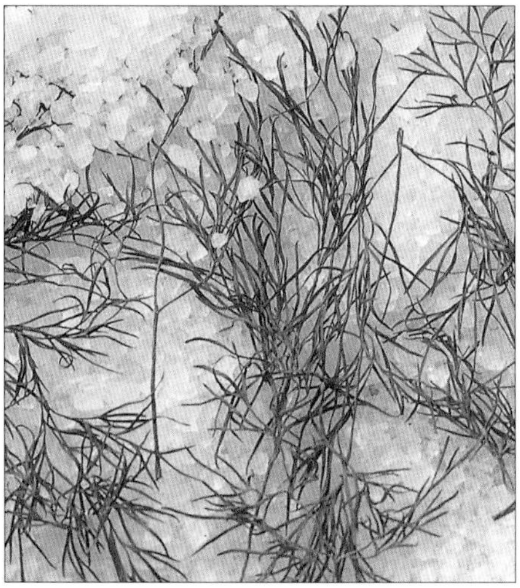

Herb salts (above)

Spread a layer of coarse salt on a sheet of baking parchment. Sprinkle the chopped fresh herbs on top of the salt and bake in a cool oven for 10–20 minutes. When the herbs are dry, let them cool and place in a jar. Chives (*Allium schoenoprasum*), oregano (*Origanum* spp), thyme (*Thymus* spp), lemon balm (*Melissa officinalis*), parsley (*Petroselinum crispum*), rosemary (*Rosmarinus officinalis*) and basil (*Ocimum basilicum*) can all be treated this way.

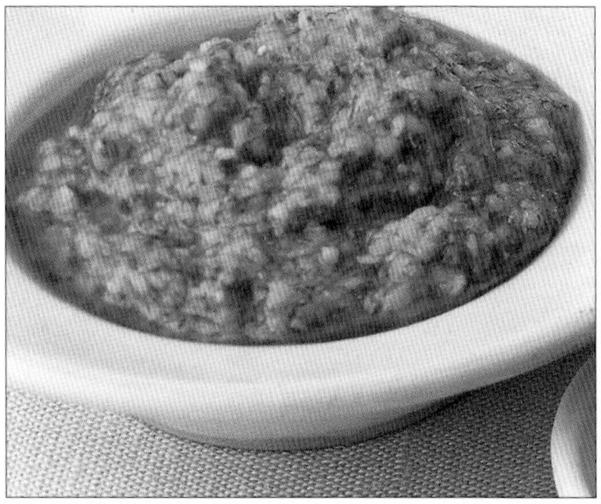

Puréeing (above)

To retain the flavour of fresh basil leaves, mix approximately 60ml/4 tbsp olive oil with 2 cups of the leaves, which have been washed and dried. Blend in a food processor to a smooth purée, then transfer to a jar. Stir each time you use it and top with a thin layer of oil afterwards. The purée should keep for up to one week in a refrigerator.

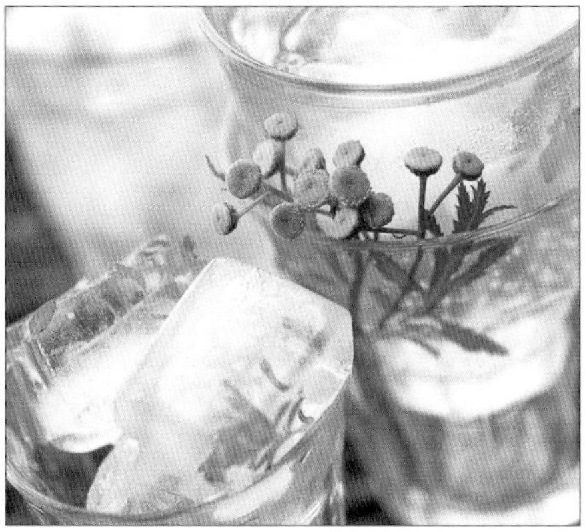

Freezing herbs (above)

Herbs such as dill (*Anethum graveolens*), fennel (*Foeniculum vulgare*), basil and parsley freeze well. The herbs should be cleaned and put into separate, labelled freezer bags. Alternatively, chop the herbs finely and half-fill each compartment of an ice cube tray, then top up with water before freezing. Transfer the frozen cubes to labelled plastic bags and freeze for up to six months. Use in cooking.

Other Herbal Remedy Ingredients

As well as the plants you grow yourself, there are a number of other ingredients you will need for making herbal preparations, some of which you may have to buy.

Dried herbs

As well as the aerial parts (leaves, stems and flowers), these ingredients may include the roots or bark of some species. Although it is useful to dry as many of your own herbs as possible, you will not be able to grow everything you need and there are times when it is more convenient to buy some. Choose a reputable supplier with a high turnover of product, and buy in small quantities, as it is not worthwhile to keep dried herbs at the back of the cupboard for years: use them within 6 months to a year.

Resins

• **Benzoin** is an aromatic resin from the styrax tree. It has preservative and antiseptic properties and is used to treat coughs and to calm the system. It is available as a tincture or in ground form.

• **Frankincense** is the gum resin produced by *Boswellia* spp, a genus of shrubby trees from the Arabian peninsula. It can be bought as grains or powder.

• **Myrrh**, the gum resin of another small tree (*Commiphora myrrha*) from the Middle East and the Horn of Africa, has antifungal and antiseptic properties. It can be bought in the form of a tincture or as grains or powder.

Below *Resins can be obtained in block or powdered form.*

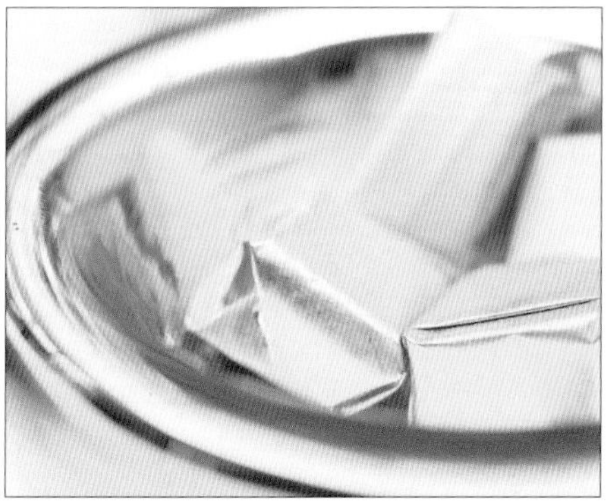

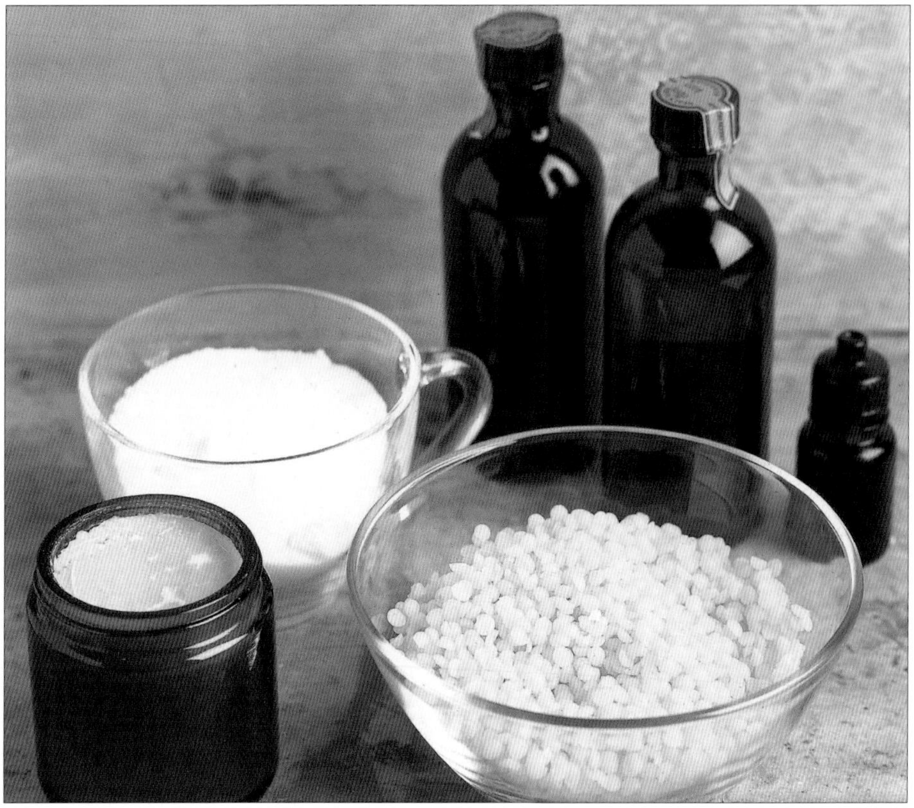

Above *Cocoa butter, borax, almond oil, lavender water and beeswax granules.*

Powders

• **Slippery elm**, the powdered bark of an elm tree (*Ulmus rubra*) native to North America, has strengthening, healing properties and is used in poultices. Slippery Elm is now threatened in the wild so only buy from a recognised responsible source.

Below *Slippery elm powder is made from the bark of several species of elm tree.*

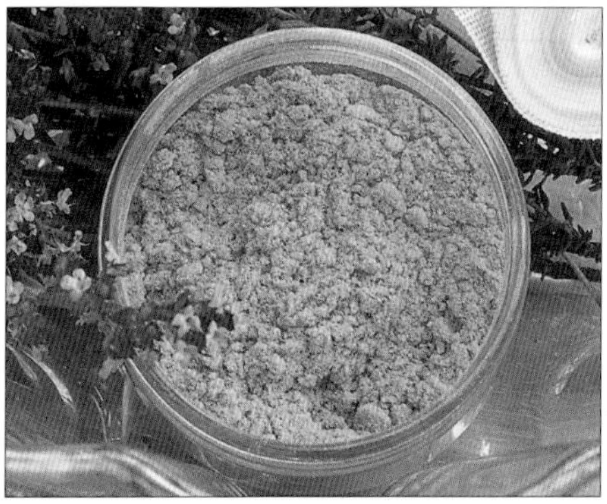

• **Borax** is a mineral deposited on the shores of alkaline lakes. It has cleansing properties and acts as an emulsifier to bind oils and water together. It is toxic if ingested in large quantities, but is safe to use in small amounts in home-made preparations.

• **Fuller's earth** is a clay-like substance, rich in minerals, used to absorb oils. It has good drawing and stimulating properties. It is an ingredient in poultices and face masks.

Below *Cayenne pepper has antibacterial properties.*

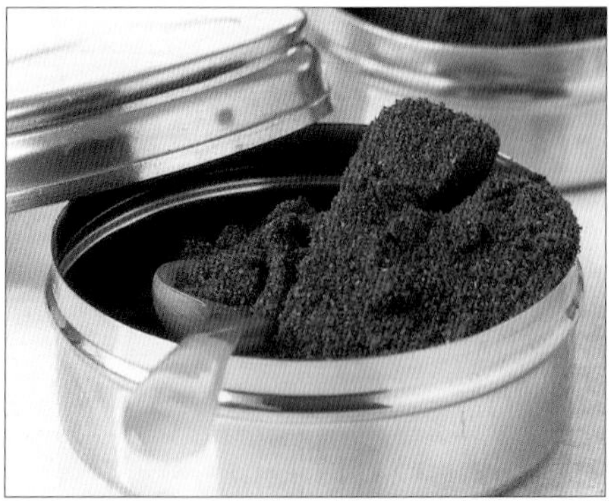

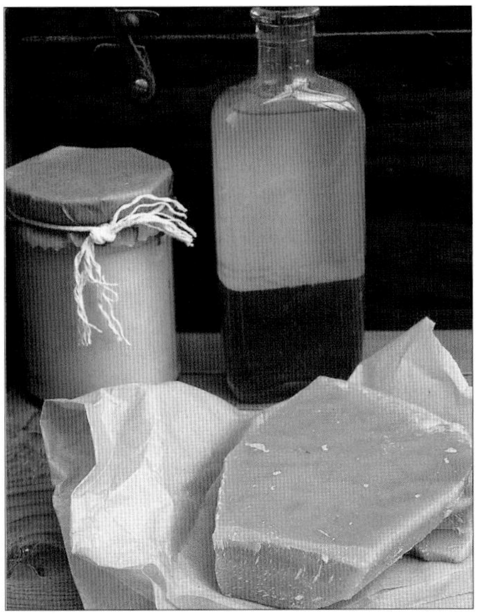

Above *Beeswax is a natural emulsifier and gives creams and ointments a firm texture.*

Spices

• **Cayenne** or chilli pepper stimulates the circulation and increases blood flow. It is harmful in excessive doses.
• **Cinnamon**, made from the rolled bark of a tropical tree (*Cinnamomum* spp), comes as "sticks" or in ground form. It is antibacterial, antifungal and has digestive properties.
• **Cloves** are the dried, immature flower buds of the tree *Syzygium aromaticum*. Stimulating and warming, they are also antiseptic and slightly anaesthetic in action.
• **Ginger** is the rhizome of a tropical plant, *Zingiber officinale*, which can be used fresh or dried, or in powdered form. It stimulates the circulation and has many uses in home remedies. High doses can be toxic and should be avoided in pregnancy.
• **Mace** and **nutmeg** both come from the fruit of the tree, *Myristica fragrans*. Mace is the outer casing of the fruit and nutmeg is the kernel. Nutmeg is a digestive and helps prevent nausea, but is harmful in large doses. The essential oil of the plant is used in anti-rheumatic remedies.

Below *Commercially available herbal tablets may contain additives.*

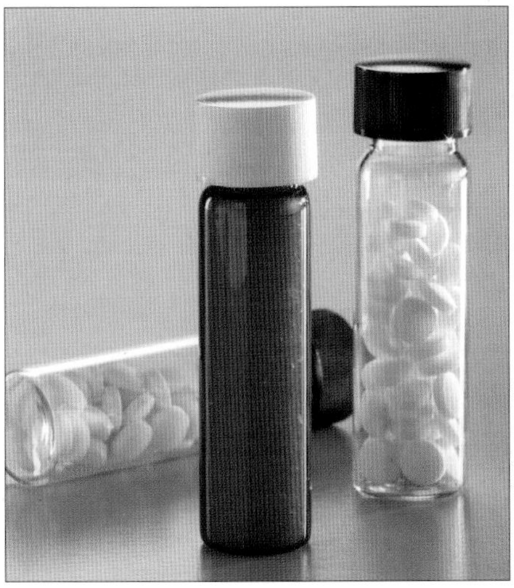

Oils and waxes

• **Beeswax** is a natural emulsifier for creams and ointments, with a high melting point and stiff texture. It is naturally yellow.
• **Cocoa butter** is the richly moisturizing fat from the cocoa bean.
• **Coconut oil** is extracted from white coconut flesh and is an excellent moisturizer for the skin. Solid at room temperature, it melts when lukewarm.
• **Emulsifying wax** is a petroleum-based wax used for binding oil and water. Although it is not an entirely "natural" product, it makes the best and simplest base for soft-textured home-made creams.
• **Petroleum jelly**, a mineral jelly, is not easily absorbed by the skin and forms a protective layer over it.

Base oils

The best base oils for use in herbal preparations are almond oil, grapeseed oil, sesame oil and jojoba oil. They are used as "carriers" to dilute essential oils.

Below *Essential oils are diluted in a base oil.*

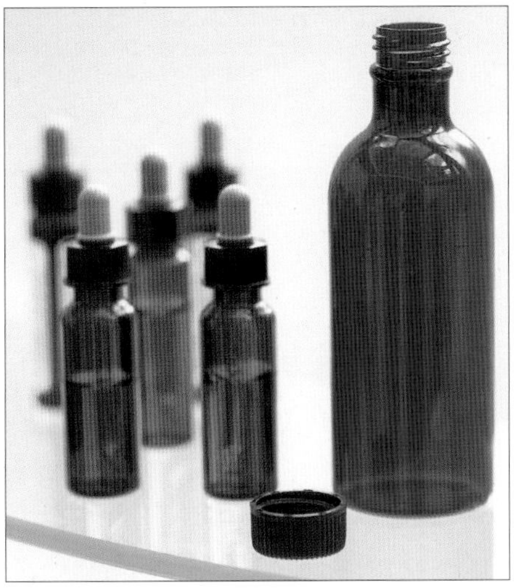

Ready-made remedies

Chosen with care, ready-made products have a valuable place in the home medicine chest.

• **Tinctures**: It is possible to make your own tinctures at home, but it is not easy to obtain all the raw ingredients necessary, and sometimes it is simply more convenient to buy a ready-made product. Manufactured tinctures vary in strength and quality, so read the labels carefully to check the contents and proportions. The proportion of herb material to liquid should be from 1:3 to 1:5, with an alcohol content of 45–50 per cent in water, depending on the herb used. The alcohol is likely to be derived from a source such as sugar beet. Tinctures provide a stronger, more concentrated way of taking a herb than infusions or decoctions. If you dilute the required dose in hot water before taking it, some of the alcohol should evaporate.
• **Herbal fluid extracts**: These are similar to tinctures, but more concentrated. They are obtainable alcohol-free. As they are so much stronger, check the labels carefully and adjust the amount you use accordingly.
• **Capsules**: Usually filled with dried, powdered herbs or a liquid extract, capsules provide a way to take an exactly measured, concentrated dose of a herb and are often standardized for quality. Follow the manufacturer's directions, or consult a qualified herbalist.
• **Tablets**: These may not be such a good choice as capsules, as they are usually made with compressed dried herbs and contain binding agents and often other additives, including artificial sweeteners and colours.
• **Macerated oils**: Herb material is steeped in a vegetable oil (preferably almond oil) to make these products. Although they are similar to the infused oils you can make for yourself, some, such as pot marigold (*Calendula*) and myrrh, are worth buying for convenience, or in order to obtain a stronger or standardized product.

Essential Oils

Essential oils are volatile liquids that are extracted from aromatic plants. They have immense therapeutic value and are often helpful in alleviating the symptoms of ill health in both physical and emotional conditions. They are used in herbal remedies in many different ways, such as diluted in a base oil and applied as a massage to relieve aches and pains, added to infusions to make compresses for sprains or bruises, incorporated into creams and ointments, mixed into decongestant steam inhalations or released into the air by vaporizing them in an essential oil burner to help improve mood.

Despite the name, essential oils are nearer to water in consistency than oil – a drop applied to paper does not usually leave any mark. They are highly volative liquids, which means they evaporate at normal air temperature. It is the essential oil in a plant that gives it its scent and it is secreted in minute glands and hairs in the leaves, stems, flowers, seeds, fruit, roots or bark. Not all plants contain essential oils.

Some plants, such as roses, contain their essential oil mainly in their flowers; others, such as lemon balm (*Melissa officinalis*), mainly in the leaves. The orange tree (*Citrus aurantium*) contains three differently named essential oils, in the flowers (neroli), the leaves (petitgrain) and the rind of the fruit (orange oil).

The organic chemical structure of plant essential oils is extremely complex. Analysis by gas liquid chromatography reveals that peppermint oil, whose 50 per cent menthol content provides its minty smell, has 98 other constituents. Flower essential oils have as many as several hundred components. For this reason it is impossible to chemically reproduce an exact copy of a naturally occurring essential oil in the laboratory.

Production of essential oils

Essential oils are soluble in fats, vegetable and mineral oils and in alcohol. For the most part they do not dissolve in water, though some of their constituents may do so. The main fragrance molecules of roses and orange flowers, for example, are soluble in water. Steam distillation is the most frequent method of extraction, and volatile solvents and alcohol are sometimes used in the process. A few fragile flower fragrances are still obtained by the centuries-old method of "enfleurage" – macerating the petals in trays of fat – and volatile oil from orange rind is extracted by expression: that is by pressing it out, now by machine, but formerly by hand. Quality is affected by varying soils, climates and harvesting conditions. Some oils may be diluted or adulterated, and it is not easy to tell, so look for a reliable source.

Essential oils in history

Plant essential oils take their name from the *quinta essentia*, or quintessence, a term coined by the Swiss physician Paracelsus, (1493–1541). He took the medieval theory of alchemy, which sought to isolate the *prima materia*, or elemental matter, of a substance, and applied it specifically to plants, to divide the "essential matter" of a plant from its "non-essential" components.

In ancient times, extracting plant fragrance by macerating it in oil or fat was common, and a technique of destructive distillation, such as that which produces oil of turpentine, was also known. At the beginning of the 11th century, steam distillation was discovered as a means of making plant-scented waters. It is usually credited to the Persian scholar and physician Avicenna, author of *The Canon of Medicine*. Arnald de Villanova, a Spanish physician

Below *Rose essential oil, distilled from highly fragrant species such as* Rosa mundi, *helps to lift depression and is good for the skin.*

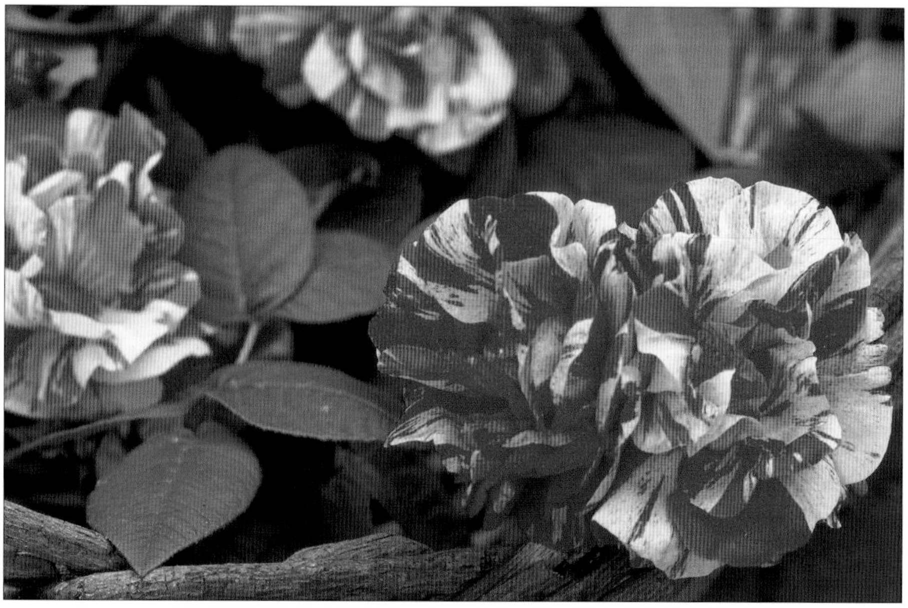

Below *Use a vegetable oil, such as almond, as a base oil for massage, to enable the essential oils to be absorbed by the skin.*

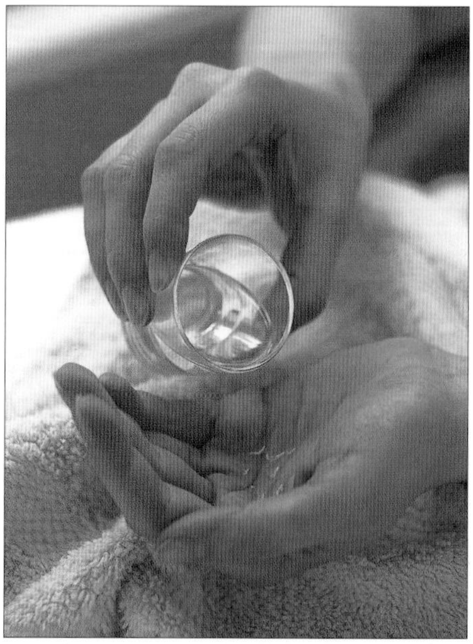

who died in 1311, popularized the use of distilled herb waters for medicinal purposes.

Distillation was seen at the time as a means of refining plant material to its purest form, through fire, and alcohol was widely used in the process because it was considered to produce the best results. It was not until the mid-16th century that the nature of essential oils was understood and the process of separating them from the distillate was put into practice.

By the beginning of the 17th century plant essential oils were available from professional pharmacies, as well as being produced on a domestic scale. Herbals and recipe books contained detailed instructions.

The power of plant fragrances

Fragrances have been revealed by many research studies to have powerful psychological effects. Some fragrances have a calming influence and others are stimulating. One six-month hospital trial found that diffusing lavender oil at night helped elderly patients to sleep better, and in Japan citrus and woody aromas are piped into offices to keep workers alert.

As well as elevating mood or acting as an aid to meditation, vaporizing plant essential oils, so that the scent molecules are dispersed through the air, has other practical benefits. Some, including tea tree, pine and eucalyptus, can destroy airborne bacteria; others, such as peppermint or lemongrass, have insect-repellent properties.

It is often claimed by scientists that synthetic plant scents are indistinguishable from natural ones, but a laboratory-made version of an essential oil replicates only its main components, perhaps five or six out of a total of more than a hundred, and cannot possibly have the same therapeutic powers.

Phototoxic oils

Most citrus oils, especially bergamot oil, make the skin more sensitive to sunlight; you should not apply them to the skin shortly before going in the sun or using a sunbed as they may cause alterations to your skin's pigmentation. It is possible to buy citrus oils that have had the offending ingredient (bergaptene) removed, but there is some question as to whether this reduces the efficacy of the oil. These treated oils are also much more expensive. You should retain a sense of proportion about this: perfumes are also phototoxic and should not be worn when sunbathing, as they can cause Berloque dermatitis, an irritating skin rash.

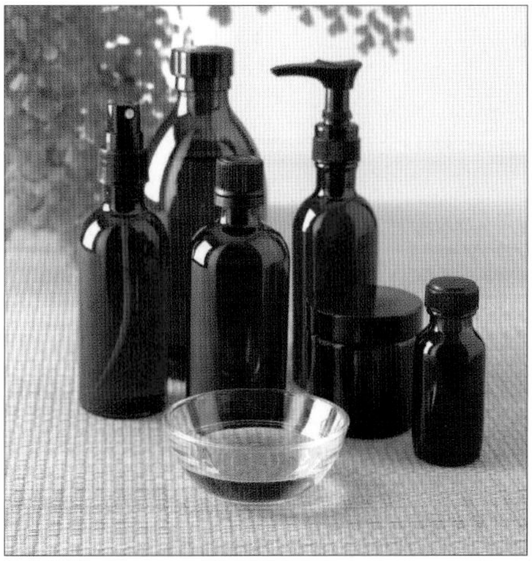

Above *Two or three essential oils can be combined to make effective blends.*

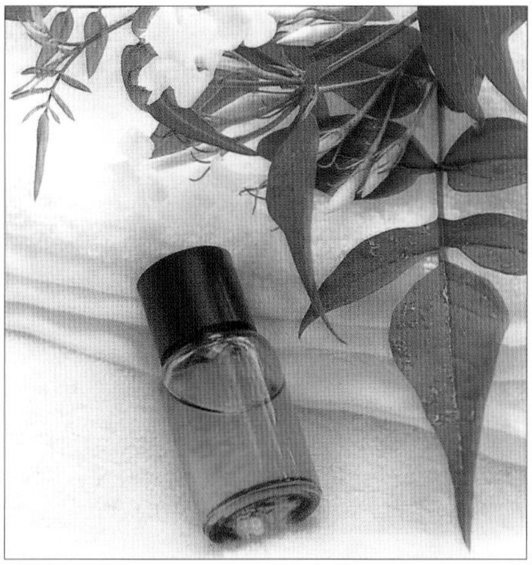

Above *Essential oil of jasmine is obtained by enfleurage, which uses fat to capture the fragrant compounds in the flowers.*

Buying essential oils

Choosing a good quality oil is not easy. You can be sure of its molecular structure and constituents only by having it analysed in a laboratory. It helps to:

- Find a reputable supplier.
- Check the price, especially for rose and other oils that are expensive to produce. Adulterated or inferior oils may be too cheap for what they purport to be.
- Look at the label – it should say "pure essential oil", not "herbal oil", which means it could be diluted in vegetable oil.
- Check that the label shows the full botanic name of the plant.

Below *A wooden box is ideal for storing a collection of essential oils, as it will protect them from the damaging effects of light.*

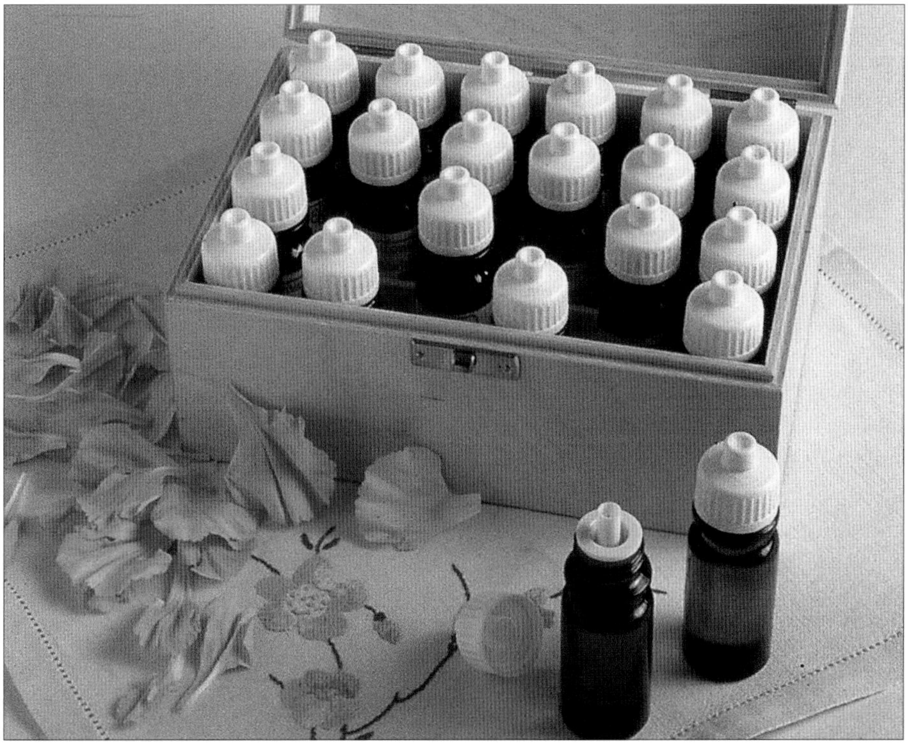

Aromatherapy

The term "aromatherapy" was coined in the early 20th century by a French chemist, René Maurice Gattefossé, who worked in his family's perfumery business. He found that essential oils are absorbed by the body from 30 minutes to 12 hours after being rubbed on to the skin, and he was among the first to recognize the therapeutic effects of essential oils. Another founder was Jean Valnet, a French army surgeon who used essential oils to good effect on the wounds of soldiers during World War II.

The concept of aromatherapy was introduced to Britain as a beauty therapy in the 1950s by Marguerite Maury, who was married to a French doctor and homeopath. It later spread to many other countries around the globe and is now widely recognized as a viable alternative therapy, with its positive benefits even acknowledged by many in the orthodox medical profession.

The healing power of fragrance has a long history, and modern research studies have confirmed its influence over mood and emotion. Essential oils are especially useful for ailments connected with the nervous system and are helpful, for example, in cases of mild depression or when feeling low.

But they have many other uses. The dividing line between aromatherapy and herbal medicine is a slim one, in the sense that essential oils have a place in many herbal home remedies. Their main applications are in massage oils, vaporizers, creams and ointments, or added to baths, foot baths, compresses and steam inhalations. They should not be taken internally without professional advice.

A MASSAGE BLEND

Vegetable oils are excellent carriers for massage. Essential oils readily dissolve in them, and they allow the hands to move continuously on the skin without dragging or slipping. Mineral oil, such as baby oil, aims to protect the skin by keeping moisture out and will not allow essential oils to penetrate, so it is not a suitable oil base. Care should be taken not to use too much of the mixed oil as it can stain sheets and clothes. To stop too much oil coming out at a time, place your fingers over the top of the bottle, tipping it against them.

Ingredients

15–20 drops essential oil (one oil or a combination of 2–3 oils of your choice)
50ml/2fl oz almond oil

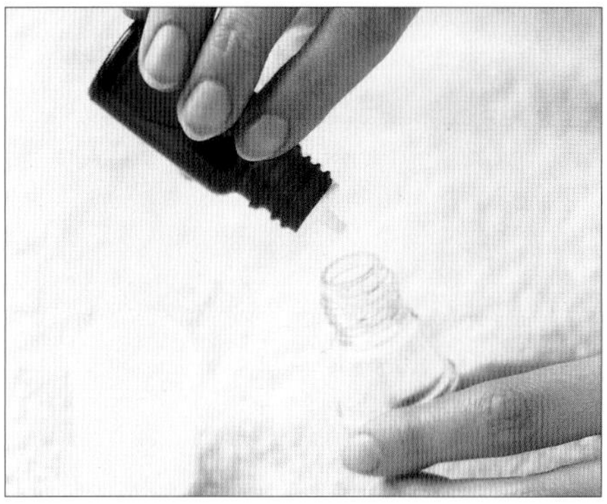

1 Measure your chosen essential oil or oils into a 50ml/2fl oz bottle. (To make a smaller amount, use a total of 8 drops in 25ml/1fl oz base oil, or 1–2 drops in 5ml/1 tsp base oil).

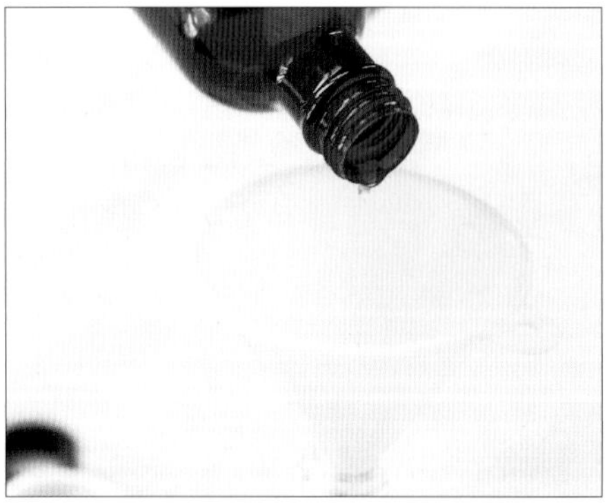

2 Fill the bottle containing the essential oil drops almost to the top with almond oil. Use a funnel, if necessary, to avoid any spillage.

3 Screw on the top securely and label the bottle with the quantity of each oil used, what the mixture is to be used for, your name and the date. Store all essential oils in a cool dark place away from direct sunlight to stop the quality deteriorating.

Safe use of essential oils

Essential oils are very powerful and should always be used sparingly. Doubling the recommended quantities will do more harm than good.

• Do not take essential oils internally without advice and guidance from a qualified aromatherapist.

• Store oils out of reach of children, in a cool, dark cupboard. When you first use an essential oil, it is sensible to do a patch test if you have reactive skin or a tendency to allergies or asthma. Mix 2 drops of essential oil with 5ml/1 tsp almond oil and apply a little to the inner arm or wrist (where skin is most sensitive). Leave for 24 hours without washing the area. If no redness or irritation develops the oil is safe to use.

• Oils should not be used undiluted – the only exception is lavender oil, which can be used on minor cuts or burns. Others must be mixed with a "base" or "carrier" oil before being applied to the skin, or they will cause irritation: in this book, almond oil is the base oil for most projects using essential oils.

• Anyone with a serious medical condition should not use essential oils without consulting their medical practicitioner and, even then, should use them only with the assistance of a qualified aromatherapist.

• Certain essential oils should not be handled by anyone who is or may be pregnant. These include cedarwood, chamomile, clary sage, frankincense, basil, jasmine, marjoram, peppermint and rosemary.

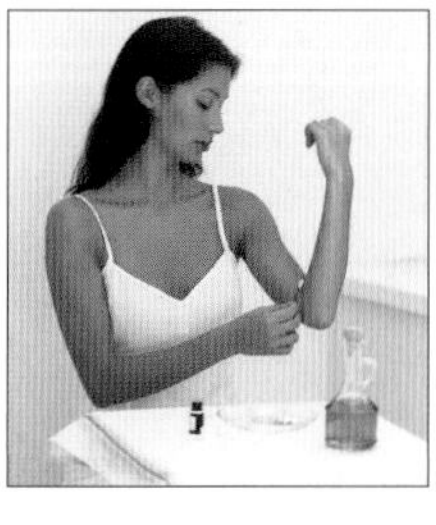

Left *Before using oils test them on a small patch of skin and leave to see if there is a reaction.*

Healing oils for home treatments

Here are some of the therapeutic properties of popular essential oils. Not all these oils will be suitable for everyone. Check the safety of any oil you use, particularly for someone who suffers from a chronic condition such as high blood pressure, or who is pregnant. Some men do not like flowery scents, but these can be combined with a citrus or woody oil to make them acceptable.

Oil	Description	Uses
• Bergamot	A flowery aroma	Antiseptic and pain-relieving; uplifting antidepressant. A good insect repellent and helpful for skin problems. Do not sunbathe for 12 hours after application.
• Chamomile	Blue oil with a gentle apple-like aroma	German chamomile relieves blisters and inflammation; Roman chamomile helps promote restful sleep and soothes aches and skin conditions.
• Frankincense	The aroma of camphor with a hint of lemon	Calms anxiety and has an uplifting effect. May relieve heavy periods. Good for mature skin and also has antiseptic properties.
• Ginger	Sweet, woody aroma	Warming: helps with aches, pains and sports injuries, arthritis, muscle spasm and poor circulation. Aids digestion and helps with travel sickness.
• Grapefruit	Tangy aroma that mixes well with flowery oils	Uplifting and works as an antidepressant. A good cleansing oil. Can help boost the immune system.
• Jasmine	Floral, slightly heady fragrance	Excellent for anxiety and menstrual problems. Considered an aphrodisiac. May be helpful in labour.
• Lavender	Slightly mossy, woody scent	Suitable for stress-related or nervous conditions. It has anti-inflammatory, antiseptic properties, and can help with skin problems and healing.
• Lemon	Sharp citrus scent that combines well with heavy floral oils	Helps aches, pains, depression, fluid retention, sluggish circulation and varicose veins. Astringent.
• Mandarin	Faintly orange aroma	Both calming and uplifting; good for anxiety, stress, insomnia and PMS. Often recommended during pregnancy.
• Neroli	Sweet floral scent with a seaweed-like note	Good for depression, shock, exhaustion and insomnia. May improve appearance of broken veins and scar tissue. Can cause drowsiness.
• Peppermint	Strong fresh minty aroma	Stimulates the circulation. Good for hot, aching feet. May cause skin reaction if overused; should not be used for people with epilepsy.
• Rose	Rich floral fragrance	Good for the skin, and may help varicose and broken veins. Helps female complaints such as PMS, as well as grief, depression and fatigue.
• Rosemary	Refreshing camphorous aroma	Soothes aches, pains, stiff muscles, increases alertness, relieves stress and exhaustion. Do not use if you have high blood pressure or epilepsy.
• Sandalwood	Warm, woody smell	Relaxing oil, with antiseptic and anti-inflammatory qualities. Good for dry skin. Helps stress and exhaustion. Said to be an aphrodisiac.
• Tangerine	Tangy, slightly sweet smell	Antispasmodic, helpful for pre-menstrual tension.
• Tea tree	Balsamic aroma	Good first-aid oil for the skin; antifungal, antiviral, anti-inflammatory. Good as an insect repellent; soothes insect bites.
• Thyme	Strong herbal scent	Antiseptic, antispasmodic, antifungal, antiviral. Stimulating oil that boosts concentration. Do not use on sensitive skin.
• Violet	Rich sweet floral	Encourages good circulation and feeds the skin. Pain-relieving and anti-inflammatory properties.
• Ylang-ylang	Powerful spicy scent	Eases tension, stress and fatigue. Over-use can cause headache or irritation.

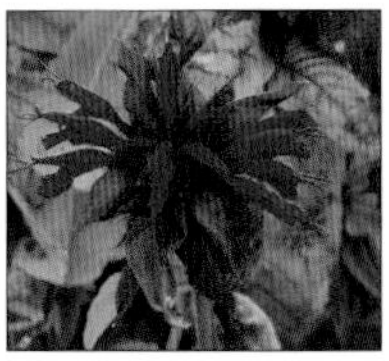
Bergamot

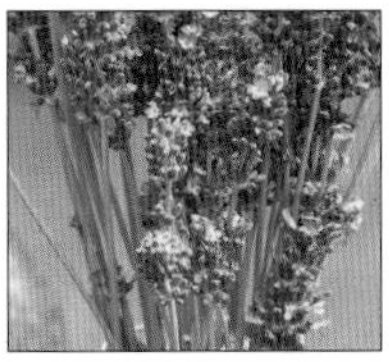
Lavender

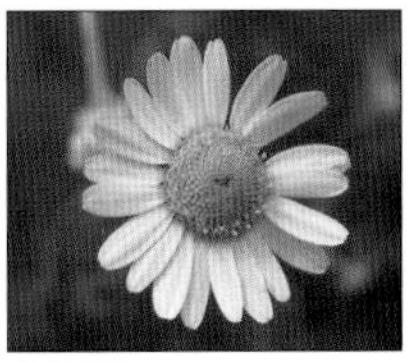
Chamomile

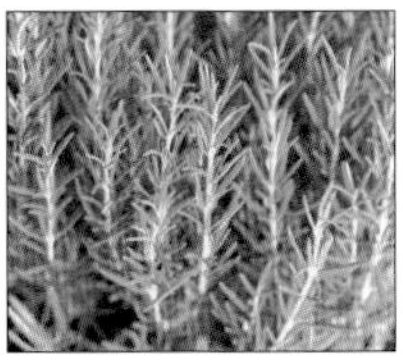
Rosemary

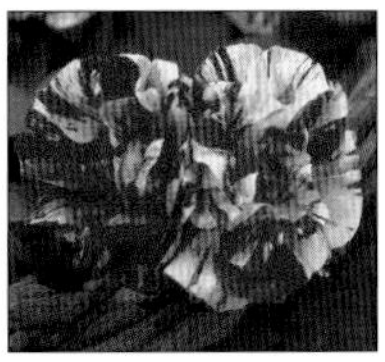
Rose

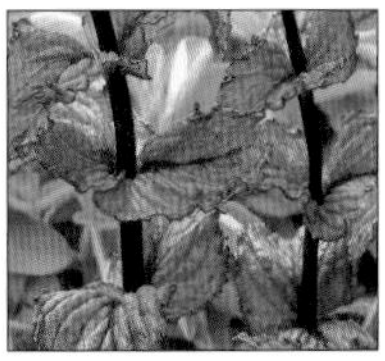
Peppermint

Making Infusions

Many of the active constituents of herbs are soluble in water, and one of the easiest ways to benefit from a herb's properties is to drink it as a tea or infusion. In principle, herb teas are made just like ordinary tea, by pouring hot water over plant material and leaving it to infuse for a short period before straining and drinking it. Many commercial brands are available, usually in the form of teabags, but the taste of teas made from fresh or home-dried garden herbs is hard to beat and ensures maximum benefit from the properties of the plant.

Herbal infusions are also useful in a number of other preparations, from creams to compresses. For these purposes they can be made a little stronger by increasing the quantity of herbs by up to one-third and leaving them to infuse a little longer. Herbal infusions for use in such preparations can be left to cool, stored in the refrigerator and used within 24 hours.

What herbs to use

Herb teas are usually made from the aerial parts of the plant: these are the leaves, stems or flowers, as appropriate. They can be used fresh or dried. Fresh herbs, such as rosemary, lemon balm and lemon verbena, provide a pleasant, lively taste, but dried herbs may sometimes be more convenient to use, especially in the winter when stocks are low.

Herbs vary in potency and when making them into teas, you will need less of a strong-tasting herb than one with a weaker flavour.

As a general rule you need twice as much fresh plant material as dried. This is because the water content has been removed from dried herbs, making them stronger and less bulky. Dried herbs that are loosely cut, or left whole (such as lemon verbena (*Aloysia triphylla*)) are bulkier than if finely cut or powdered.

When making any herbal preparation from fresh material, correct identification of the plant you are using is crucial. If in doubt, do not use the plant.

A FRESH HERB TEA

Leafy fresh herbs cannot be measured by volume as they are too bulky, so they must be weighed. Wash them before use, especially if they have been picked from the wild. A cafetière is convenient, but you can also use an ordinary teapot or a jug with a lid, then strain the tea into a cup to drink. For a single cup, use 10g/⅓oz fresh herb (or two small sprigs).

Ingredients

30g/1oz fresh herb
600ml/1pint/2½ cups boiling water

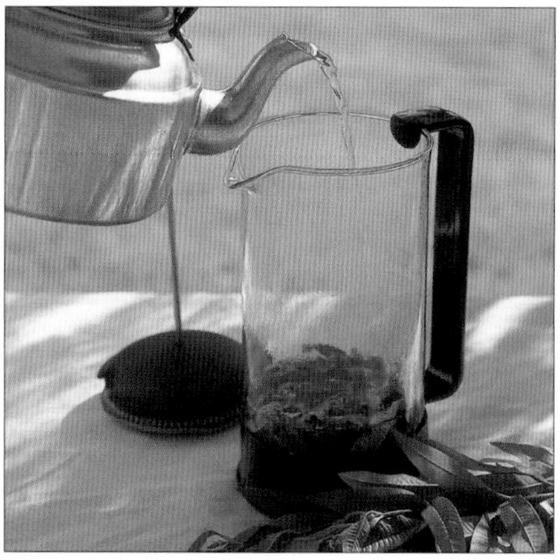

1 Warm the cafetière or pot and put in the herbs. Pour on boiling water and replace the lid to prevent the vapour dissipating.

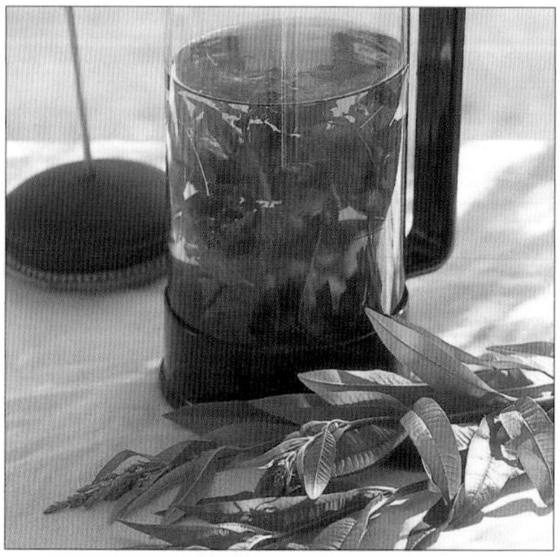

2 Leave to brew for 3–4 minutes, then depress the plunger or strain the tea into a cup for a refreshing drink.

A DRIED HERB TEA

When finely cut or powdered, dried herbs can be measured by volume, in the same way that you would measure out coffee. But when they are bulky, loose-cut leaves, such as home-dried lemon verbena (*Aloysia triphylla*), it is not possible to measure them in a spoon, and they must be weighed.

Ingredients

15ml/1tbsp finely cut dried herb, or 15g/½ oz loose-cut dried herb
600ml/1pt/2½ cups boiling water

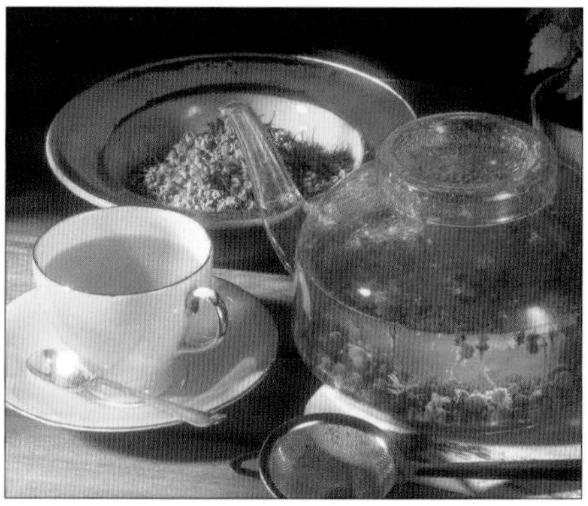

Make the infusion in the same way as for fresh herb tea. For a single cup use 5ml/1 tsp finely cut herb, or 5g/⅙oz loose-cut dried herb.

Below *A tea infuser is useful for making a herbal infusion in an individual cup, and saves having to strain out the herb.*

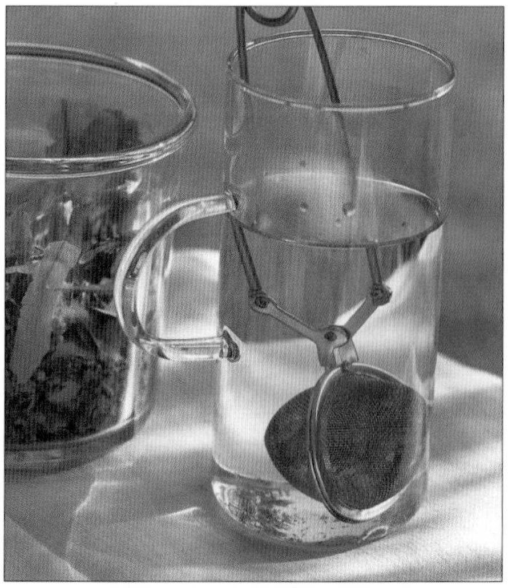

Making Decoctions and Syrups

Infusing in boiling water works well with the aerial parts of herbs, but is not enough to extract the active constituents from roots or bark, the parts used in herbs such as valerian (*Valeriana officinalis*), ginger (*Zingiber officinale*) and cramp bark (*Viburnum opulus*). This harder plant material needs to be simmered in water. The resulting liquid is strained off and is called a decoction.

MAKING A DECOCTION

Decoctions are used for similar purposes as herbal infusions: they can be taken internally to relieve a variety of conditions, such as cold symptoms, or applied externally as lotions or compresses.

Ingredients

30g/1oz herb material (roots, rhizomes or bark), freshly harvested or dried
1 litre/1½ pints/3¾ cups water

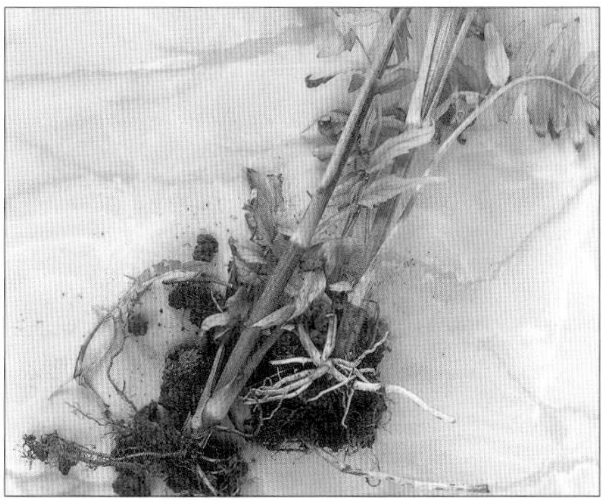

1 Roots and barks need to be prepared for use when harvested in the autumn.

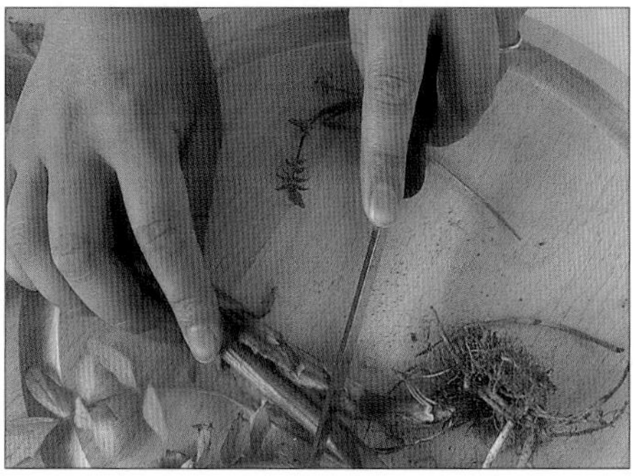

2 Trim the aerial parts of the plant away from the root.

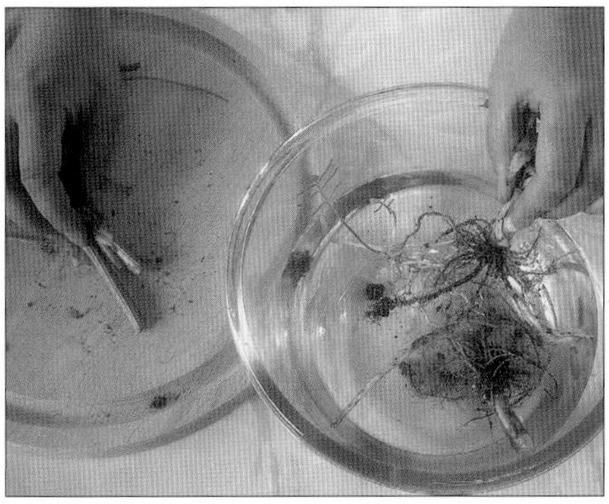

3 Wash the roots thoroughly in clean water, then chop into small pieces.

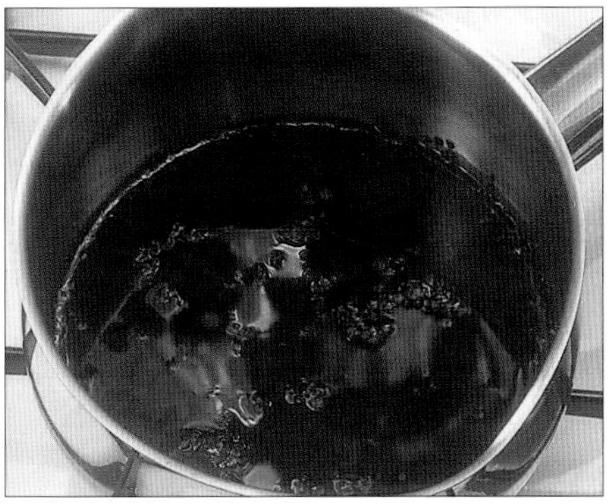

4 Put 30g/1oz of the herb material into a pan (not aluminium), and add the water. Bring to the boil and simmer for 15–20 minutes or until the liquid has reduced to 600ml/1pt/2½ cups. Remove from the heat.

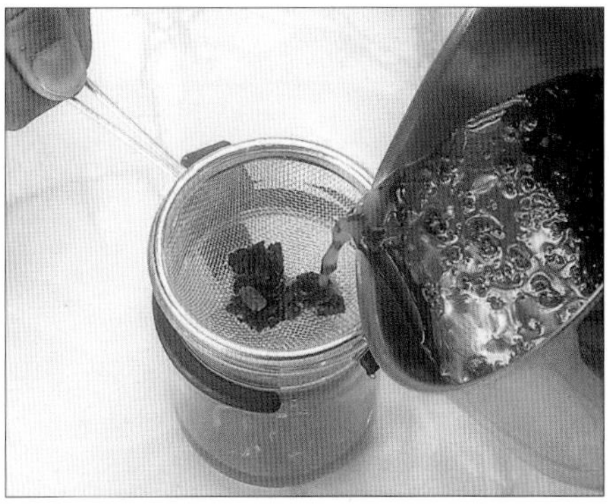

5 Strain the liquid and allow to cool before drinking, or cover and chill for to 24 hours. Decoctions can be drunk hot or cold.
They can also be used as ingredients in other herbal products.

MAKING A SYRUP

Herb syrups conserve the active constituents of plants and are useful for preserving items such as elderberries for winter coughs and colds. A syrup is also a useful way to improve the flavour of bitter herbs such as mugwort (*Artemisia vulgaris*) and vervain (*Verbena officinalis*).

Ingredients

500g/1¼lb sugar or honey
1¾ pints/4 cups water
150g/5oz plant material

1 Place the sugar or honey in a pan. Add the water. Heat gently, stirring, to dissolve. Add the herbs and heat gently for 5 minutes.

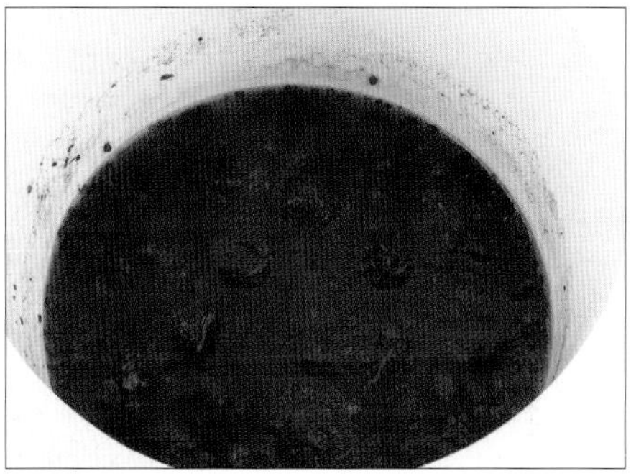

2 Turn off the heat and allow to steep overnight. Strain and store in a sterilized airtight container in the refrigerator.

Below *Syrups will keep for 18 months.*

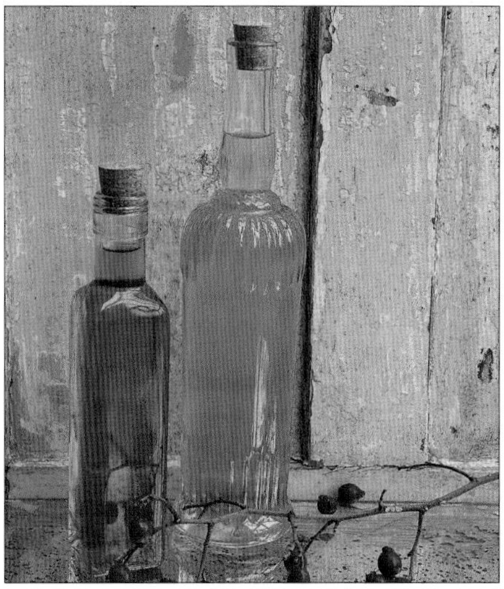

Making Tinctures

A tincture provides a more concentrated herbal product than either an infusion or a decoction. It is made by steeping the prepared herb material in a mixture of alcohol and water for several weeks: this extracts both the non-water-soluble and water-soluble active constituents.

Fresh or dried herb material can be used to make tinctures. Leaves, stems, flowers, berries, even roots, may all be suitable, depending on the plant.

Storing tinctures

The alcohol used to steep the herbs acts as a preservative, so tinctures will keep for up to 2 years. Strain them into sterlized dark glass bottles with tight-fitting stoppers to prevent deterioration of the contents. If you do need to use clear glass, keep the tinctures in a dark cupboard to protect them from light.

A TINCTURE

Useful tinctures include lavender for headaches, raspberry leaf for mouth ulcers, elderflower for colds, juniper for rheumatism, and sweet violet for insomnia. Vodka is the most appropriate alcohol for home-made tinctures, since it is a pure spirit containing few additives. In order to make the tincture strong enough, the herb material has to be soaked in the alcohol and water in batches, as there is not enough liquid to cover all the herbs at once.

Ingredients

100g/4oz dried herbs or 300g/11oz fresh herbs
250ml/8fl oz/1 cup vodka
100ml/4fl oz water

CAUTION Under no circumstances use industrial alcohol or white spirits to make tinctures, as they are highly toxic.

Right *Tinctures are an effective way to extract the active ingredients of plants and are easy to prepare. They can be used in compresses and lotions or diluted and taken internally for various conditions.*

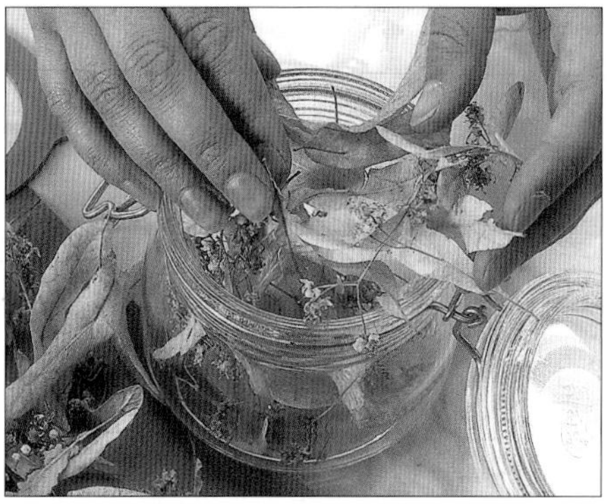

1 Place one third of the given quantity of dried or fresh herbs in a jar.

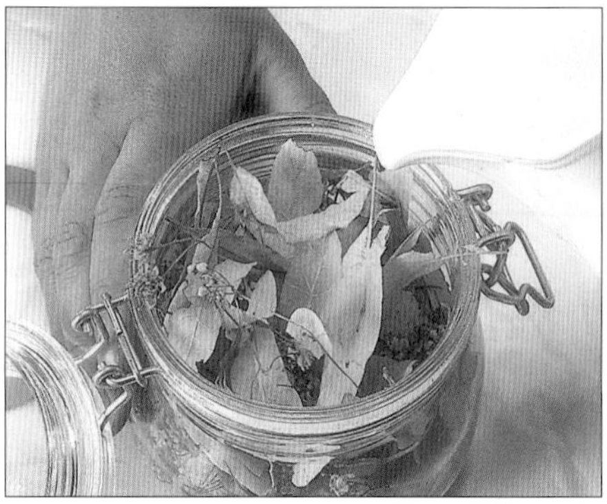

2 Stir the alcohol and water together and pour the mixture over the herbs. Leave the herbs to steep in the liquid for one week, preferably in a warm, dry place.

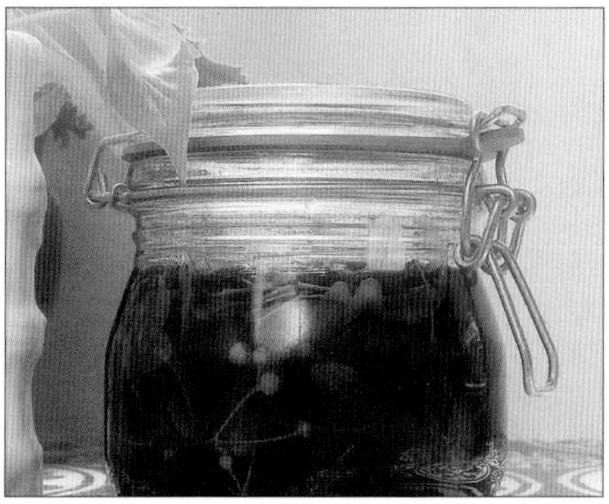

3 Gently shake the jar once a day.

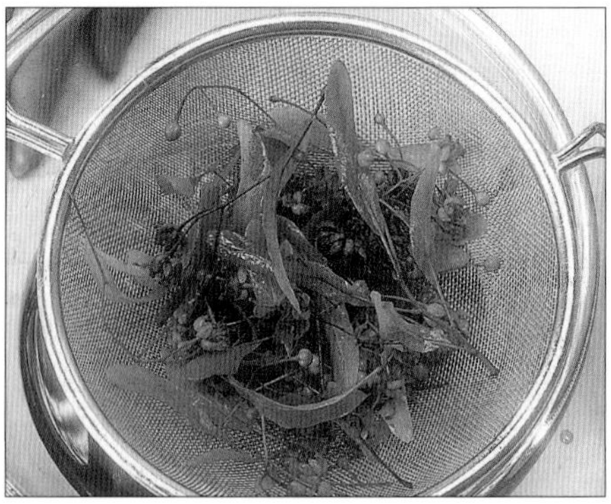

4 Strain and discard the herbs. Substitute a fresh batch and leave for a further week. Repeat with the final batch of herbs, before straining and storing the liquid in a cool dark place.

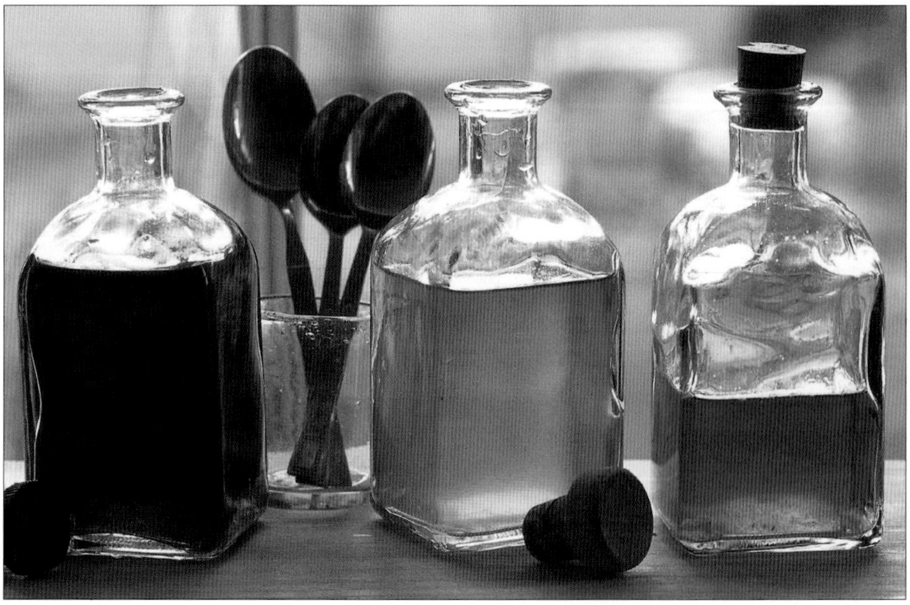

Making Cold-infused Oils

Cold infused oils, also known as "macerated oils" or herbal oils, are simple to prepare and are an effective way to infuse herb material in a vegetable oil base. They are suitable for external use in massage, as bath oils or for conditioning the hair and skin.

It pays to use a good quality oil for massage and therapeutic purposes – such as almond or grapeseed. Sunflower oil can be used, but is more suitable as a culinary oil. It is best not to leave any of the fresh herb in the oil once the infusion is complete, as after a couple of weeks it will start to decay and adversely affect the keeping properties of the oil.

Which herbs to use

Fresh herbs are best for this purpose, but dried ones may also be used. Delicate flower heads, such as chamomile (*Chamaemelum nobile*), marigold (*Calendula officinalis*) or St John's wort (*Hypericum perforatum*), work well, as does more robust herb material, including rosemary, marjoram, thyme, sage and lavender, garlic and spices.

Exact quantities cannot be specified, as the method depends on covering plant material with oil and, depending on which herb you use, you may need to steep several batches in the oil to suffuse it sufficiently with the desired fragrance.

Do not put St John's wort oil directly on to the skin before going out into bright sunlight as it can cause a reaction.

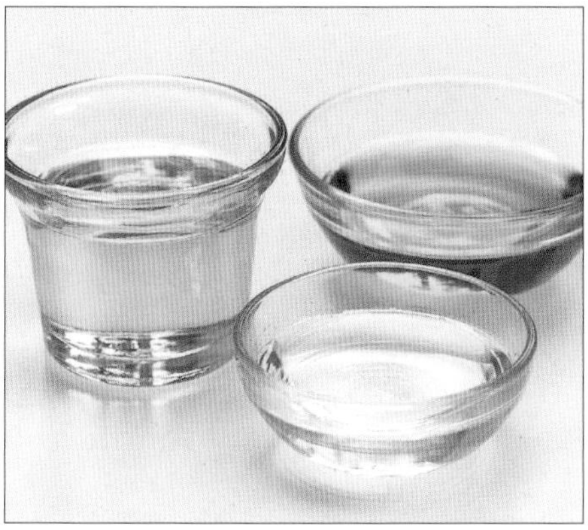

Above *Almond and grapeseed oils are best when making herbal oils for massage.*

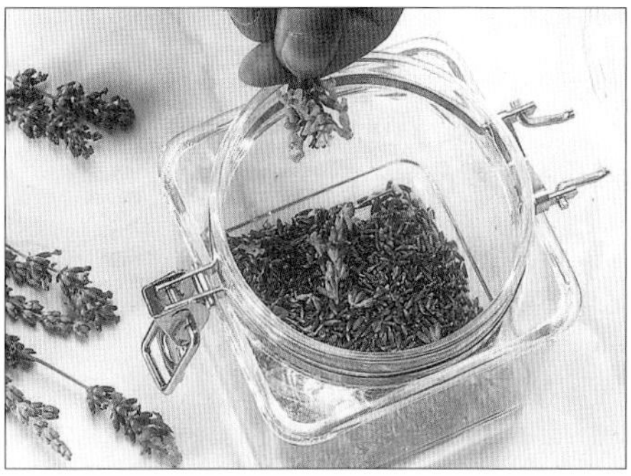

1 Fill a glass storage jar with the flowers or leaves of your chosen herb.

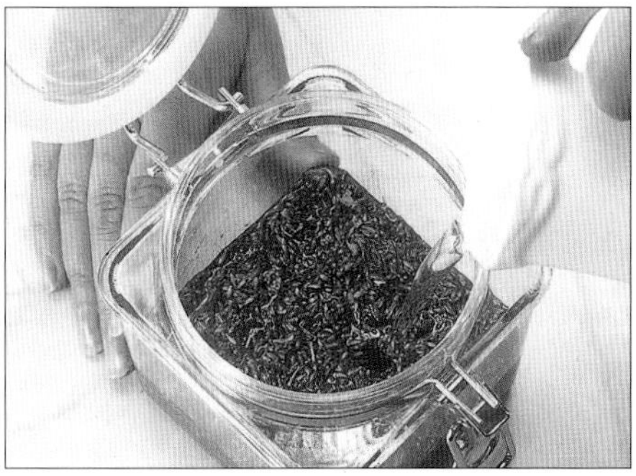

2 Pour in a light vegetable oil to cover the herbs – try sunflower or grapeseed oil.

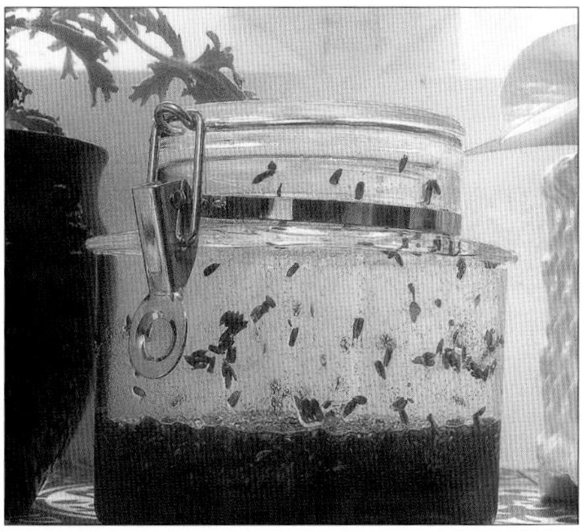

3 Leave the jar to stand on a sunny windowsill for a month to steep. Give it a shake every day.

Right *Massaging the head and hair with herbal oils relieves stress and conditions the scalp at the same time. Ensure that there is time to relax after the massage to fully feel the benefit of it.*

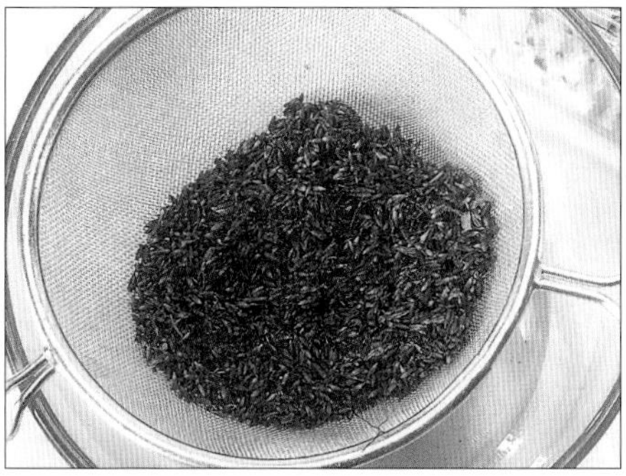

4 Strain the flowers or leaves and discard them. For a stronger infusion, renew the herbs in the oil every 2 weeks.

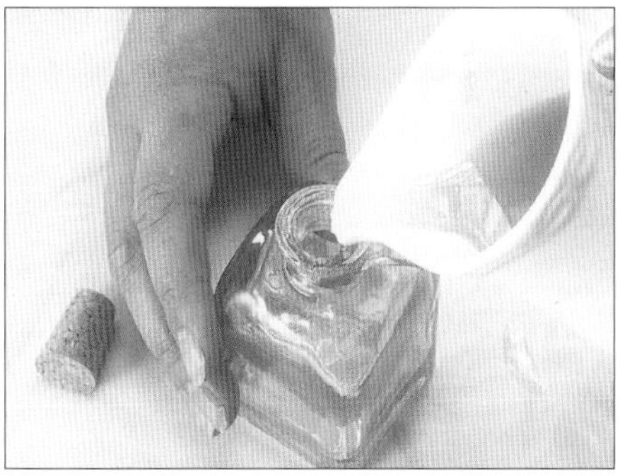

5 Pour the finished infused oil into sterilized stoppered bottles and keep in a dark, dry place for up to 6 months.

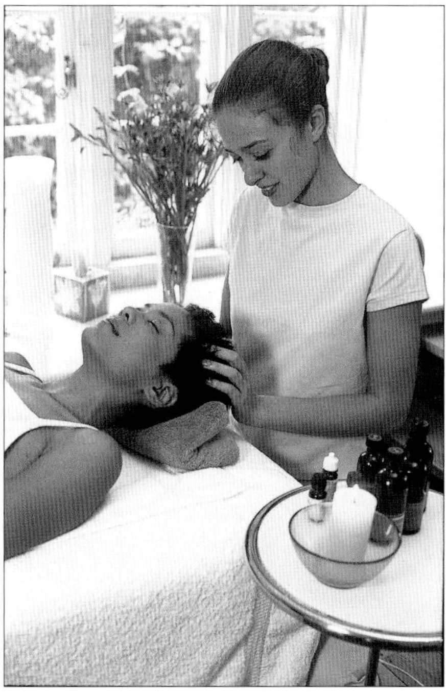

Making Poultices and Compresses

Poultices are made with solid herb material and compresses with liquid preparations. They are applied to the area to be treated using gauze bandaging, or a similar soft material. Both poultices and compresses are helpful in easing general aches and pains, including headache, backache, stomach and period pain, stiff muscles, joint pains and strains, as well as relieving spots, boils, itchy skin and insect bites. They may be used cold or hot, according to the condition being treated.

A HERBAL POULTICE

A poultice is made using the fresh herb applied to the skin at the point of pain or injury and held in place with a bandage. Dried leaves can also be used for convenience, or when no fresh material is available.

Ingredients

handful of fresh herbs or
30–45ml/2–3 tbsp of dried herbs
boiling water to cover

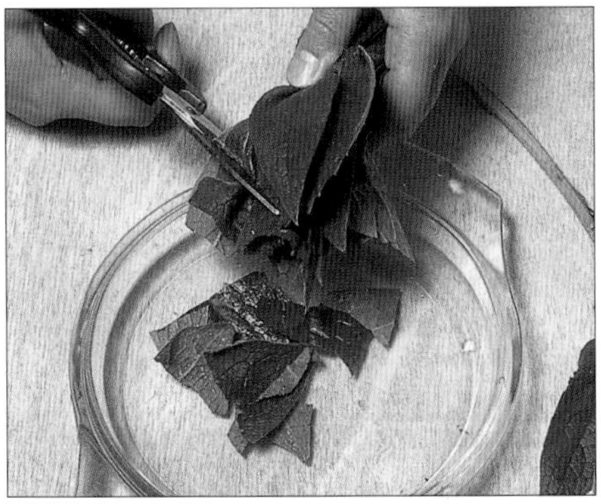

1 Place a handful of roughly chopped clean and freshly picked herb leaves in a bowl and cover with boiling water. Leave to stand for 5–10 minutes. Mash with a fork.

CAUTION Do not use herbal poultices or compresses on broken skin. They may exacerbate the problem.

Right *Essential oils can be used to soak fabric to make a compress or a poultice.*

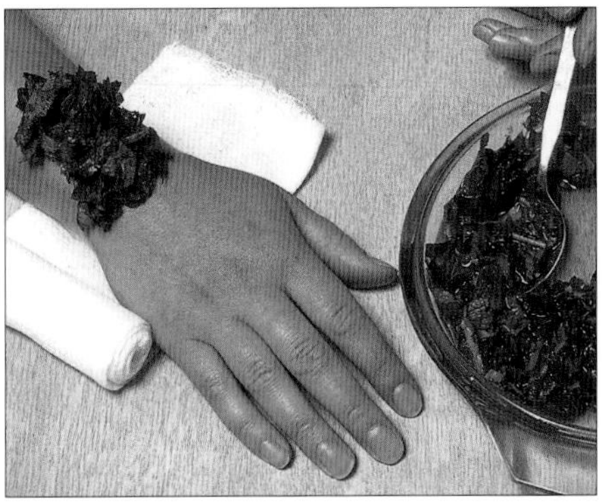

2 Squeeze out the excess liquid and apply the herbs directly to the skin, or place between two layers of gauze. Bind the herbs loosely with a bandage to hold it in place.

A HERBAL COMPRESS

A compress is made by soaking a piece of fabric in a liquid herbal preparation and applying it to the skin of the affected area. For a cold compress, place a sealed plastic bag of frozen vegetables or crushed ice cubes wrapped in fabric over the treatment area and hold in place. For a warm compress, wring out a pad or cloth in the hot liquid and hold it on the area until it cools, then repeat as necessary.

Ingredients

handful of fresh herbs or
30–45ml/2–3 tbsp dried herbs
or 2–3 tsp/10–15ml tincture
or 5–8 drops essential oil
600ml/1pt/2½ cups boiling water

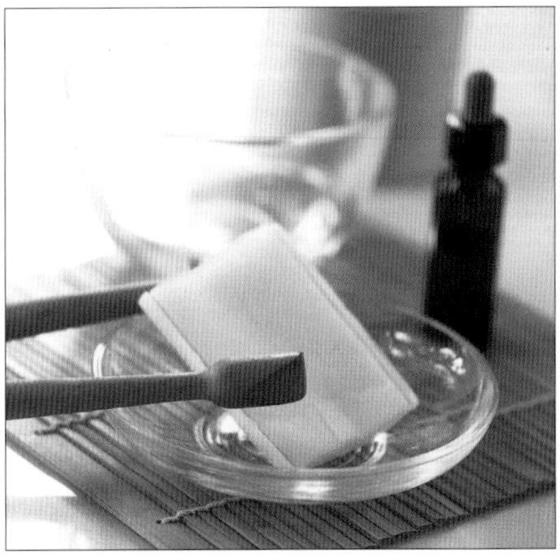

1 To make a herbal infusion, put the fresh or dried herbs in a bowl and pour over the measured amount of boiling water. Leave to stand for 30 minutes to one hour. Alternatively, dilute the herbal tincture or essential oil in hot or cold water.

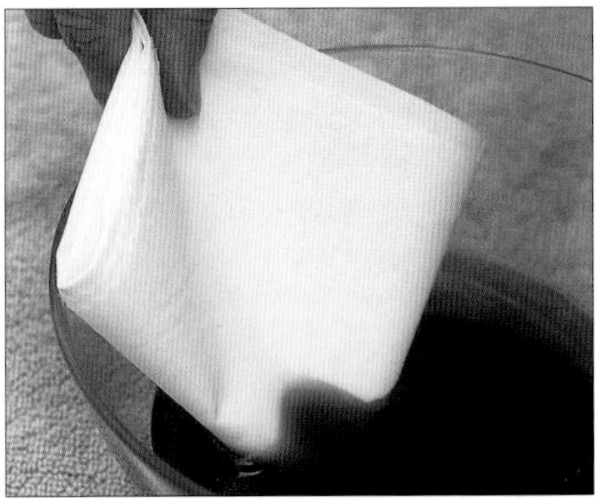

2 Fold a piece of clean, soft cotton fabric into a loose pad, and soak it in the infusion, diluted tincture or essential oil. Wring out the excess liquid.

3 Apply the pad directly to the affected area, holding it in place and repeating as necessary.

Below *A hot compress soothes aching joints and muscles.*

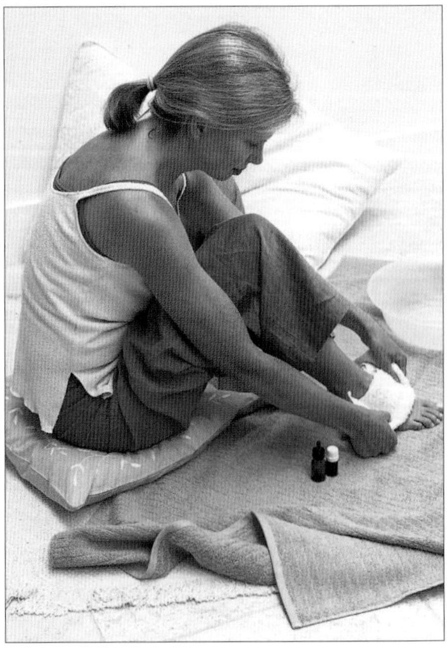

Making Creams and Ointments

Herbal creams and ointments have many uses for soothing and conditioning the skin, or as liniments and rubs for aches and pains.

Though both are used in similar ways their composition is different. A cream is a mixture of oils or fats with water, which softens on the skin and is absorbed into it. An ointment is made of oils or fats but contains no water and is not intended to be absorbed into the skin; instead it provides a barrier or protective layer over it, keeping out dirt and moisture and helping to retain the skin's natural oils.

Making your own creams and ointments is not difficult. You can also buy simple, unperfumed base creams or lotions, to which you can add essential oils, herbs or herbal tinctures as appropriate.

Whether you buy ready-made base creams or make your own, the addition of any plant material, including essential oils and tinctures, will shorten the shelf life of the products and most should be used within 2–3 months.

A HERBAL OINTMENT

Protective barrier ointments were once made from animal fats, but petroleum jelly or paraffin wax makes a longer-lasting base that is more pleasant to apply.

Ingredients

200g/7oz petroleum jelly
30g/1oz fresh herbs, finely chopped, or
15g/½oz dried herbs

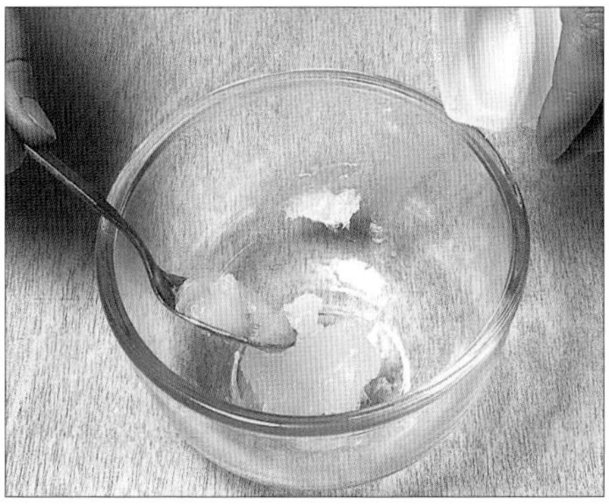

1 Put the petroleum jelly into a bowl and set it over a pan of simmering water to melt.

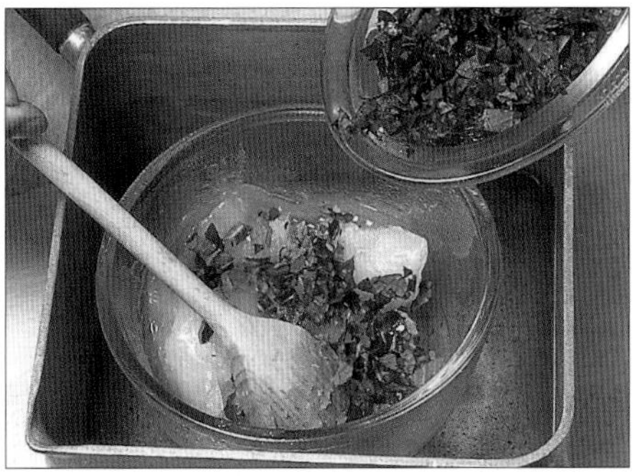

2 Stir in the chopped fresh or dried herbs and continue to heat gently over simmering water, stirring occasionally, for about 1 hour. Strain the mixture through muslin (cheesecloth) or a jelly bag, and pour into a sterilized jar immediately. Seal and label.

CAUTION Do not add more herbal content, essential oil or tincture than specified.

A HERBAL CREAM

Skin creams made from natural ingredients have many uses and are soothing and moisturizing. If you are using essential oils instead of an infusion, lavender, rose and neroli have beneficial properties, and smell delicious. Emulsifying ointment, a product that readily mixes with water, is available from pharmacies and is the standard base for home-made skin creams. It is easy to use and provides the right texture, though it is not an entirely natural product. Natural ingredients that can be used to make creams in the same way include beeswax, coconut oil and cocoa butter, and they are used in some of the recipes for beauty treatments later in this book.

Ingredients

300ml/½ pint/1¼ cups water
30g/1oz fresh herbs or 15g/½oz dried herbs
or 5–6 drops essential oil
or 5ml/1 tsp herbal tincture
60ml/4 tbsp emulsifying ointment
15ml/1 tbsp glycerine

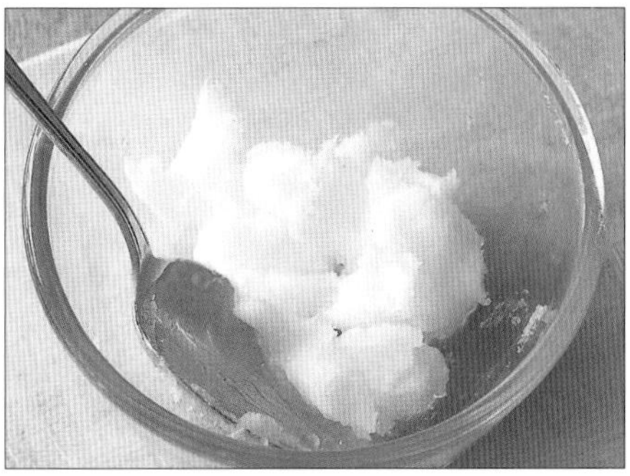

1 Boil the water and pour it over the fresh or dried herbs. Leave to infuse until cool, then strain. Place the emulsifying ointment with the glycerine in a bowl and set it over a pan of simmering water. Heat gently, stirring, until the ointment has melted, then remove the bowl from the heat.

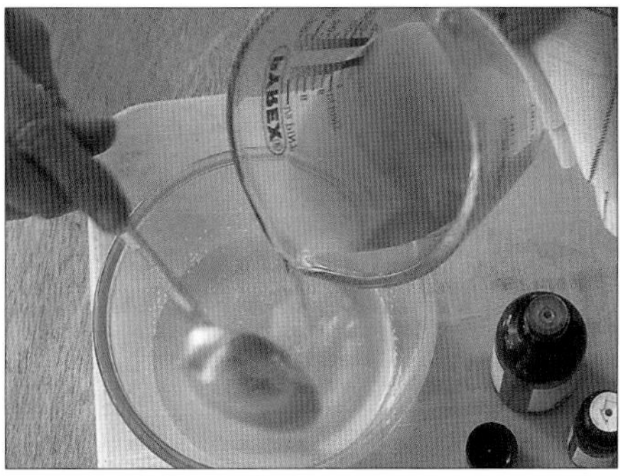

2 Add the cooled herbal infusion (or 300ml/½ pint/1¼ cups plain water to which you have added the essential oil or herbal tincture), and stir until the mixture starts to thicken. Before it has set completely, pour it into a small sterilized jar. Seal, date and label. Keep the cream in a cool place and use it within 2 months.

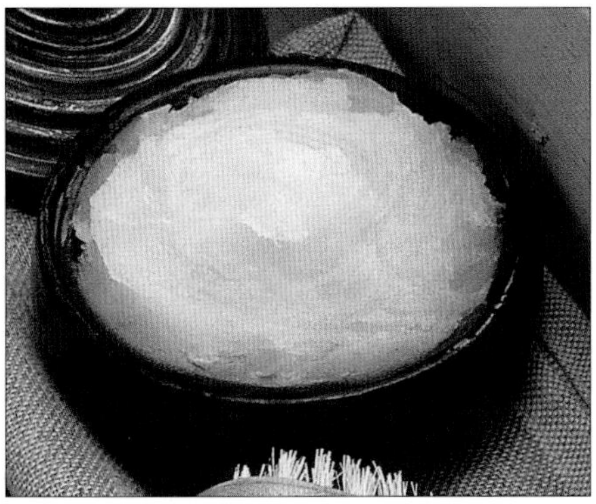

Right *Herbal creams should be used soon after making.*

Making Inhalations

Breathing in herbal vapours can be beneficial both for physical and mental conditions. Steam inhalations are an effective way of bringing temporary relief for catarrh and blocked sinuses, and can also be used in facial beauty treatments to open the pores and cleanse the skin. Inhaling just the fragrance of plant essential oils has a powerful effect on mood and mental states. It is simple to do using a vaporizer or essential oil burner to scent the air, which works more subtly than breathing in steam.

A STEAM INHALATION

This old-fashioned treatment remains highly effective as a decongestant. You can use an appropriate essential oil or strong herbal infusion to scent the steaming water, but for the gentlest effect use the fresh herbs themselves.

Ingredients

600ml/1pt/2½ cups water
large handful of fresh herbs
or 200ml/7fl oz/1 cup strong herbal infusion made from fresh or dried herbs
or 6–8 drops essential oil

1 Boil the water, pour it into a bowl and add the herb material appropriate to the condition you are treating. Add a little cold water.

2 Lean over the bowl, place a towel over both your head and the bowl to retain the steam and aroma, and inhale the steam for a few seconds at a time. Continue for up to 10 minutes overall.

Below *Inhaling steam infused with herbs helps to clear the nasal passages. Allow the water to cool sufficiently first.*

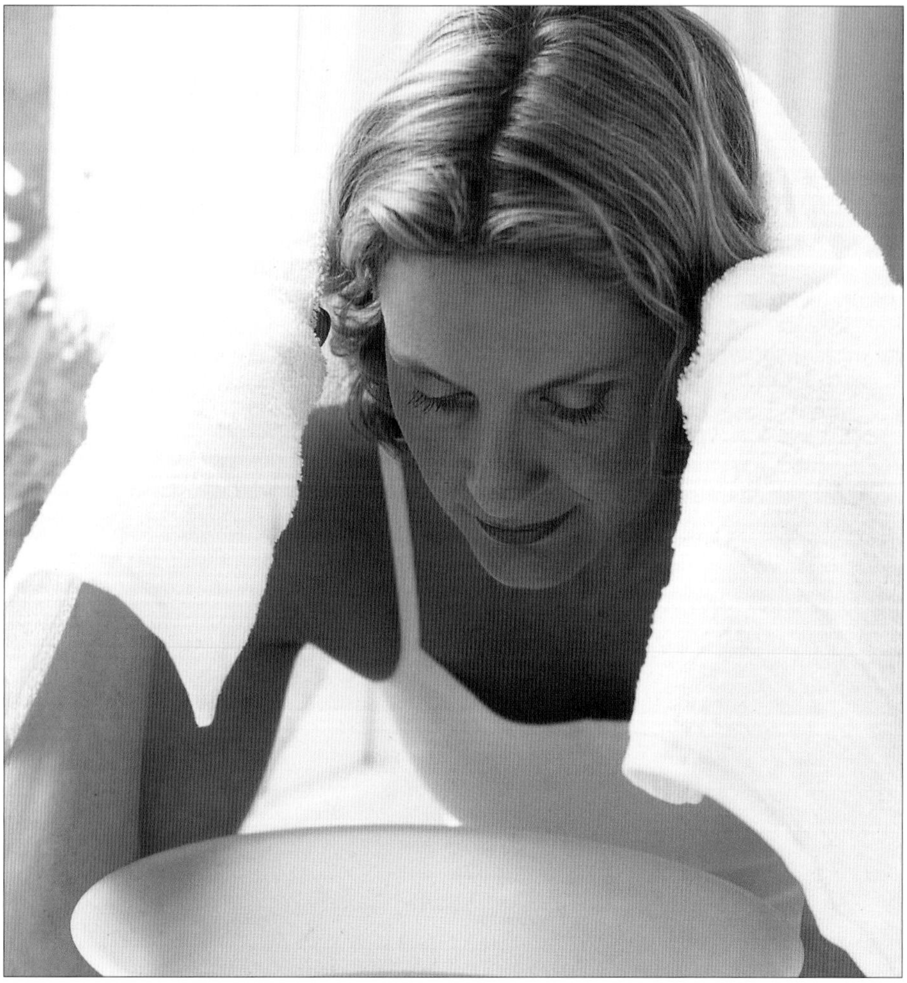

AN ESSENTIAL OIL BURNER

Breathing in essential oil vapours can be relaxing, restorative or uplifting. One way to inhale the scent is simply to put a few drops on a handkerchief and keep it on your pillow overnight. But for a more controlled and concentrated method, which is also longer lasting, an essential oil burner is the answer.

There is a wide range of styles to choose from, but they all work by heating the essential oil in water so that it vaporizes as steam, which can be inhaled. The heat is usually supplied by any candle or nightlight (tealight). Always treat an essential oil burner as you would a candle: do not leave it unattended or with an unsupervised child, and never leave one burning overnight.

Put 6–8 drops of essential oil into the filled water chamber of the burner.
Top up the water as it evaporates, adding another 1–2 drops of oil as necessary.
A few drops of oil in a bowl of hot water will also scent a room.

CAUTION If you have either high blood pressure or asthma you should seek medical advice before using steam, and in any case do not overdo an inhalation.

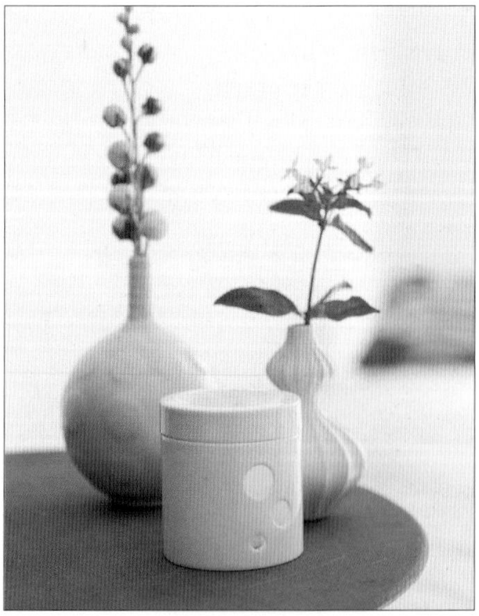

Above *An essential oil burner is a good way to inhale beneficial vapours.*

Making Bath Mixes and Sleep Pillows

Other ways to benefit from the scent of herbs include putting them into bath bags to hang over the taps, allowing the warm water to release a restorative, relaxing steam, or adding them to sleep pillows to help induce a restful night.

A HERBAL BATH MIX

- **Relaxing:** Chamomile (*Chamaemelum nobile*) flowers and foliage.
- **Revitalizing:** Rosemary (*Rosmarinus officinale*), peppermint (*Mentha* x *piperita*), lemon thyme (*Thymus* x *citriodorus*), pine needles.
- **To improve circulation:** Nettles (*Urtica dioica*). These will lose their sting once they have been soaked in hot water.
- **For aches and pains:** Comfrey leaves (*Symphytum officinale*) with 15ml/1 tbsp powdered ginger (*Zingiber officinale*).
- **For colds:** Lavender (*Lavandula*), thyme and a 2.5cm/1in piece of grated fresh ginger.
- **For itchy skin:** Comfrey, houseleek (*Sempervivum tectorum*), lady's mantle (*Alchemilla mollis*), marshmallow (*Althaea officinalis*). Add a cup of cider vinegar to the bath as well.

Below *For a restorative, invigorating bath, hang a herb-filled bath bag over the tap while the water is running, then stir 1kg/2¼lb sea salt into the bath. Soak in it for 10 minutes before scrubbing the skin with the bath bag, to which you have added some grated soap. Finish with a cool shower to leave the skin feeling soft and refreshed.*

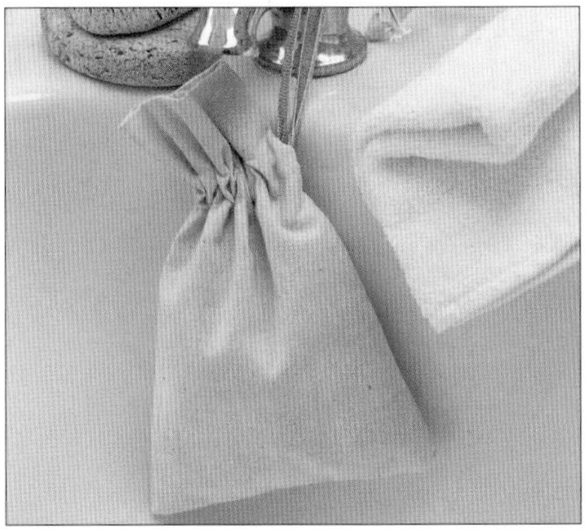

A SLEEP PILLOW

To fill this pillow use a mixed rose pot-pourri incorporating sleep-inducing herbs such as hops (*Humulus lupulus*), chamomile and lavender. Alternatively fill with hops alone.

You will need

40 x 25cm/16 x 10in cotton wadding (batting)
pins
sewing machine
matching sewing thread and needle
rose and herb pot-pourri
2 pieces of fabric, 24 x 29cm/9½ x 11½in
1m/1yd gathered broderie anglaise edging
tacking (basting) thread
22cm/8½in strip self-adhesive fabric tape

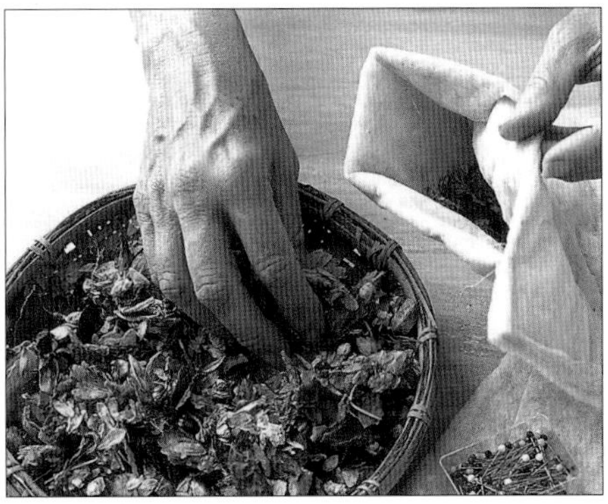

1 To make the inner pad, fold the wadding (batting) in half with the shorter edges together. Pin, then stitch together, leaving an opening at one end. Turn through and fill with pot-pourri. Slip-stitch the opening.

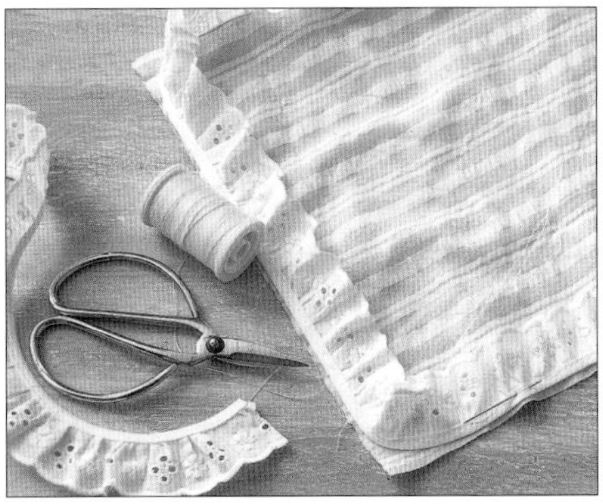

2 To make the decoration on the outer casing, place one cover piece right side up on a flat surface. Pin and baste the broderie anglaise all around the edge, with the frill facing inwards.

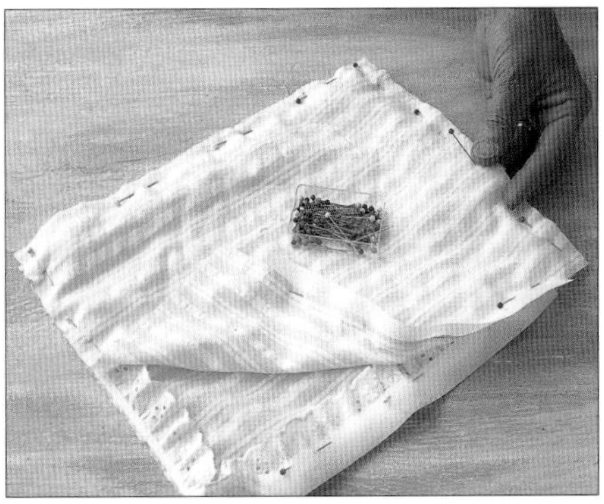

3 Separate the fabric tape and centre the two strips on matching edges of the right side of two cover pieces. Stitch in place. Stitch the covers together around the remaining sides.

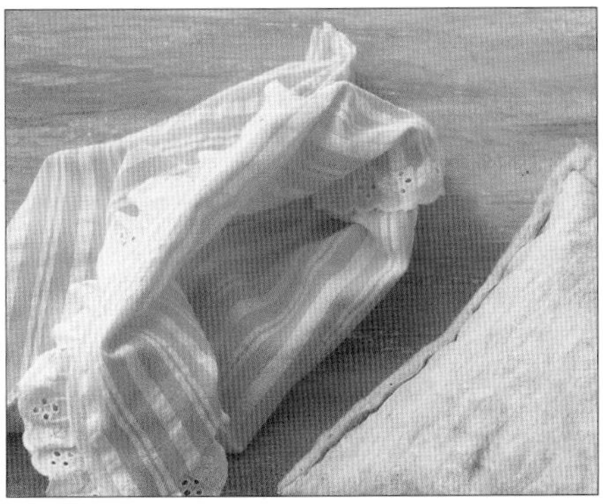

4 Turn the cover through and insert the filled pad. Fasten the fabric tape.

Below *Herbal pillows can aid sleep.*

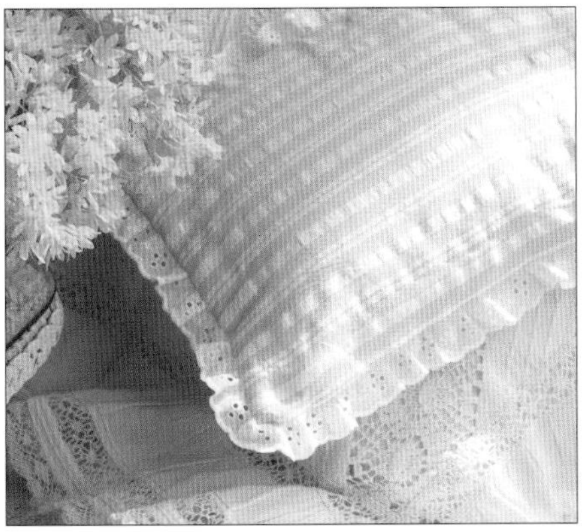

Healing Herbs in Food

There are many health benefits to be gained from adding plenty of herbs to food. Herbs add interest and flavour to bland foods, and are rich in vitamins and minerals: although it may be argued that they are only used in small amounts in many dishes, the effect is cumulative. In some dishes, where a specific herb is the main ingredient – such as basil in pesto sauce or nettles in soup – it will be eaten in more than adequate amounts. Some herb seeds aid digestion and certain familiar food items, such as garlic and oats, have useful herbal applications. Spices are also valuable in the diet for their medicinal properties as well as for flavour.

Reducing fat and salt in the diet

There is no doubt that fat makes food more palatable, and it is all too easy to acquire a taste for over-salty food, but excess salt in the diet has been linked to high blood pressure. If you are trying to cut down on your intake of fat and salt, herb and spice seasonings are a healthy alternative way to add extra flavour to food. Mix dried herbs into soups and casseroles, stir-fries and pasta sauces, or sprinkle them over lightly cooked vegetables. Nothing beats fresh herbs as seasoning. Tie them in small mixed bunches and use as required as a bouquet garni.

Herbs to use in place of salt

- Bay (*Laurus nobilis*)
- Coriander (*Coriandrum sativum*)
- Hyssop (*Hyssopus officinalis*)
- Lovage (*Levisticum officinale*)
- Pot marjoram (*Origanum onites*)
- Rosemary (*Rosmarinus officinalis*)
- Sage (*Salvia officinalis*)
- Summer savory (*Satureja hortensis*)
- Thyme (*Thymus* spp)
- Winter savory (*Satureja montana*)

CAUTION Spices should never be ingested in large quantities, or taken as medicines without medical or professional healthcare advice – turmeric can interact with some pharmaceutical drugs, and nutmeg is dangerous in high doses.

A HERBAL SEASONING

Make this seasoning with home grown herbs in early summer when they are plentiful.

Ingredients

Dried lovage (*Levisticum officinale*)
Marjoram (*Origanum* spp)
Summer or winter savory (*Satureja hortensis* or *S.montana*)
Parsley (*Petroselinum crispum*)
Bay leaves (*Laurus nobilis*)
Sage (*Salvia officinalis*)
Thyme (*Thymus vulgaris*)
Rosemary (*Rosmarinus officinalis*)

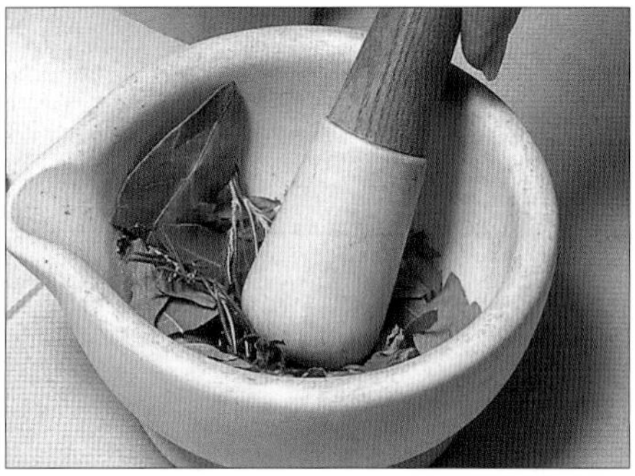

1 Pound equal quantities of dried lovage, marjoram, summer or winter savory and parsley, with half quantities of bay leaf, sage, thyme and rosemary with a mortar and pestle. Pour into airtight jars to store.

Below *Store dried herbs in dark containers.*

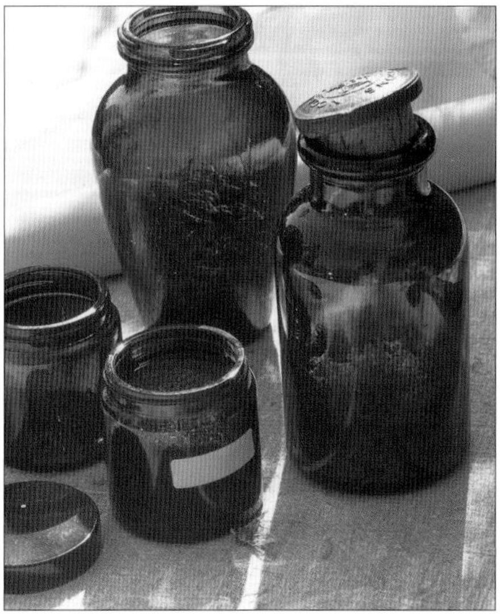

A HOT AND SPICY SEASONING

All these spices stimulate the appetite as well as acting as digestives. Cayenne and ginger help to boost circulation, and cayenne is antibacterial. Add cumin as an optional extra.

Ingredients

Ground mace (*Myristica fragrans*)
Ground coriander (*Coriandrum sativum*)
Ground ginger (*Zingiber officinale*)
Cayenne pepper
Nutmeg (*Myristica fragrans*)

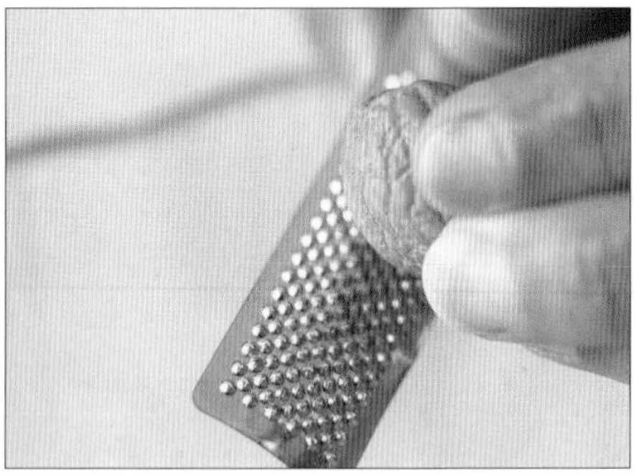

1 Mix together equal quantities of mace, coriander and ginger with one-third as much cayenne pepper and freshly grated nutmeg.

2 Store the mixture in a dark glass jar.

Below *Spices have beneficial properties as well as adding flavour to food.*

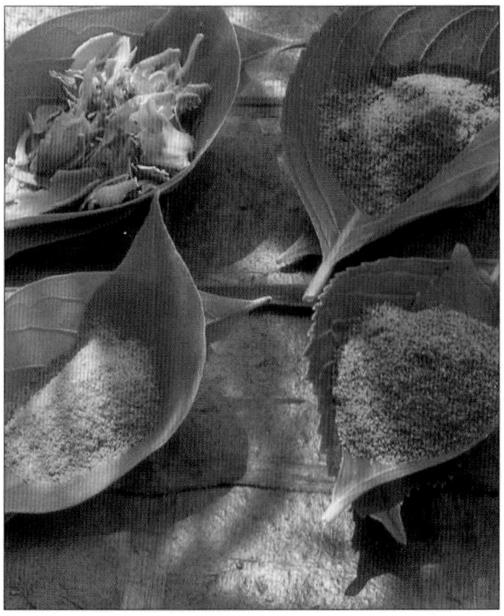

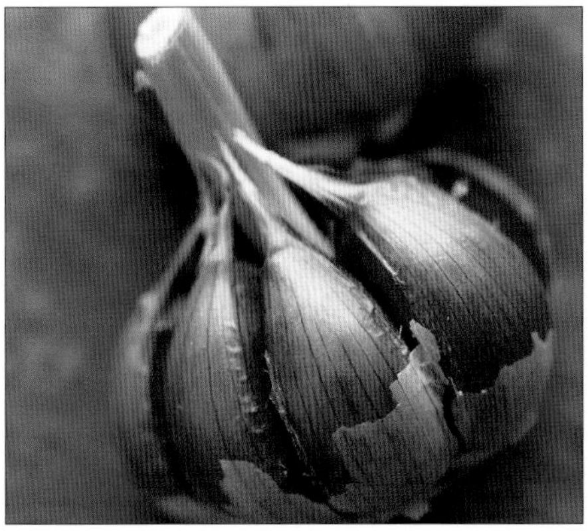

Above *Garlic is good for the circulation.*

Health benefits of garlic

Nature's antibiotic, garlic (*Allium sativum*) has powerful antibacterial and anti-inflammatory properties, and helps the respiratory and other bodily systems to fight infections. It works on the digestive system by supporting beneficial bacteria in the gut, stimulating the secretion of digestive enzymes and aiding absorption of nutrients. It also boosts the circulation and has an effect on lowering blood pressure and cholesterol levels.

For maximum benefit, it should be eaten raw, but it is also efficacious when cooked.

As garlic has a blood-thinning action, it should not be eaten in large quantities if taking anticoagulant medication, or taken as a medicinal extract without medical advice.

Nutritional properties of some herbs

Herb	Constituents
• Chicory	Potassium, folic acid
• Dandelion	Vitamin A
• Garlic	Potassium, vitamins A, B, C
• Kelp	Calcium, iron, iodine, vitamins B_1, B_2, B_{12}
• Nettle	Calcium, iron, vitamins A, C
• Parsley	Calcium, copper, iron, potassium, vitamins A, C
• Watercress	Calcium, folic acid, vitamins A, B_2, C
Fruit	
• Elderberry	Vitamins A, C
• Raspberry	Calcium, vitamin C

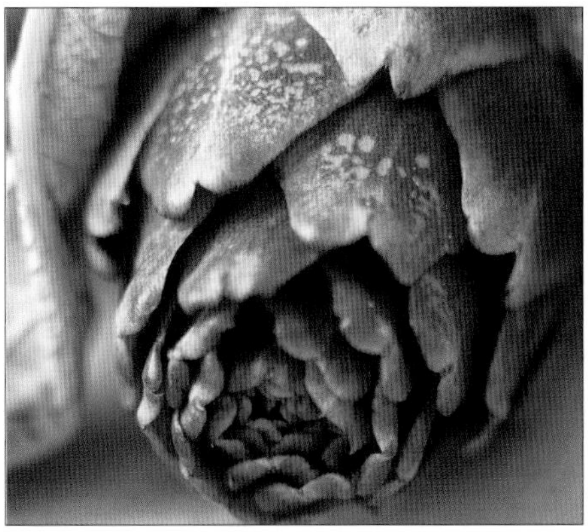

Above *Globe artichoke benefits the liver.*

Health benefits of other foods

• **Globe artichoke** (*Cynara scolymus*) flower heads stimulate the appetite, detoxify the liver and act as a digestive. (The leaves are used in medicinal preparations, but they can be harmful if suffering from gallstones or liver disease and should only be taken on medical advice.)

• **Shiitake mushrooms** are a traditional Japanese remedy, taken in the form of an extract as a restorative tonic and anti-tumour agent. The mushrooms make a useful addition to the diet, helping to boost the immune system.

• **Alfalfa sprouting seeds** contain vitamins C, E, K and beta-carotene. They make an excellent food supplement and can be added to salads or stir-fries.

Below *Seeds, ground and sprinkled on salads, breakfast cereals and cooked dishes, bring health benefits.*

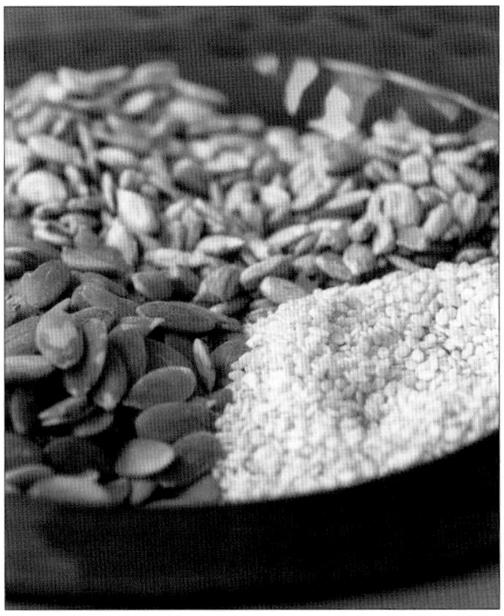

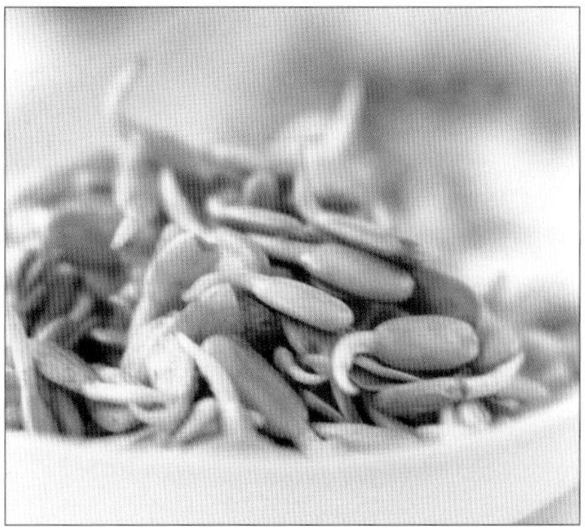

Above *Sprouting seeds are full of vitamins. Add a range of seeds to your cooking whenever possible for their health-boosting attributes.*

• **Safflower oil, olive oil, nuts and avocados** are all good sources of vitamin E, and help to support the immune system.

• **Cloves, nutmeg, cayenne pepper and turmeric** all have antibacterial properties.

• **Cinnamon** helps stabilize blood sugar levels.

• **Caraway, fennel, cardamom and dill** aid digestion.

• **Pumpkin seeds** contain zinc and other trace elements.

• **Sunflower seeds** are rich in B vitamins.

Below *Cinnamon is warming and has been shown to have health benefits particularly for diabetics. Enjoy it in curries, tea and sweet cakes. Even when spices are added sparingly to food, they do more than just provide flavour.*

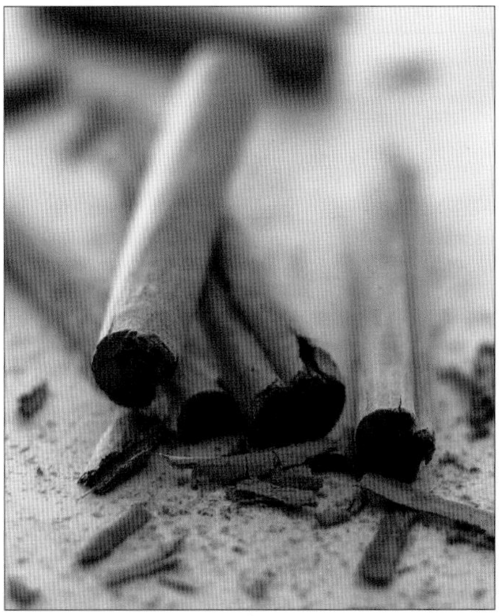

DANDELION VITALITY SALAD

Salads are an essential part of a healthy diet, and are especially nutritious when they include lavish quantities of fresh herbs. Try new and unusual combinations to add colour and variety to meals. Dandelion leaves are rich in potassium, iron and other minerals as well as vitamins A, B, C and D. Many herbalists use them to stimulate the liver, aid digestion and combat fluid retention, and they have a reputation for lifting the spirits into the bargain.

Ingredients

Serves 4

1 yellow (bell) pepper
mixed salad leaves: dandelion, baby spinach, rocket (arugula), lamb's lettuce (corn salad)
small bunch of spearmint
a few lemon balm (*Melissa officinalis*) leaves
borage flowers
pot marigold (*Calendula officinalis*) petals
vinaigrette dressing, to serve

1 Slice the pepper and mix it with the salad leaves in a large bowl.

2 Snip in the mint and lemon balm, and top with borage flowers and marigold petals. Toss the salad gently in a vinaigrette dressing just before serving.

Below *Dandelion salad is packed with vitamins and minerals to promote vitality. Edible flowers add appetizing colour. Borage has many uses in herbal remedies. Infusions of the flowers make a stress-relieving tea but here they add decorative value. Spearmint adds a strong and refreshing taste to this salad dish.*

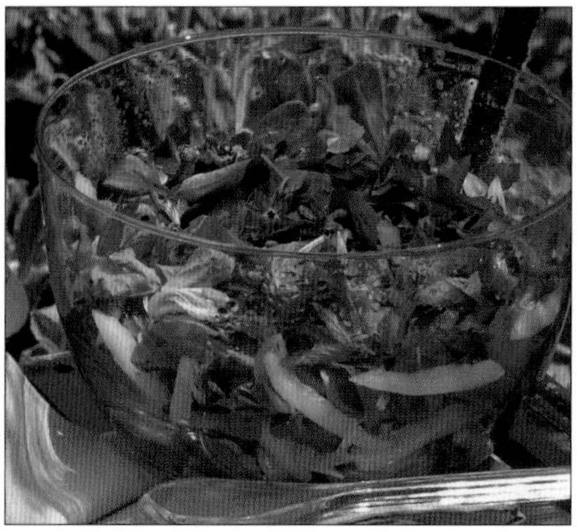

NASTURTIUM AND WATERCRESS SALAD

Mix peppery nasturtium leaves with watercress and parsley to make an energizing and decorative salad to help boost the immune system. Orange flower water, which is used in the dressing, is a by-product of the steam distillation of neroli oil, a natural antidepressant.

Ingredients

Serves 4

6–8 nasturtium flowers and leaves
bunch of watercress, stalks trimmed
25g/1oz parsley (*Petroselinum crispum*), chopped
lettuce leaves
cucumber slices
1 large orange, peeled, sliced and quartered

For the orange flower dressing

2.5g/½ tsp garlic salt
5ml/1 tsp Dijon mustard
45ml/3 tbsp safflower oil
15ml/1 tbsp orange flower water
5ml/1 tsp lemon juice
small bunch of chives, finely snipped
ground black pepper

1 To make the dressing put all the ingredients in a screw-topped jar. Shake thoroughly to mix before use.

2 Reserve some nasturtium flowers for decoration. Separate the petals of the rest, shred the leaves, and put them in a bowl with the other salad ingredients.

3 Drizzle the salad with the dressing and toss. Serve garnished with the reserved whole nasturtium flowers.

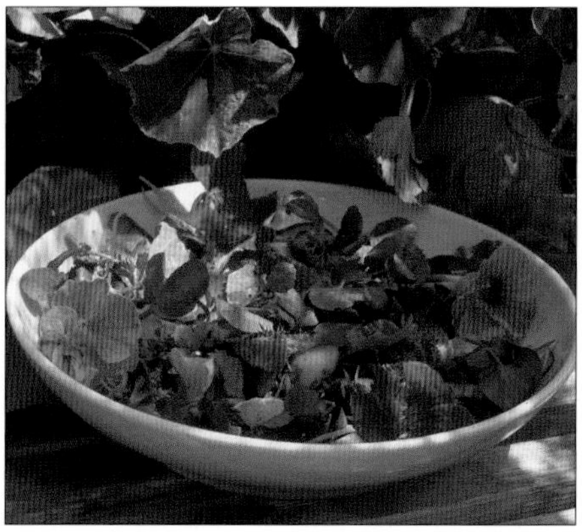

MIXED GREEN LEAF AND HERB SALAD

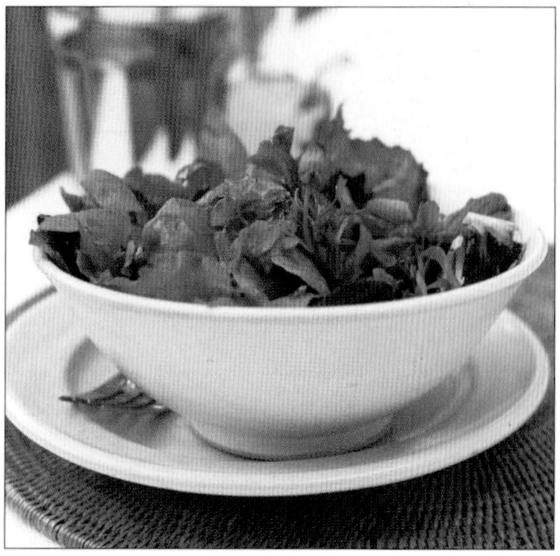

This delicious salad makes a light lunch full of vitamins and minerals.

Ingredients

Serves 4

15g/½oz/½ cup mixed fresh herbs, such as chervil, tarragon (use sparingly), dill, basil, marjoram (use sparingly), flat leaf parsley, mint, sorrel, fennel and coriander (cilantro)
350g/12oz mixed salad leaves, such as rocket (arugula), radicchio, chicory (Belgian endive), watercress, frisée lettuce, baby spinach, oakleaf lettuce, dandelion

For the dressing

50ml/2fl oz/½ cup extra virgin olive oil
15ml/1 tbsp cider vinegar
ground black pepper

1 Wash and dry the herbs and salad leaves in a salad spinner, or use two clean, dry dish towels to pat them dry.

2 In a small bowl, blend together the olive oil and cider vinegar and season with freshly ground black pepper to taste.

3 Place the mixed salad leaves and herbs in a large bowl. Pour over the dressing and mix well, using your hands to toss the leaves. Serve the salad as soon as you have added the dressing to prevent the leaves wilting.

Serve with new potatoes in their jackets, crumbled hard-boiled egg yolks and sprouted bean sprouts, or with cooked chickpeas, asparagus tips and green olives.

MIXED SALAD WITH TOASTED SUNFLOWER AND PUMPKIN SEEDS

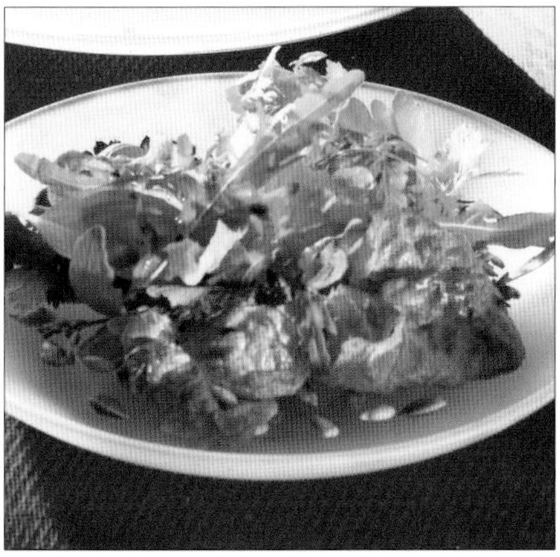

The fusion of coriander (*Coriandrum sativum*), parsley (*Petroselinum crispum*), basil (*Ocimum basilicum*) and rocket with sunflower and pumpkin seeds gives this salad its crunchy, crisp textures. Toasting the seeds brings out their flavours. The seeds contain minerals and vitamin E, while coriander stimulates appetite.

Ingredients

Serves 4

25g/1oz/3 tbsp pumpkin seeds
25g/1oz/3 tbsp sunflower seeds
90g/3½oz/3 cups mixed salad leaves
50g/2oz/2 cups mixed salad herbs, such as coriander (cilantro), parsley, basil and rocket (arugula)

For the dressing

60ml/4 tbsp extra virgin olive oil
15ml/1 tbsp balsamic vinegar
2.5ml/½tsp Dijon mustard
salt and ground black pepper

1 To make the dressing, put the ingredients in a bowl and whisk together with a fork.

2 Toast the seeds in a dry frying pan over a medium heat for 2 minutes, or until golden, tossing frequently to prevent them burning. Allow to cool slightly.

3 Put the salad and herb leaves in a large bowl and then sprinkle with the cooled seeds. Pour the dressing over the salad and toss carefully until the leaves are well coated, then serve.

SPRING TONIC NETTLE SOUP

The consumption of nettles as a springtime tonic goes back many centuries. They are rich in iron, contain calcium and other minerals, and vitamins A and C. Research studies show that nettle extract helps to flush away uric acid, an excess of which causes arthritis.

Chicken stock is not essential – you can use water or vegetable stock instead – but it has long been claimed to be a mild antibiotic and it is helpful if you are fighting a cold or bacterial infection.

Ingredients

Serves 4

large handful of nettle tops
25g/1oz/2 tbsp butter
1 onion, chopped
2 garlic cloves, crushed
450g/1lb potatoes, peeled and diced
5–6 juniper berries, crushed
25g/1oz parsley
600ml/1 pint 2½ cups chicken stock
600ml/1 pint 2½ cups milk
salt, pepper and cayenne pepper
yogurt or fromage frais, to serve

Below *Young nettle tops make a delicious tonic soup with a refreshing flavour.*

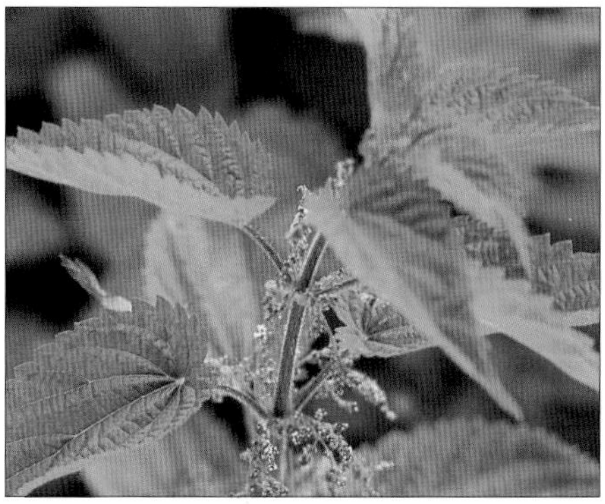

1 Wearing gloves, pick the young central nettle leaves from the tip of each plant.

2 Melt the butter in a large pan, and add the onions, garlic, potatoes and crushed juniper berries. Cook gently for 4–5 minutes.

3 Stir in the nettle tops and parsley and cook for another minute until they have wilted. Add the stock and simmer for about 15 minutes, until the potatoes are tender.

4 Blend in a food processor or blender until smooth. Return the soup to the rinsed-out pan and stir in the milk. Reheat gently, season to taste with salt, pepper and cayenne and serve, adding a swirl of yogurt or fromage frais to each bowl.

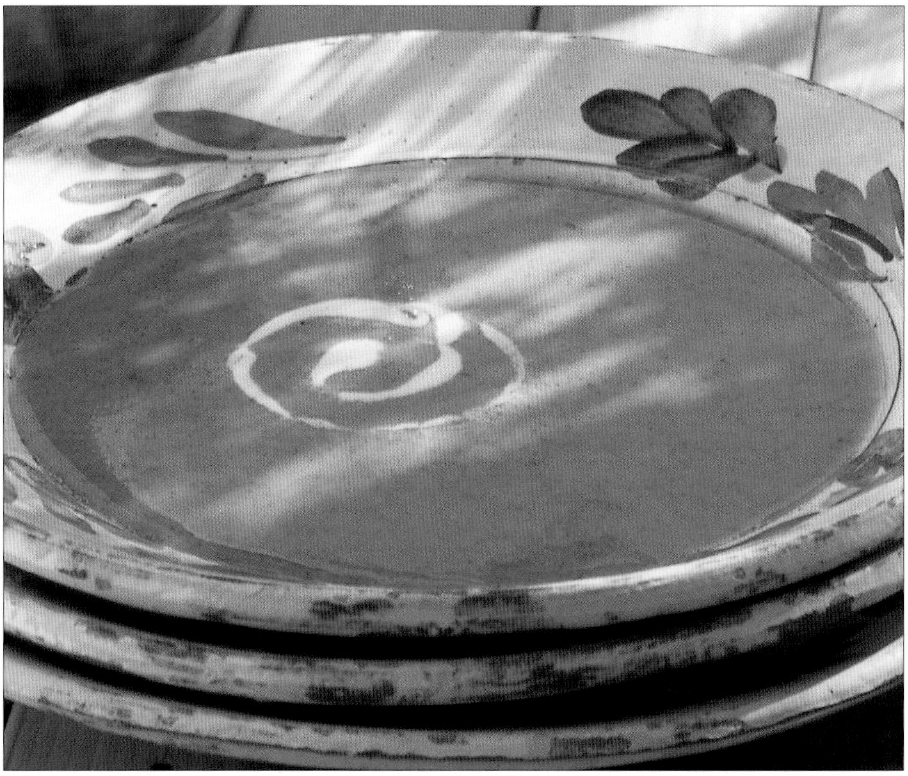

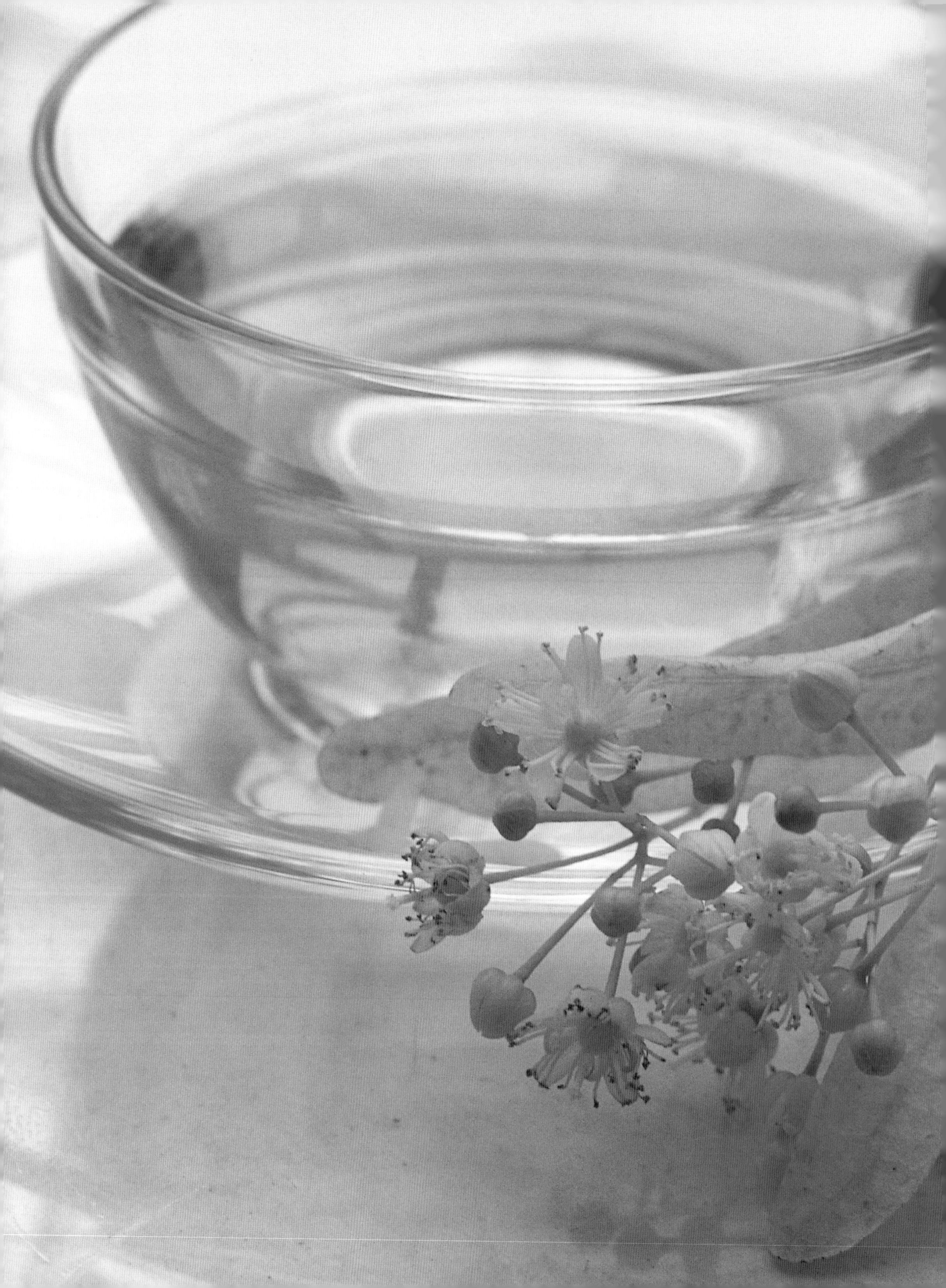

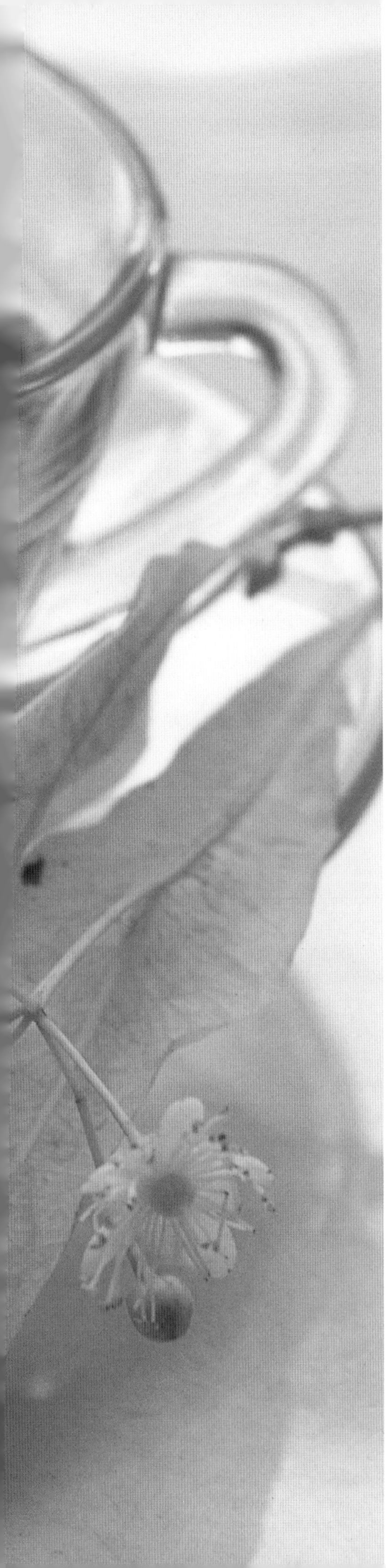

Herbal Remedies for Common Ailments

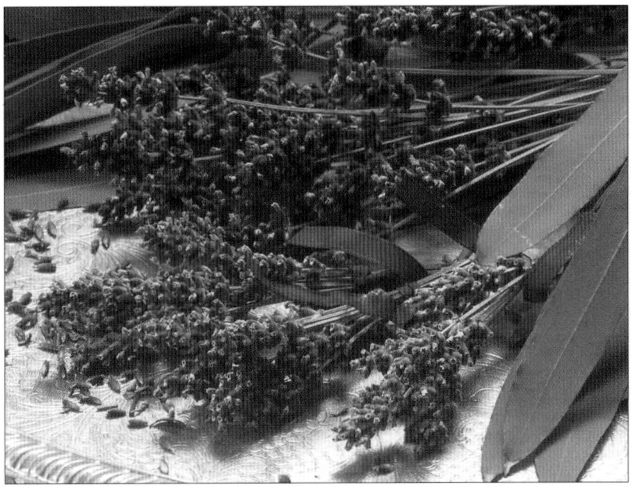

Herbs have great healing potential and there are many ways of using them to relieve minor ailments. They can also be invaluable for alleviating the discomfort of long-term or recurrent conditions, from anxiety and stress to headaches and skin irritations, and as first aid for simple cuts and bruises, stings, sprains and strains. However, for serious conditions, or where symptoms cause concern, self-diagnosis and self-treatment can be dangerous, and it is essential to consult your general practitioner. The recipes, remedies and general advice given in the following pages are not intended to replace professional medical advice or guidance.

Above *Lavender and eucalyptus are powerful decongestants.*

Left *Simple infusions, or teas, made with herbal ingredients provide a convenient way to benefit from their healing properties.*

Anxiety

There are many situations where some level of anxiety is perfectly normal, and a natural response to a stressful situation. Anxiety becomes a problem only when its degree is out of proportion to the problem, or when there is no objective, external reason for it.

Symptoms of anxiety

When anxiety is out of control, some of the symptoms that may be suffered are:

- Constant feelings of tension
- Sweating
- Palpitations
- Irritability
- Sleeplessness.

Herbal preparations cannot deal with a deep-seated psychological problem, but they can be a great help in calming general over-anxiety and nervous tension.

Herbal teas

Try one of the following calming infusions:

- **Chamomile** (*Chamaemelum nobile*) is relaxing and good for the digestion. Teabags are widely available, or you can make your own infusion using the fresh flowers.
- **Lemon balm** (*Melissa officinalis*) is a traditional herb for mild anxiety. Always use the fresh leaf; just gather a few sprigs to make an infusion and drink a cup two or three times a day.
- **Skullcap** (*Scutellaria laterifolia*) has a more strongly relaxing effect and can also be taken as a tincture or tablet.

Below *Lime blossom (*Tilia europaea*) makes a very good evening drink, to soothe the mind and calm the digestion and heart rate. Make it from the dried flowers. To increase the effect, combine it with passion flower (*Passiflora incarnata*).*

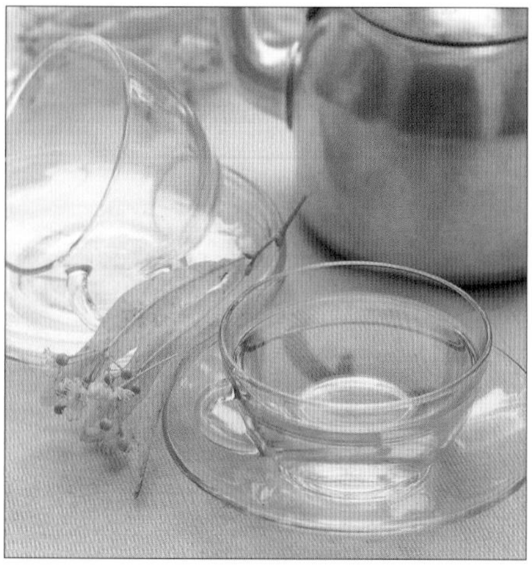

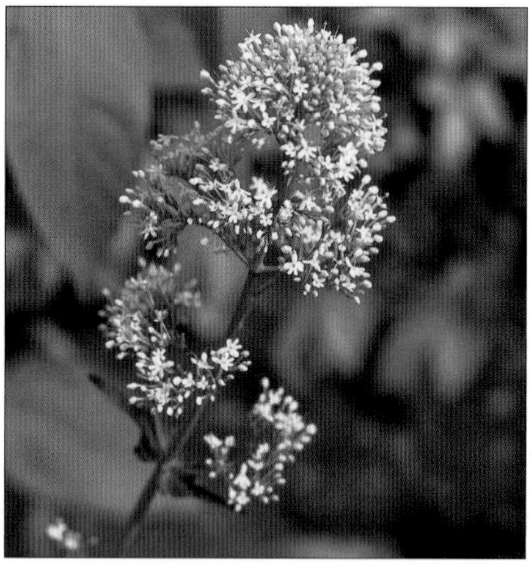

Above *Valerian (*Valeriana officinalis*) has a powerfully sedative effect. High doses may cause headaches. Make a decoction of the dried root. Drink one cup at bedtime.*

CAUTION If you are taking medication speak to your doctor before using valerian.

Below *Relaxing in a herb-scented bath can be very soothing. Fill a bath bag, to hang over the taps, with chamomile flowers, lavender and oatmeal, or add 8 drops of essential oil of lavender to the water.*

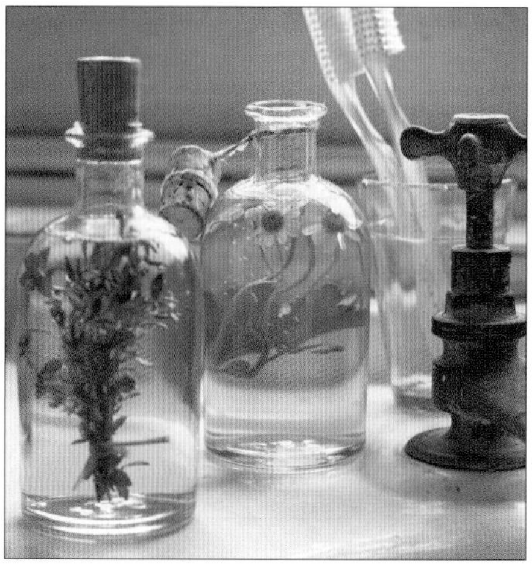

Calming oats

An excellent tonic for the nervous system, oats provide both nourishment and energy. They contain vitamin E, iron, zinc, manganese and protein and help to lower cholesterol levels. *Avena sativa*, often referred to in traditional herbal medicine as "wild oats", is the same plant as cultivated oats. The seed, or grain, and stalks are the parts used, and commercial preparations include tinctures and tablets. Oats are not suitable for those with a gluten sensitivity.

Below *Porridge, flapjacks and oatcakes are good ways to incorporate oats in your diet.*

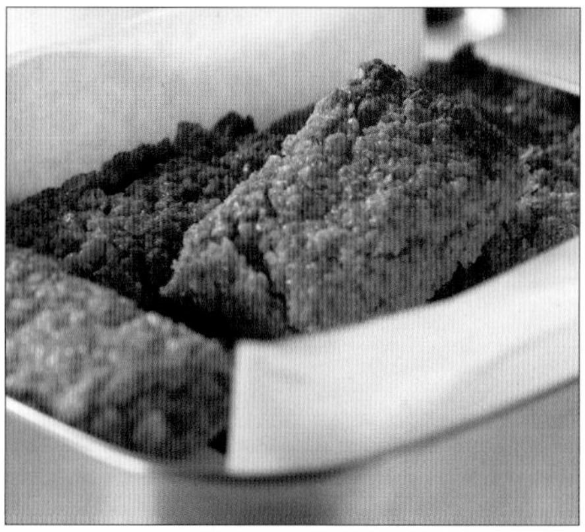

Below *Rescue Remedy is a Bach Flower Remedy, readily available over the counter. It is a combination of five Bach remedies for different aspects of shock, and can be used if you feel frightened or anxious – just put 2 drops on your tongue.*

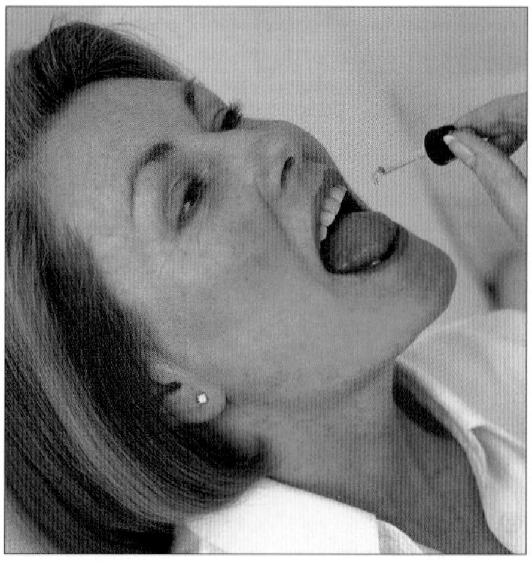

Stress

Although the condition is frequently cited as being prevalent in modern life, stress is one of those rather vague terms that is very difficult to define. It is also important to say that stress is not in itself harmful, and a certain amount can be necessary to get motivated and enjoy life. Only when the amount of stress is too much for the system to cope with does it become a problem.

Most people have a marvellous capacity to adapt to and cope with various sources of stress in their lives, but someone who is never able to relax can get overloaded, and if nervous exhaustion sets in, they can become seriously ill.

Symptoms of stress

The symptoms of stress vary, but if you experience some or all of the following, you may be overstressed:

- Constantly on edge, with a very short fuse and ready to explode for no real reason.
- Feeling on the verge of tears much of the time.
- Difficulty in concentrating, decision-making or with memory.
- Always tired, even after a full night's sleep.
- Sleep itself is disturbed and unrefreshing.
- A feeling of not being able to cope, of everything being too much.
- Poor appetite, or nibbling without hunger.
- No sense of fun or enjoyment in life.

Below *The demands of modern life all too often lead to an overload of stress.*

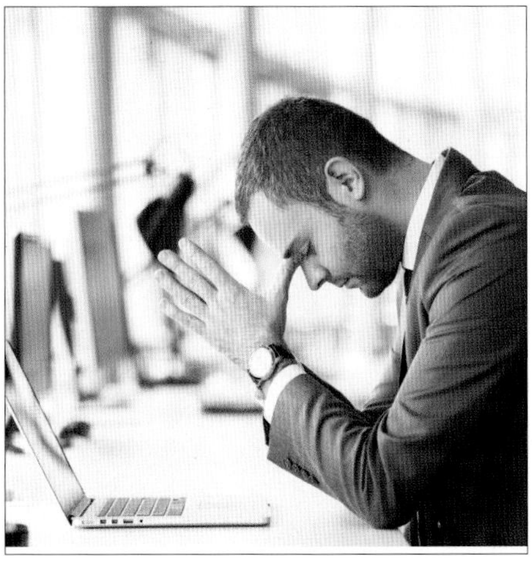

- Mistrustful of everybody, unable to enjoy being in company.
- Inability to relax or unwind even if not working.
- Problems in personal relationships, no interest in sex.
- Always fidgeting or having a nervous habit such as biting your nails or chewing your hair.

The first step to improving the situation is to recognize that you are stressed, and to know what your limits are. Taking active steps to reduce the amount of external stress will of course be helpful, as well as looking at methods for easing the effects of the stress on your system. Other steps might include trying a class in relaxation techniques, yoga or tai chi, or having professional massage treatments. Making sure you take regular breaks from a stressful lifestyle will help you to cope better and avoid the situation reaching a crisis point.

Herbal tea

Lemon balm *(Melissa officinalis)* and lime blossom *(Tilia cordata)* Lime blossom has a scent of honey and is one of the best antidotes for stress. Lemon balm has a gently sedative effect, helpful in calming both stress and anxiety. It is much better to use the freshly gathered herbs whenever possible, as most of the scent, flavour and therapeutic properties are lost when the leaves are dried and stored. Lime blossom teabags are widely available commercially.

Put 30g/1oz fresh lemon balm and 10g/⅓ oz dried lime blossom into a teapot and pour 600ml/1pint/2½ cups boiling water. Allow to infuse for 5–10 minutes, strain, sweeten with honey to taste and drink one cup three times a day.

Below *Lemon balm promotes relaxation.*

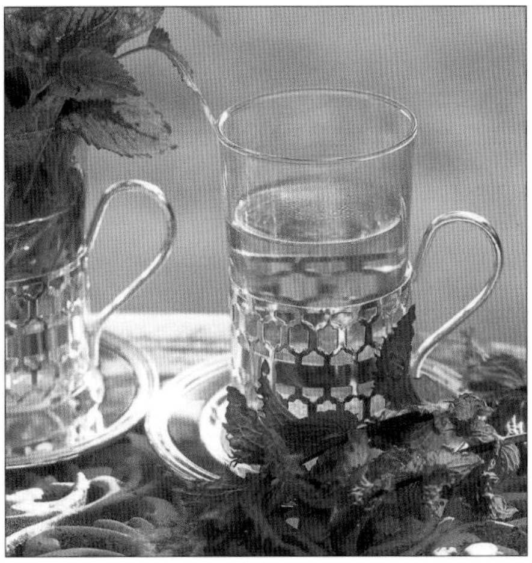

Massage to relax tense muscles

Muscles can become tense as a result of anxiety; this often causes slightly raised shoulders or contracted back muscles. The effort of maintaining your muscles in this semi-contracted state is tiring and may eventually result in perpetual spasm and bad postural habits. Your neck will feel stiff and your back may ache. Tight neck muscles can also prevent adequate blood flow to your head and cause tension headaches.

Massaging the neck and shoulders on a daily basis with a relaxing oil can help relieve muscular discomfort. Try 2–3 drops in total of cedarwood, juniper, lemon balm, neroli or lavender essential oils in a base of 20ml/4tsp almond oil. Using three fingers, work in a circular movement with firm pressure.

Vaporizing essential oils for their calming fragrance is also soothing. Choose from the oils above, adding 6–8 drops in total to an essential oil burner.

Below *Massage can help to ease aching muscles and calm the nervous system.*

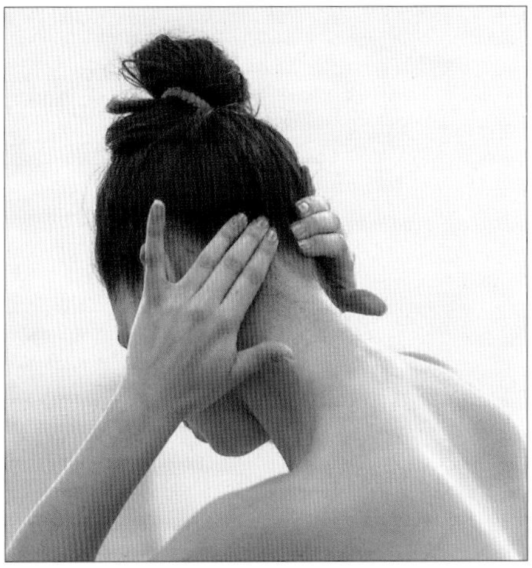

Depression and Feeling Low

Just as with anxiety, depression may have a variety of causes and symptoms. It can be a very serious illness, and for a continued state of depression at any level professional advice should always be sought. But many people have periods of "feeling low", which is a different matter, and at such times herbal teas and tinctures can provide a welcome boost for the spirits.

Symptoms of depression

Depression affects people in different ways and varying degrees. Common symptoms include:

- Low mood.
- Feeling listless.
- Losing interest in everyday pleasures.
- Loss of appetite or overeating.
- Constant tiredess.
- Insomnia or oversleeping.
- Feeling irritable.
- Feeling helpless.

Herbal teas

Teas provide a gentle way to benefit from the properties of herbs, especially if the depression is mild and transient.

• **Borage *(Borago officinalis)* flower tea** is traditionally associated with courage and strengthening the system. Borage can lift the spirits at stressful times.

To make one cup infuse 10g/⅓ oz fresh borage flowers and 2.5ml/½ tsp dried passion flower in 250ml/8fl oz/1 cup boiling water. Sweeten to taste and drink three times a day.

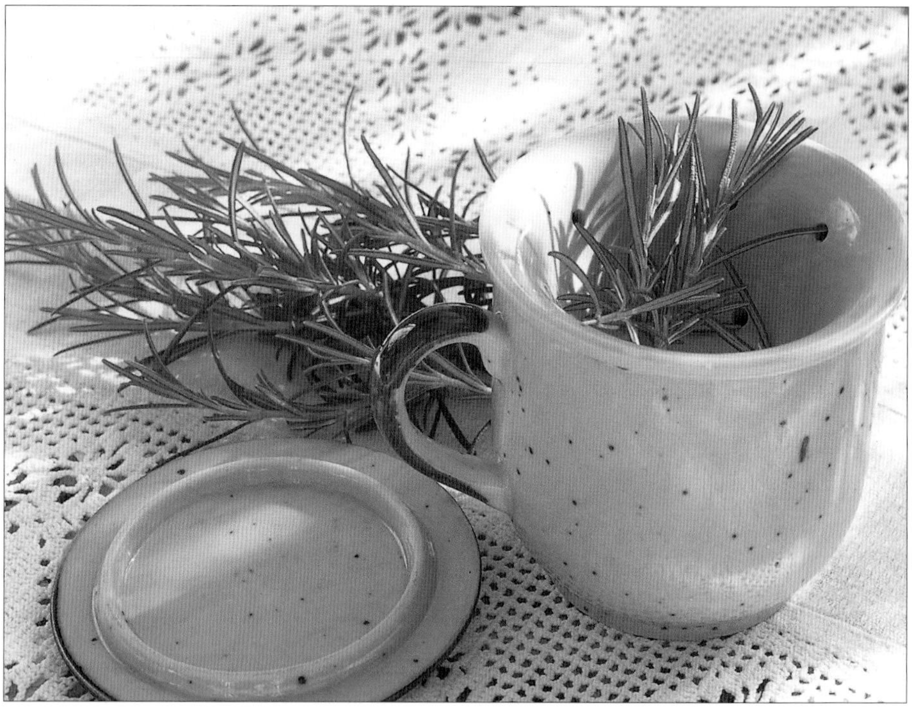

Above *A tea infuser is convenient for making a single cup of tea. Rosemary is uplifting.*

• To make a **restorative tea** try this powerful combination of herbs. Mix equal parts of dried vervain (*Verbena officinalis*), dried wood betony (*Stachys betonica*), dried mugwort (*Artemisia vulgaris*) and dried rosemary (*Rosmarinus officinalis*). Put 10ml/2 tsp of the mixture into a teapot and fill with boiling water. Allow to steep for 10 minutes and then strain off and discard the dried herbs. Sweeten if preferred with a little honey, and drink one cup of this tea three times a day, but for not more than one week at a time and occasional use only.

CAUTION Wood betony and mugwort are both uterine stimulants and should be avoided during pregnancy and breastfeeding.

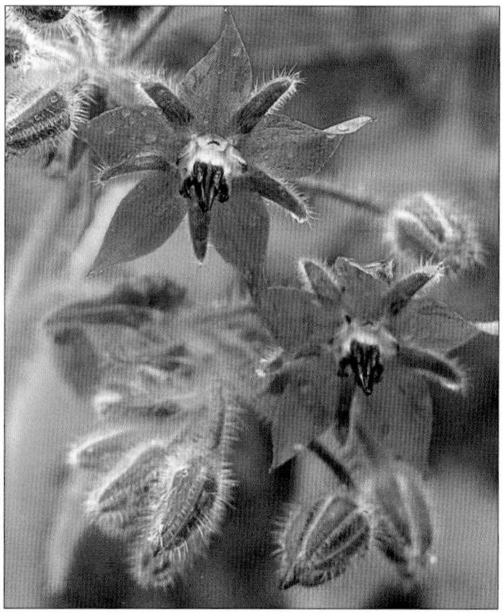

Left *Borage flowers make a soothing tea for any time of day.*

Tincture

A tincture of wild oats (*Avena sativa*), taken in a standard dose, three times a day, is a traditional treatment for mild depression.

Essential oil

Add 6–8 drops essential oil of rose (relaxing) or rosemary (uplifting) to the bath. Or blend 1 drop each essential oil of marjoram, lavender and sandalwood with 5ml/1 tsp almond oil and use as a bath oil.

A healthy diet

Depression illustrates well the connection between body and mind: physical and emotional energy are both depleted when you are in a depressed state. Both will benefit from a healthy diet with plenty of raw, vital foods, nuts, seeds and B vitamins. A multivitamin and mineral supplement may be useful until you feel energetic enough to prepare good food. Try also to cut down on stimulants, such as caffeine, which tend to exhaust both body and mind.

Poor Memory and Concentration

Both memory and concentration can be affected by stress, tiredness and general ill-health. Short-term memory loss is also associated with the ageing process.

Symptoms of poor memory

Losing the memory can be a worrying experience for many people as:

- Levels of alertness may drop.
- Attention span and focus may lessen.
- Memory function may become poor.

Making time for relaxation, taking exercise and eating a nutritious diet will all help to minimize the problem, and herbal treatments can help to make you feel more invigorated and alert. Ginseng (*Panax ginseng*) and ginkgo (*Ginkgo biloba*) are two powerful herbs with a long tradition of use in China and the Far East for enhancing mental performance. Modern research studies have confirmed their reputation for strengthening the memory, particularly in the case of ginkgo. Both ginkgo and ginseng are available as ready-made remedies to take on the advice of a qualified practitioner.

Gotu kola (*Centella asiatica*) has been used in India since ancient times for strengthening memory and concentration. It is available in the form of a tincture or tablets, but should only be taken on the advice of a qualified herbal practitioner.

CAUTION Ginseng and ginkgo are associated with various possible side effects and contra-indications, and they can interact with prescription medicines. For example, ginseng should not be taken by anyone who is suffering from high blood pressure or diabetes, and ginkgo must not be taken while on anticoagulant medication (such as aspirin and warfarin). Only take these remedies under strict medical supervision.

Herbal teas

Favourite teas for improving concentration and general alertness are lemon verbena and rosemary. Use the fresh herb for better taste.

- **Lemon verbena tea** is made using the fresh or dried leaves of the plant and makes a pale golden, lemony tea, which will help to wake up your system. The essential oil of this plant is used by the perfume industry for its invigorating scent. Pour 250ml/8fl oz/1 cup boiling water over a few fresh leaves or 5g/⅛oz dried lemon verbena (*Aloysia triphylla*). Leave to infuse before drinking.
- **Rosemary** Add a small fresh sprig or 5ml/1 tsp of the dried herb to 250ml/8fl oz/1 cup boiling water to make a reviving tea.

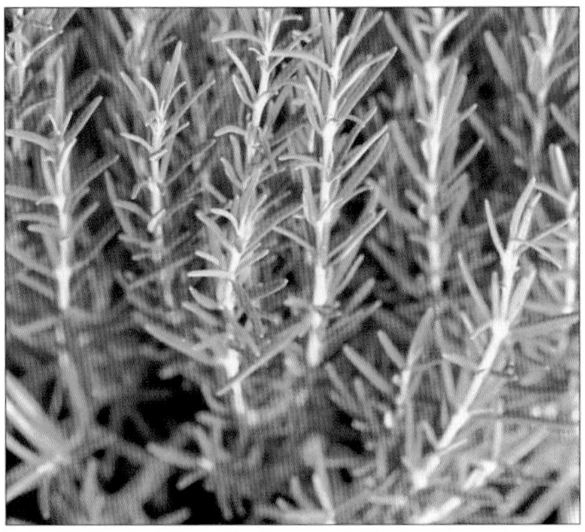

Above *Rosemary contains several active, aromatic oils. Its action is stimulating, as it increases the supply of blood to the brain, keeping the mind clear and aiding concentration. It will also relax nervous tension and combat fatigue.*

Essential oils

Oils to aid concentration include basil, cardamom, peppermint, rosemary, lemon, lemon grass, eucalyptus and cedarwood. Use them singly or in blends of two to three essential oils at a time in a base oil. Use the oil to dab on to a handkerchief or to rub into the pulse points on the wrist, and at the temples.

Below *Ginkgo biloba is a powerful herb with mind-enhancing properties.*

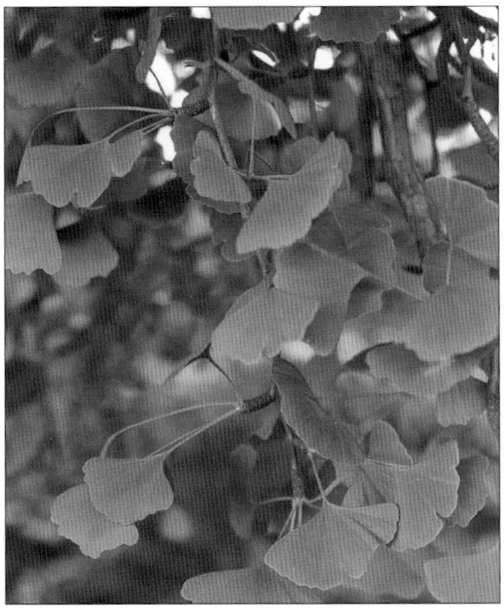

Below *Ginseng is said to stimulate the nervous system and increase stamina.*

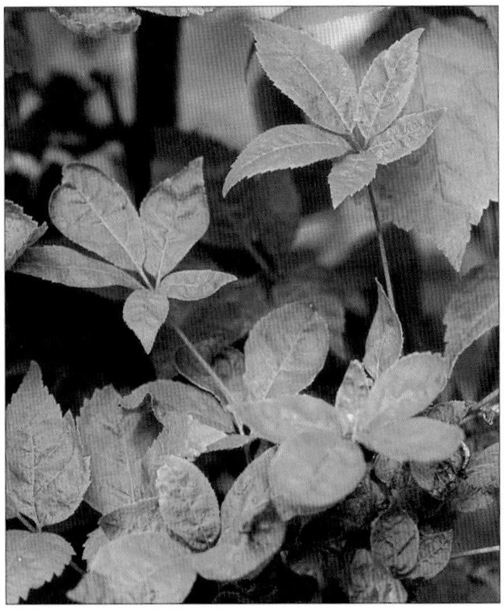

Below *Essential oils can be vaporized on an essential oil burner, or sprinkled on a handkerchief and the fragrance inhaled.*

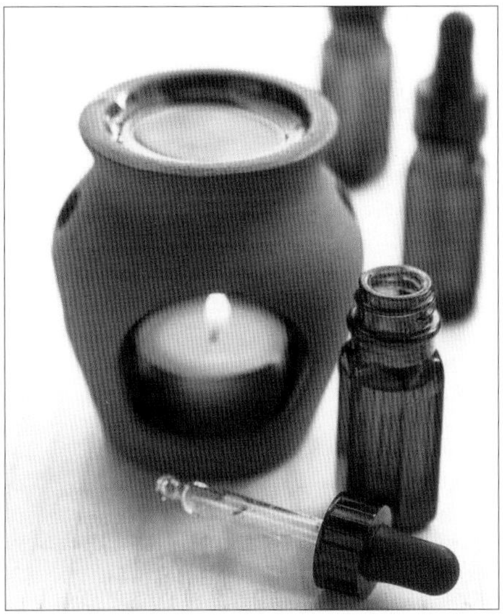

Tiredness and Low Energy

A hectic pace of life, overwork, prolonged stress, illness and even the ageing process can all lead to a constant feeling of tiredness and lack of energy. A healthy diet, high in vitamins (especially A, C, E and B complex), minerals (iron, calcium, magnesium and zinc) and low in refined carbohydrates and sugars, will help boost energy. Alcohol and caffeine drinks are also best avoided and replaced with herb teas and fruit juices.

Causes of tiredness and low energy

Constant feelings of fatigue should make us reassess our lifestyles:

- Eating the wrong foods and drinking too much alcohol can deplete our energy levels.
- A cycle of working too many hours with inadequate time for rest and recuperation can leave us tired or with anxiety, which drains energy.
- Not taking enough exercise makes us feel sluggish. Exercise raises energy levels.

Herbal tea

The gentle action of a herbal infusion provides an uplifting way to start the day. In the early morning, the fresh or dried leaves of lemon verbena (*Aloysia triphylla*) make a cheering drink with a lively flavour to wake up the system. Peppermint also has a gently stimulating effect when taken first thing in the morning.

Revitalizing juice

If you have a juicer, make fresh fruit juices to revitalize the system; they are a good way to increase vitamin content in the diet.

KIWI AND STEM GINGER SPRITZER

A single kiwi fruit contains more than one day's vitamin C requirement. Ginger is a circulatory stimulant that will give your body a much needed boost.

Ingredients

Makes 1 tall glass

2 kiwi fruit

1 piece preserved stem ginger, plus 15ml/1 tbsp syrup from the ginger jar

sparkling mineral water

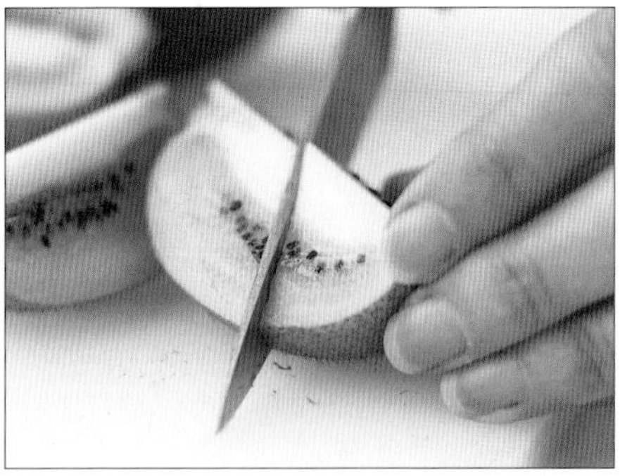

1 Using a sharp knife, roughly chop the kiwi fruit and the ginger.

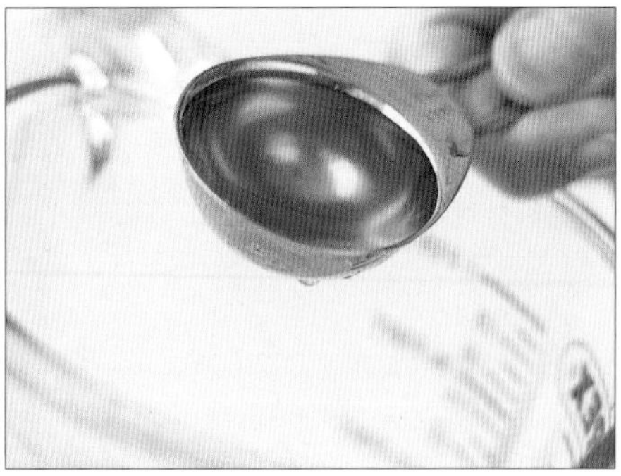

2 Push the ginger and kiwi fruit through a juicer and pour the juice into a jug (pitcher). Stir in the ginger syrup.

3 Pour the juice into a glass, then top up with sparkling mineral water.

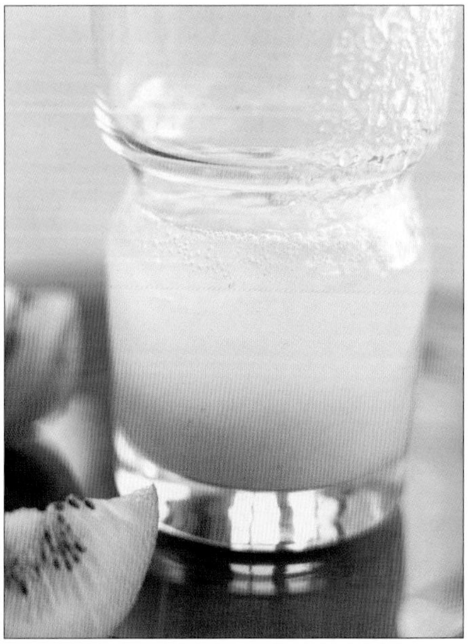

Essential oils

Basil, black pepper, cardamom, pennyroyal, peppermint, pine and rosemary essential oils are re-energizing when used in an oil burner. Use them singly, or experiment with combinations of two or three together, using 8–10 drops in all.

Bath oil

To make an invigorating bath oil, blend
3 drops essential oil of rosemary and
2 drops essential oil of camphor with
5 drops essential oil of peppermint.
Add this blend to 30ml/2 tbsp almond oil. Keep in a stoppered bottle and add 8–10 drops to the water when running a bath.

Bath bag

For a revitalizing mix put equal quantities of dried rosemary (*Rosmarinus officinalis*), peppermint (*Mentha* x *piperita*), lemon thyme (*Thymus* x *citriodorus*) and pine needles into a bath bag to hang over the taps.

Below *A small bag of herbs mixed with essential oils will revive flagging spirits. For a sachet to hang in the car, this pot-pourri mix will help to maintain a clear head. Stir 4 drops each camphor and lemon essential oils into 30ml/2 tbsp ground orris root, then add 25g/1oz each dried lemon verbena (*Aloysia triphylla*), mint, rosemary and thyme and 25g/1oz dried orange and lemon peel. Mix the ingredients together well. Use to fill small sachets. Refresh from time to time with a few drops of essential oil.*

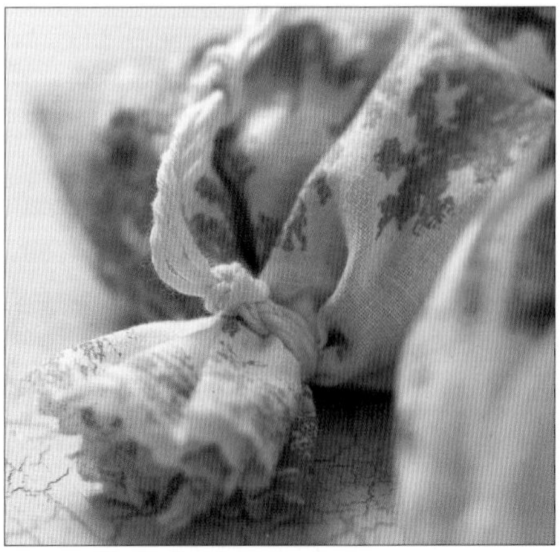

Sleep Disturbances

It is important to distinguish between habitual sleeplessness and a temporary problem, which may be due to some specific worry or anxiety. It would also be sensible not to become obsessed with trying to get a certain amount of sleep, as not everyone needs a full eight hours. But if you are going through a phase of restless nights, there are many ways in which herbs can help. For chronic insomnia seek medical advice.

Causes of sleep disturbances

Many medical conditions can produce sleep disturbances, so too can:

- Anxiety.
- Pain and discomfort.
- External noise.

Herbal teas

An infusion of one or more of these relaxing herbs can help to restore a natural sleep pattern if it has been disturbed by temporary stress and anxiety.

- Chamomile (*Chamaemelum nobile* or *Matricaria chamomilla*) is calming to the nervous system as well as a digestive, and is one of the best bedtime drinks for those who have difficulty dropping off. If the tea is made with dried chamomile flowers (rather than a ready-made teabag), it can be combined with an equal quantity of sweet marjoram (*Origanum majorana*).
- Lime blossom (*Tilia europaea*) and elderflower (*Sambucus nigra*) make a pleasant-tasting tea that is gently soporific. For maximum effect, add a dash of nutmeg and sweeten with honey.
- Passion flower (*Passiflora incarnata*) is known for its sedative properties, and for relieving nervous conditions such as palpitations. It makes a relaxing tea. You can also mix it with an equal quantity of other sedative herbs, including wood betony (*Stachys officinalis*), vervain (*Verbena officinalis*) and mugwort (*Artemisia vulgaris*).
- Put 5ml/1 tsp each dried passion flower (*Passiflora incarnata*), vervain (*Verbena officinalis*) and wood betony into a pot and pour in 600ml/1 pint/2½ cups boiling water water. Leave to infuse for 5 minutes. Strain.

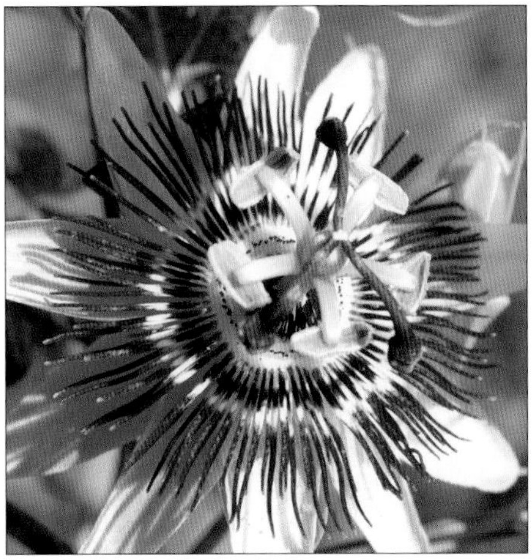

Above *Passion flower is easy to grow. The flowers have gently sedative properties.*

CAUTION Wood betony and mugwort are uterine stimulants, and should not be used during pregnancy or while breastfeeding.

Drink 1–2 cups of this gently sedative mixture daily, for not more than 2 weeks.

Tincture

A tincture made with the flowers of sweet violet (*Viola odorata*) taken in a standard dose, helps induce restfulness.

Essential oils

Chamomile, juniper, lavender, marjoram, neroli, sandalwood and lemon essential oils can be used in an oil burner, singly or in combinations of two or three together.

- For a massage oil to help you sleep, add 4 drops each of chamomile, lemon and sandalwood to 30ml/2 tbsp base oil.
- A simple way to promote restful sleep is to sprinkle a few drops of essential oil of lavender on to your pillow or handkerchief.
- A small cushion filled with sleep-inducing hops and lavender, placed behind your head, or under your main pillow, is a gentle way to encourage a restful night.
- Adding a few drops of lavender oil to a warm, not hot, bath taken just before going to bed will also have a calming effect on the body.

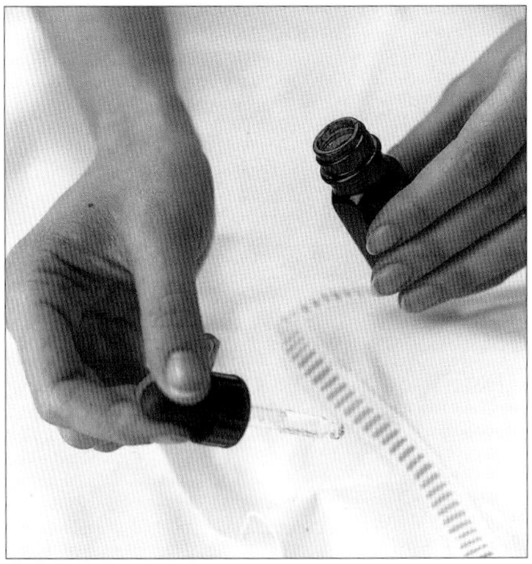

Above *A few drops of essential oil of lavender on the pillow should ensure a restful night.*

SLEEP TIME OIL SPRAY

Spray the room before you go to sleep with this relaxing fragrance. You can also use it at any time to provide a calming atmosphere. Once mixed, keep the oils in a cool dark place away from a source of heat.

Ingredients

25ml/5 tsp grapeseed oil
25ml/5 tsp almond oil
25ml/5 tsp jojoba oil
10ml/2 tsp rosewater
10ml/2 tsp glycerine
20 drops each lavender and chamomile essential oils

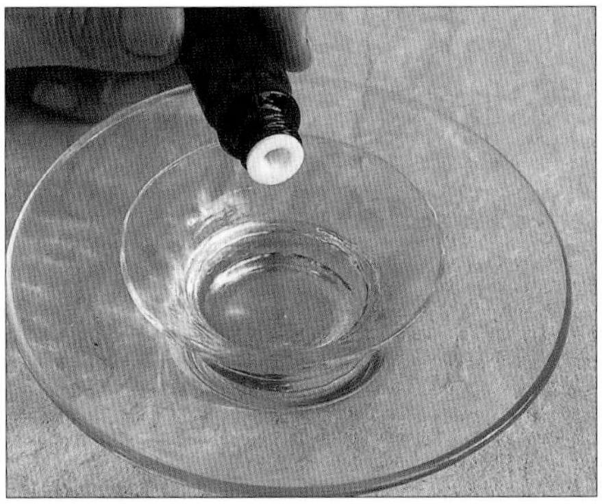

Mix the first five ingredients together, then stir in the essential oils, mixing well. Transfer to a clean 100ml/3½fl oz spray bottle. Shake before use.

Headaches

Ranging in severity from mild and bearable to severe and debilitating, headaches can be very disruptive to life. Herbs may be helpful in relieving headaches that are brought on by anxiety or tension. Fresh or dried herbs can be made into teas; or a lavender infusion can be used for a compress.

Causes of headaches

Headaches can develop for a number of reasons; usually they are related to some obvious cause such as:

- Nasal congestion or sinusitis.
- Eye strain, fatigue or tension.
- Stress or worries, with muscle spasms in the neck leading to head pains.
- Poor posture – many jobs create special problems: for instance, computer operators often suffer from eye strain and stiff, aching shoulders or neck muscles, and consequently headaches.

Herbal teas

At the earliest signs of a headache, taking a tea made from one of the following herbs can stop it in its tracks.

- **German chamomile** (*Matricaria chamomilla*) is good for bilious headaches stemming from over-eating, or indigestion, where there is a dull, throbbing pain on top of the head.
- **Lime blossom** (*Tilia europaea*) soothes the nerves and is very helpful for tension headaches; it can be mixed with peppermint for a more uplifting effect.
- **Peppermint** (*Mentha piperita*) works well for digestive or sinus headaches, especially where the head feels hot.
- **Rosemary** (*Rosmarinus officinalis*) is good for headaches related to exhaustion or depression, and also for bilious heavy heads.
- **Hangover remedy** Put 5ml/1 tsp dried vervain (*Verbena officinalis*) and 2.5ml/½ tsp lavender (*Lavandula*) flowers in a teapot and pour over 600ml/1 pint/2½ cups boiling water. Allow to steep for 10 minutes, then strain. Sweeten with a little honey, if you like. Sip this tea as often as you like throughout the day until you start to feel better, but remember that prevention is better than cure!

Severe headaches

Persistent headaches can be debilitating and if they become a recurrent problem, you should get medical advice. Conditions such as very high blood pressure, meningitis or even brain tumours are relatively rare causes of headaches, but they need professional treatment. Severe, unexplained or persistent headaches should be checked out carefully by a medical practitioner, but most headaches and their causes can be identified and cured at home. Where some kind of accident has resulted in, say, a whiplash injury, professional help is required, and you could consult a manipulative therapist such as a chiropractor or an osteopath for treatment.

Compress

Headaches are often caused by tension in the neck and upper back muscles. This can prevent adequate blood supply to the head and thus lead to pain. Both massage and exercise can be a great help in easing this kind of headache. A cool compress may also help. An infusion of a cooling herb such as mint can be used to make a compress. Lavender is also popular, but if you find the fragrance too strong, leave out the essential oil content in the recipe below.

LAVENDER COMPRESS FOR A HEADACHE

Place a cool lavender compress across the forehead to relieve a tension headache. Sit and relax with the compress in place. As soon as the compress gets warm, soak it again in the infusion and reapply.

Ingredients

25g/1oz dried lavender (*Lavandula* spp)
600ml/1 pint/2½ cups boiling water
3–4 drops lavender essential oil
10ml/2 tsp lavender tincture

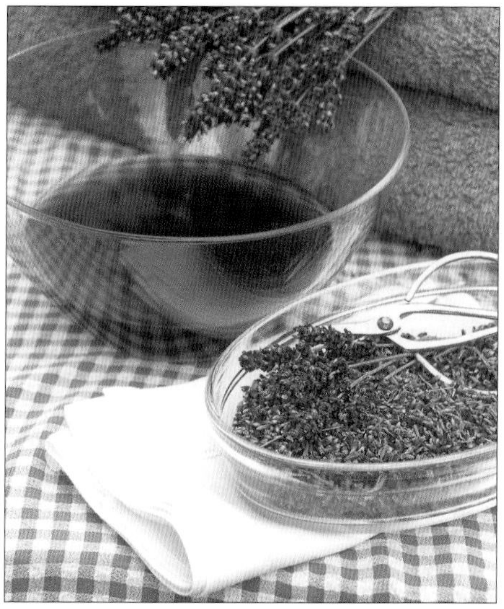

1 Put the dried lavender in a bowl and pour the boiling water over it. Leave to stand for 1 hour, then strain. When cool, mix in the essential oil and tincture.

2 Fold a piece of soft cotton fabric into a loose pad. Soak it in the lavender infusion and wring it out lightly.

Below *Holding a pad to your head with a few drops each of sweet marjoram and lemon balm essential oils can relieve a tension headache. If the headache persists, try adding a few drops of chamomile (*Chamaemelum nobile*). While using a compress it is better to try and relax than to continue with your usual daily activities.*

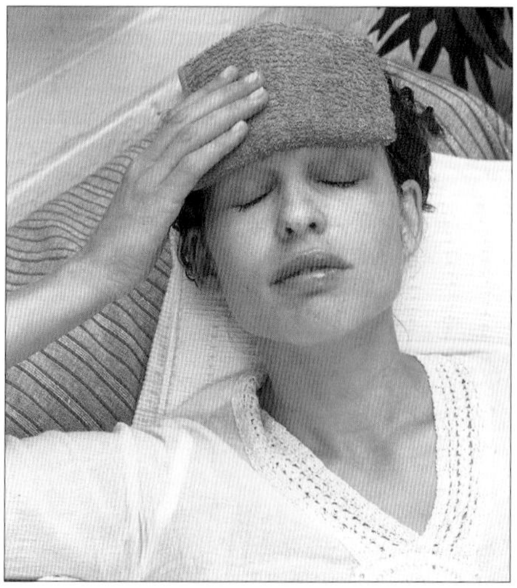

Migraine

Anyone who has experienced migraine will know that it is more than a severe headache. Diet may be a key factor. Tea, coffee, alcohol (especially red wine), cheese, chocolate, tomatoes and eggs have all been implicated as triggers.

Symptoms of migraine

- Intense and uncomfortable headache.
- Acute pains, often over one eye.
- Disturbed vision or flashing lights.
- Nausea or vomiting.
- Sensitivity to bright light.

Massaging the neck, in between attacks, may help, and herbal teas are soothing and comforting.

Herbal teas

Taking a herbal tea in the early stages may help reduce the effects of a migraine. You could also try drinking one of these infusions regularly in place of tea or coffee.

- **German chamomile** (*Matricaria chamomilla*) for dull, throbbing headache with a feeling of queasiness – add a little ginger (*Zingiber officinalis*) to relieve more severe nausea.
- **Rosemary** (*Rosmarinus officinalis*) is good where stress is a trigger for migraines, and where local warmth gives relief.
- For a **soothing tea** drink 1 cup of this herbal tea a day for up to one week. Put 5ml/1 tsp dried wood betony and 2.5ml/½ tsp dried lavender (*Lavandula*) or rosemary (*Rosmarinus officinalis*) in a cup. Top up with boiling water and steep for 10 minutes, then strain.

Below *Feverfew is an age-old migraine cure.*

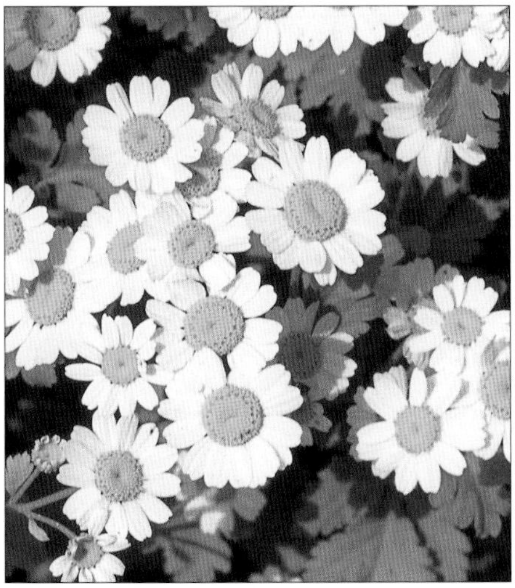

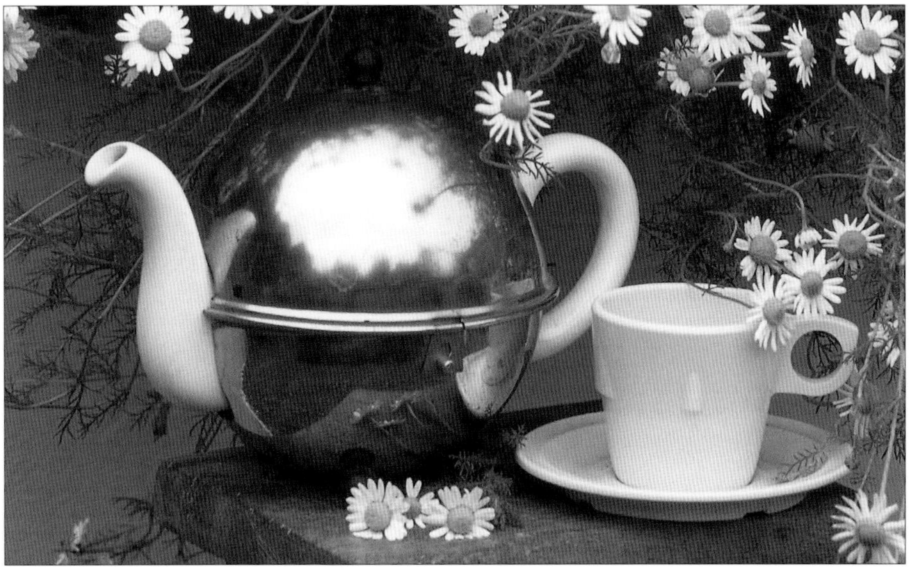

Above *Chamomile tea makes a soothing drink at any time of day for those prone to migraine.*

Feverfew

This is one of the herbal remedies of which most people have heard, as it was hailed as a "wonder cure" for migraine in the 1970s after a Welsh doctor's wife found that it put a stop to her chronic migraine attacks. Since then the use of feverfew (*Tanacetum parthenium*) has undergone much scientific research, which has largely confirmed its effectiveness but also revealed its side effects and risks. It should be used with caution.

CAUTION It was once considered safe to eat one or two fresh small leaves of feverfew a day, with food, as a preventive measure, but it has now been established that feverfew is potentially toxic and can cause allergic reactions, mouth ulcers and stomach upsets. It also interacts with prescription blood-thinning medication, such as aspirin and warfarin, and should not be taken without medical advice and supervision.

Compress

A cool compress placed across the forehead may be helpful. It is probably best to use plain water for this, as the sense of smell is often heightened or altered during a migraine, and any strongly scented herb is likely to make matters worse. You could try adding a few fresh mint leaves to the water for the compress, for a hint of fragrance.

Treating migraine

A migraine can be triggered by hormone changes, stress, stuffy atmospheres, noises, smells and certain foods. Repeated attacks call for professional help: self-help treatments are largely for preventive use.

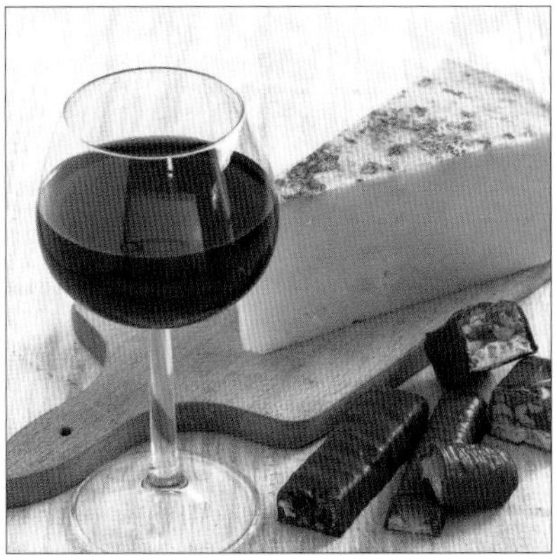

Colds and Influenza

Once a cold has developed it generally has to run its course, but herbal treatments can help to relieve symptoms and also stop the cold leading on to persistent catarrh or a deeper infection. Influenza is a much more serious complaint than a bad cold, as anyone who has suffered it will know, but some of its symptoms may also be eased by preparations appropriate for colds.

Symptoms of colds and flu

Everyone is familiar with the symptoms of a cold. At their worst, colds can leave us feeling low and disinterested in life and with:

- Sore throats
- Coughs
- Headaches
- Blocked sinuses or runny nose.

Herbal teas

One of the herbalists' most traditional standbys for colds is still one of the best: make an infusion of equal amounts of peppermint (*Mentha* x *piperita*), elderflower (*Sambucus nigra*) and yarrow (*Achillea millefolium*). Taken hot just before going to bed, it will induce a sweat. You could also add a pinch of **cayenne powder**, a favourite North American Indian remedy: it stimulates the circulation.

- **Ginger** (*Zingiber officinalis*) – use a ginger herbal tea bag or make an infusion from grated fresh root.

Below *Ginger tea is warming and ideal for relieving the symptoms of colds.*

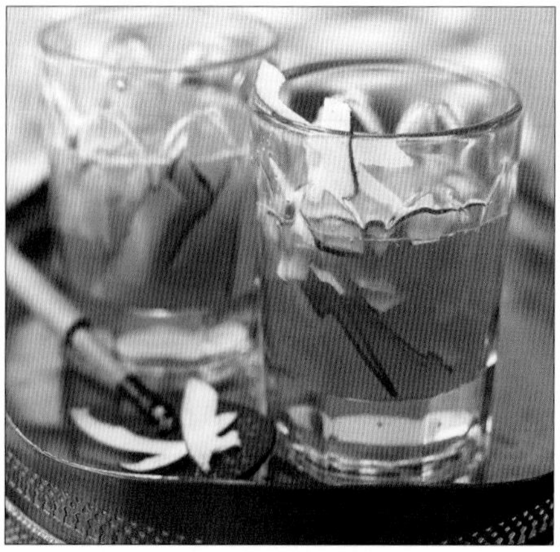

GARLIC COLD SYRUP

The health-giving properties of garlic have been recognized since ancient Egyptian times, when it was thought to bestow strength. Modern research confirms that garlic has antibacterial properties.

It is also antiviral, a decongestant and may help the body combat infection. Combine it with honey, which is soothing and mildly antiseptic, in a syrup to prevent or relieve the symptoms of colds and flu. Take 10–15ml/2–3 tsp three times a day.

Ingredients

1 head of garlic (*Allium sativum*)
300ml/½ pint/1¼ cups water
juice of ½ lemon
30ml/2 tbsp honey

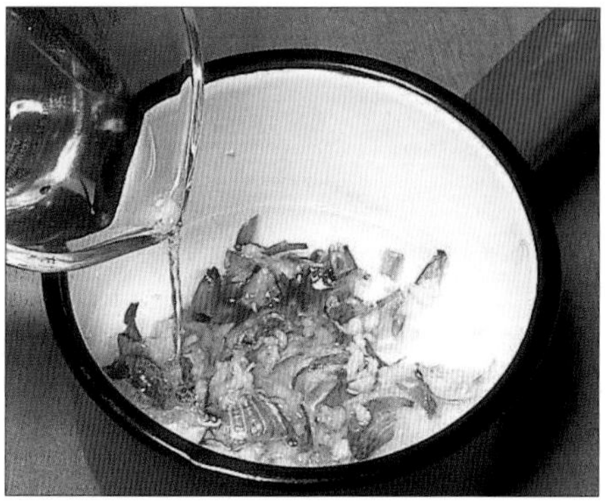

1 Crush the garlic cloves – there is no need to peel them – and put them in a pan with the water. Bring to the boil and simmer gently for 20 minutes. Cover the pan to prevent the liquid evaporating.

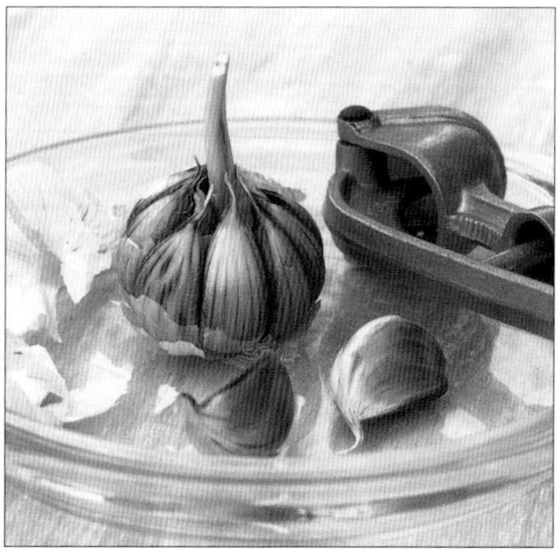

TIP Make the most of garlic's beneficial properties by adding it to food on a daily basis. You could also consider taking it in capsule form.

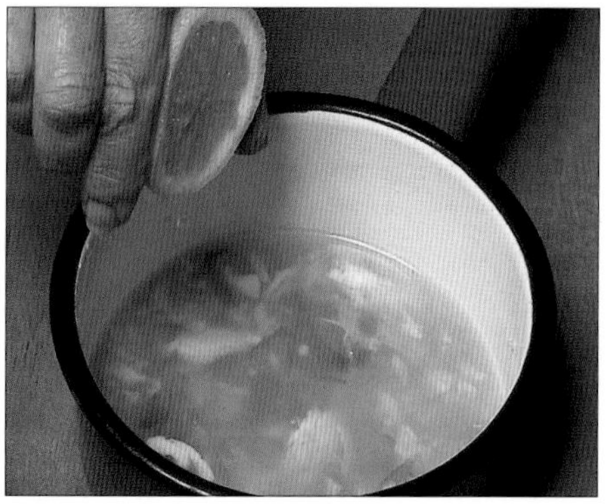

2 Add the lemon juice and honey and simmer for a further 2–3 minutes. Allow the mixture to cool slightly, then strain it into a clean, dark glass jar or bottle with an airtight lid. Keep for 2–3 weeks in the refrigerator.

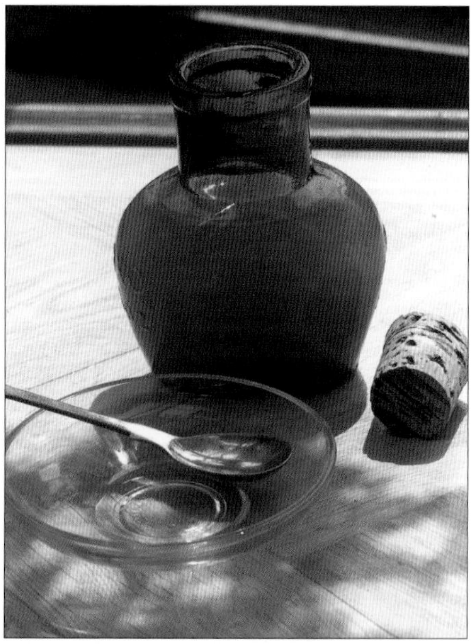

Above *Garlic syrup, made with honey and lemon, makes an excellent cold cure.*

Left *Look for plump fresh cloves when buying garlic. Its beneficial properties are most potent when it is eaten raw, but when cooked it still has some potency.*

CAMPHOR AND EUCALYPTUS VAPOUR RUB

This ointment contains decongestant oils to relieve blocked nasal cavities. It should be rubbed on to the throat or chest or used as an inhalant.

Ingredients

50g/2oz petroleum jelly
15g/1 tbsp dried lavender (*Lavandula* spp)
6 drops eucalyptus essential oil
4 drops camphor essential oil

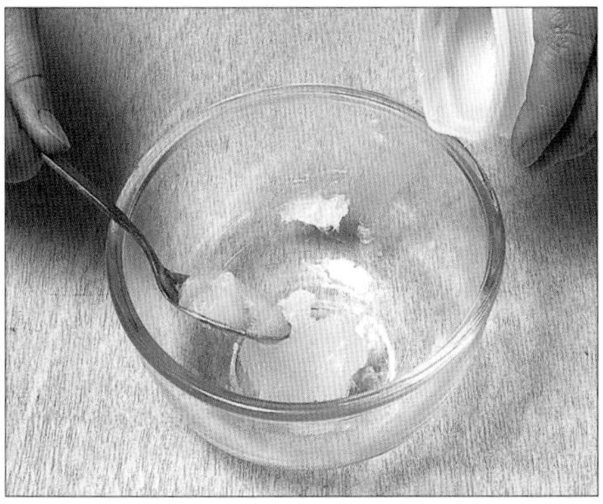

1 Melt the petroleum jelly in a bowl over a pan of simmering water, stir in the lavender and heat gently for 30 minutes.

2 Strain the liquid jelly through muslin, leave to cool slightly, then add the essential oils. Pour into a clean jar and leave until set. This will keep for 6 months.

3 Rub on to the chest or melt 15ml/1 tbsp in a bowl of hot water and inhale the steam.

Essential oils

The warmth and steam of a scented bath at bedtime will clear a stuffy head and help you sleep. Add 3–4 drops each of eucalyptus, thyme and lavender essential oils.

- Alternatively fill a bath bag with lavender (*Lavandula* spp), thyme and a 2.5cm/1in piece of fresh ginger (*Zingiber officinale*), grated, and hang it under the running tap to scent the bath water.
- Vaporizing essential oils in a burner will help with breathing difficulties when you are suffering from a cold. Try one of the following combinations: 3 drops each eucalyptus, tea tree and lavender, or 4 drops eucalyptus, 2 drops hyssop and 2 drops thyme.

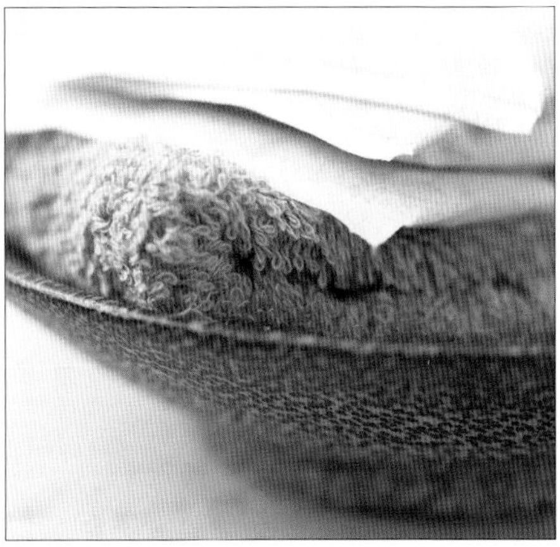

Above *A bath bag filled with head-clearing herbs relieves a stuffy nose. Make your own small cotton bag and add your choice of fresh or dried herbs.*

MUSTARD FOOT BATH

This has long been a popular treatment for colds and chills. It has a warming effect and is extremely comforting.

Ingredients

15g/1 tbsp mustard powder
2.2 litres/4 pints/9 cups hot water

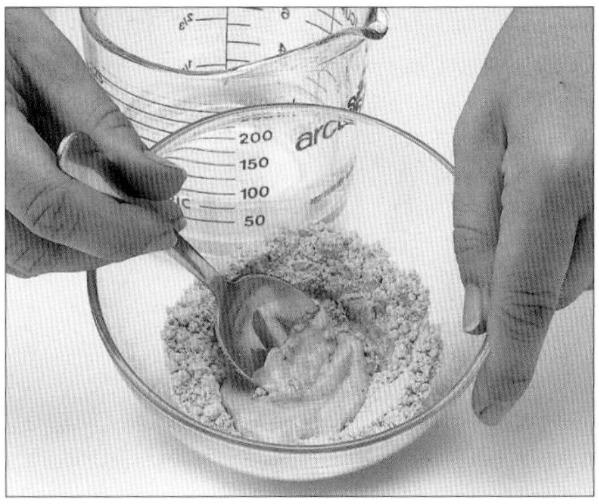

1 Stir the mustard and a small quantity of water together in a small bowl, stirring until the mustard dissolves.

2 Put the remaining hot water in the foot bath and add the dissolved mustard. Stir well.

3 Immerse the feet while the water is still hot. Re-heat the water if required.

Below *A mustard foot bath is a traditional treatment for colds. You could also try adding stimulating herbs such as rosemary (*Rosmarinus officinalis*) to the water.*

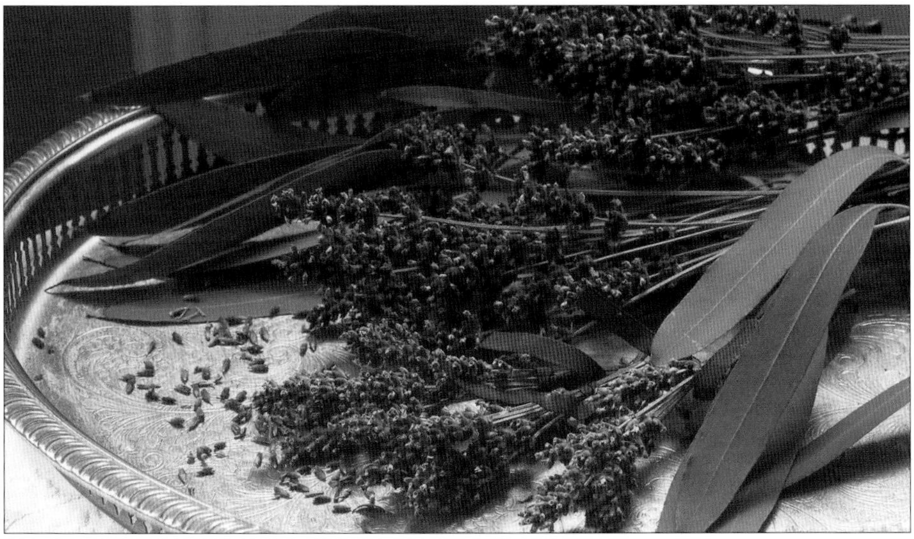

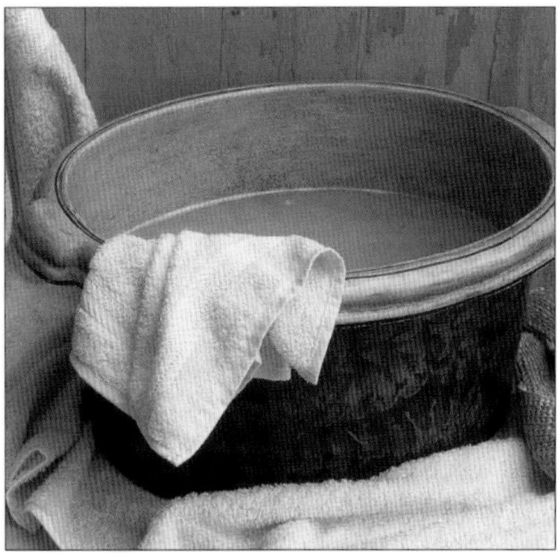

Left *Lavender and eucalyptus have a decongestant action.*

Coughs

A cough is a natural reflex reaction to any irritation, inflammation or blockage in the airways and is nature's way of keeping the bronchial tubes open and clear. It often accompanies an infection such as a cold but may also be due to breathing in dust or some other pollutant or allergen and will be self-limiting.

Causes of coughs

- Coughs often accompany colds, when we are run down and feeling low.
- Coughs can be a response to a much more serious underlying medical issue such as asthma, bronchitis or cancer.

CAUTION The herbal treatments recommended here are for the type of cough associated with common colds. Self-treatment is not appropriate for more serious or persistent coughs, or for one that accompanies a chest infection such as bronchitis. Always seek medical advice under these circumstances.

Herbal teas

A herbal infusion can be very soothing for troublesome, tickly coughs.

- **Coltsfoot** (*Tussilago farfara*) is a traditional herb for a cough, particularly for one that is irritating and spasmodic, and is recommended by many herbalists. It has a soothing effect, loosens mucus and reduces the spasm of a cough. Use the dried leaf of coltsfoot to make an infusion or buy as a standardized extract. Not to be taken during pregnancy or while breastfeeding.
- **Hyssop** (*Hyssopus officinalis*) is calming and relaxing and a gentle expectorant. Use the fresh or dried leaf, or the flower heads, to make a tea. As hyssop tastes quite bitter, honey and a little freshly squeezed orange juice (which also adds valuable vitamin C) will make it more palatable.
- **Marshmallow** (*Althaea officinalis*) is a herb whose demulcent properties make it highly soothing to inflamed bronchial tubes. It is especially useful for a harsh, dry cough to ease the soreness. It is best taken as an infusion, made from the fresh or dried flowers, or as a decoction of the dried roots.
- **Thyme** (*Thymus vulgaris*) is well known for its antiseptic properties; an infusion of fresh or dried thyme helps relieve a dry cough linked with a respiratory infection. Lemon thyme (*T. citriodorus*) can also be used.
- **White horehound** (*Marrubium vulgare*), used as an expectorant, helps free up thick, sticky mucus when you have a chesty cold. Make a tea with the fresh or dried herb. Sweeten with honey to taste and add a dash of lemon juice for a burst of vitamin C.
- **Chamomile** (*Chamaemelum nobile*), **elderflower** (*Sambucus nigra*) and **peppermint** (*Mentha* x *piperita*) make a palatable, soothing tea that will help to ease a troublesome cough. Put 2.5g/½ tsp each of dried peppermint, elderflower and chamomile in a small teapot. Add a pinch each dried lavender and ginger and pour over 250ml/8fl oz/1 cup boiling water. Infuse for 2–3 minutes, then strain into a cup. Stir in 5ml/1 tsp honey. Add a slice of lemon.

Below *If you are susceptible to coughs, make up a batch of linctus at the onset of winter. Drink plenty of herb teas to keep the throat moist. This will also help relieve the discomfort of a sore throat.*

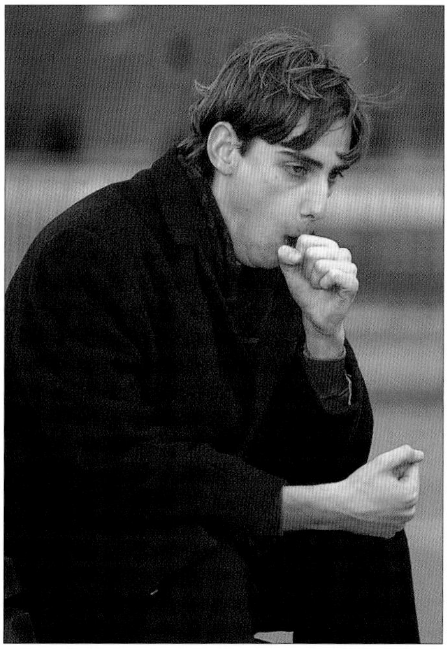

THYME AND BORAGE COUGH LINCTUS

Borage and thyme combine well to make a pleasant-tasting linctus.

Ingredients

25g/1oz fresh or 15g/½oz dried thyme (*Thymus* spp)
25g/1oz fresh or 15g/½oz dried borage (*Borago officinale*)
2 x 5cm/2in cinnamon sticks
600ml/1 pint/2½ cups water
juice of 1 small lemon
100g/4oz/½ cup honey

1 Put the herbs into a pan with the cinnamon and water. Bring to the boil, cover and simmer for 20 minutes.

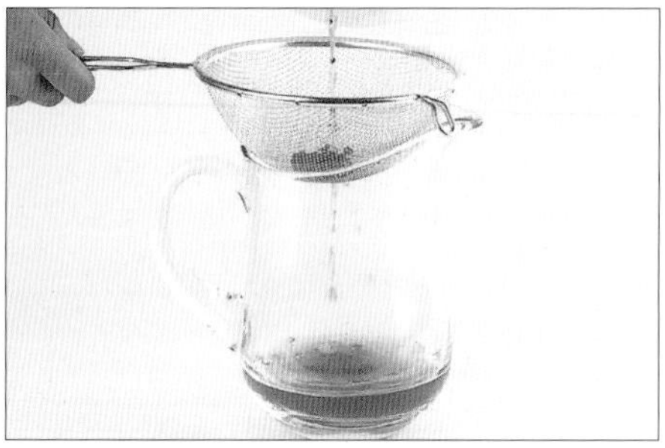

2 Strain off the herbs. Return the liquid to the pan. Simmer, uncovered, until reduced by half. Add the lemon juice and honey and simmer for 5 mintues. Bottle and store for up to 2 months. Take 5ml/1 tsp, as required.

Below *The antiseptic properties of thyme make it ideal for treating coughs.*

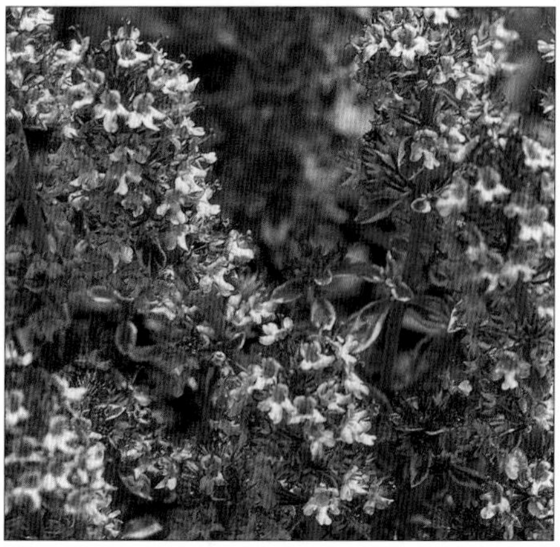

Sore Throats

With increased airborne pollution and the dry atmosphere in air-conditioned offices, sore throats are becoming more common throughout the year, and not just in the winter months. The irritation can range from an annoying tickle to a rasping soreness that makes speech difficult. Gargling with a strong herbal infusion or sipping a warming decoction will help ease the discomfort.

CAUTION A sore throat may be linked to another infection or be a symptom of a serious health problem, and if it persists for more than a week, seek medical advice.

HYSSOP AND HOREHOUND GARGLE

Both hyssop (*Hyssopus officinalis*) and white horehound (*Marrubium vulgare*) have been considered by herbalists to be effective remedies for sore throats. They also combine well to make a strong gargle. Make an infusion of the leaves and flowering tops of both herbs, following the directions given here for thyme and sage gargle. Sipping herb teas can also bring relief for a sore throat. Choose from any you find palatable.

Below *Lemon offers vitamin C, which can be taken in drinks to soothe a sore throat.*

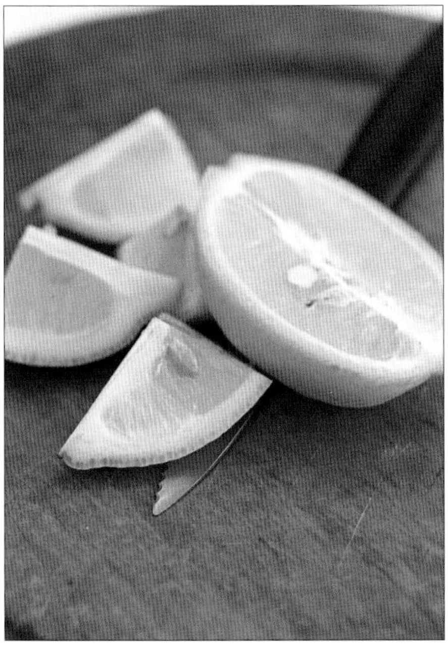

THYME AND SAGE GARGLE

Gargling with a strong herbal infusion or sipping a warming decoction will help ease the discomfort of a sore throat. When fresh herbs are not available, dried ones can be substituted, using 30ml/2 tbsp in 600ml/1 pint/2½ cups water.

Gargle with this mixture at the first sign of a sore throat. It can also be taken internally, 10ml/2 tsp at a time, 2–3 times a day. Use within 2 days.

Ingredients

small handfull each fresh sage (*Salvia officinalis*) and thyme (*Thymus* spp) leaves, roughly chopped
600ml/1 pint/2½ cups boiling water
30ml/2 tbsp cider vinegar
10ml/2 tsp honey
5ml/1 tsp cayenne pepper

Put the chopped leaves into a pot, pour in the boiling water, cover and leave to steep for 30 minutes. Strain off the liquid and stir in the cider vinegar, honey and cayenne.

Below: *Hyssop (*Hyssopus officinalis*) (with blue flowers) and horehound (*Marrubium vulgare*) (far right) combine well in a gargle for sore throats.*

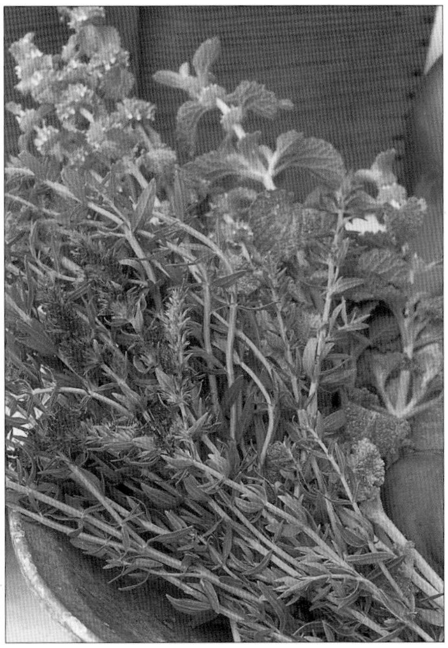

GINGER AND LEMON DECOCTION

Lemon provides vitamin C, while ginger is warming and stimulating and encourages sweating to eliminate toxins and dispel mucus and catarrh. This decoction will keep for 2–3 days.

Ingredients

115g/4oz piece of fresh root ginger
600ml/1 pint/2½ cups water
juice and rind of 1 lemon
pinch of cayenne pepper

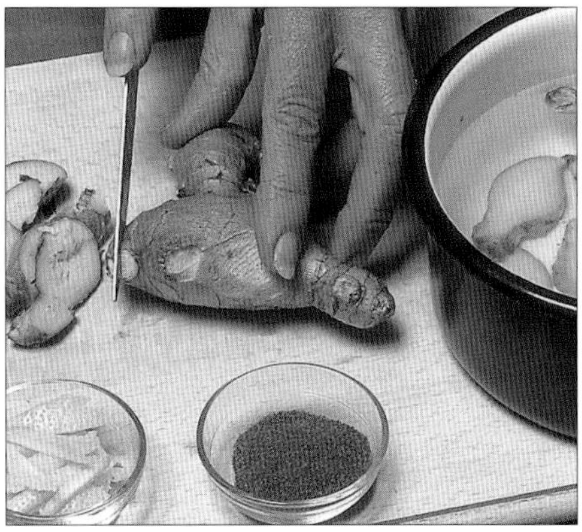

1 Slice the ginger root – there is no need to peel it – and put it in a pan with the water, lemon rind and cayenne. Always use an enamelled rather than an aluminium pan.

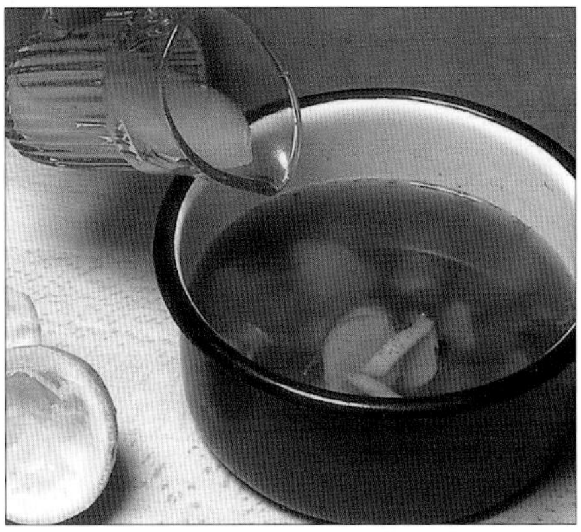

2 Bring to the boil, cover the pan and simmer for 20 minutes. Remove from the heat and add the lemon juice.

3 Drink a small cupful at a time, sweetened with honey.

Catarrh

Irritation of the membranes of the nose and throat encourages the production of mucus as a defence mechanism; where this becomes excessive or prolonged, for example after a cold, then catarrh is the result. Sinusitis is the name for inflammation of the sinus membranes.

Symptoms of catarrh

Like those of a heavy cold, the symptoms of catarrh are:

- A runny nose or a blocked and stuffy nose.
- Headaches.
- A persistent cough.

Simple herbal treatments, which help provide some relief from the symptoms of both catarrh and sinusitis, include steam inhalations and a decongestant rub (*see page 55*).

Herbal tea

A blocked nose is a misery when you are suffering from a cold, and it often stops you getting a sound night's sleep.

- **Elderflower (*Sambucus nigra*), yarrow (*Achillea millefolium*) and peppermint (*Mentha* x *piperita*) tea** This warming tea has a soothing action. Put 5ml/1tsp dried elderflower, 5ml/1tsp dried yarrow and 1 sprig of fresh peppermint in a teapot. Add 600ml/1 pint 2½ cups boiling water and leave to steep. Strain before serving. Take one cupful before bedtime at the onset of a cold but not for more than two consecutive days.

An infusion of yarrow taken internally can cause light sensitivity. Do not drink this tea before going into sunlight.

Decongestant essential oils

Essential oils provide a convenient way to inhale healing plant fragrance, as you can keep a stock always to hand. Add a few drops to a bowl of hot water and breathe in the steam, or sprinkle some on a handkerchief to sniff throughout the day. Use in place of fresh herbs. Essential oils to try include cinnamon, eucalyptus, lavender, lemon, marjoram, peppermint and pine.

ESSENTIAL OIL INHALANT

This combination of oils could also be sprinkled on a tissue to tuck under a pillow.

Ingredients

5 drops eucalyptus essential oil
2 drops camphor essential oil
1 drop citronella essential oil

Add the essential oils to 600ml/1 pint/ 2½ cups boiling water in a bowl. Breathe in the steam, leaning over the bowl.

FRESH HERB INHALANT

Inhaling steam scented with freshly picked aromatic herbs is an excellent way to relieve the congestion of a cold or blocked sinuses. It is one of the simplest and most effective methods to treat catarrh. Use a combination of herbs and spices from the list below:

Ingredients

Herbs: Eucalyptus leaves, basil (*Basilicum ocimum*), hyssop (*Hyssopus officinalis*), juniper (*Juniperus communis*) foliage, lavender (*Lavandula* spp), lemon balm (*Melissa officinalis*), mint (*Mentha* spp), rosemary (*Rosmarinus officinalis*), sage (*Salvia officinalis*), thyme (*Thymus* spp).
Spices: Cayenne pepper, cinnamon stick, juniper berries, ground ginger, dried lemon rind.

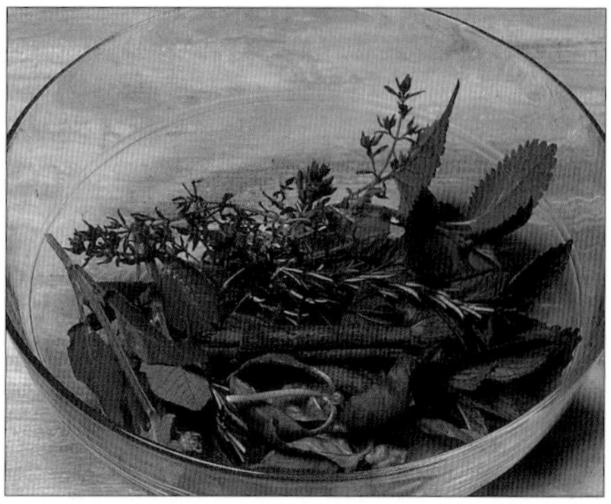

1 Put a large handful of herbs and spices, selected from the lists supplied, in a bowl. Crush them lightly.

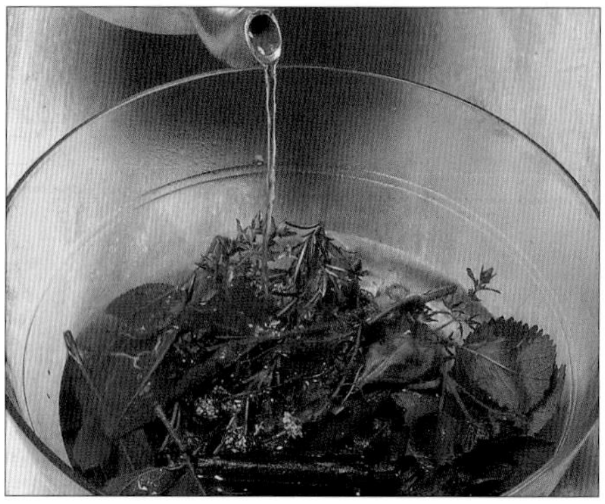

2 Pour in about 1 litre/1¾ pints/4 cups boiling water and lean over the bowl, covering both it and your head with a towel. Breathe in the steam.

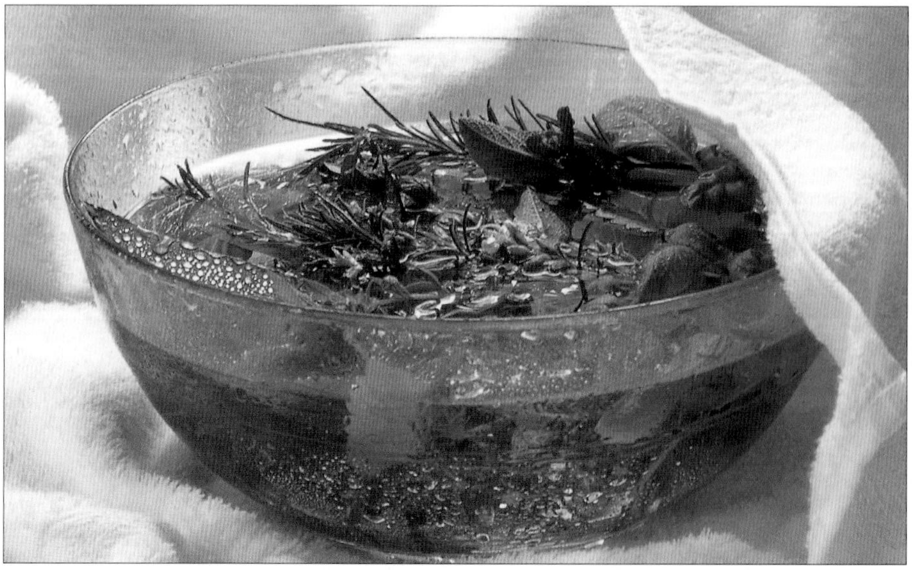

Hayfever

Hayfever is an allergic reaction, which can be triggered in some people not just by grass pollens, but also by tree or flower pollens. It is often seen together with other allergic reactions such as asthma and/or eczema.

Symptoms of hayfever

- Sneezing and a blocked or runny nose.
- Itchy eyes, throat, mouth, ears.

Although it is best to seek medical advice for its treatment, the preventive measures suggested below can sometimes help, and there are a number of ways in which herbs can be used to ease the distressing symptoms on a day-to-day basis.

Preventive measures

Two to three months before the onset of the hayfever season, take:

- **Elderflower (*Sambucus nigra*) tincture** made with dried or fresh flowers, in a standard dose of 5ml/1 tsp diluted in water three times daily.
- **Echinacea tincture**, useful for boosting the immune system. Buy it as a ready-made product and take 15 drops in water twice a day over several periods of 2–3 weeks at a time, with breaks of 2–3 weeks in between and not continuously.
- **Honey** – if made locally, the pollens it contains may be the same as those that trigger your hayfever. Taking 10–15ml/ 2–3 tsp daily for two months before the start of the season, can help acclimatize your system to the allergens. Local honey is also the best to use as a sweetener for herb teas.

Herbal teas

Comforting as well as helpful, herbal teas are a good antidote to hayfever.

- **Plantain** (*Plantago major*) has anti-catarrhal and astringent properties to help tone the membranes and clear congestion. Take it as a strong infusion, in combination with elderflower (*Sambucus nigra*) for maximum effect. Ribwort (*Plantago lanceolata)* can also be used but is less effective medicinally.
- **Chamomile** (*Chamaemelum nobile*) or lemon balm (*Melissa officinalis*), combined with an equal part of yarrow (*Achillea millefolium*), and taken as a standard tea, help reduce allergic reactions.
- **Nettle** (*Urtica dioica*) in a strong infusion, taken regularly over a period of a few weeks, can help to reduce inflammation, excess mucus and sensitivity to pollen. The infusion is not very palatable. Try also nettle soup.

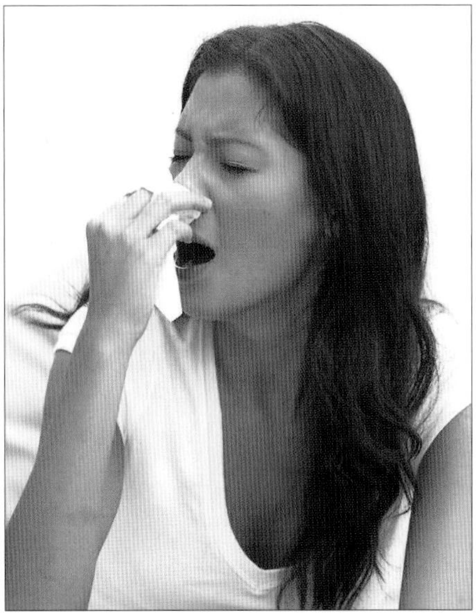

Above *Herbal teas and tinctures can ease the misery of summer hayfever. It's best to start taking them before the onset of the season when the pollen causing the reaction is shed.*

Compress

Soak small cotton wool pads in an infusion of chamomile (*Chamaemelum nobile*) or eyebright (*Euphrasia officinalis*) and place over closed eyelids for 10–15 minutes to relieve sore, itchy eyes.

Below *Eyepads soaked in a gentle herbal infusion help relieve soreness and itching.*

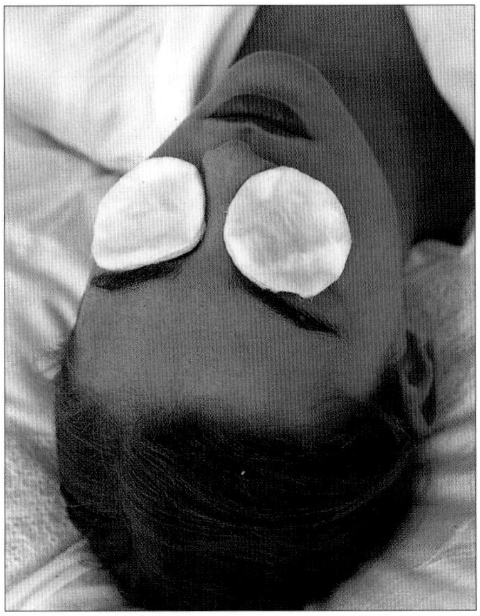

Below *Local honey may be helpful in acclimatizing the system to allergens.*

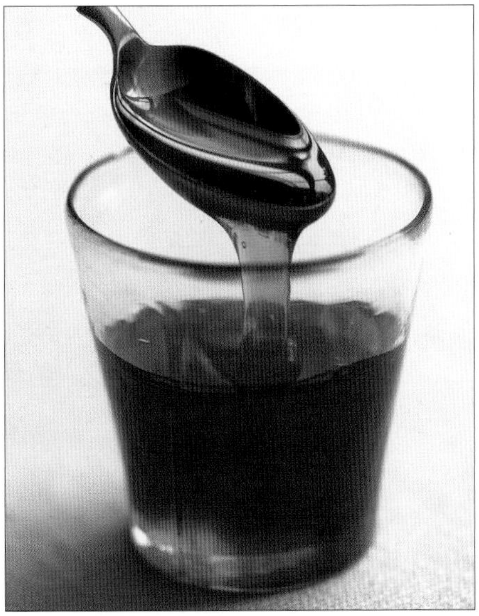

Below *Chamomile flowers provide the raw material for both soothing teas and eyepads.*

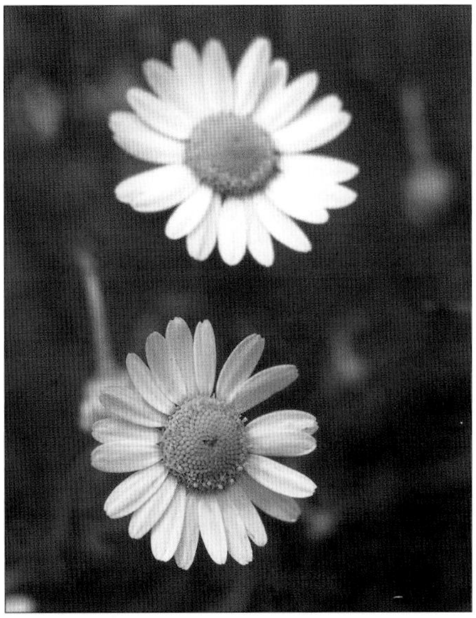

Indigestion

Indigestion is a general term for the discomfort caused by digestive disturbances. Usually it is a temporary problem brought about by eating too much or the wrong kind of food or from drinking excess alcohol. It can also be stress related. Short-term digestive problems of this kind generally respond quite well to herbal treatment. Longer-term digestive pains may have more serious causes for which medical advice should always be taken.

Symptoms of indigestion

• Abdominal discomfort and flatulence.
• Upset stomach.
• Heartburn.

Herbal teas

Infusions can be very helpful in easing indigestion. Choose from the following.

• **German chamomile** (*Matricaria chamomilla*) is calming and is good for the effects of over-eating and for stress-related indigestion.

• **Lemon balm** (*Melissa officinalis*) settles a churning stomach and is a good herb for nervous indigestion. Make with fresh leaves.

• **Peppermint** (*Mentha* x *piperita*) is good for indigestion accompanied by flatulence and a bloated abdomen.

• **Dill** (*Anethum graveolens*) acts gently to ease indigestion and can even be given to babies and young children. Allow 5ml/1 tsp lightly crushed dill seed to 250ml/8fl oz/ 1 cup of water and boil for 10 minutes. Strain and allow to cool before drinking.

• **Fennel seed** (*Foeniculum vulgare*) is good for flatulence and acid indigestion. See the recipe for fennel seed tea opposite.

• **Marigold** (*Calendula officinalis*) and **lemon verbena** (*Aloysia triphylla*) make a refreshing digestive. This tisane is reputed to be excellent for purifying the blood and aiding digestion. The verbena gives an intense lemon flavour and the marigold adds a peppery note. Mix 50g/2oz dried marigold petals with 25g/1oz dried lemon verbena leaves. Store in an airtight container. Prepare an infusion using 15g/½oz herb to 600ml/1 pint/ 2½ cups boiling water.

GINGER JUICE WITH PINEAPPLE

Fresh root ginger is one of the best natural cures for indigestion. It also helps to settle upset stomachs, whether caused by food poisoning or motion sickness. In this unusual fruity blend, it is mixed with fresh, juicy pineapple and sweet-tasting carrot. It can be juiced up in seconds and tastes delicious. Make one for breakfast for general indigestion. For an upset stomach take weak ginger tea on its own.

Ingredients

Makes 1 glass
½ small pineapple
25g/1oz fresh root ginger
1 carrot
ice cubes

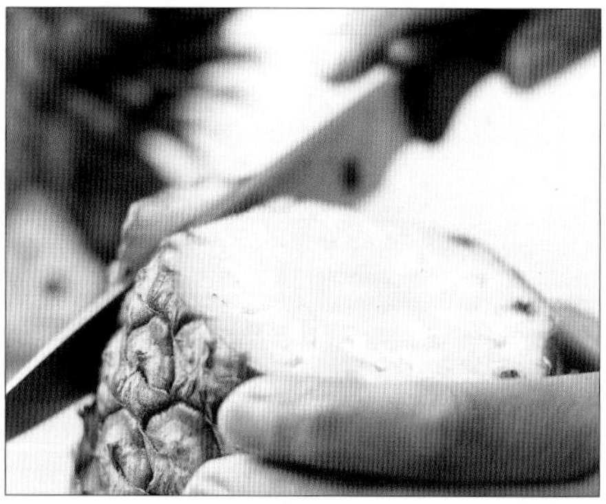

1 Cut away the skin from the pineapple, then halve and remove the core. Roughly slice the pineapple flesh, reserving half for another use.

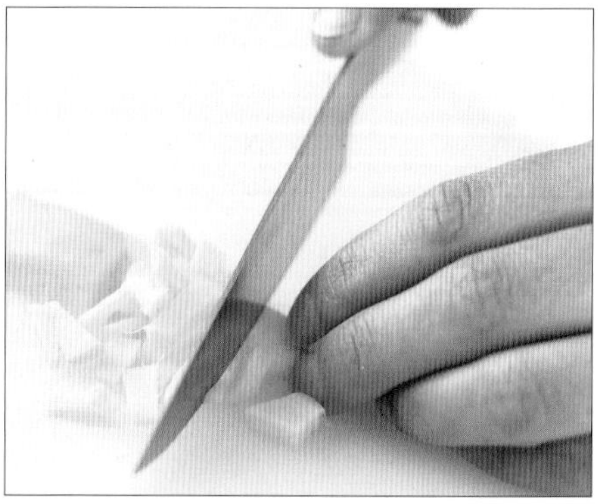

2 Peel and chop the ginger and chop the carrot into large chunks.

TIP Before preparing a pineapple for juicing or cutting it into chunks or rings, cut off the leafy top, turn the pineapple upside down in a dish and leave it for half an hour – this makes it juicier.

The quickest and easiest way to cut up a pineapple is to cut off the top and bottom edges. Then slice the skin away from the sides using a sharp knife. Carefully trim away the eyes, without discarding too much of the fruit.

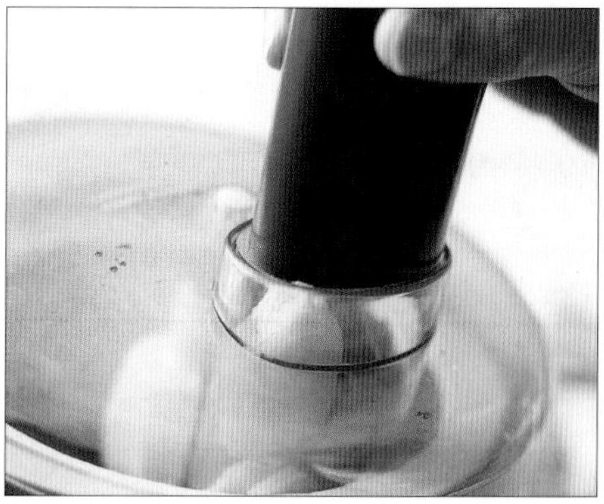

3 Push the carrot, ginger and pineapple through a juicer and pour into a glass. Add ice cubes and serve immediately.

Below *Ginger is a well known cure for many everyday ailments.*

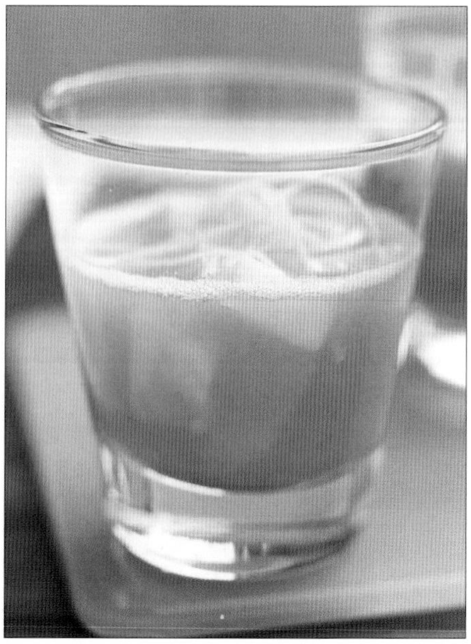

Acidity and Heartburn

Many people get occasional bouts of acid dyspepsia, as this kind of indigestion is known, usually related to a temporary problem such as having eaten rich, spicy foods or having eaten too quickly. If the symptoms happen very regularly, you may need to look more carefully at what you eat and how fast you eat it. If there is persistent discomfort, seek professional treatment. When excess acid leaks back up into the gullet, this inflames and irritates the lining of the oesophagus and the feeling of heartburn is produced. Taking antacid tablets regularly may not only mask underlying problems, but can also be counterproductive as the stomach tries to compensate by creating more acid.

Symptoms of heartburn

- A burning sensation near the breastbone.
- Mild discomfort.

Herbal teas

To relieve a temporary bout of heartburn, choose from the following teas. For repeated symptoms of acidity and heartburn, make the infusions stronger by increasing the quantity of herb used (by half as much again) and leaving to steep for a few minutes longer.

- **German chamomile** (*Matricaria chamomilla*) is an anti-inflammatory remedy and relaxant that helps the whole digestive tract; if acid symptoms are related to stress and/or over-eating of rich foods, this herb makes an excellent choice.

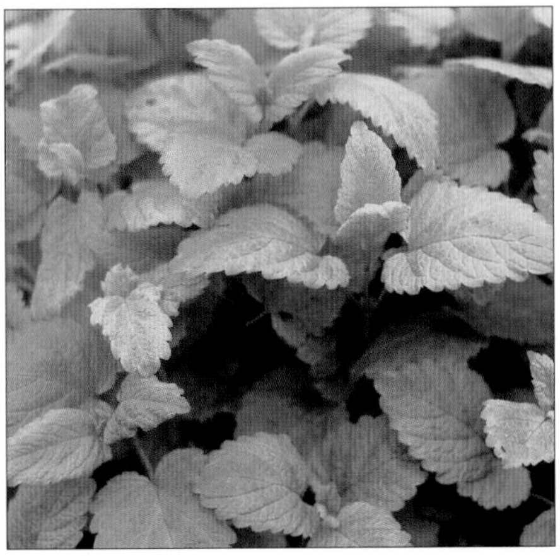

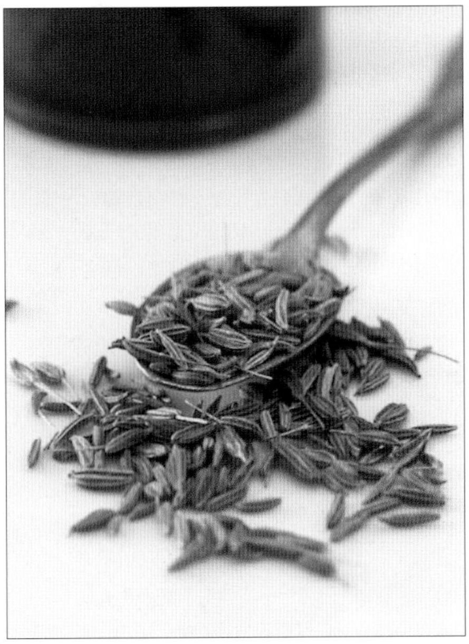

Above *Known for their digestive properties, fennel seeds, along with caraway seeds, are often handed round after meals in eastern countries as aids to digestion. They may be in their natural state or coated in sugar.*

- **Lemon balm** (*Melissa officinalis*) is another excellent herb where the condition is caused by stress; always use the fresh leaves.
- **Meadowsweet** (*Filipendula ulmaria*), although chemically related to aspirin, it is soothing for an inflamed stomach. It may need to be avoided by those who have a hypersensitivity to salicylates such as aspirin. It also reduces acidity.
- **Slippery elm** (*Ulmus fulva*), the powdered bark of a native North American elm tree, is highly soothing to the inflamed gullet or stomach. It may be taken by mixing 5ml/1 tsp of the pure powder in a little warm water. Slippery elm is now threatened in the wild so only buy from a responsible source.
- **Fennel seed** (***Foeniculum vulgare***) **tea** With a mild aniseed flavour, fennel is a diuretic and has a calming effect on the stomach, easing flatulence and indigestion. Caraway seeds can be prepared in the same way, or combined with fennel in equal quantities. Put 5ml/1 tsp fennel seeds in a small pan with 250ml/8fl oz/1 cup of water and boil for 10 minutes. Strain and allow to cool before drinking. Add a slice of orange or a sliver of orange rind for extra flavour.

Left *Lemon balm makes a soothing tea for reducing stress.*

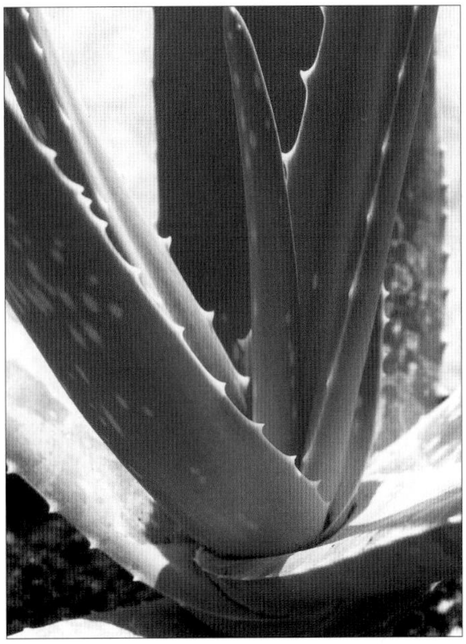

Above *Aloe vera, a traditional digestive remedy, should be used with medical advice.*

Aloe vera juice

The juice of the aloe vera plant has a long history of use as a remedy for digestive problems. While this, and its positive effect on the immune system, have been confirmed by research studies, some species used in medicinal products are potentially toxic. It is therefore essential, if taking aloe vera internally, to do so with professional advice and under medical supervision.

Digestive herbs in food

- **Sage** (*Salvia officinalis*), like many culinary herbs, aids digestion. It has a robust flavour, which stands up to long cooking processes and goes well with cheese and meat dishes.
- **Parsley** (*Petroselinum crispum*) and **chervil** (*Anthriscus cerefolium*) are also helpful to the digestion when used in cooking.
- **Caraway** and **fennel seeds**, well known for their digestive properties, can be added to dishes or chewed after a meal.

Nausea and Vomiting

There are many causes for feelings of nausea, or actual vomiting. Most of them will be "self-limiting", which means they will settle without the need for further treatment or investigation. If you are in any doubt as to the cause you should of course seek professional advice first, but mild nausea can usually be treated safely with natural remedies.

Nausea or vomiting can usually be linked to a specific situation such as eating too much rich food, drinking too much alcohol, travel or motion sickness, and anxiety.

CAUTION If symptoms are persistent and do not settle down in one to two days, or for more serious conditions, including food poisoning and gastric infection, seek medical help.

Herbal tea

Herbs to take as teas include peppermint, chamomile (*Chamaemelum nobile*) and lemon balm (*Melissa officinalis*). They are all soothing to the digestion and will help to settle the stomach.

Below *Ginger cookies are a useful standby for relieving symptoms of travel sickness. Crytallized (candied) ginger may also help, but has a much stronger flavour.*

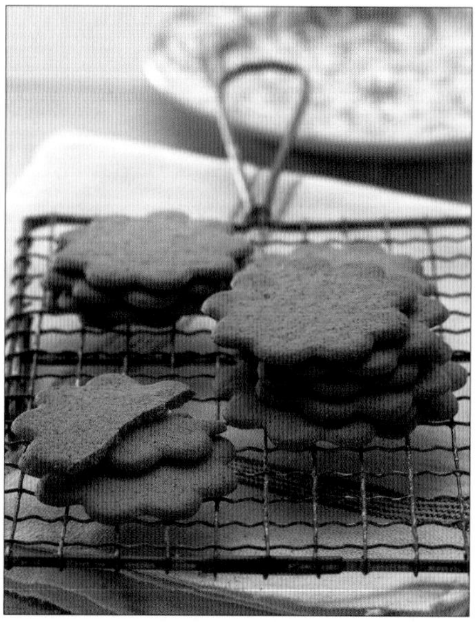

The benefits of ginger

The first choice remedy for most cases of mild nausea is ginger (*Zingiber officinalis*). It can be taken as a tea, made with a bought teabag or as a homemade infusion using the fresh or dried grated root (5ml/1 tsp fresh, or 2.5ml/½ tsp dried to 250ml/8fl oz/1 cup water). Take one cup three times a day. For travel sickness, chewing a piece of crystallized ginger, nibbling a ginger biscuit (cookie) or even drinking a little flat ginger ale will often relieve the symptoms.

Morning sickness

Ginger, taken in the ways suggested above, may be helpful in alleviating the effects of morning sickness, suffered by many during pregnancy. Do not take ginger in medicinal or large doses without medical advice. Smaller quantities of ginger used in cooking do not generally pose a problem.

Essential oil

Vaporizing essential oils may reduce feelings of nausea. Essential oils of lemon, ginger and basil – 2–3 drops of each – work for some, although others develop an antipathy to any strong smell.

Below *Essential oils of lemon and ginger help counteract feelings of nausea with their fresh and distinctive fragrances.*

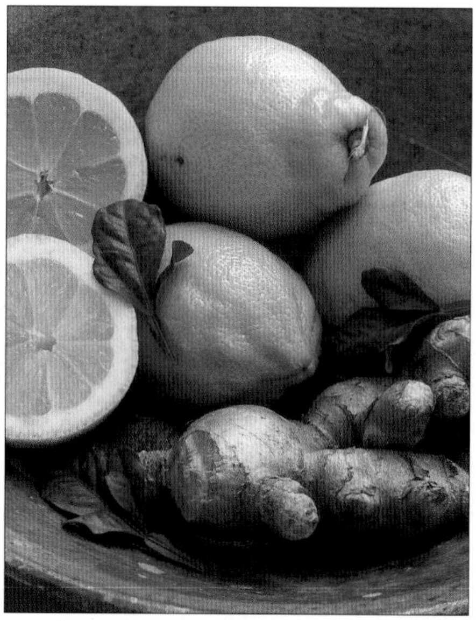

Preparing fresh root ginger

This spice is one of the oldest cultivated and most popular medicinal herbs. Its unmistakable hot, fragrant and peppery taste is used in a huge variety of sweet and savoury dishes, such as tisanes, soups, stir-fries, curries, desserts and cakes. Ground ginger is often used in recipes, but finely grated ginger can also be used.

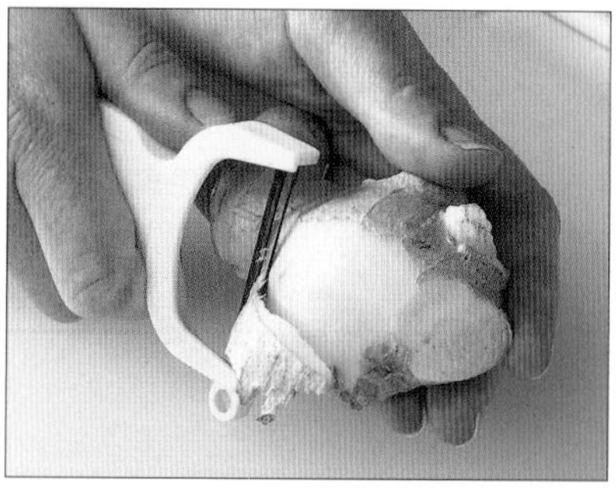

1 Peel fresh root ginger using a vegetable peeler.

2 Chop ginger using a sharp knife to the size specified in the recipe.

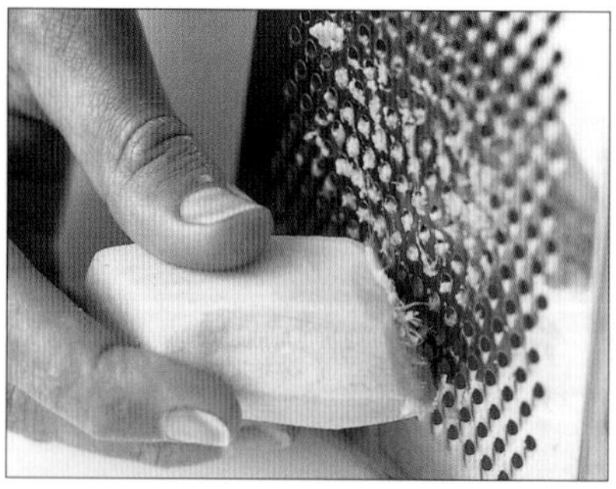

3 Grate ginger finely – a box grater works well. Freshly grated ginger can also be squeezed to release the juice.

CAUTION Ginger may interact with anti-coagulant drugs if taken in large doses. The maximum per day is 2g dried or 4g fresh ginger. If you are taking any other medication seek professional advice.

Mouth Ulcers

Small ulcers can occur on the tongue, gums and lining of the mouth. These are sometimes due to local trauma, for instance biting your cheek or wearing ill-fitting dentures, but often reflect a state of generally being run-down. Recurrent "crops" of mouth ulcers may therefore indicate a need for more general treatment, perhaps to relieve stress.

Tinctures

Herbal tinctures, applied locally, may relieve the discomfort of mouth ulcers. They should be diluted in water and used as a mouthwash, swishing them around the affected area. Pay attention to general health, and seek professional treatment if the ulcers are persistent or recurrent.

- **Myrrh** (*Commiphora myrrha*) is the strongest and most effective tincture for combating mouth ulcers. Buy a commercial product and use 8–10 drops, diluted in a little warm water.
- Others to try are **marigold** (*Calendula officinalis*), **sage** (*Salvia officinalis*) and **thyme** (*Thymus vulgaris*) – all are gently astringent and antiseptic. They can be made into tinctures at home, following the recipe for raspberry leaf tincture.
- **Echinacea tincture** – buy this ready-made and follow the manufacturer's instructions. *Echinacea* helps boost the immune system and can be taken for a few weeks at a time when you are feeling generally run down.

Below Echinacea *may ward off infections.*

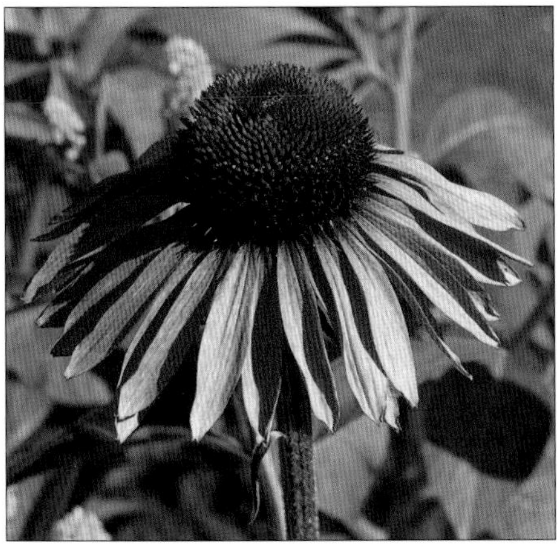

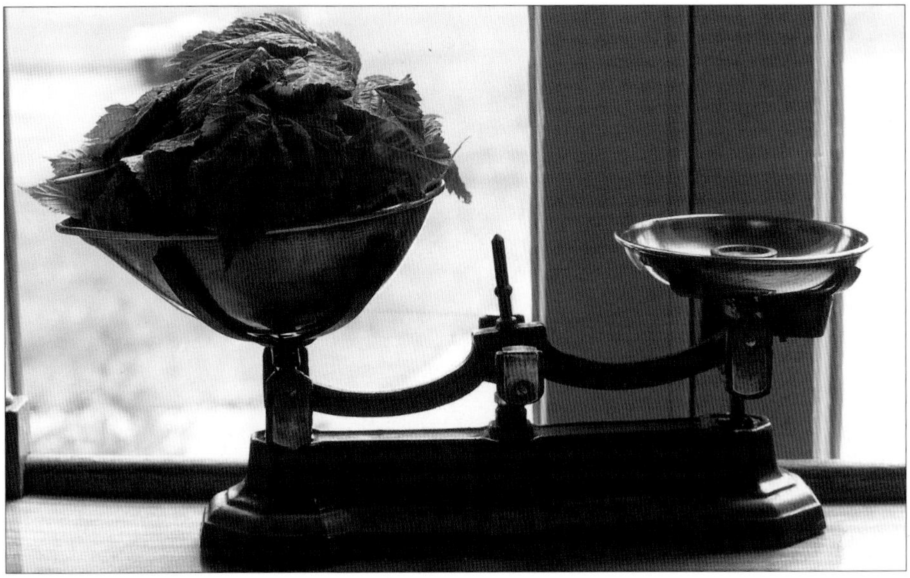

Above *Raspberry leaves contain vitamins and minerals beneficial for good health.*

RASPBERRY LEAF TINCTURE

A traditional remedy for mouth ulcers and inflamed gums. Use 10ml/2 tsp diluted in a little warm water to rinse the mouth.

Ingredients

50g/2oz fresh raspberry leaves, coarsely chopped
250ml/8fl oz/1 cup vodka, made up to 300ml/½ pint/1¼ cups with water

1 Put the fresh leaves into a large glass jar and pour in the vodka and water mixture. If the liquid does not quite cover the leaves, top up with a little extra vodka and water.

2 Put a lid on the jar and leave in a cool place for 7–10 days. Shake the jar occasionally and keep the leaves immersed.

3 Strain out the herb material through muslin (cheesecloth) before pouring the tincture into a sterilized glass bottle and sealing. Fresh leaves soak up more liquid than dried, so squeeze them out by pressing with a wooden spoon when straining. Store in a cool dark place, preferably in dark glass bottles.

Right *Mouth ulcers can be painful and are generally a sign of feeling at a low ebb, when the body's resources are depleted.*

Sage and myrrh infusion

A strong infusion of sage (*Salvia officinalis*), combined with tincture of myrrh, makes a powerful rinse to combat mouth ulcers.

Pour 300ml/½ pint/1¼ cups boiling water over 15ml/1 tbsp dried sage in a jug (pitcher). Leave to stand for 20 minutes. Strain through a sieve lined with muslin (cheesecloth) and mix with 20 drops tincture of myrrh. Use to rinse the mouth.

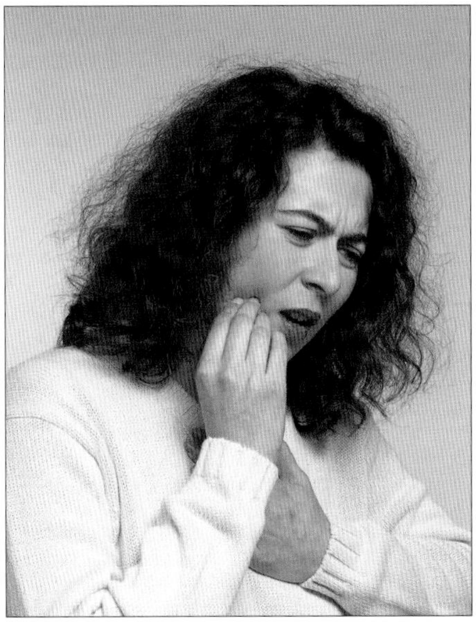

Constipation

Diet and lifestyle are a major factor in causing constipation; too many refined foods and inadequate dietary fibre, too little exercise and too much stress may all be contributory factors to the condition. Digestive and liver problems, piles and the ageing process could also be responsible. Herbal laxatives can be useful in providing a solution where the problem is temporary, but if constipation continues, or becomes painful, it is important to consult your doctor immediately.

Types of constipation

There are essentially two types of constipation. Where there is inadequate fibre and a sluggish digestive system, treatment should be aimed at toning up the bowel; when the constipation is linked to high levels of stress and spasm, treatment may need to focus on relaxation and even reducing excessive fibre such as bran. If in doubt seek professional treatment, as the regular use of laxatives may be completely counterproductive.

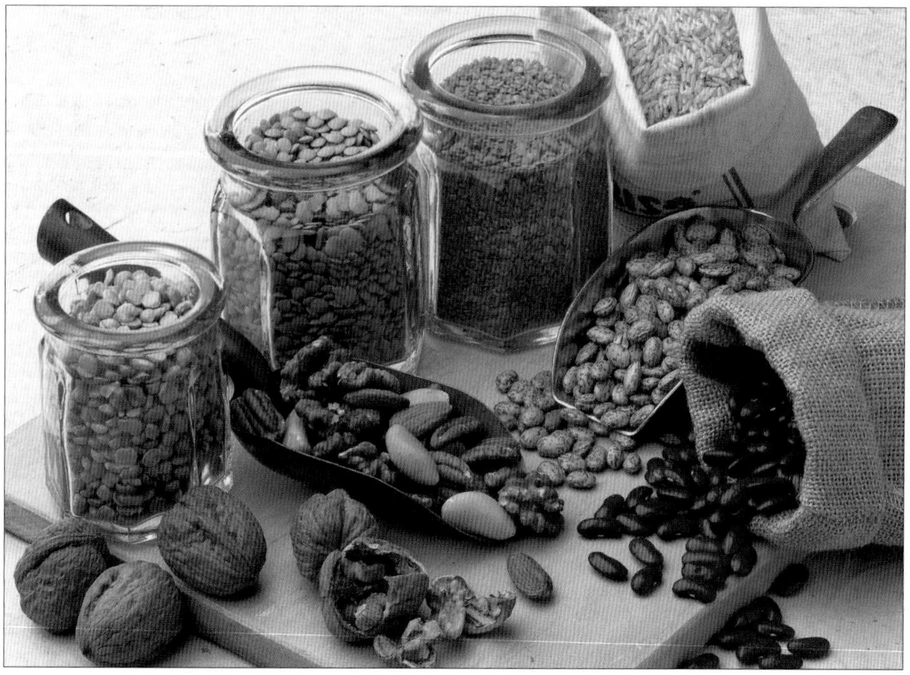

Below *Pulses, including beans, peas and lentils, are high in fibre and help to promote regular bowel movements.*

Herbal laxatives

Always start with gentle laxatives or aperients, which increase bowel tone without giving griping. One of the best is dandelion root (*Taraxacum officinale*), ideally taken as a decoction – although you may get a gentle action from one of the dandelion coffee drinks on the market.

If the constipation persists, switch to another herb that works in quite a different way. Linseed (*Linum usitatissimum*) absorbs liquid and creates a soft bulk internally that aids the peristaltic wave movements that propel faeces through the bowel. Take 10ml/2 tsp linseed at breakfast, with at least 300ml/½ pint/1¼ cups) of water. Ideally soak the linseed overnight in a little water to start the swelling process. It may look like frogspawn but it can relieve constipation. Make sure you take plenty of liquids, however.

Decoction

Cramp bark (*Viburnum opulus*) has been found to reduce intestinal spasms and ease the symptoms of irritable bowel syndrome. It may be taken as a standard decoction of the bark in the standard dose of one cup three times daily.

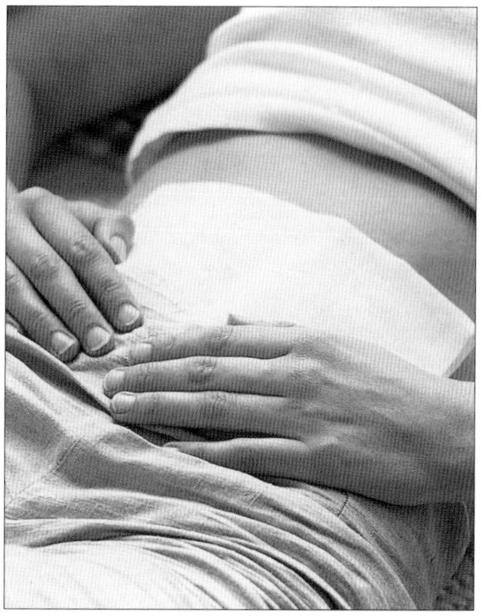

Above *Gently massage a mixture of rosemary, marjoram and chamomile essential oils (5 drops of each) diluted in a little almond oil, into the area around the navel. A warm compress, applied to the abdomen, may also help to ease the discomfort of constipation.*

Liquorice

As a herbal remedy for digestive problems liquorice root (*Glycyrrhiza glabra*) has a long history and is widely used in Chinese traditional medicine. It has often been recommended in the past for relieving constipation and forms the basis of many proprietary laxatives.

However, scientific research studies have now established that it can have some serious side effects, especially when taken over a long period, and in particular that it causes high blood pressure and water retention. It has also been found to interact with many medical drugs prescribed for a whole range of serious illnesses. It should, therefore, only be taken on medical advice and under professional supervision.

Diet

Too many refined foods and not enough fibre in the diet may lead to constipation. Eating plenty of fresh fruit, vegetables and wholegrains should help.

Diarrhoea

Loose, frequent bowel movements can happen as a short-term reaction to infection, inflammation or food poisoning, and as such are quite a positive, cleansing action. A common experience is holiday diarrhoea, and this is usually a response to exposure to unfamiliar bacteria.

CAUTION Always seek medical advice for persistent diarrhoea lasting more than a few days and for serious food poisoning.

Causes of diarrhoea

Some foods have a natural laxative effect, for instance prunes or figs, so over-indulgence will give temporary diarrhoea. Stress and anxiety often increase peristalsis and hurry bowel contents through. Repeated episodes of diarrhoea may indicate more complex digestive problems and should be treated professionally.

Prolonged diarrhoea, especially in young children, can be quite serious as it causes dehydration; ensure adequate fluid intake and seek professional advice. A simple yet dramatically effective rehydration drink can be made by dissolving 5ml/1 tsp salt and

Below *It's important not to become dehydrated when suffering from diarrhoea, so drink plenty of water, sipped slowly.*

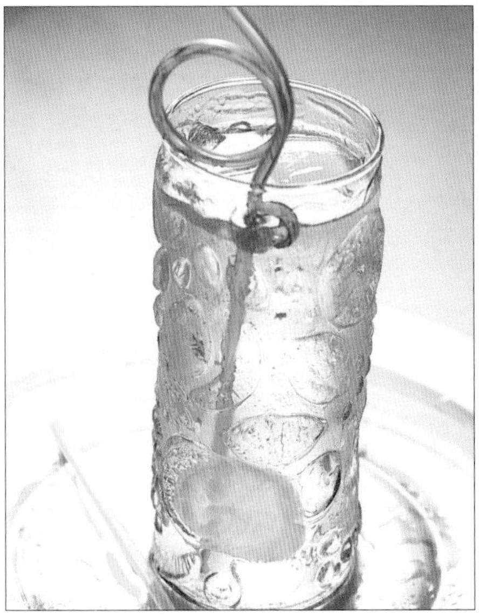

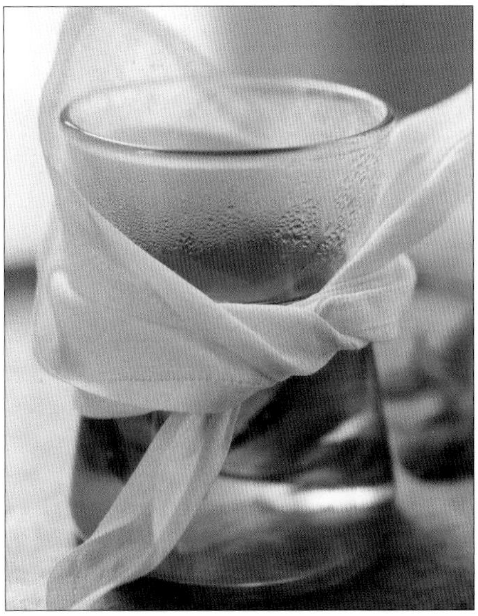

Above *Herbal teas are helpful in settling an upset stomach.*

15ml/1 tbsp sugar in 600ml/1 pint/2½ cups boiled water. Keep in the refrigerator in a screw-topped bottle and give small amounts frequently. Use for a short time only. Alternatively, buy electrolyte supplements from a pharmacist.

Herbal teas

An infusion made from the choice of herbs listed below may help to soothe the bowels and calm griping discomfort. If mild food poisoning or infection has been the cause of the upset, you could also try eating garlic as a natural gut disinfectant.

- **Agrimony** (*Agrimonia eupatoria*) is astringent and healing to the inflamed and swollen membranes lining the gut, and helpful in mild gastro-enteritis.
- **German chamomile** (*Matricaria chamomilla*), which is calming and anti-inflammatory, reduces the impact of tension on the digestive tract. This is one of the first herbs to think of in many digestive disorders.
- **Meadowsweet** (*Filipendula ulmaria*) will help to settle an acidic stomach, as well as being mildly astringent.
- **Ribwort** (*Plantago lanceolata*) has excellent toning, soothing and healing properties, and is useful in cases of diarrhoea from many causes where there is inflammation.
- **Thyme** (*Thymus vulgaris*) will fight infections and improve digestion generally, settling churning, loose bowels and killing harmful bacteria.

GINGER AND CINNAMON TEA

This is a tea to relieve a griping sensation in the bowel, and could be taken once the worst symptoms have subsided. It also helps combat infection.

Ingredients

small piece of fresh or dried ginger, finely grated
1 small cinnamon stick
pinch of ground cinnamon
250ml/8fl oz/1 cup water
honey to taste

1 Put the ginger in a pan, with the water and cinnamon stick, over a gentle heat, bring to the boil and simmer for 10 minutes.

2 Strain, stir in a little honey and sprinkle with ground cinnamon before drinking.

Below *Comforting, spicy ginger and warming cinnamon tea helps to calm the bowel as well as an upset stomach. Sweeten with a little honey, if you like.*

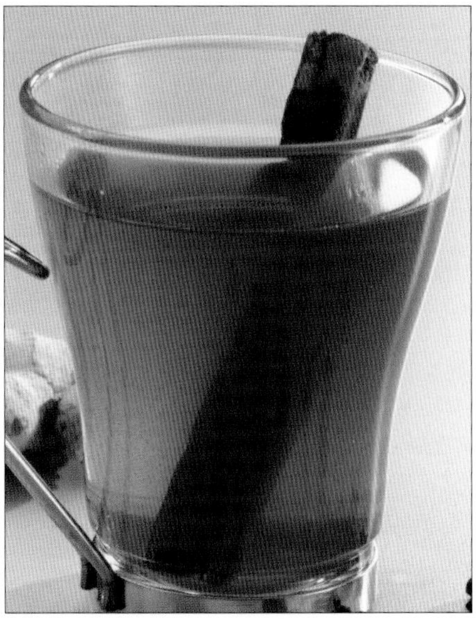

Poor Circulation

Sluggish circulation is quite common in cooler climates and particularly in elderly people or those who do little exercise. Tension and stress may also contribute. Those who suffer from it are likely to feel the cold, particularly in the extremities, and may have a tendency to chilblains. Where it is not the symptom of a serious health problem, there are many ways that herbs can help.

Since the bloodstream transports nourishment in the form of oxygen and nutrients from food around the body, good circulation is essential for overall health and vitality. Waste matter from all the cells is carried away in the bloodstream for elimination, and white blood cells form an essential part of the immune system. Keeping circulation flowing well, therefore, should be a priority for everyone.

Exercise

Regular exercise is the best way to help yourself in improving circulation. It stimulates the flow of blood and keeps the heart and lungs in good condition. As you get older, circulation tends to slow down, and this is exaggerated if you stop exercising or being active. With increasingly sedentary lifestyles in many countries, it is very important to move as much as possible at work or at home, to combat the effects of reduced circulation.

Below *Daily exercise is a good way to boost circulation; it also lifts the spirits.*

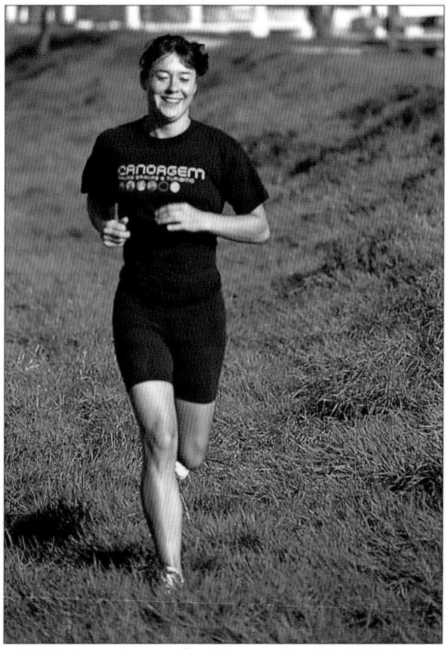

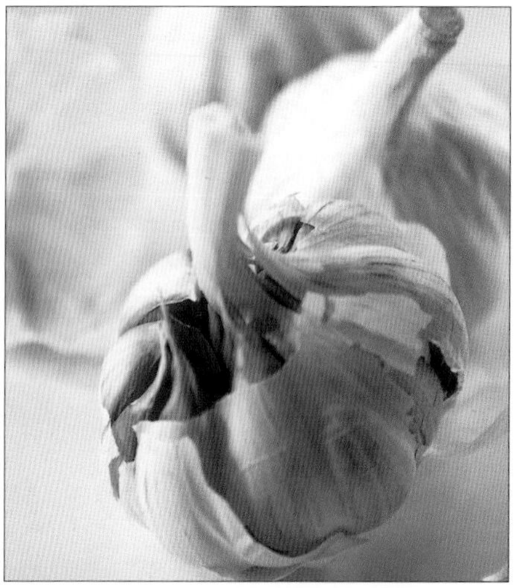

Above *Add plenty of garlic to the diet for its health-giving attributes and beneficial effects on the circulation.*

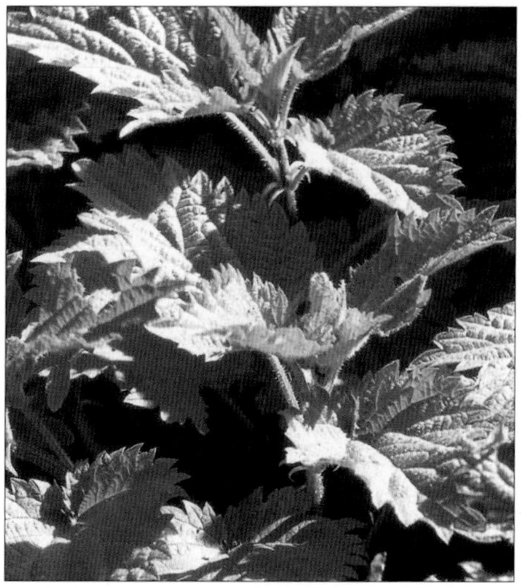

Above *Nettles make an invigorating ingredient for bath bags, and the young tips can be made into a tonic spring soup.*

Herbal teas

Hot herbal infusions, taken regularly, aid peripheral circulation and are a great way to start the day.

• **Ginger** (*Zingiber officinalis*) is especially good at dilating the blood vessels and boosting circulation. Use a bought teabag, or for a more powerful effect, make ginger tea by infusing fresh, grated ginger in hot water. (Do not take ginger in large doses if pregnant or on prescribed medication, when you should talk to your doctor first.)

Other teas to improve circulation include lime blossom, nettle or yarrow.

• **Rosemary** (*Rosmarinus officinalis*) – a familiar plant containing several active, aromatic oils, this sturdy shrub is often found in gardens, providing a convenient remedy close to hand. It increases the supply of blood to the head and with its generally relaxing, antidepressive action, is an appropriate herb for many problems associated with poor circulation. As well as being taken as a tea or tincture, it can be used externally in the form of essential or infused oil for massaging hands or feet.

CAUTION Poor circulation may be a sign of a serious condition, such as phlebitis, thrombosis or a heart disorder, and as such should be referred to a doctor.

Herbs in food

• **Garlic**, eaten daily, stimulates blood flow. Incorporate it in cooked dishes or add a little raw garlic to salads.

• **Spices** – cayenne pepper is the strongest circulatory stimulant; use it regularly in cooking, along with other warming spices, such as cinnamon, cumin, coriander and ginger. (Large doses of garlic and spices should not be taken if on prescribed medication, seek professional advice first.)

Nettle bath bags

Take advantage of the circulation-boosting properties of these common weeds by putting them, cut up into small pieces, into a fabric sachet or bag that has been fastened with a drawstring, and add them to your bath water. Nettles lose their sting once they have been soaked in hot water. Wear gloves to pick them from the wild.

Cold Hands and Feet

If the circulation is sluggish, the supply of blood to the hands and feet will be slow, making them feel especially cold. Anything you can do to boost the body's circulation will help combat this. Foot and hand baths and massage with herbal oils are also warming and comforting.

Essential oils

Massage the hands or feet with essential oils, diluted in a base oil, such as almond, or use an infused lavender oil, or warm infused rosemary oil. You could also add essential oils to a warm hand or foot bath. Oils of rosemary, marjoram, lavender and black pepper are all warming and invigorating.

WARM INFUSED ROSEMARY OIL

Warming the oil helps to extract the fragrance of the rosemary's tough leaves, but ensure it doesn't get too hot and cook.

Ingredients

2–3 large sprigs fresh rosemary (*Rosmarinus officinale*)
300ml/½ pint/1¼ cups sunflower oil

1 Put the rosemary in a pan with the oil. Heat very gently, without boiling, for up to 10 minutes. Remove from the heat.

2 Leave until lukewarm and remove the rosemary. Use as a massage oil. Do not keep for more than 2–3 days.

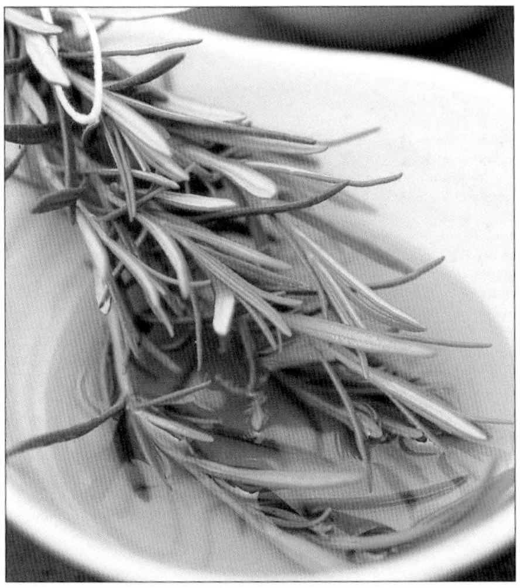

HAND MASSAGE

A professional massage is always beneficial but massaging your own hands and feet is also effective. Soak them first for 10 minutes in warm water to which essential oil or fresh herbs have been added, then dry carefully with a soft towel. Three drops each of sandalwood and geranium essential oil and 2 drops of rosemary, in 30ml/2 tbsp almond oil, makes a good massage oil.

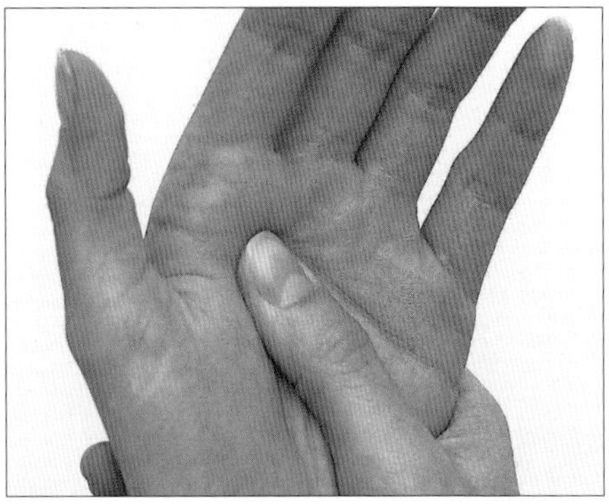

1 Place some base oil in a bowl, with essential oils added. Massage into palms of hands with a steady circular movement.

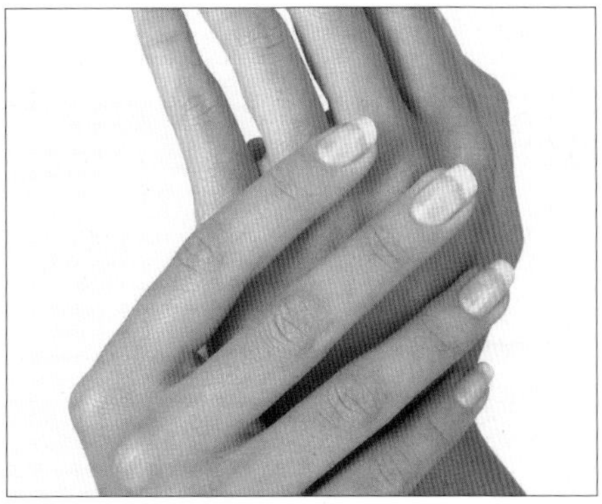

2 Squeeze down the fingers to stretch and loosen them, pushing towards the palm. Repeat steps 1 and 2 several times.

Right *Soaking hands in hot water infused with herbs is beneficial.*

Left *Rosemary is a robust herb suited to a warm oil infusion process. It is also an evergreen perennial so you can cut fresh sprigs all year round.*

FOOT MASSAGE

Soak feet first in a warm herbal foot bath. Then give them a fast friction rub to boost circulation and warm them up. Start with one hand beneath the arch and the other across the top of the foot, moving down to the toes. Rub heels briskly with palms on each side of the ankle. Continue massaging. Use 3 drops each of eucalyptus, ginger and rosemary essential oil in 30ml/2 tbsp base oil.

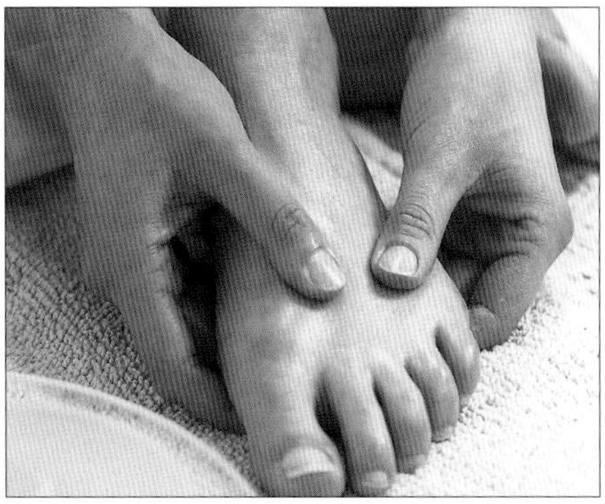

1 To stretch the feet, place hands with thumbs on top of the foot, keeping a firm grip with both of the hands.

2 Move thumbs outward, as if breaking a piece of bread; repeat the movement several times.

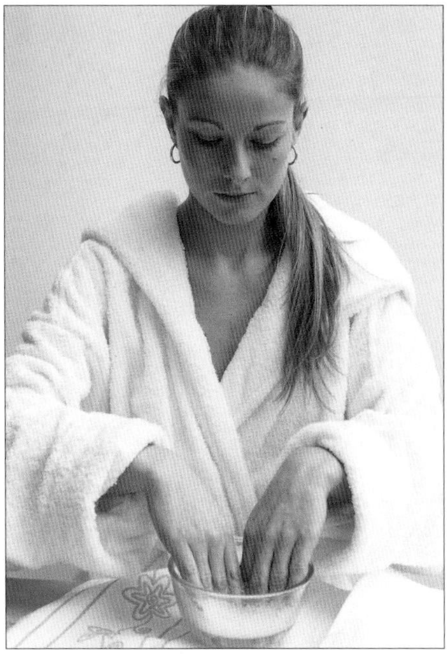

Chilblains

People with poor peripheral circulation living in cool, damp climates are often prone to chilblains. In cold weather, when circulation is reduced, the oxygen supply to the fingers and toes can become restricted to the point of damaging skin cells, resulting in swelling, redness and itching. Warmer weather improves the condition. As well as the measures below, any of the suggestions given for boosting circulation will help prevent chilblains.

Herbal foot baths

• **Ginger** – If the skin is unbroken, use the ginger decoction recipe for a foot bath. Make a double quantity and top it up with warm water if necessary, to give sufficient depth of liquid to submerge the feet. Soak for 10–15 minutes at a time.

• **Yarrow** (*Achillea millefolium*) – For gentle action, a strong infusion of yarrow, made with the fresh or dried herb, may be used in a foot bath; it dilates the tiny blood vessels in the hands and feet, helping them to warm.

• **Rosemary** (*Rosmarinus officinalis*), **thyme** (*Thymus* spp) and **cinnamon** – Make this with fresh herbs. Gather a small handful each of rosemary and thyme and put them in a large bowl with a good sprinkling of cinnamon powder. Cover with hot water and leave to steep for 20 minutes before soaking feet.

Below *Using radiant heat, such as warming by the fire, will aggravate the swelling and burning itchy sensation of chilblains.*

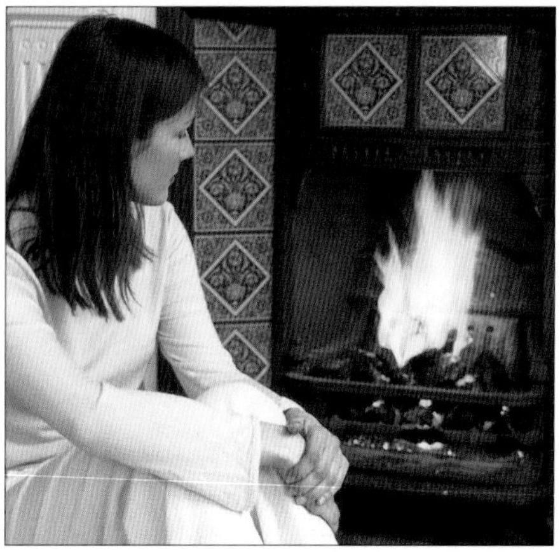

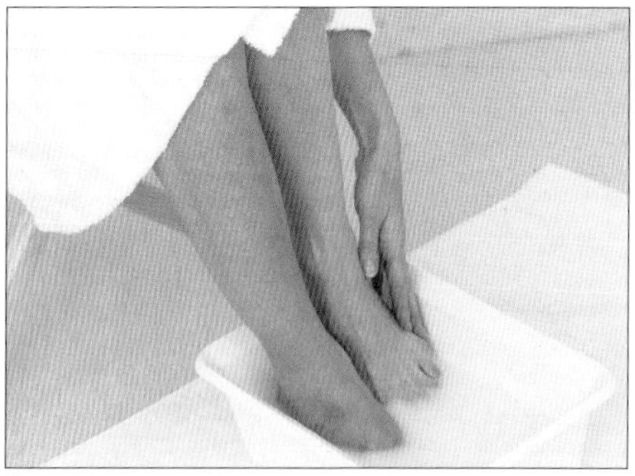

Above *A warm herbal foot bath will relieve the pain of chilblains.*

Essential oils

These should only be applied locally, in baths or with massage, if the skin is unbroken, otherwise they may cause further inflammation.

For a foot bath, add warming essential oils such as black pepper, ginger, rosemary or marjoram, either singly or in combination, using a total of 10 drops to a small basin of water.

To massage the affected areas, the same essential oils may be used. Dilute them in vegetable oil, in the proportion of 5 drops essential oil to 10ml/2 tsp carrier oil.

In the bath, for longer-term treatment during the winter months, add 6–8 drops of oils of cypress, juniper, pine or rosemary to the water.

Below *Mix essential oils with a base oil for gently massaging into chilblains, provided the skin is unbroken.*

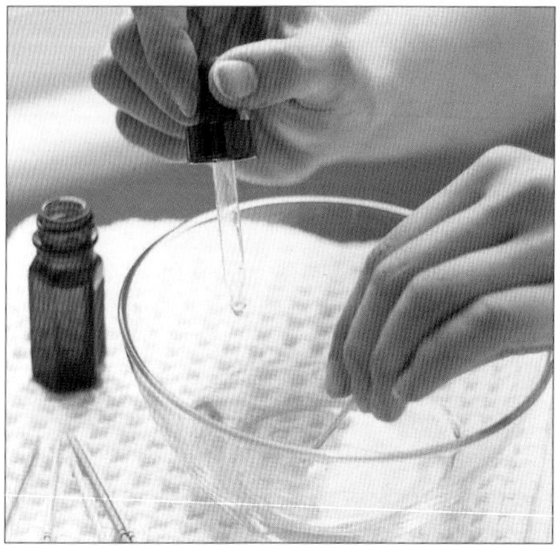

GINGER DECOCTION

Taking ginger internally as a decoction, rather than as an infusion, is one way to kick-start the circulation.

Ginger can be made into a tea, but a stronger medicine is made from a decoction.

Ingredients

15g/½oz fresh root ginger
750ml/1¼ pint/2⅔ cups water

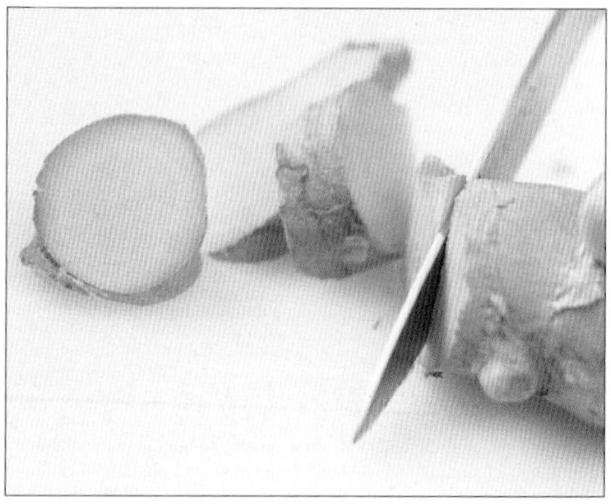

1 Chop the ginger and put it in a pan with the water. Bring to the boil and simmer until the liquid is reduced to about 600ml/1 pint/2½ cups.

2 Strain into a jug (pitcher). Give in doses of 5–20ml/1 tsp–1½ tbsp, three times a day. It will keep in the refrigerator for 3 days.

Below *Do not take ginger in large doses (maximum per day 2g dried, 4g fresh). If pregnant, on prescribed medication or any pharmaceutical drugs seek medical advice.*

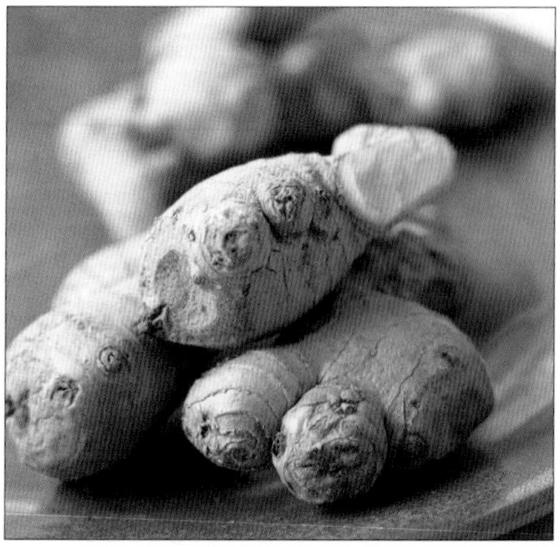

Cramp

The condition known as cramp occurs when a muscle goes into a painful spasm and feels rock hard. It commonly affects the calves of the legs, but can also happen in other muscles. It frequently occurs after exercise, when you are dehydrated, and may also strike in the night. Initial measures should be to use the muscle by walking around, or stretching and massaging it, and drinking plenty of water.

A major factor to be considered when someone has cramp is inadequate circulation to the muscles, especially if cramp comes on with exercise or effort; with athletes or those doing hard physical work there may be a problem of salt deficiency from excessive sweating. Repetitive movements, such as typing, can provoke cramping and lead to inflammation – repetitive strain injury is a potential consequence of overuse of a set of muscles in this way. Night cramps may be due to a combination of reduced circulation, tiredness and stress, and the whole person needs to be treated.

Herbal teas

Drinking hot tea made with rosemary (*Rosmarinus officinalis*), elderflower (*Sambucus nigra*), lime flower (*Tilia cordata*), peppermint (*Mentha* x *piperita*) or thyme (*Thymus* spp) can help to ease the problem of cramp by stimulating the circulation.

Below *Cramp is a painful condition which often affects the calf muscles.*

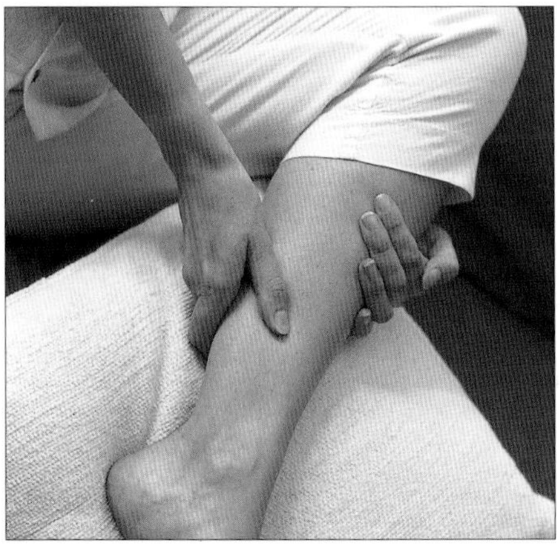

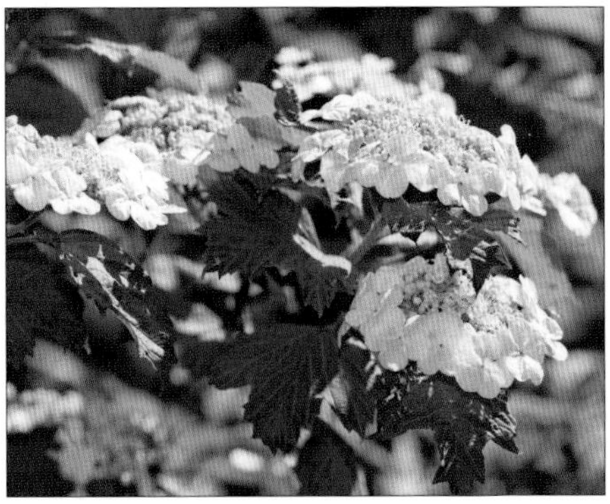

Above *Guelder rose (*Viburnum opulus*) has clusters of white flowers.*

Essential oils

Massage the affected area vigorously with 2 drops essential oil of rosemary, basil or marjoram diluted in 5ml/1 tsp almond oil.

Herbs in food

Add plenty of oatmeal and nettles to the diet, in the form of porridge and nettle soup, and increase the amount of chopped herbs used in food, especially thyme and parsley, which are both rich in calcium.

Cramp bark preparations

As it has an efficient antispasmodic action and helps to relax tense muscles, cramp bark (*Viburnum opulus*) is a first-choice herbal treatment for cramp. Also known as the guelder rose, it is a deciduous shrub with flat-topped clusters of tiny white flowers in summer, followed by oval red fruits. It is found in the wild in woodland and hedges, and there are various garden cultivars with less potent medicinal properties. The bark is the part used, and it is not therefore sustainable to harvest it regularly from your own plant, but you can buy the bark in dried form from a herbal supplier in order to make your own decoctions.

CAUTION Little research has so far been carried out on the possible adverse effects of cramp bark. As with all herbs, if you are pregnant or taking prescription drugs, do not take it without medical advice.

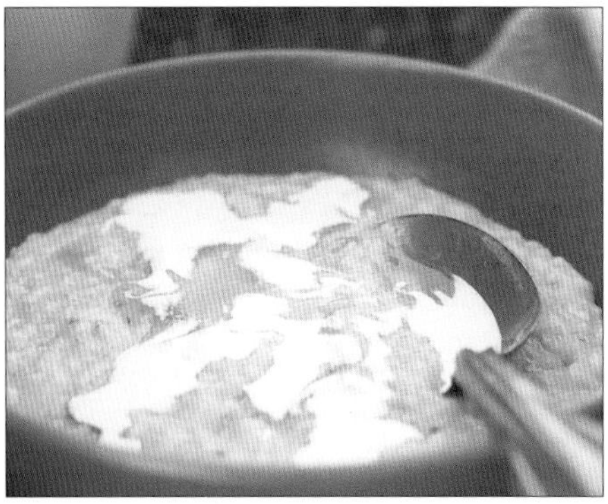

Above *Porridge eaten with milk boosts calcium levels.*

- **Decoction** – Take 2 tbsp/30ml, diluted in a little water, 2–3 times a day. It can be sweetened with honey.
- **Tincture** – You can make your own and take 5ml/1 tsp, diluted with water, 2–3 times a day as necessary, or buy a ready-made product and take it according to the manufacturer's instructions.
- **Compress** – To apply cramp bark locally, make a warm compress by soaking a pad of fabric in the tincture diluted in the proportion 1:4 with hot water.
- **Cream** – Cramp bark can also be made into a cream incorporating the tincture or decoction, and massaged into the affected area. Use 5ml/1 tsp tincture, or 300ml/ ½ pint/1¼ cups cramp bark decoction in the standard cream recipe.

Below *Fresh parsley (*Petroselinum crispum*) is rich in calcium and other minerals.*

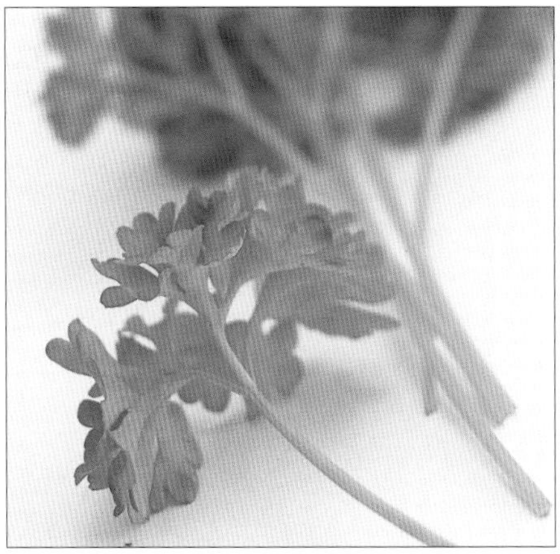

Skin Irritations

There are many reasons why the skin should become inflamed or develop a rash. There may be a serious underlying cause, or the symptoms may be too varied or complex for self-diagnosis and treatment – if in doubt always seek medical attention. But for general itchiness and for mild cases of nettle rash (also known as hives and urticaria) simple home remedies may provide some relief.

Causes of nettle rash

An allergic skin condition, characterized by an itchy, often lumpy, red rash, as when stung by nettles, nettle rash can take an acute form – when it is just a temporary reaction to an irritant – or be more persistent and recur regularly. Locally, it can be caused by irritants such as plants, chemicals, latex or insect bites. It can also be a reaction to some foods or medicines, follow a viral infection, or be triggered by heat, cold, pressure or even sunlight.

Herbal teas

Teas are calming to the system. If the skin is irritated, try drinking one with anti-allergenic properties: choose from nettle, lemon balm, chamomile and dandelion.

Plant first aid and lotions

Applying a cool, soothing lotion or the juice of an appropriate plant to the affected area is one of the best ways to reduce itchiness and provide temporary relief, breaking the itch-scratch cycle and giving the skin a chance to recover.

- **Aloe vera** – Break open a leaf and squeeze the juice directly from the plant on to the skin, or apply a ready-made lotion based on aloe vera.
- **Houseleek** (*Sempervivum tectorum*) can be used in the same way as aloe vera.
- **Rosewater** – Buy a good quality product and use to bathe the itchy area.
- **Yarrow** (*Achillea millefolium*) and **pot marigold** (*Calendula officinalis*), made into an infusion using 15g/½oz each dried yarrow and marigold petals to 600ml/1 pint/2½ cups water, make a soothing lotion.

MARIGOLD SKIN SALVE

Calendula cream is recognized for its ability to soothe all manner of skin irritations, from insect bites and sunburn to eczema and other itchy rashes brought on by allergic reactions. Calendula oil, which you can buy from specialist outlets, can be omitted, but it adds to the therapeutic action of the cream. Tincture of benzoin is an antiseptic and preservative.

Ingredients

300ml/½ pint/1¼ cups boiling water
15g/½oz dried pot marigold (*Calendula officinalis*) petals or 30g/1oz fresh petals
60ml/4 tbsp emulsifying ointment
15ml/1 tbsp glycerine
4 drops tincture of benzoin
4–5 drops calendula oil

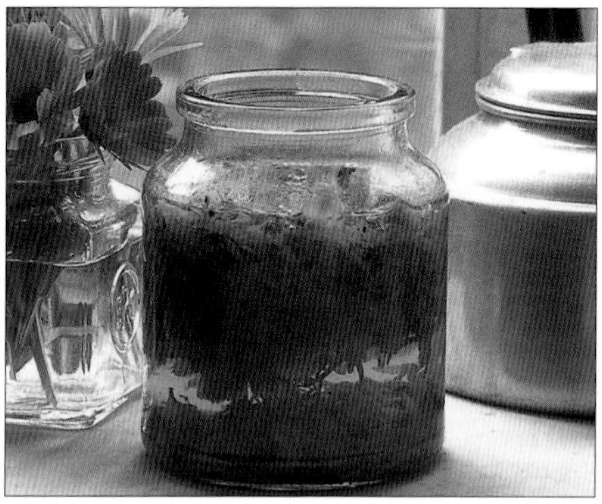

1 First make a strong marigold infusion by pouring the boiling water over the marigold petals in a jar. Cover and leave until cool before straining.

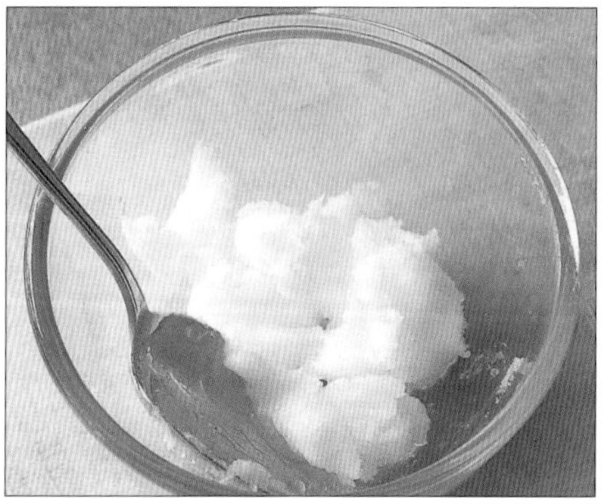

2 Put the emulsifying ointment and glycerine in a bowl set over a pan of gently simmering water and stir continuously until melted. It will take about 10 minutes to melt the emulsifier.

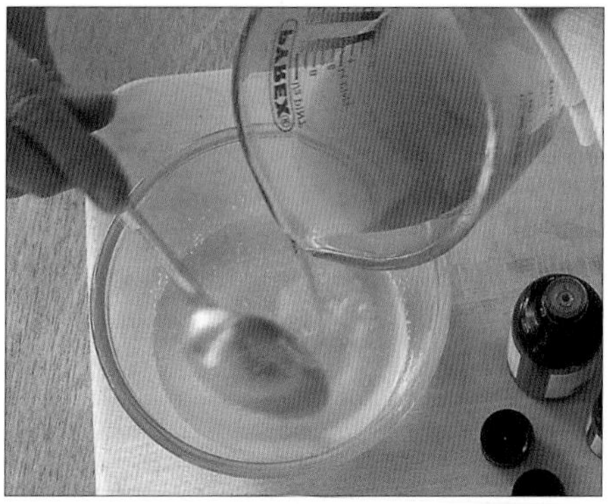

3 Remove from the heat and mix in 150ml/¼ pint/⅔ cup of the marigold infusion, with the tincture of benzoin and calendula oil. Stir the mixture until it has cooled and reached a consistency similar to double (heavy) cream. Pour into a small jar to set.

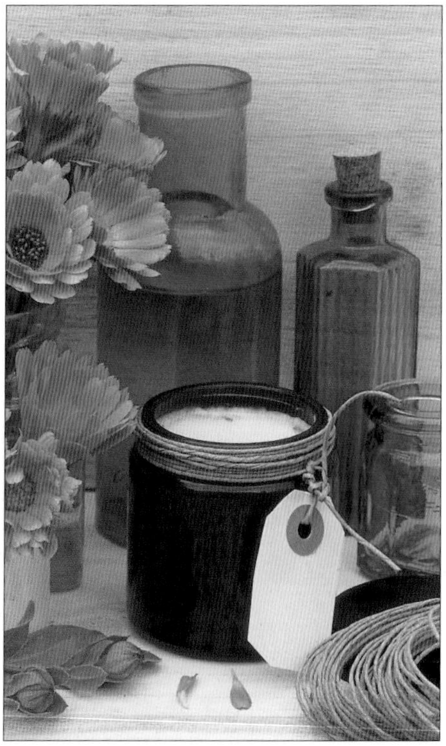

Right *Marigold skin salve will keep for at least 6 months. A dark glass jar maximizes its keeping quality. Make one large batch and store in a cool, dark place.*

Eczema

This is a complex skin condition, with many causes and triggers, and in most cases will need professional treatment. Some people find it responds well to natural therapies and that herbal remedies provide relief for the distressing symptoms and intense itchiness.

Herbal teas

- Red clover (*Trifolium pratense*) and nettle (*Urtica dioica*) have blood cleansing properties and may be taken singly, or in combination, as a tea.

Decoction

A decoction of the roots of burdock (*Arctium lappa*) and dandelion (*Taraxacum officinale*), made with equal quantities of each, is a traditional detoxifying treatment for skin conditions and eczema. Take no more than a small cupful 2–3 times daily for up to one week at a time.

CAUTION It is best to start with a smaller dose initially, and wait before repeating, as burdock sometimes causes a flare-up of symptoms. As with all herbal remedies, do not take in pregnancy or while breast-feeding, or if taking other medication.

Below *The flowering tops of red clover are used for many herbal treatments. Red clover, taken as a tea, cleanses the system and helps reduce chronic toxicity associated with skin problems.*

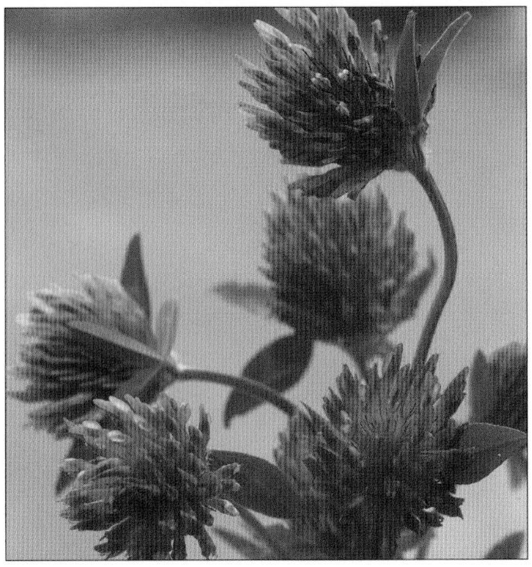

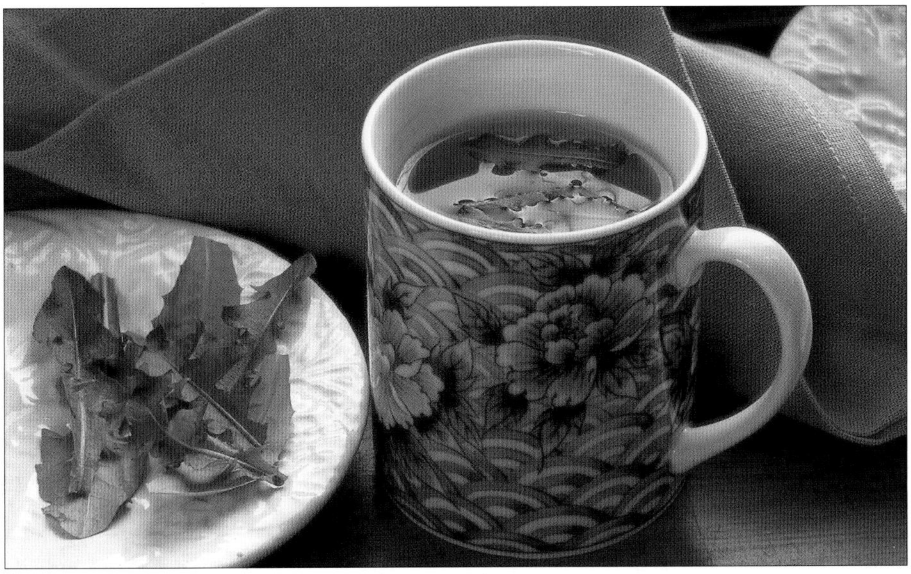

Above *Dandelion (*Taraxacum officinale*) tea can be made from the leaves and the roots.*

Lotions and compresses

Infusions of herbs applied directly to the skin or as cool compresses can be very soothing. Make them in the same way as herbal teas.

- **Chickweed** (*Stellaria media*) has a cooling action that helps relieve itchiness.
- **Heartsease** (*Viola tricolor*), **red clover** (*T. pratense*) and **nettle** (*U. dioica*) all have anti-inflammatory properties, and combine well together as an infusion.

Creams and ointments

Applying a soothing herbal ointment to the skin may help to relieve the intense itchiness that is a symptom of eczema, reducing inflammation and speeding up healing.

Below *Heartsease (*Viola tricolor*) should be used in small quantities only.*

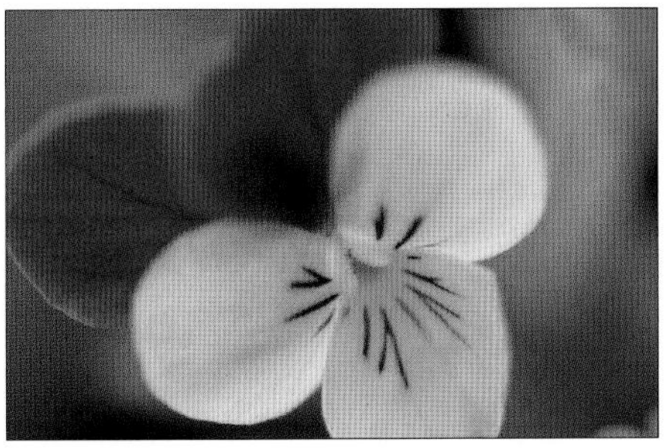

- **Marigold** (*Calendula officinalis*) is a good choice for a healing cream. Use the skin salve recipe on the opposite page.
- **Chickweed** has soothing, cooling properties and can also be made into a cream, following the marigold skin salve recipe, and substituting a chickweed infusion for the marigold one.
- **Evening primrose oil** is well known for its anti-inflammatory properties; the oil can be applied locally to affected skin. It can also be taken internally, but this should be done on professional advice only.

Below *A soothing cream calms inflamed skin, reducing soreness and itching.*

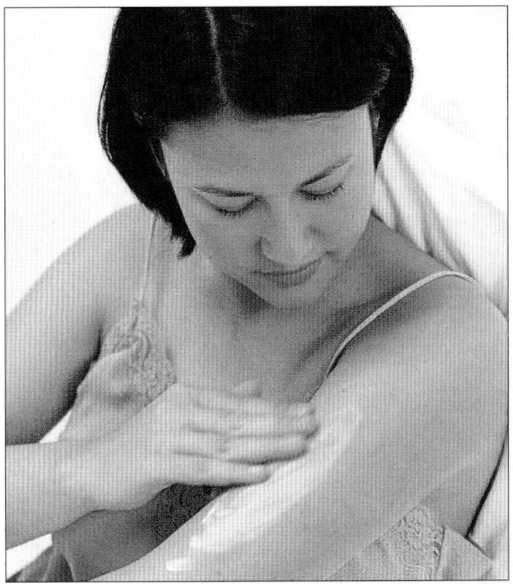

Acne

This skin condition is very common during puberty, and may continue into later life for some people. Increasing levels of hormones during adolescence lead to greater activity of the skin's sebaceous glands, and if this becomes too great, excessive amounts of sebum, the skin's natural oily lubricant, are produced. This in turn can cause the glands and hair follicles to become blocked and infected. Diet is an important factor in treating acne, and herbal remedies should be aimed at cleansing the whole system as well as the skin.

The most common reaction of most people who suffer from acne is to squeeze the spots; this almost always serves to spread the infection into the surrounding tissues, and if done repeatedly can damage the local skin areas, producing scarring. Any programme of treatment therefore needs to include a lot of self-help to be successful.

The natural therapies offer the most successful and sensible ways to improve the condition and rebalance the skin. The best approach is to combine local, external cleansing with internal treatment; all therapies are likely to emphasize the importance of diet in treating acne. Where acne persists for years after adolescence, there may be an abnormal imbalance that needs to be addressed, and again there are natural remedies that may be used – seek professional treatment if necessary.

Below *Milk thistle (*Silybum marianum*) is a detoxifying herb with antioxidant properties that is often recommended for treating acne.*

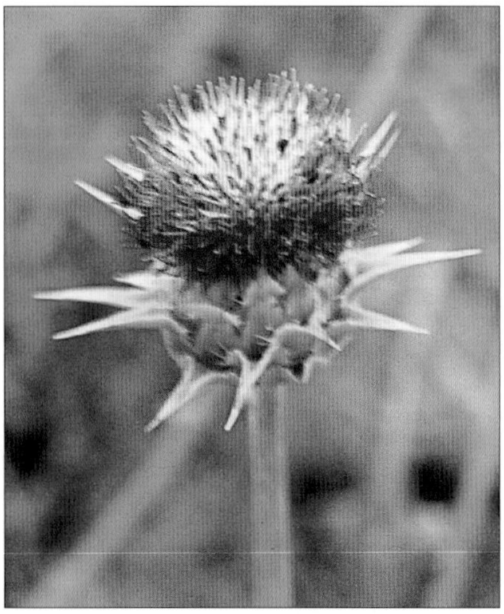

Herbal teas

Drinking teas made from detoxifying herbs will help to reduce inflammation. Choose from the following and drink three or four cups during the day: red clover (*Trifolium pratense*), nettle (*Urtica dioica*), cleavers (*Galium aparine*) and milk thistle (*Silybum marianum*), singly or in combination.

Infusion

Instead of using soap, which removes the acid mantle of the skin and thus increases the susceptibility to infection, rinse the face with a herbal infusion.

Red clover is an excellent blood and tissue cleanser and has a gentle action: as well as drinking it as a tea, an infusion of red clover can be used externally to carefully bathe inflamed spots.

Decoction

Dandelion root (*Taraxacum officinale*), taken as a decoction, is helpful in improving the detoxifying action of the liver, which can help to clear the skin. It also has a gentle laxative action, taking pressure away from the skin as an organ of elimination.

Tincture

Echinacea (*E. purpurea*) is one of the best all-purpose immune stimulants, aiding resistance to infection. It can be taken in conjunction with the herbal treatments suggested above, to help the detoxification process. It is best taken in the form of a ready-made tincture, following the manufacturer's directions on dosage. Do not take for more than 2–3 weeks at a time and do not resume taking it within a month.

Steam inhalation

Regular steam inhalations with juniper can help clear blocked pores or blackheads. Add 3–4 drops juniper oil or fresh juniper leaves and berries to a basin of water.

HERBAL CLEANSING RINSE

This rinse is best made fresh each day. For early morning use, make it the night before and keep it in a cool place, in a covered container. Elderflower and marigold have soothing, anti-inflammatory properties and lavender is antiseptic in action. Witch hazel is an astringent, to help tone the skin.

Ingredients

15ml/1 tbsp each dried elderflower, lavender and marigold petals
5ml/1 tsp distilled witch hazel
600ml/1 pint/2½ cups boiling water

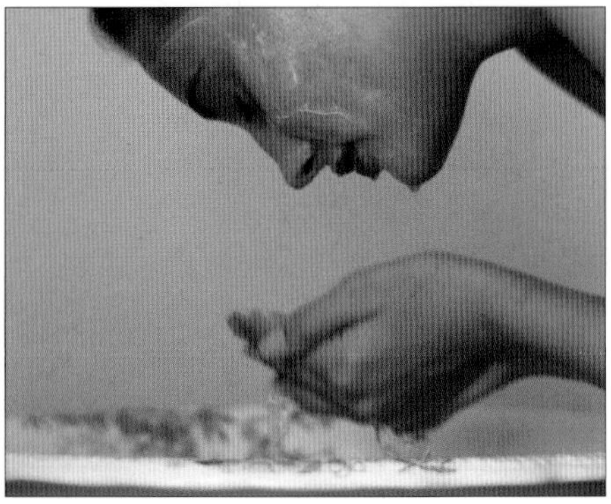

Put the dried herbs into a bowl and pour in the boiling water. Leave for 20 minutes before straining into a larger bowl. Stir in the witch hazel and use to rinse the face.

Below *Dandelion has a detoxifying action.*

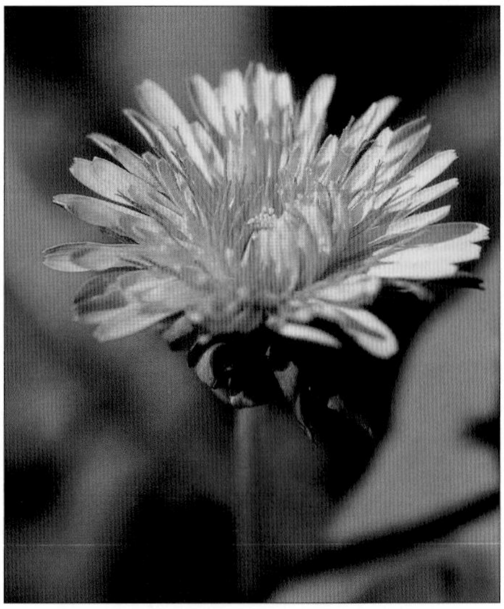

Athlete's Foot

Athlete's foot is a common fungal infection that affects the skin of the foot (not just those of athletes). It is highly contagious and thrives in warm, moist environments, such as swimming pool changing rooms and showers. Symptoms are an itchy, red rash between the toes, which may then blister and become sore. It can also spread to toenails, making them flaky and yellow. Self-treatment with herbal remedies may help to clear it. If it persists it is best to seek professional advice.

It is most important to keep the affected area cool and dry. Pay scrupulous attention to hygiene as the fungus can accumulate under the nails, causing the infection to spread between the toes.

Prevention

- Do not share towels.
- Wear plastic shoes in communal changing areas and around swimming pools.
- Wash feet daily and dry thoroughly between the toes.
- Do not wear shoes without socks or tights.
- Change your socks or tights daily.

Tinctures

- Marigold (*Calendula officinalis*) and myrrh (*Commiphora myrrha*) have antifungal properties and can be applied directly to the skin as tinctures. Buy them as ready-made products, or make your own tinctures following the instructions on page 34.

Internal treatments

To prevent recurrent infection, it may help to take internal remedies to bolster the immune system. Take garlic regularly, either in food, or in capsule form (but not without first seeking professional healthcare advice if you are taking other medication), and perhaps a short course of echinacea tincture (see opposite). Aloe vera juice may be helpful, but should only be taken with professional advice. Drink plenty of herbal teas with antifungal and digestive properties, including thyme (*Thymus* spp), chamomile (*Chamaemelum nobile*), marigold (*Calendula officinalis*) and rose (*Rosa* spp).

ANTIFUNGAL FOOT BATH

Make a strong infusion of marigold (*Calendula officinalis*) and thyme (*Thymus vulgaris*), or ginger and cinnamon, and soak your feet in it twice a day for 15 minutes, taking care to dry them well afterwards and dust with antifungal foot powder. The cider vinegar in this foot bath helps to restore the pH balance of the skin, which becomes over-alkaline when suffering from athlete's foot. Both myrrh and tea tree oil have antifungal properties.

Ingredients

25g/1oz dried sage (*Salvia officinalis*)
25g/1oz dried pot marigold (*Calendula officinalis*) flowers
1 large aloe vera leaf, chopped
15ml/1 tbsp myrrh granules
2¼ pints/9 cups water
10 drops tea tree essential oil
60ml/4 tbsp cider vinegar

1 Simmer the herbs and myrrh in the water for 20 minutes.

2 Leave to cool a little, then strain and add the tea tree oil and the cider vinegar.

Below *Soaking the feet in a decoction of antifungal herbs and oils helps combat this contagious condition and can provide instant relief to itching feet.*

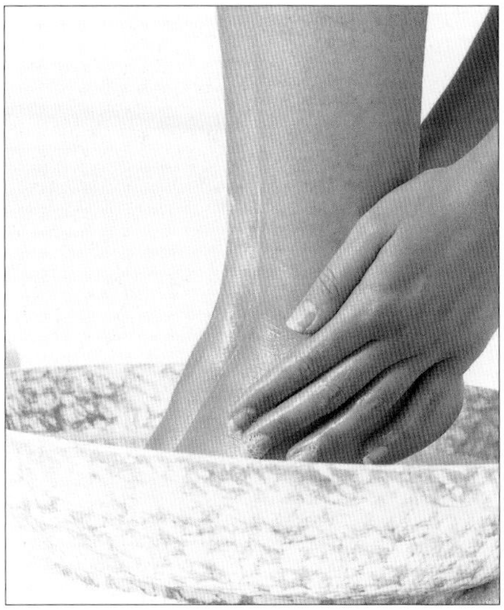

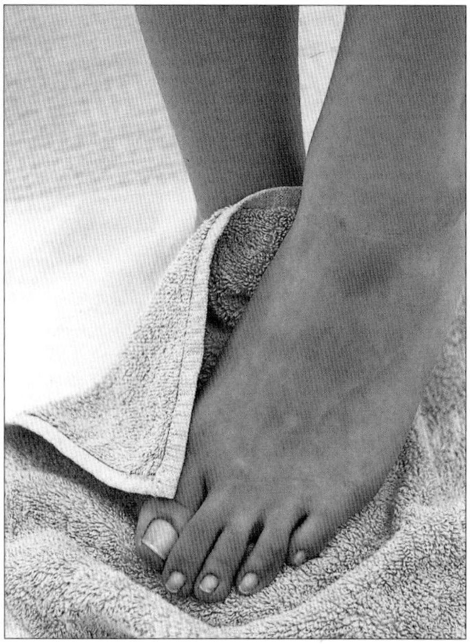

Above *Keeping feet clean and dry helps to prevent athlete's foot.*

MARIGOLD AND MYRRH FOOT POWDER

Talcum powder helps keep feet dry and sweat-free, and a mixture incorporating antifungal ingredients, such as marigold petals and myrrh grains, is doubly effective.

Ingredients

30ml/2 tbsp dried marigold petals
small tin of simple, preferably unperfumed talcum powder
30ml/2 tbsp fine grains or powdered myrrh

1 Grind the marigold petals to a powder, using a pestle and mortar or electric grinder, and mix them into the talcum powder with the myrrh.

2 Return the new mixture to the talcum powder tin, or it may be easier to keep it in a wide-necked jar or pot with a lid. Keep the lid closed to stop contamination of the contents.

3 After drying the feet carefully use cotton wool balls to dust the feet with the powder, paying special attention to the areas between the toes.

Boils and Abscesses

A boil, also known as a skin abscess, is a localized infection under the skin, which forms a tender, hard swelling. As the body fights the infection, the swelling softens and fills with pus, which is then expelled, sometimes spontaneously and sometimes by lancing. Most small, simple boils can be treated at home, but any that become painful, or do not respond rapidly, should be referred to a doctor. You should also seek medical attention if you are taking any other medication, if there is any fever, or if the boils are associated with diabetes or a damaged immune system illness.

Causes of boils

Boils frequently occur as a result of being run down, either by stress or through poor diet and hygiene. Specific causes include:

• An ingrown hair.
• A splinter or other foreign body in the skin.
• Plugged sweat glands that become infected (acne boils).
• A break in the skin, such as a cut or graze, which becomes infected.
• Depressed immune system, diabetes or other serious illness.

Generally, treatments are geared initially to bringing the boil to a head and allowing it to burst and discharge the pus. It is important that all external applications are as clean as possible – for example, use sterile dressings for applying any poultices. In the medium to longer term, the natural therapies are ideally suited to cleaning the system as a whole, building up immunity to further outbreaks and restoring health and vitality.

Internal treatments

These are aimed at strengthening the immune system.

• **Garlic** may be helpful, for its antibiotic properties and as an immune system booster. Take it regularly in food or as capsules. (Do not take in medicinal doses without professional healthcare advice if on blood-thinning or other medication.)
• **Burdock** (*Arctium lappa*) and **dandelion root** (*Taraxacum officinale*), taken together as a decoction, have blood-cleansing properties.
• **Cleavers** (*Galium aparine*) or **red clover** (*Trifolium pratense*) can be taken as teas.

Poultices

Many herbs are soothing and anti-inflammatory when used as a hot poultice; two excellent herbs to use in this way are slippery elm (*Ulmus rubra*) and marshmallow (*Althaea officinalis*).

• Marshmallow poultice is made by either pouring boiling water on to some fresh leaves or mixing the powdered root with hot water to make a paste. It may be helpful to use a little oil on the skin first to stop the poultice sticking. The herb should then be placed on the boil or abscess and covered with a clean gauze or strips of cotton, to hold it in position. It can be kept in place until cool, then replaced.
• Slippery elm (*Ulmus rubra*) has been called the "herbalist's knife" for its ability to bring a boil to bursting point. Simply thicken the powder with a little boiling water and apply the paste, as hot as you can bear. Alternatively, combine slippery elm and thyme as in the recipe below: thyme is a good herb to use for its antiseptic, antibacterial properties.

Below *The healing powers of slippery elm powder are combined with the antiseptic properties of thyme in this poultice.*

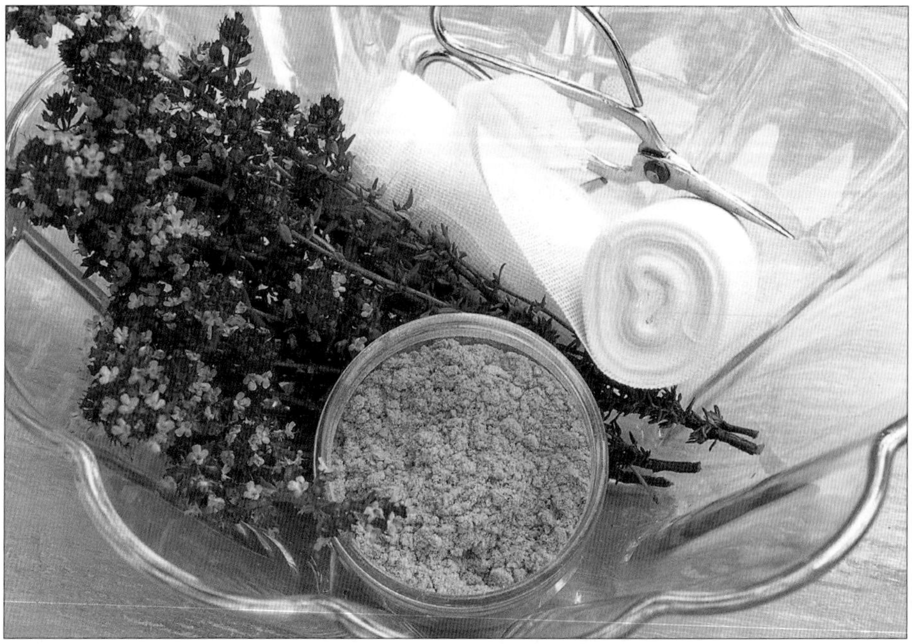

SLIPPERY ELM AND THYME POULTICE

Lay this soothing poultice on the boil while it is still warm, applying a little base oil to the skin first. When the boil has burst, wash the area with a cooled lavender infusion.

Ingredients

small handful of thyme (*Thymus vulgaris*)
boiling water
30ml/2 tbsp slippery elm powder (*Ulmus rubra*)

1 Strip the thyme leaves from the stalks (there should be about 15g/½oz), put them on a saucer and cover with boiling water. Mash thoroughly and leave to cool.

2 Pour off some of the liquid, then add the slippery elm powder and mix thoroughly to make a coarse-textured paste.

3 Apply directly to the skin or enclose in gauze, and hold in place with a bandage.

Cold Sores

These are caused by the *Herpes simplex* virus and occur on the lip or just above or below it. They can only be caught through close contact with someone else who has the condition. It is thought that most people carry the virus responsible for cold sores, which is acquired in childhood then lies dormant indefinitely until triggered, though many never have more than one attack. When activated, it causes a tingling sensation on the lip before the itchy, painful sore erupts.

Attack triggers

The virus inhabits the nerves supplying the skin, awaiting an opportunity to become active when the body's defences are lowered or compromised. Common triggers include the following:

- The common cold, flu and other respiratory infections.
- Being generally run down or over-tired.
- Stress and emotional upsets.
- Extremes of temperature.
- Overexposure to cold wind.
- Overexposure to bright sunlight.

When an attack does occur, one or more small blisters erupt on the lips or at the corners of the mouth. These form a crust and remain moist underneath for up to 10 days or so before drying out. They are highly contagious during the moist and weeping stages, and contact with others, especially young children, should be avoided.

Avoid known triggers and keep the immune system strong by eating a healthy diet, rich in vitamins A, C and E, zinc and iron.

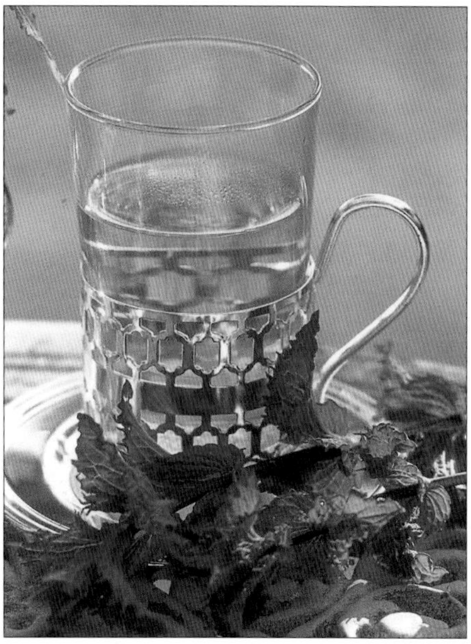

Above *A tea made with freshly picked lemon balm (*Melissa officinalis*) leaves is helpful for relieving the discomfort of cold sores.*

- **Garlic** (*Allium sativum*) also strengthens the immune system, and can be included in food or taken as capsules.
- **Lemon balm** (*Melissa officinalis*) has antiviral properties and is a first-choice herb for dealing with cold sores. Take it as a tea made with the fresh herb, or make a strong infusion and use it to bathe the affected area. (Always wash your hands after touching a cold sore).

Tinctures

Local applications of herbs are most effective when applied in tincture form, dabbed on to the cold sores frequently to dry and heal the area. Lavender, marigold and myrrh are all good for this purpose. You can also use distilled witch hazel.

Compress

A cold compress helps relieve any pain and encourages healing of the skin. Use any of the above tinctures, or distilled witch hazel, diluted in a little water.

You could also make a compress with a strong infusion of rosemary, thyme and peppermint: use 5ml/1tsp of each herb and infuse in 300ml/½ pint/1 cup boiling water for 10 minutes, then strain the liquid off the herbs and cool before applying to the cold sore.

Below *A healthy diet, rich in vitamins and minerals, strengthens the immune system and makes the eruption of cold sores and other problems less likely.*

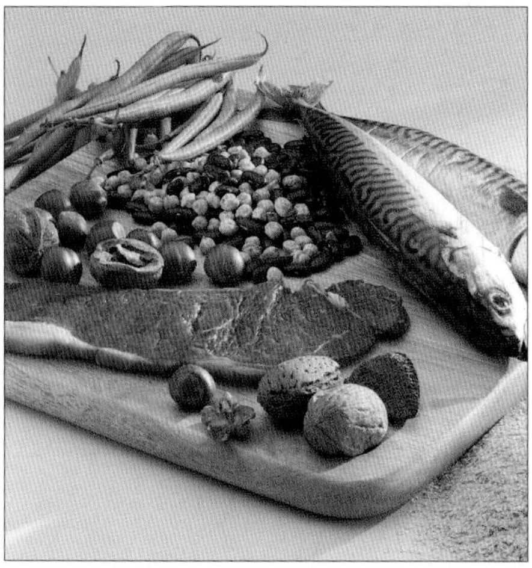

Below *Tinctures can be applied to the affected area on cotton wool (cotton balls) or as cold compresses.*

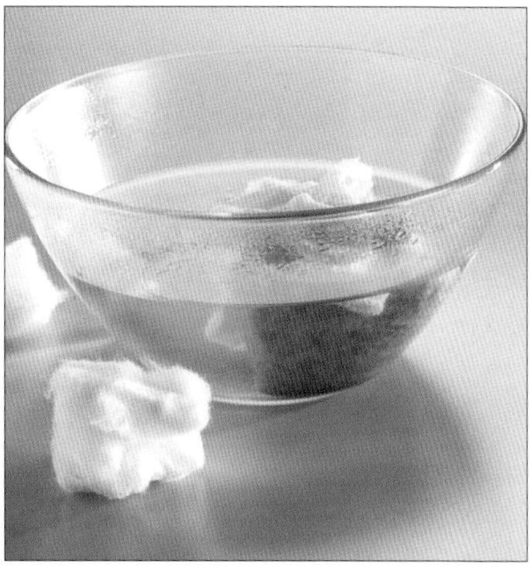

Below *Healing lavender oil tincture is simple to prepare at home. It can be dabbed directly on to a cold sore or applied in a compress.*

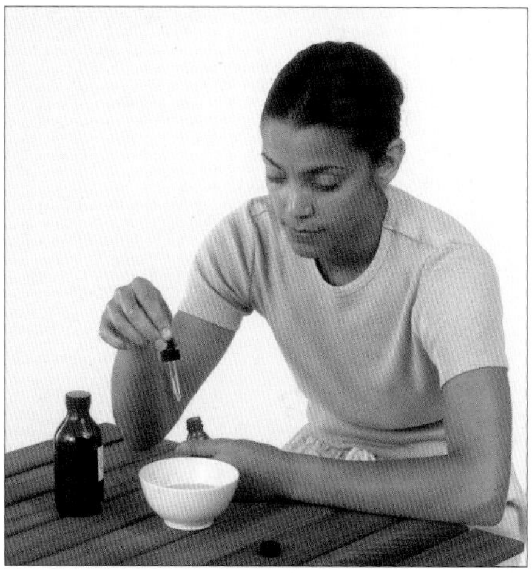

Eye Strain

Tired eyes are a common problem for those who have to spend long hours in front of computer screens or who work in air-conditioned offices under artificial light. Prolonged spells of close work, including reading and writing, can also strain the eyes, and there are a number of simple herbal treatments that will revive and revitalize them. All these treatments involve lying down with your eyes covered for at least 15 minutes, and this enforced relaxation is probably almost as important a part of the treatment as the compresses.

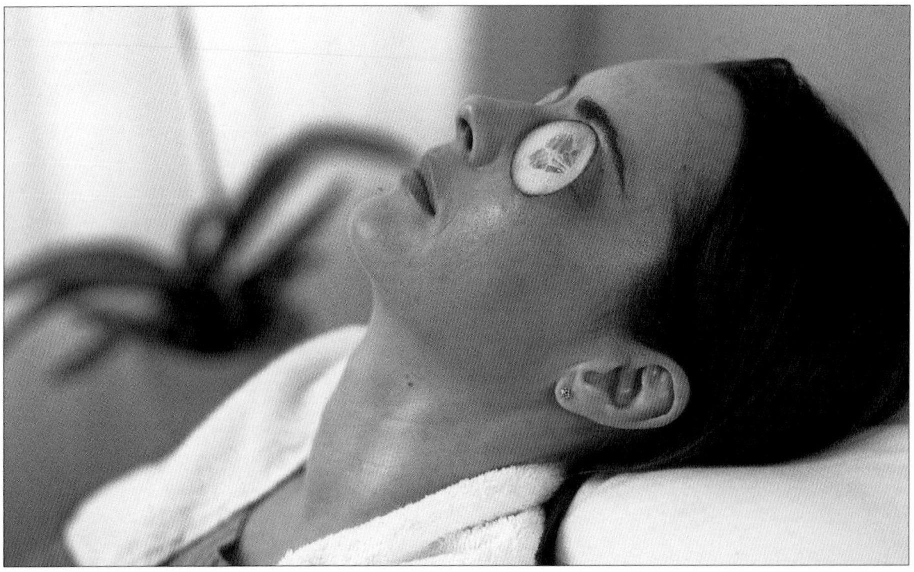

Above *This is the simplest treatment of all. Place a slice of cucumber over each eye while you relax for 15 minutes. The cucumber will very gently tone the skin around the eyes and help restore tired eyes. A rest from close work always helps.*

Compresses

Placing a cool herbal compress over the eyes will refresh them, reduce puffiness and relieve itchiness. Keep decoctions or infusions in the refrigerator for an hour before use, to make sure they are cold. Lie down for 15–20 minutes with the pads over the eyes.

- **Fennel** (*Foeniculum vulgare*) – Make a decoction of fennel seeds by boiling 10ml/2 tsp seeds in 300ml/½ pint/1¼ cups purified water in a covered pan for 20 minutes. Strain and leave to cool, then use to soak cotton wool pads.
- **Chamomile** (*Chamomaelum nobile*) – Use chamomile teabags to make an infusion, or the fresh flowers. In either case, leave to steep for 20 minutes before straining off the liquid and discarding the flowers.
- **Rosewater**: Soak cotton wool pads in an infusion of scented rose petals made with purified water.
- Tea contains tannin, which is astringent and will firm the skin. Place two teabags on a saucer and pour hot water over them. Leave to cool, then refrigerate until cold. Squeeze the excess moisture from the teabags and lie down with them covering your eyes for 10–15 minutes. Remove and gently pat the skin dry before dabbing on moisturizer.

Below *Potatoes, cucumber and herbal teabags make useful eye pads.*

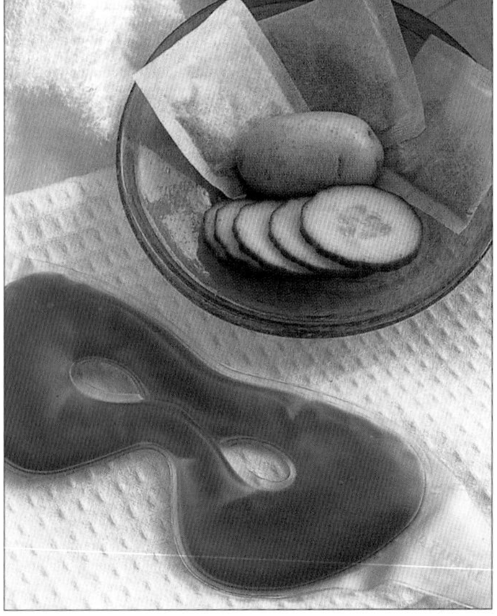

Below *Everyday teabags make good compresses for sore eyes.*

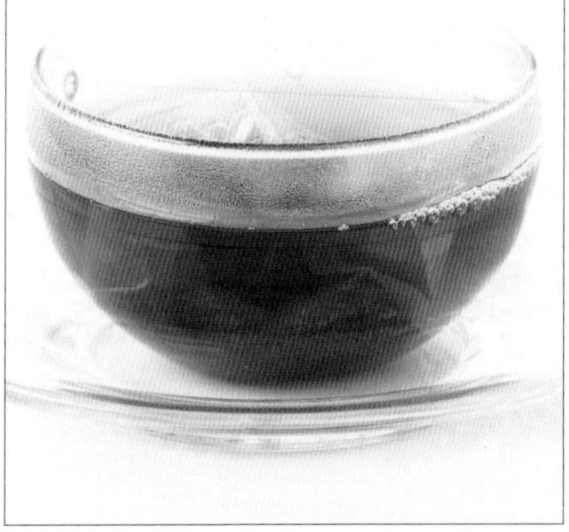

Below *An old country remedy for tired skin around the eyes is to grate potato finely and place it between two layers of muslin (cheesecloth) before applying it as a compress over the eyes. Certainly, the starch in the potatoes seems to tighten the skin, so it may be more than an old wives' tale.*

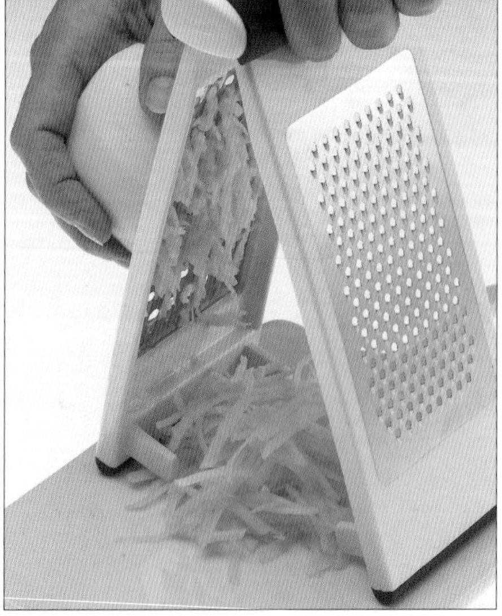

Styes

A stye develops when the root of an eyelash becomes infected. It starts as a tender, red area and then forms a small painful abscess. Repeated attacks may occur if the infection is spread from one lash to another, or if the immune system is depressed, increasing vulnerability to infection. Recurrent styes are occasionally a symptom of diabetes. Always seek medical attention if they are very painful or recur frequently.

Preventive measures

- Eat a healthy diet rich in vitamins and minerals.
- Make sure you get plenty of restful sleep.
- Try to reduce stress.
- Do not share towels, eye make-up or applicators, as styes are contagious.
- Pay scrupulous attention to hygiene.
- Try not to rub the eyes as this will spread the infection.

Herbal tea

- Red clover (*Trifolium pratense*) and fresh red rose petals is a combination that makes a pleasant-tasting, detoxifying drink. Red clover is recommended to boost the body's immune system, helping to defend against infections such as styes.

Put 20g/⅔oz fresh or 10g/⅓oz dried red clover flowers and 10g/⅓oz fresh red rose petals into a pot. Pour over 600ml/1 pint/ 2½ cups boiling water and leave to infuse for 5 minutes; strain before drinking.

Below *Rose petals are gently soothing.*

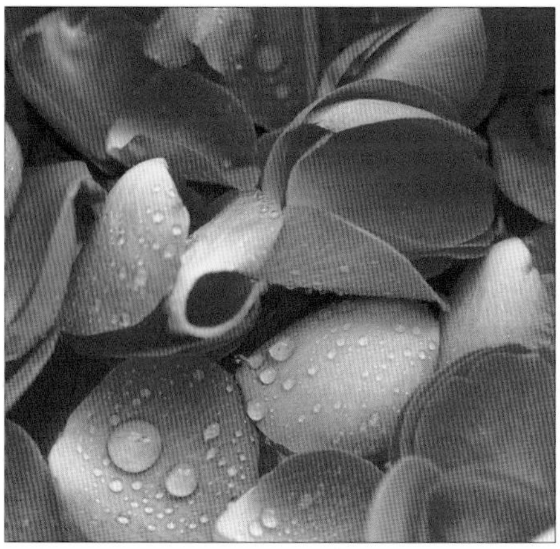

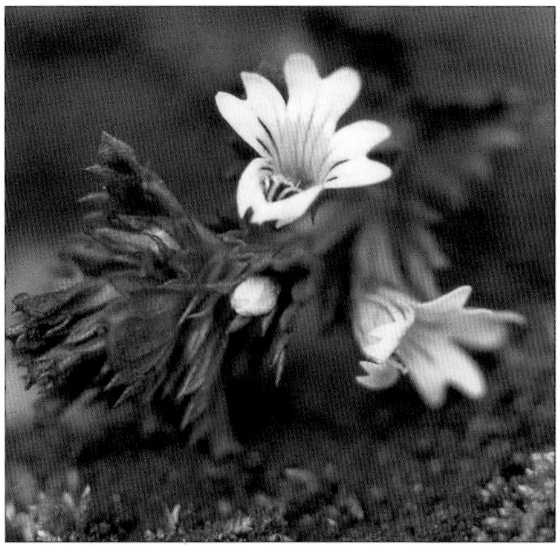

Above *Eyebright (*Euphrasia officinalis*) is a herb traditionally used in eye washes and treatments for styes and conjunctivitis.*

Compress

Applying a warm compress – a piece of gauze dipped in a hot herbal infusion of eyebright (*Euphrasia officinalis*), German chamomile (*Matricaria chamomilla*) or elderflower (*Sambucus nigra*) – helps reduce discomfort, and should bring the stye to a head, releasing the pus.

To make a soothing rose and elderflower compress, mix 5ml/1 tsp tincture of elderflower with 150ml/6fl oz distilled rosewater and 150ml/6fl oz purified water, warm it gently and apply to the eyelid on gauze or a cotton wool pad.

Below *Getting enough sleep has many health benefits and is essential if you are feeling run down due to a depressed immune system.*

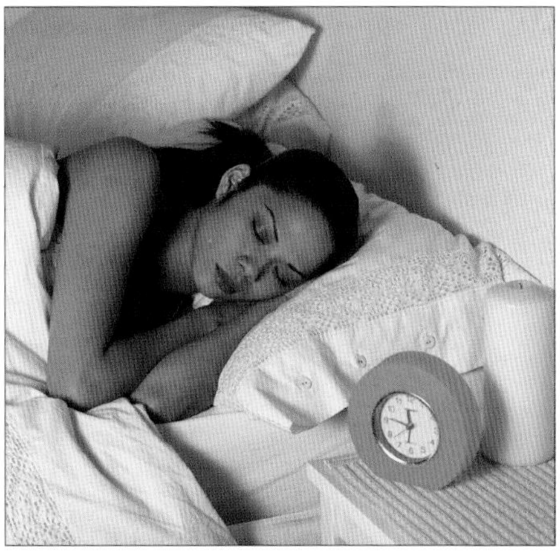

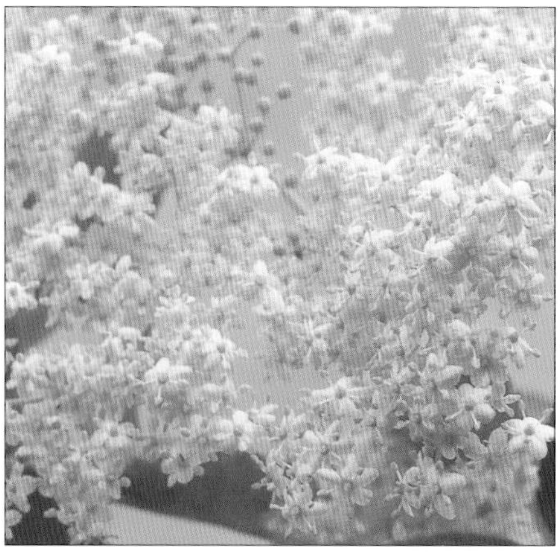

Above *Elderflower (*Sambucus nigra*) has a gentle action when used in a warm compress to reduce the discomfort of a stye.*

Tincture

Echinacea tincture, bought as a ready-made product and taken for a week or two only, may help to give the immune system a general boost.

Steam inhalation

Fill a basin with boiling water, add 2 drops tea tree essential oil, close the eyes and lean over the steam for a minute or two with the head and the basin covered by a towel. Repeat for 5–10 minutes in total at any one time and then on a daily basis until the problem clears.

Below *Tea tree oil is a powerful antiseptic. Add it to a bowl of steaming water as a treatment for styes.*

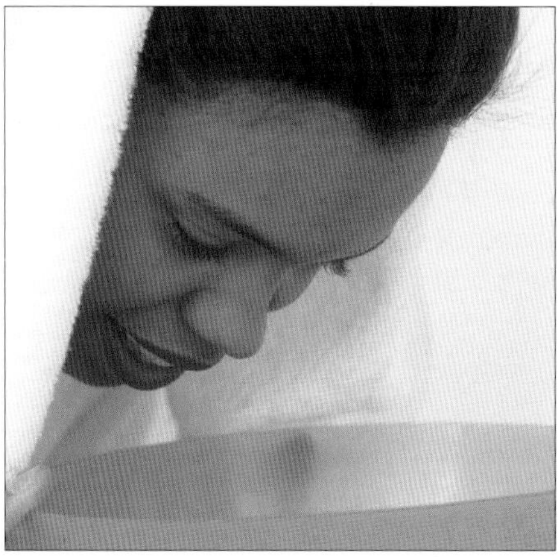

Menstrual Problems

There are many different kinds of menstrual disorder and they may be due to a variety of causes. Natural remedies can often be effective and appropriate. Many herbs have a hormonal action and this, coupled with a holistic approach, helps restore overall balance better than if synthetic hormones alone are used. For serious and persistent problems, or if self-help does not improve matters, seek professional medical advice. When hormonal imbalances are the cause of symptoms, it is also best to seek professional guidance before taking herbal remedies.

Types of menstrual problems

Complete lack of periods (amenorrhoea) can be a result of emotional traumas, excessive exercise, or sharp changes in weight such as loss brought on by anorexia or physical debility. Irregular periods may result from similar causes, and of course both disturbances can happen when going into the menopause.

A more common problem for the majority of women, periods may become far more painful (dysmenorrhoea). This may be due to a hormonal imbalance and you should seek medical advice. Pain during or just before periods is due to contraction in the muscles of the womb, which reduces blood flow causing the muscles to ache. Exercise and heat will increase the circulation and lessen the pain. A hot water bottle can be comforting, but for added benefit try using a hot, aromatic compress. Excessively heavy menstrual bleeding (menorrhagia) may happen without obvious cause, but can also indicate disorders such as fibroids or pelvic infection. A potential problem with menorrhagia is the risk of becoming anaemic.

Self-help measures

A major factor in disturbances of the menstrual cycle for many women is excessive stress. This can cause irregular, scanty or painful periods. Changes in lifestyle, to include more opportunities for relaxation, increased exercise and an improved diet, can have a dramatic effect on hormone levels and menstrual patterns.

Another potential cause of irregular periods is sudden and drastic dieting or yo-yo dieting. Extreme dieting is never a good idea, and can result in the temporary loss of periods altogether. If you need to lose weight, do it gradually and under the guidance of a dietician or your doctor. Natural forms of treatment may be required alongside self-help, but don't neglect the latter.

Herbal teas and decoctions

Infusions of lemon balm (*Melissa officinalis*) or chamomile (*Chamaemelum nobile*), or weak ginger tea, may ease painful periods. For more severe cramping, a decoction of cramp bark (*Viburnum opulus*), or valerian (*Valeriana officinalis*) may ease the discomfort. As these are not very palatable, they may be sweetened with honey, or perhaps taken in tablet form, following the manufacturer's directions for dosage.

- Heavy periods may be regulated by **infusions of yarrow** (*Achillea millefolium*), or for a stronger action, by lady's mantle (*Alchemilla mollis*).
- **Nettle tea** (*Urtica dioica*) is helpful in counteracting the possibility of anaemia, which may result from a heavy flow.

CRAMP BARK AND ROSEMARY COMPRESS

As its name implies, cramp bark reduces spasm, and rosemary is a circulatory stimulant, particularly associated with the womb and head. Its aroma is cheering and relaxing in bouts of period pain.

Ingredients

10ml/2 tsp cramp bark (*Viburnum opulus*)
600ml/1 pint/2½ cups water
10ml/2 tsp dried rosemary (*Rosmarinus officinalis*) or 1 small sprig fresh rosemary

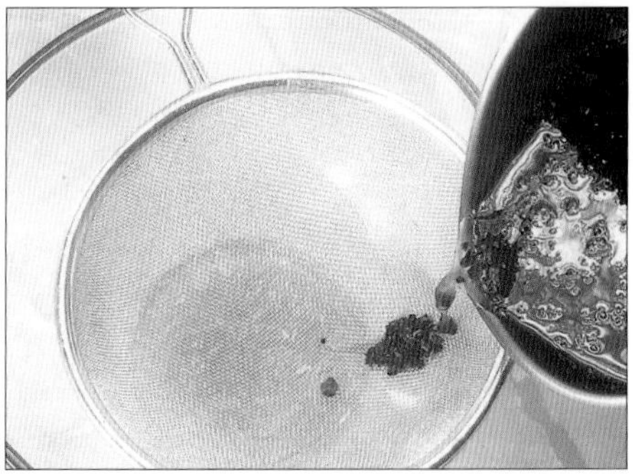

1 Put the cramp bark in a pan with the water and boil for 10–15 minutes. Add the rosemary. Leave to steep for 15 minutes, then strain.

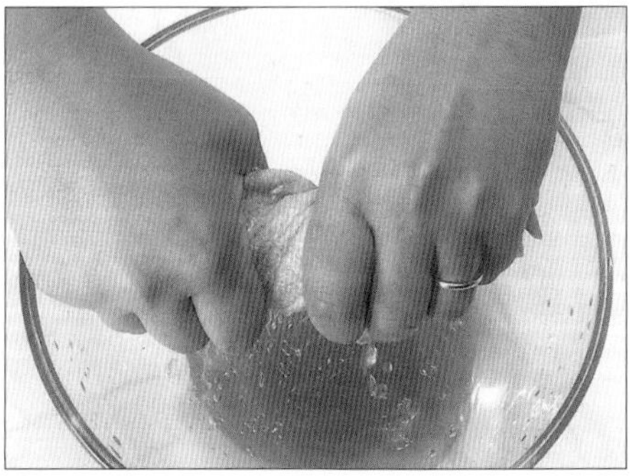

2 Soak a clean cotton cloth or bandage in the liquid. When cool enough to handle, wring out the cloth. Place the hot compress on your abdomen and relax.

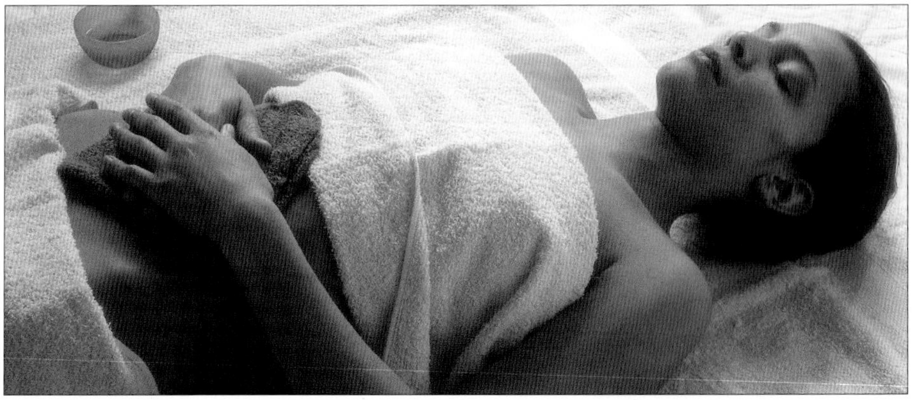

Pre-menstrual Symptoms

A number of symptoms can occur in the second half of the menstrual cycle leading up to the period, due mostly to imbalances in hormone production. These symptoms are known collectively as "pre-menstrual syndrome" (PMS), but not all women experience them in the same combination or in the same way. Herbal treatments may relieve some of the discomfort or distress suffered, but it would be best to seek advice from a qualified herbalist first.

Common symptoms include mood changes, with irritability and/or weepiness, headaches and sometimes migraine, fluid retention, tender breasts, and deep aching in the low abdomen or thighs before and at the start of the period. This half of the cycle can also be when creativity and energy, including sexual energy, can be higher, so do not automatically assume that the pre-period phase has to be awful.

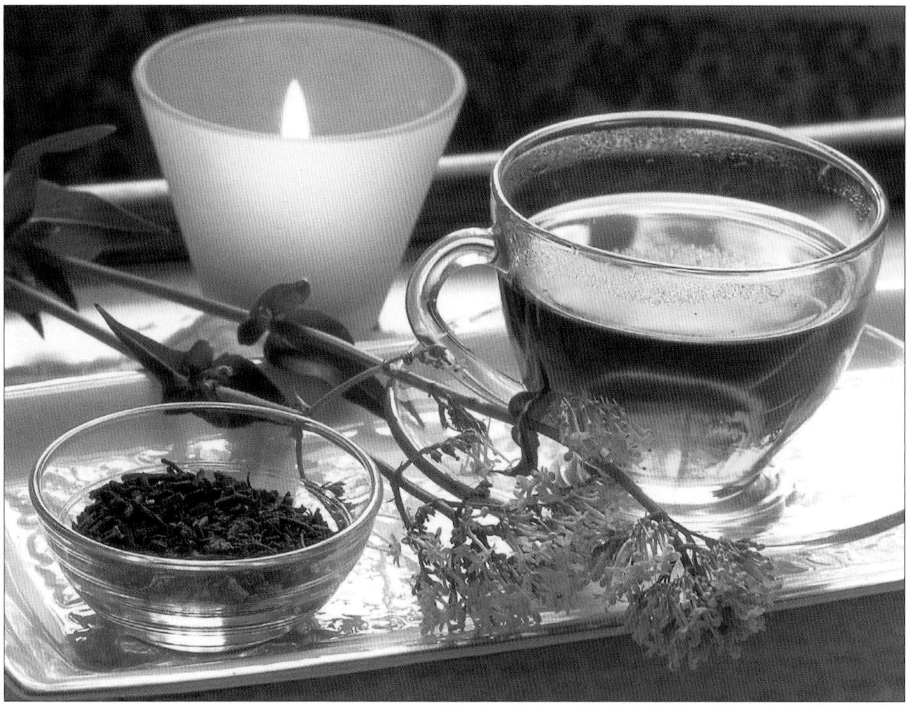

Above *Herbal infusions are a comforting way to benefit from plant properties and relieve stress.*

Stress and PMS

It can be easy to label all physical and emotional upsets as PMS, and overlook other causes or problems. Try to keep a check on whether symptoms definitely occur in monthly cycles. A good way of doing this is to keep a diary as a record of mood swings and general discomfort and note any pattern. Tension and irritability can be due to excess stress or genuine relationship problems, which need to be sorted out. Trying to relax can also help if in a stressful situation.

Below *Chaste tree (*Vitex agnus-castus*) is an aromatic wayside bush native to southern Europe.*

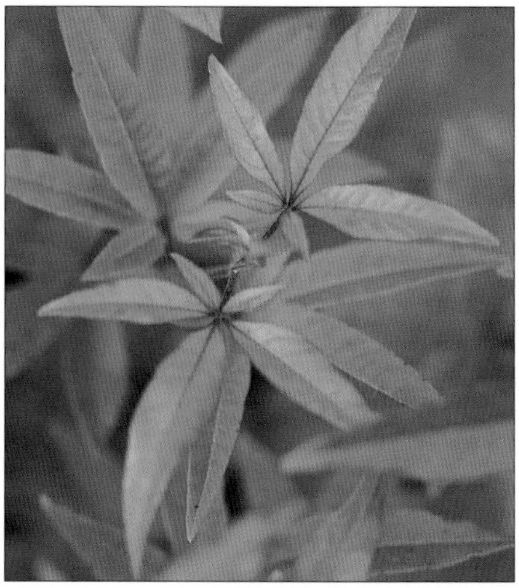

Chaste tree and evening primrose

Also known as monk's pepper, the common names of chaste tree (*Vitex agnus-castus*) reflect its slight anti-oestrogen effect, which can cool passion. Many menstrual problems are a result of an excess of oestrogen, and small doses can rebalance the hormones and may reduce some symptoms of PMS.

The berry is the part used, and chaste tree is probably best taken as a tincture, following the advice of a medical herbalist. They are also available in tablet form, which should be taken according to the manufacturer's directions.

CAUTION Chaste tree should not be taken in conjunction with HRT, the contraceptive pill or fertility treatment. Avoid in pregnancy. In rare cases it may cause headache or upset stomach. It is best taken on the advice of a qualified healthcare professional.

Evening primrose oil also has a reputation for balancing hormonal swings and provides essential fatty acids, which are often lacking with PMS. It can be taken in capsule form, as directed on the packet.

Herbal teas

Herbs with gentle diuretic effects, such as cleavers (*Galium aparine*), may be useful in giving some relief when taken as teas. Two other helpful herbs are chamomile (*Chamaemelum nobile*), for its slightly diuretic and relaxant properties, and lemon balm (*Melissa officinalis*), which may help to ease emotional swings.

• **Vervain and lady's mantle tea** This is a traditional tea for PMS and menstrual problems such as headache and abdominal pain. Put 5ml/1 tsp dried vervain (*Verbena officinalis*) and 5ml/1 tsp dried lady's mantle (*Alchemilla vulgaris*) in a pot and pour on some boiling water. Steep for 5–6 minutes. Strain and sweeten to taste. Take one cup twice a day from day 14 of the cycle.

Menopausal Problems

The change of life, when periods cease, is a variable experience. For some women there is very little disturbance to their lives, except for the relief of no longer having monthly bleeding, although the majority probably suffer at least some degree of discomfort. For others, symptoms such as hot flushes, anxiety, depression, insomnia, heavy periods or severe vaginal dryness make their lives miserable for a considerable time. Everyone is different. Don't hesitate to get advice suited to your individual needs.

Hormone replacement therapy

The risks and benefits of taking HRT as a conventional treatment are constantly under review, and different recommendations emerge as new studies are carried out. Clearly there are pros and cons, and it does not suit everyone, so it is worth looking at other ways of helping the process.

Herbs that help

Many herbs have quite powerful hormonal effects (the contraceptive pill itself was originally derived from a species of Mexican yam) and it is always best to seek professional healthcare advice before deciding which ones to take.

All the herbs mentioned here are effective because they are potent, so treat them with respect and follow the safety guidelines given in this book. Do not exceed recommended doses, and if in doubt speak to your doctor before taking them.

• **Sage** (*Salvia officinalis*) is not only a tonic for the nervous system but also has oestrogenic activity and can ease the dramatic drop in hormone levels that can upset the whole system. It helps to reduce excessive sweating.

Make it as a standard tea and drink two small cups daily for 3 weeks, then avoid for at least a week. It is pleasanter sweetened with a teaspoon of honey and will help to reduce night sweats if taken just before going to bed.

Purple sage can be used as well as the common form, but avoid other ornamental varieties of sage.

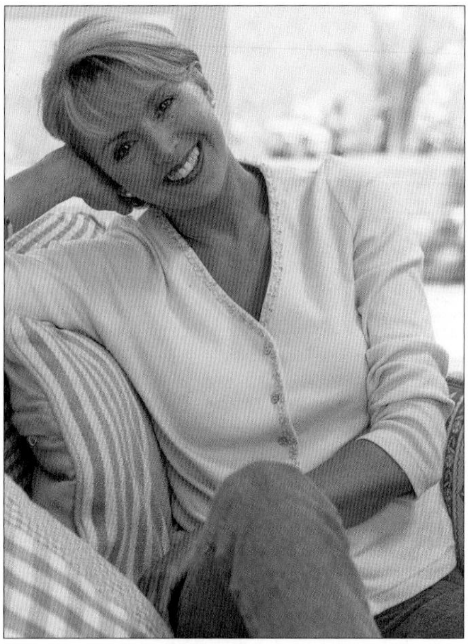

CAUTION Sage can be toxic at high doses or if taken over long periods. It should be avoided if pregnancy is a possibility.

• **Motherwort** (*Leonurus cardiaca*) is a stately plant with delicate mauve flowers. It has a calming action, improving and toning the circulation and helping to relieve menstrual and menopausal symptoms. It may help to reduce blood pressure, and following one set of clinical trials was said to strengthen the heart. Motherwort can be made into a syrup: take 5ml/1 tsp daily for a week or two, or use it to sweeten sage tea.

• **Chaste tree** (*Vitex agnus-castus*) is another powerful herb with hormonal effects, which may help to relieve symptoms such as hot flushes and night sweats.

CAUTION Chaste tree may interfere with other medication, including HRT. Too high a dose can induce an itching sensation on the skin. Always seek professional advice immediately if you suffer any adverse reaction, are on other medication or if in any doubt as to the suitability of this herb for your needs.

Left *Herbal remedies offer a way to reduce menopausal discomfort.*

CAUTION In high doses motherwort can be a uterine stimulant and should be avoided if pregnancy is a possibility.

Below *Motherwort has a calming action.*

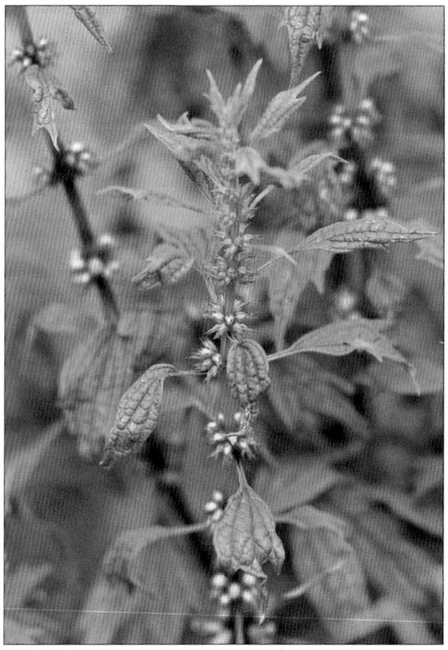

Below *Sage is oestrogenic in action.*

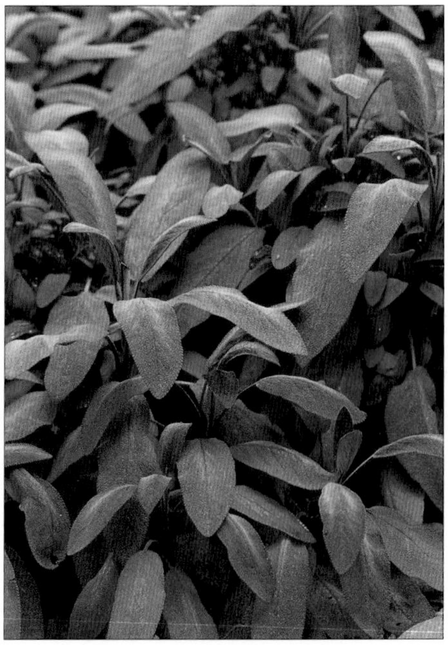

The berry is the part used and it acts on the pituitary gland. Chaste tree is best taken as a ready-made tincture or tablet, when periods first become irregular. Follow the manufacturer's directions or consult a qualified herbalist for advice on dosage to suit your individual requirements.

Herbal teas

Simple relaxants such as German chamomile (*Matricaria chamomilla)* common chamomile (*Chamaemelum nobile*) and lime blossom (*Tilia europaea*), taken as teas 2–3 times a day, may help to reduce the emotional swings that can occur during menopause.

• For alleviating night sweats try sage (*Salvia officinalis*) and motherwort (*Leonurus cardiaca*) tea. Put 5ml/1 tsp each of dried motherwort and dried sage in a pot and pour on 600ml/1 pint/2½ cups boiling water. Leave to steep for 5–6 minutes then strain and sweeten with honey.

Essential oils

Geranium and rose essential oils seem to have a regulating, balancing effect on the female hormone cycle. Bergamot, neroli and jasmine are all uplifting aromas and can help a great deal with the emotional swings and other life changes that may occur around the time of menopause, which can result in a general sense of upheaval and loss.

All these oils can be used either by adding a few drops to the bath or by diluting them in a base oil and massaging into the skin. They can also be vaporized in an essential oil burner.

Try ringing the changes and do not use one oil exclusively for more than a week or so. If you are drawn to the scent of a particular essential oil, then it is most likely to be what you need at that time.

Aromatherapists also recommend the use of clary sage to alleviate hot flushes and night sweats.

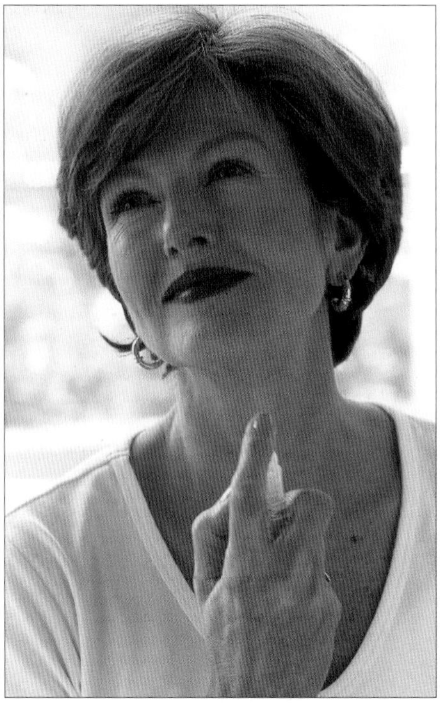

Right *Rose otto, peppermint and cypress oils are useful for hot flushes. Make up a mix and use it in an atomizer during the day whenever you need to cool down.*

Rose otto spray

A cooling spray is handy to counteract the discomfort of hot flushes, which can strike at any time. Rose otto is considered the queen of all essential oils. It has a gentle action and also helps with loss of libido. Put 8–10 drops rose otto essential oil and 300ml/½ pint/1¼ cups spring water in a screw top bottle. Fit the lid, shake well and transfer some to a small purse-size atomizer that you can carry with you. For a more invigorating mix, use 5 drops peppermint and 3 drops cypress oil.

Below *Switch to drinking herbal teas. Chamomile and lime blossom are relaxing and help regulate mood swings.*

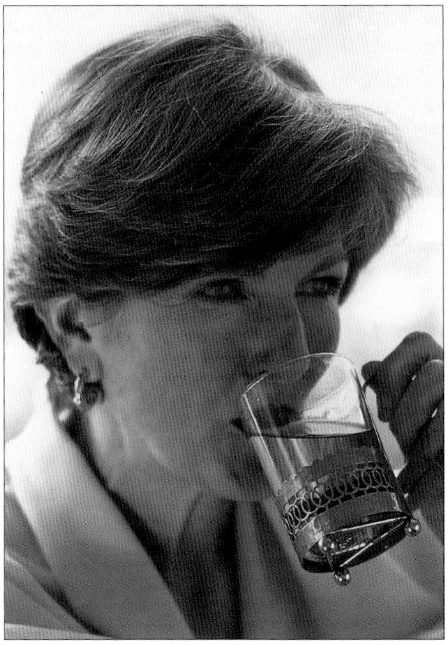

Below *Roses have a gentle action on the skin and a soothing fragrance that can lift the spirits at a difficult time.*

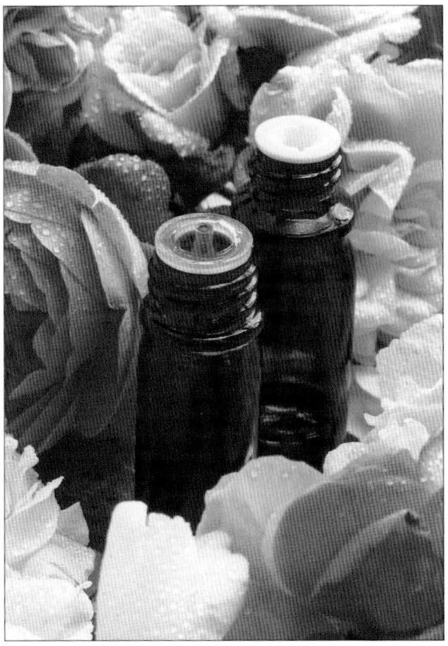

Below *The exquisite scent of jasmine is uplifting and balancing. Use the essential oil to boost your confidence.*

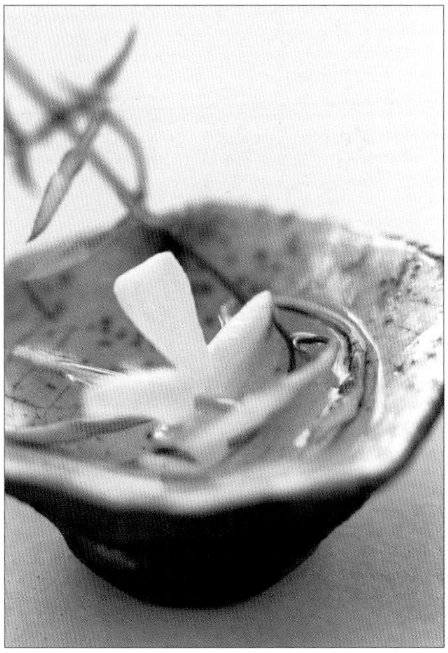

Rheumatism and Arthritis

The general term "rheumatism" is used to describe any pain or inflammation of the muscles, joints and bones. Arthritis, of which there are many different, identifiable conditions, refers more specifically to inflammation of the joints. The herbal preparations and suggestions below are intended to relieve the general muscular aches and pains, and stiffness in the joints, commonly suffered by most people.

CAUTION Any serious, frequent or persistent rheumatic symptoms, including back pain, swellings and injuries, should be referred to your doctor.

Arthritis

There are many kinds of arthritis, each with different symptoms and causes. Two major divisions are osteo and rheumatoid arthritis:

Osteoarthritis is related to wear and tear of the joints, and thinning of the cartilage surrounding them, which commonly occurs with aging. Other factors that may cause it include previous injuries as well as occupations that put a strain on the joints on a daily basis or over a period of time. Osteoarthritis is also sometimes associated with an excess of acid waste matter in the body, accumulating around the joints. (For mild cases of osteoarthritis, home treatments may help.)

Rheumatoid arthritis is a totally different problem. Sometimes defined as an auto-immune disorder, it is caused when the body's defence system attacks its own cells, in this case the soft tissue in the joints. The result is swollen, painful, often deformed joints and a general feeling of being unwell, due to the chemicals released into the body. Self-treatment is not appropriate for this chronic condition, and a doctor should always be consulted.

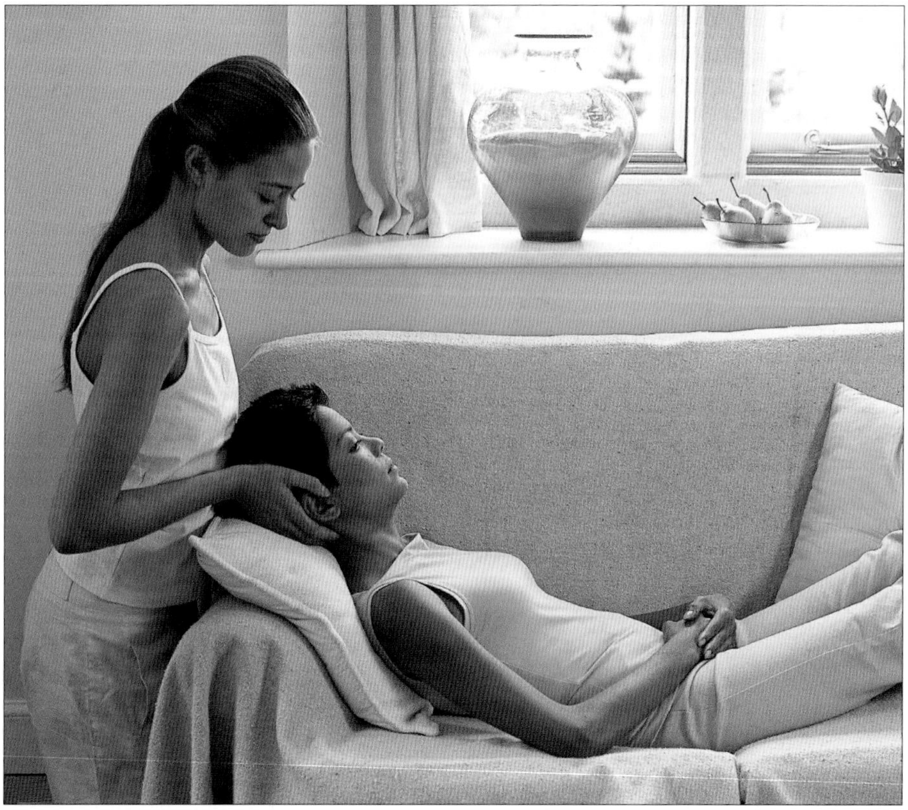

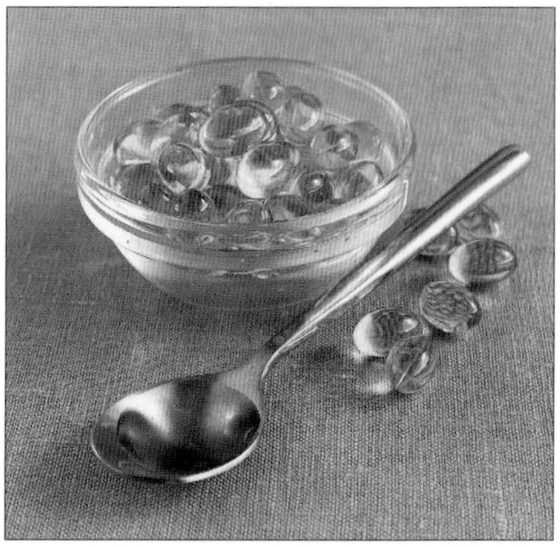

Right *Cod liver oil capsules contain vitamins A and D, and taking them daily can help to keep joints and bones healthy. As well as helping stiffness of joints, cod liver oil is beneficial for the skin, bones, hair and nails.*

Self-help measures

An active lifestyle and a sensible diet are important for overall health, and will minimize muscular aches and pains and stiffness in the joints.

- **Exercise** – Moderate exercise, within limits of comfort, such as walking or swimming, improves muscle tone and helps keep joints working well.
- **Diet** – As with most conditions, it helps to eat a healthy, balanced diet, rich in vitamins and minerals, which includes plenty of fruit, vegetables and oily fish, high in essential fatty acids.
- **Cod liver oil** – A daily dose of up to 5ml/ 1 tsp can be beneficial for the joints and reduce stiffness.

Herbal teas and decoctions

Detoxifying the system and eliminating irritant waste material is often advised for reducing the effects of muscular aches and pains. Stiff joints and mild osteoarthritic conditions also benefit from detoxifying the system and stimulating the circulation. Herbs for these purposes, taken as teas or decoctions, include the following:

- **Dandelion** (*Taraxacum officinale*) is a good choice for home use and can be used in two ways. The leaf, taken as an infusion, has diuretic properties, to increase output from the kidneys. The root, made into a decoction, acts as a gentle liver tonic and mild laxative. Take one cup of each daily for up to a week at a time.
- **Nettle** (*Urtica dioica*) is not only rich in

minerals, including iron, but acts as a "blood cleanser", helping to provide the means for tissue repair and renewal.
It can be taken as a tea on its own, or in combination with dandelion.

- **Meadowsweet** (*Filipendula ulmaria*) is a useful herb for easing the discomfort of muscle pain. It can be taken as an infusion of the dried leaves for 1–2 weeks. For persistent pain seek professional treatment.
- **Celery seed** (*Apium graveolens*) helps remove acidic toxins and has an alkaline effect on the system. For the maximum effect use it in conjunction with parsley, which increases elimination via the urine.
- **Ginger** (*Zingiber officinale*) has a warming effect and may be taken as a tea or decoction, or a little may be added in powdered form to other herbal teas recommended for rheumatism, to stimulate restricted circulation. Ginger should not be taken in high doses. Seek professional healthcare advice before taking it if pregnant or on any other medication.
- **Celery seed and parsley tea** This tea may be taken hot or cold with a slice of lemon. It has an invigorating, cleansing effect. This quantity may be taken daily for no more than 1 week at a time. Put 5ml/1 tsp lightly crushed celery seed in a small teapot, pour in 300ml/½ pint/1¼ cups boiling water and leave to infuse for 5 minutes. Strain and sprinkle with 5ml/1 tsp chopped fresh parsley before drinking.

CAUTION Celery seed should not be taken during pregnancy, or if suffering from kidney disease. It may also cause an allergic reaction. If in doubt, seek professional advice before taking it.

Compress

Pain and stiffness is eased by warmth, and a hot compress will provide extra topical relief. Use 5 drops of any of the essential oils recommended above in 300ml/½ pint hot water; dip in a cloth, wring it out and apply to the affected area.

Essential oils

A warm bath helps to relax stiff and aching muscles, and is especially effective with the addition of a few drops of cypress, juniper, pine and rosemary essential oils. Add 5 drops each of any two in combination. For a greater degree of relaxation, 3–5 drops essential oil of lavender may be added to the water.

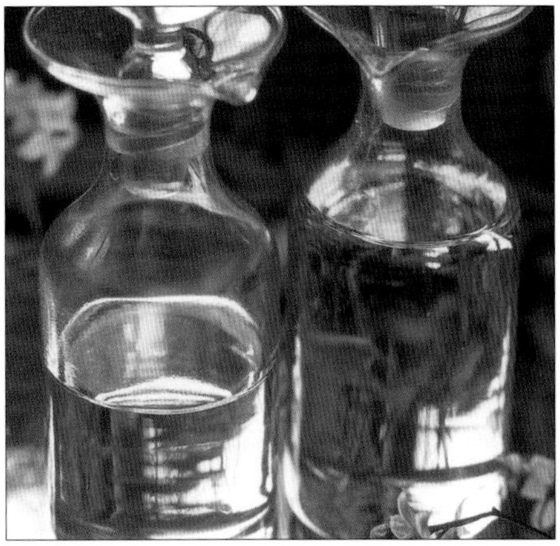

Above *Lavender and rosemary oils together (5 drops of each in the bath) have a slightly analgesic effect, to bring relief from pain and stiffness. Use them to add to a bath or to a massage oil for gentle relief from aches and pains.*

Massage

Gently rubbing the affected areas with anti-inflammatory, painkilling essential oils, such as juniper, lavender and rosemary, eases muscular aches and stiffness of joints. Essential oils of black pepper, ginger and marjoram stimulate the circulation and are also suitable for massage.

Dilute 3 drops of any one, or 1–2 drops of any two oils in combination, in a base of 5ml/1tsp sesame oil.

RHEUMATISM LINIMENT

A liniment is a liquid preparation, often made by mixing a herb oil with a tincture. Some liniments have an alcohol or vinegar base instead of oil.

For rheumatic pains, aching joints and tired muscles, rub this liniment gently into the affected areas. It should be applied to the skin at body temperature.

Right *The healing properties of garlic and juniper are harnessed to make a liniment for massaging aching joints and muscles.*

Ingredients

6 garlic cloves
300ml/½ pint/1¼ cups olive oil
30ml/2 tbsp tincture of juniper

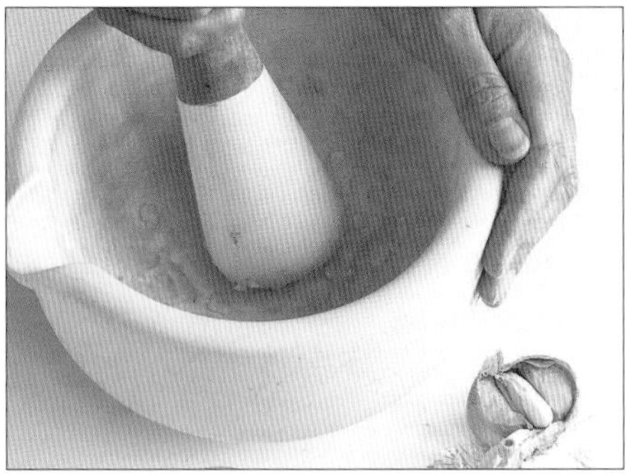

1 Crush the garlic cloves, without peeling them, and put them in a bowl. Pour the olive oil over the crushed garlic cloves. Cover the bowl with a piece of foil and stand it over a pan of simmering water. Heat gently for 1 hour. Check the water level in the pan regularly and top up as necessary.

2 Strain the oil, leave until lukewarm, then stir in the tincture of juniper and pour into a stoppered bottle. This liniment will keep for several months.

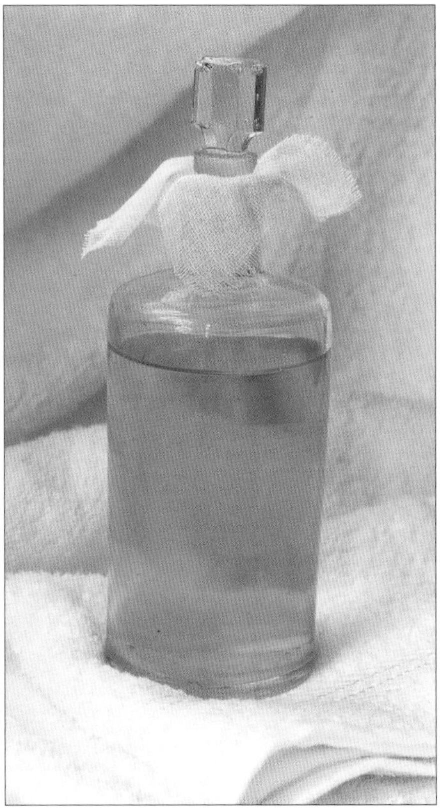

Bites and Stings

Herbal preparations and essential oils can be very effective as first aid for insect bites and stings. These can result from contact with many different insects and vary greatly as to the degree of pain or reaction caused.

CAUTION If a bite or sting affects the mouth or throat, and if there are any signs of an allergic reaction, or difficulty in breathing, get medical help immediately.

Prevention

Cover skin to prevent being bitten by mosquitoes, especially at dawn and dusk when they are most active.

To make a natural insect repellent lotion, mix 5 drops each lavender, rosemary and citronella essential oils in 25ml/5 tsp almond oil and rub on to exposed skin.

Fresh plant material

For immediate relief, it is sometimes enough to rub the fresh leaves of suitable herbs

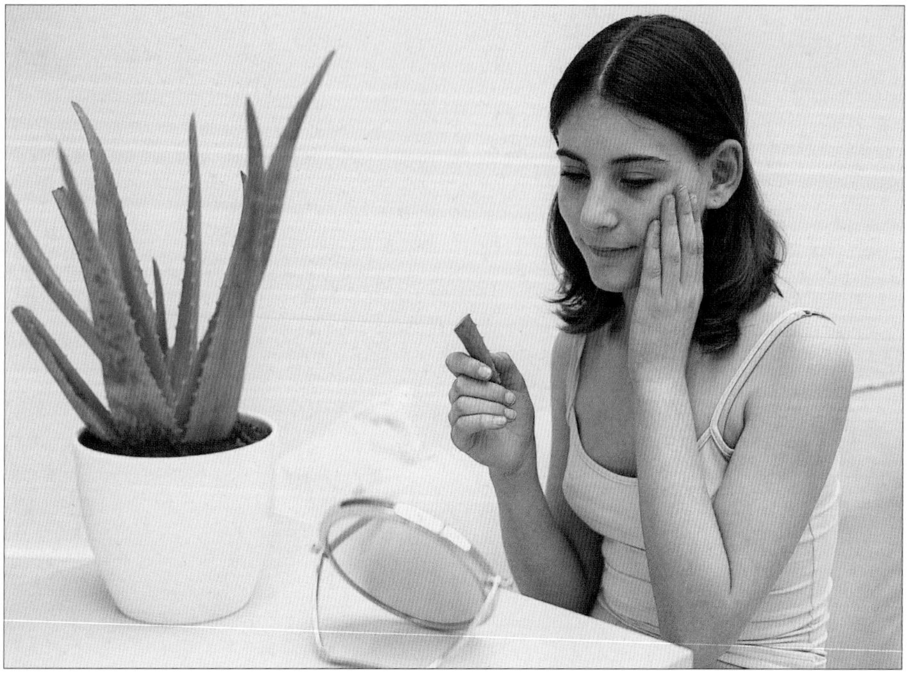

Below *The leaves of aloe vera contain a soothing gel. Break off a leaf, slit it open with a sharp knife and apply the gel that seeps out to the bite or sting.*

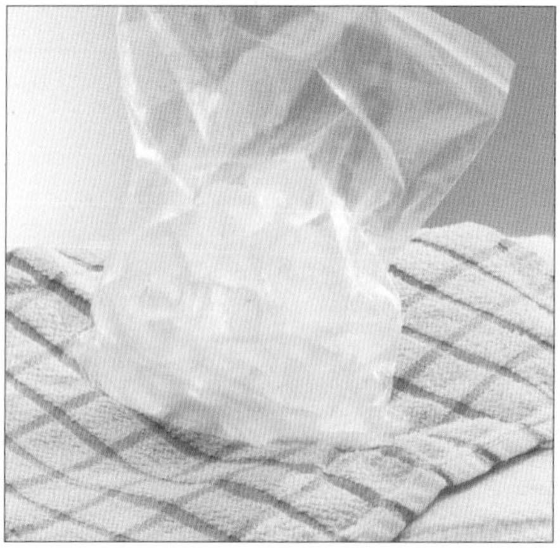

Above *Applying ice to the area as soon as possible reduces inflammation.*

directly on to the skin. Remember herbs are powerful, so always try a small test patch on the skin if you are using a herbal infusion as an insect repellent for the first time, in case of allergies. Do not use insect-repellent lotions near the eyes. Do not use if pregnant or for children under five.

- **Lemon balm** (*Melissa officinalis*) is an anti-allergenic, with insect repellent properties.
- **Basil** (*Ocimum basilicum*) is antiseptic and cleansing in action.
- **Plantain** (*Plantago major* or *P. lanceolata*)

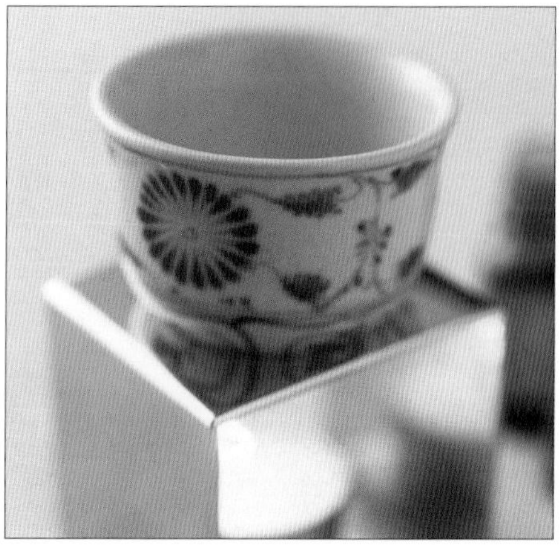

Above *Burn citronella, lavender and rosemary essential oils in an essential oil burner when you are sitting outside, to keep biting insects away.*

is a traditional treatment for wasp stings.

- **Yellow dock** (*Rumex crispus*) is commonly used for easing nettle stings.

For a bee sting, there may be some value in using diluted bicarbonate of soda (baking soda) on the area.

Cold compresses

A cold compress helps reduce the pain and swelling of an insect bite. An infusion of lavender (*Lavandula*), made with fresh or dried flowers, is ideal for this. Infusions of chamomile (*Chamaemelum nobile*), red clover (*Trifolium pratense*) or sage (*Salvia officinalis*) are also suitable.

- A compress could be made using tinctures of St John's wort (*Hypericum perforatum*) or myrrh, diluting 5ml/1 tsp in 15ml/1 tbsp cool water. Or you could apply 1–2 drops of either of these tinctures directly to the bite.
- Use distilled witch hazel as a compress.

Essential oils

A few drops of tea tree oil, diluted in a little iced water, may be applied to the area.

For wasp stings, bee stings and mosquito bites, lavender essential oil is effective when applied directly to the skin, provided it is a good quality, pure essential oil. This may be applied every 10 minutes or so until the pain and irritation have subsided.

Cuts and Grazes

The first thing to do is to remove any dirt and ensure that the area is thoroughly clean by gently washing it in cool water. For minor cuts and wounds, herbal remedies can be a great help, but if the cut is deep it may need stitches and treatment against tetanus, so it is important to get medical assistance. Medical advice should also be sought if inflammation or swelling develops or there are any signs of infection.

• Distilled witch hazel (*Hamamelis virginiana*) has astringent, anti-inflammatory properties and helps stop bleeding. It is useful for washing the area around cuts and grazes or can be applied diluted (15ml/ 1 tbsp to 300ml/½ pt/1¼ cups of water) on a dressing.

• Calendula or myrrh tinctures (which have antiseptic properties), similarly diluted, are alternatives for use on a dressing.

• Yarrow (*Achillea millefolium*) is an astringent herb that helps stop bleeding; an infusion can be used.

• Marigold (*Calendula officinalis*) salve is an ideal soothing healer to apply to minor cuts and grazes.

• Comfrey (*Symphytum officinale*) ointment is a powerful tissue healer, so much so that it should be used only on clean cuts as it can seal dirt inside a wound. (See Bruises for directions on how to make it.)

Below *Lavender is one of the few essential oils it is safe to use undiluted on the skin.*

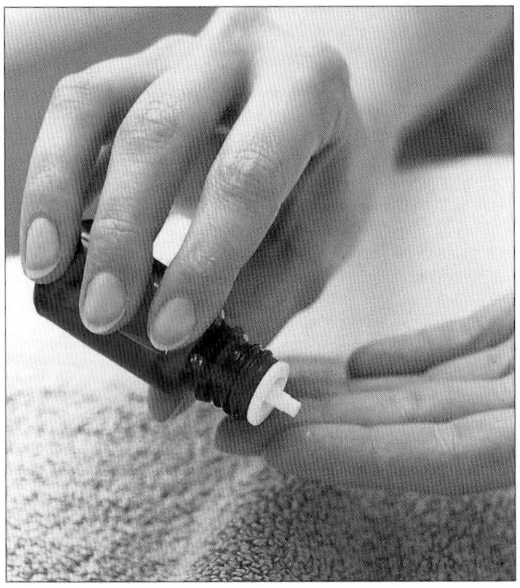

• Aloe vera – The fresh gel in the leaves is soothing and healing, and may be applied 2–3 times a day, until the cut is fully healed.

Essential oils

The two oils of choice are probably lavender and tea tree. These may be used neat on small cuts and scratches; they will sting temporarily but this soon passes. They can be added to a bowl of water for bathing and cleaning the affected area initially, or a couple of drops may be placed on a plaster or other clean dressing and applied over the site of the injury. Both these oils fight any infection as well as stimulating healing, and are generally very safe to use undiluted in this way.

Below *The antiseptic action of essential oils of tea tree and lavender makes them useful for cleaning minor wounds.*

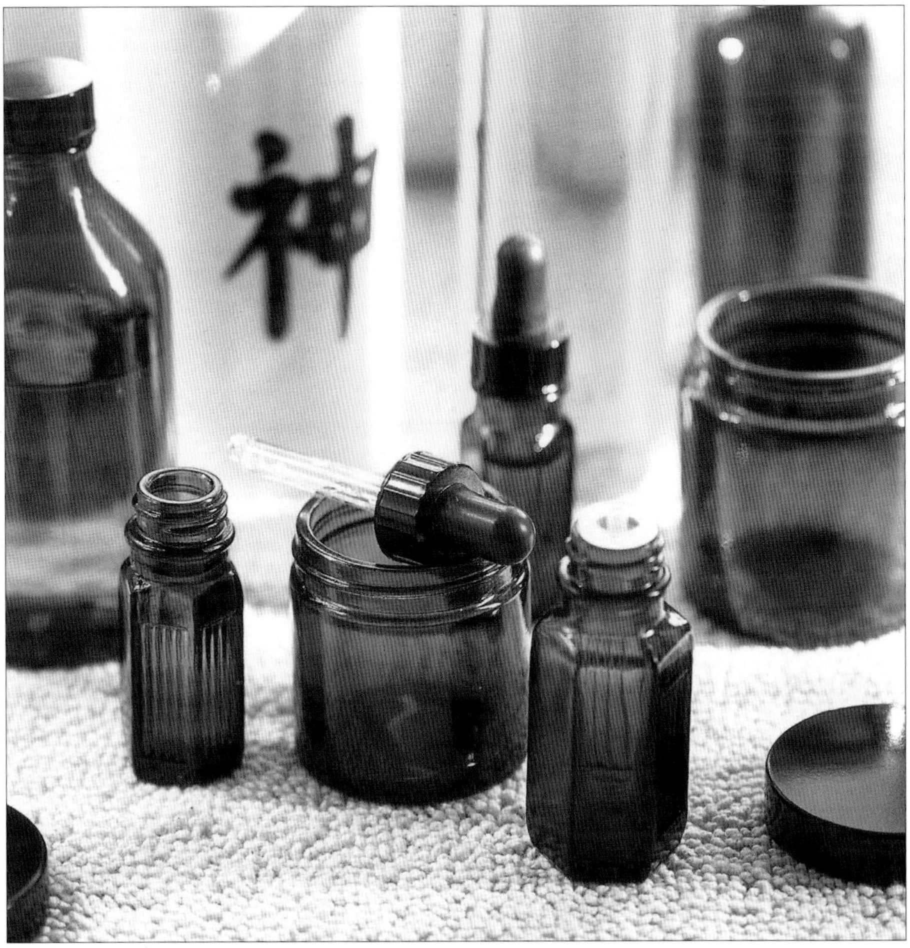

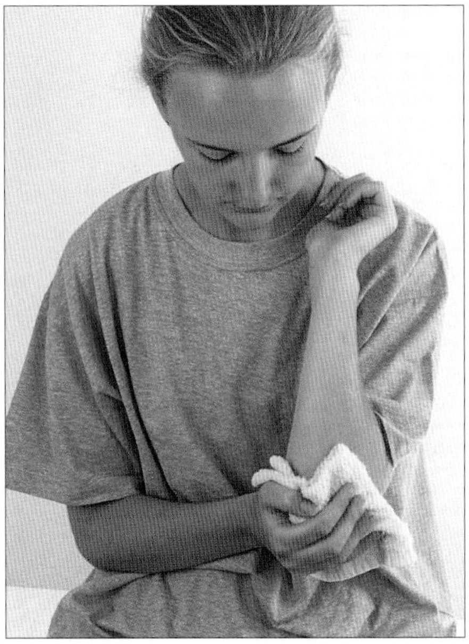

Above *Add 2–3 drops of lavender oil to a cool compress as a powerful antiseptic.*

Bruises

A bruise happens when capillary blood vessels burst beneath the skin. Minor bruises, which occur as a result of a knock, crushed finger or toe, sprain or other injury, respond well to herbal first aid. However, bruises without an obvious cause could be the sign of a dangerous condition, such as cancer, and serious bruising could mean there is an underlying grave injury, such as a broken bone. All such cases should be referred to a doctor.

Compress

Ice-cold compresses, applied immediately to the affected area, are one of the best home treatments for bruising.

Dilute 15ml/1 tbsp distilled witch hazel in 300ml/½ pint/1¼ cups cold water and use as a compress. To save time when accidents happen, keep some ice cubes made with witch hazel in a separately labelled bag in the freezer to put on bruises (a useful policy if you have children).

Essential oil

Immediate use of oil of lavender in an ice-cold compress can be the most effective treatment to avoid swelling and widespread bruising. If a bruise has developed, at a later stage when it is changing colour and resolving, use rosemary essential oil diluted in a vegetable oil base to massage gently into the tissues to increase local circulation and speed up the healing process.

Poultice

Comfrey contains a substance called allantoin, which stimulates the growth of the body's soft tissue cells. It provides a soothing, anti-inflammatory mucilage that is ideal for alleviating the discomfort of bruises and sprains. In cases of bruising it is best applied cold.

Ointment

Arnica ointment is widely available from pharmacists and makes a useful standby for applying to bruises, but it should never be applied if the skin is broken, as it can be an irritant.

COMFREY BRUISE OINTMENT

Comfrey had many traditional uses in herbal medicine. Knitbone, was once a common name for this herb, so called because of its value in 'mending' the body. This ointment forms a protective layer over the skin. It will keep for 3–4 months in a cool dark place and makes a useful addition to the first aid cabinet, especially if you are prone to bruising easily.

Ingredients

200g/7oz petroleum jelly or paraffin wax
30g/1oz fresh comfrey (*Symphytum officinale*) leaves, roughly chopped

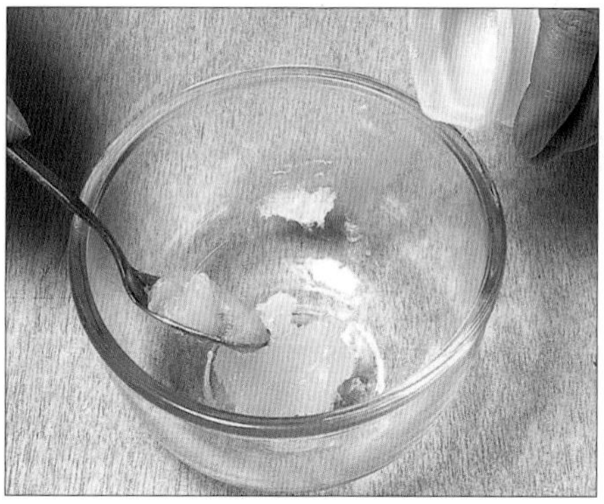

1 Put the petroleum jelly or paraffin wax into a bowl and set the bowl over a pan of gently simmering water. Allow to melt slightly.

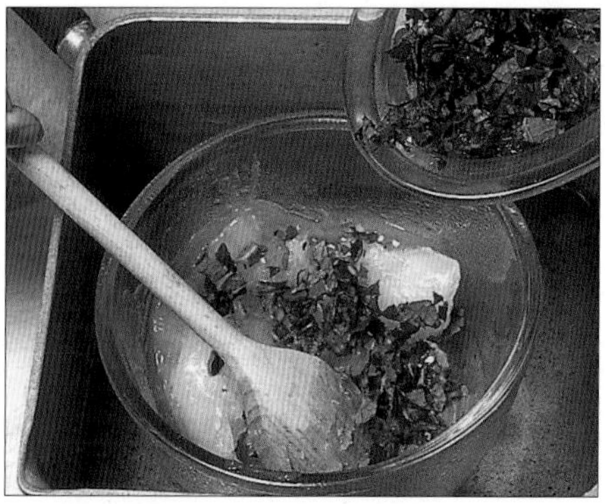

2 Add the chopped comfrey leaves and stir well to combine the ingredients. Heat over gently simmering water for about 1 hour until the petroleum jelly is liquid and the active contituents from the comfrey have permeated the liquid.

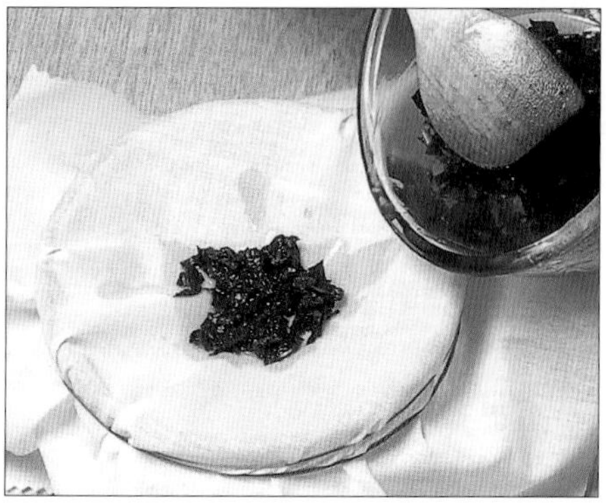

3 Strain the mixture through muslin (cheesecloth) secured to the rim of a jug (pitcher) with an elastic band. Pour immediately into a clean glass jar, before it has a chance to set.

Variations

Bruise ointments can also be made with houseleek (*Sempervivim tectorum*), which has a soothing, astringent effect and is useful for many skin conditions, or arnica flowers (*Arnica montana*). Follow the instructions given for comfrey ointment, substituting a similar quantity of plant material.

Below *Bruises and cuts respond to the healing power of comfrey.*

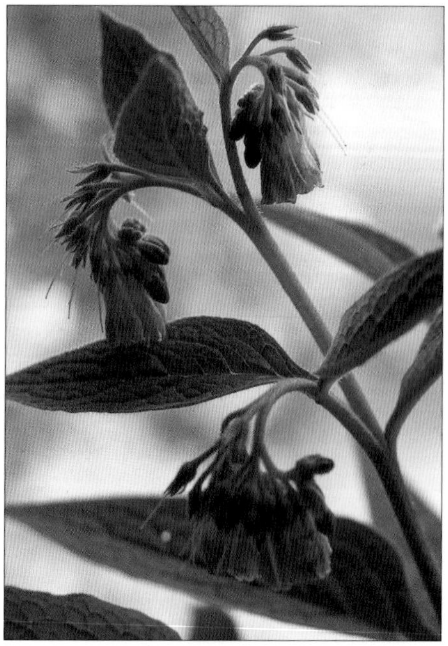

Sprains and Strains

A sprain is an injury affecting a joint, with the tendons that attach muscles to the bones being overstretched and often torn. A strain is an injury to the muscles themselves, usually caused by excessive or inappropriate exercise, such as lifting weights. The first thing to do, for such injuries, is to apply a cold compress; massage of the area is not helpful at this stage, but can be used if the after-effects linger on.

The ICE approach

The immediate treatment is to apply the "ICE" approach: ice, compression and elevation. For example, a pack of frozen peas, held firmly around a sprained ankle, with the leg raised and supported, will help a good deal in reducing internal bleeding and joint swelling.

After the symptoms have subsided there may be a case for using alternate hot and cold compresses (3 minutes hot followed by 1 minute cold, repeated for about 15 minutes) to improve local circulation to the relevant muscles, and later treatment may include massage to relieve muscular aches. Diluted oil of lavender (about 2 per cent in a base oil) is helpful for this.

Compresses

Applying a cold compress to a sprain or strain will help to reduce the pain and inflammation. The colder the infusion for the compress, the more effective it will be, so it is a good idea to cool the liquid by adding ice cubes.

- **Comfrey** (*Symphytum officinale*) is one of the most effective herbs for the purpose. You could also use pot marigold (*Calendula officinalis*) or yarrow (*Achillea millefolium*). The compress can be made with infusions of the leaves or petals, but as these take time to cool down, it may be easier to use a tincture of the herb, diluted in the proportion of 15ml/1tbsp tincture to 300ml/½ pint/1¼ cups of cold water.
- **Lavender** is the best essential oil for a sprain compress; use 8 drops oil to 30ml/2 tbsp iced water.

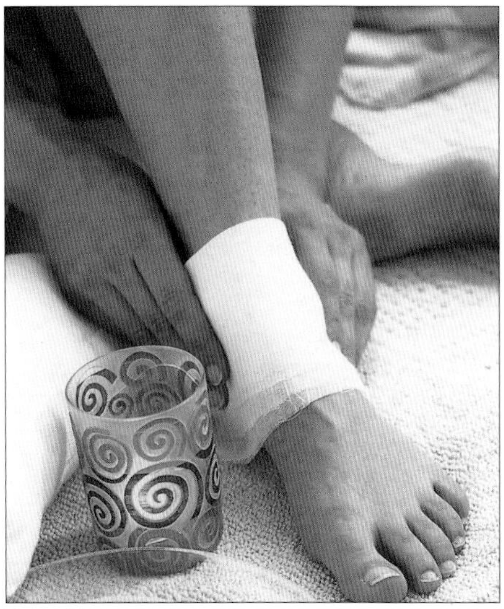

Above *A cold compress applied to a sprain as soon as possible after the injury helps to reduce swelling.*

- **Chamomile** essential oil may be used in the same way; where there is a sprain, try to keep the affected joint as still as possible initially to reduce internal bleeding and allow healing to start as quickly as possible.

Ointment

When the swelling has subsided, gently rub in comfrey bruise ointment to speed up healing of the damaged fibres. If muscles ache through over-exercise, this ointment is a good home treatment, with massage of the surrounding area twice a day.

Below *Elevating and supporting the leg is helpful for a sprained ankle. Other measures include applying an ice-cold compress, followed by one made with a herbal infusion. For strained muscles, gentle massage of the area with a herbal oil is effective.*

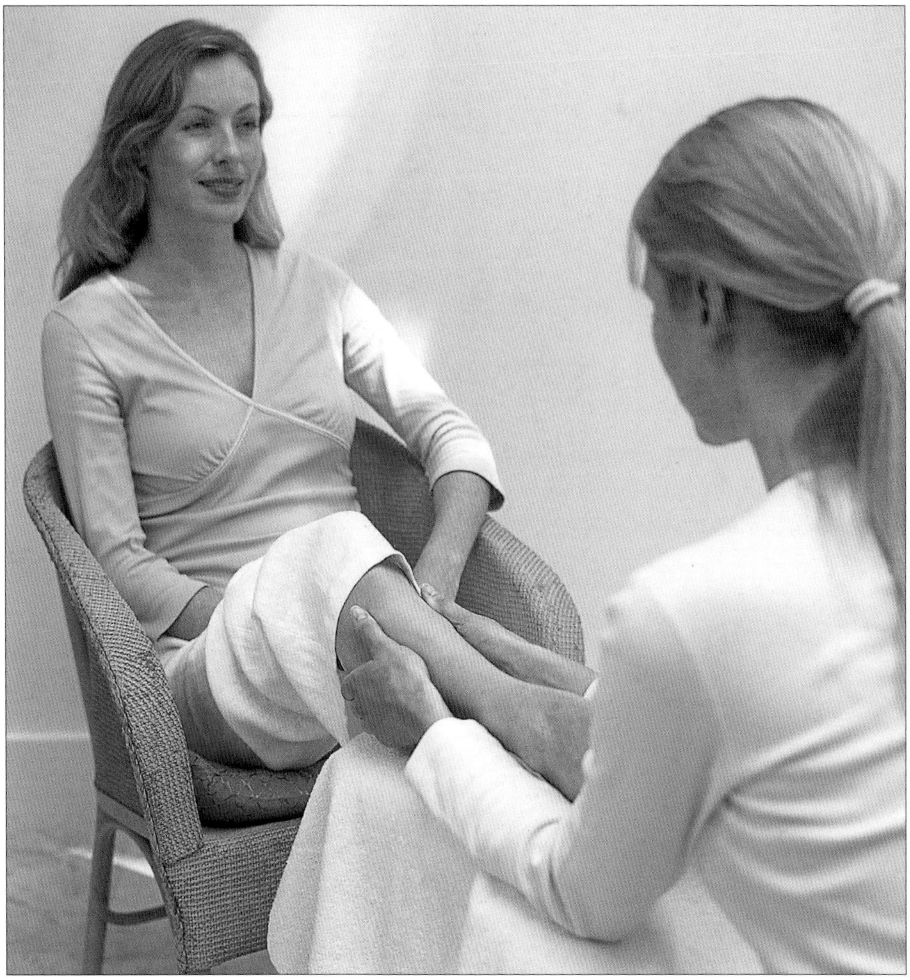

Burns

Herbal first aid is appropriate for minor burns and scalds only, when it can be used to minimize pain and encourage healing. The immediate treatment, before using any herbal preparations, should be to apply cold water for 5–10 minutes, to reduce the heat in the affected tissue. Severe burns require urgent medical assistance, with no delay in getting treatment, especially for children or babies. If the burn is from a chemical, affected clothing can be removed, but if clothing is stuck to the burn, it is better not to remove it before seeking treatment as this might do more damage.

CAUTION Burns larger than the palm of your hand should be seen by a doctor immediately, regardless of any self-help treatment that has been advised here.
All burns are painful and should be touched as little as possible.

Tips for treating burns

Remember, do not use greasy ointments, butter or other fats on new burns as all this does is fry the skin. Always cool the area thoroughly as the first treatment.

Below *Lavender essential oil, applied directly to the affected skin, has been found to be very effective in healing burns.*

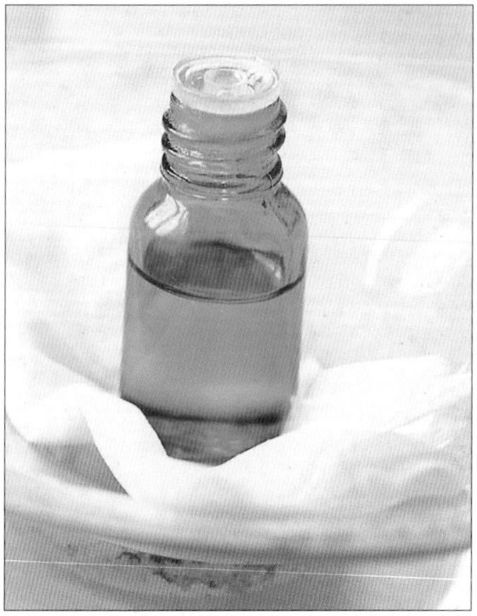

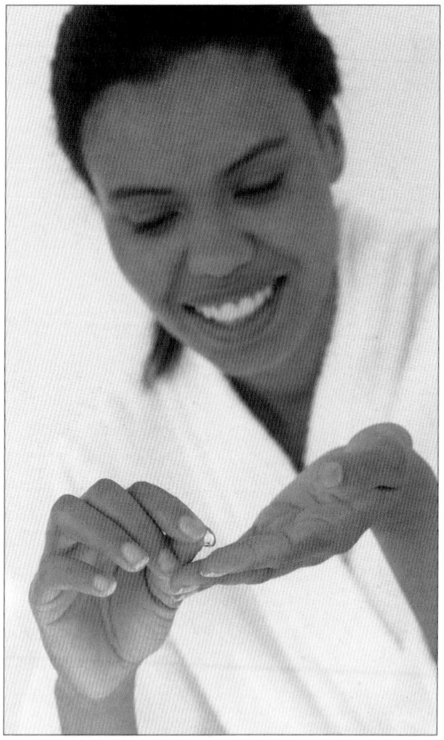

Above *Vitamin E oil, squeezed from a capsule and applied to a burn, supports the skin and reduces scarring.*

Once the skin has been cooled a valuable home remedy is honey: this is both antiseptic and promotes healing. Once healing has started, a vitamin E cream can aid restoration of tissue elasticity and reduce scarring. Do not give hot drinks to someone who has a burn; frequent small sips of cool water can help to replace lost fluids in more serious cases.

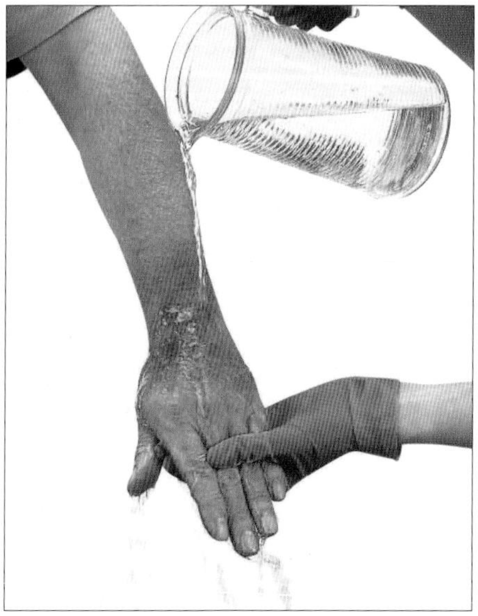

Essential oils

Lavender essential oil has anti-inflammatory, analgesic properties and promotes healing of the tissues. It has been used as an effective first-aid treatment for burns since the early years of the 20th century, when René Gattefossé, the founding father of aromatherapy, fortuitously discovered its miraculous healing powers following a laboratory accident.

Provided – and this is crucial – you use a top quality, unadulterated, pure lavender essential oil, a few drops can be applied directly to the skin. If a larger area is affected, the oil can be put on to sterile gauze or smooth lint first.

Tea tree oil may help to prevent blistering of the skin: dilute 1–2 drops of the oil in 5ml/1tsp water and apply it to a minor burn, after first cooling it with plain water.

Other herbal treatments

An aloe vera plant is an invaluable source of first aid for minor burns and scalds. (The plant is easy to care for provided it is kept frost-free and given a sunny spot, such as a kitchen windowsill.) Simply break open one of the leaves and spread the thick gel that seeps out directly on to the burn. If this is done as soon as possible it will promote scar-free healing. Alternatively, an infusion of chamomile (*Matricaria chamomilla* or *Chamaemelum nobile*) or pot marigold (*Calendula officinalis*) can be applied to a burn on a smooth dressing.

Marigold skin salve (see Skin Irritations) may be used after some time has elapsed and the skin is beginning to heal, to ease continuing inflammation and soreness.

Left *Pouring cold water over a burn to reduce the heat is the first step to take when applying first aid. If the burn is in a suitable area such as a hand or arm it can be held under a cold running tap.*

Sunburn

Sunlight produces a sense of well-being and we all need a little exposure to sun in order to metabolize vitamin D. Too much, however, is not only ageing, but increases the possibility of developing skin cancer. Prevention is always better than cure, and strong sunshine should be avoided at all costs. Some people burn more easily than others (those with fair skins are particularly at risk) and if mild sunburn does occur, herbal preparations can be used to soothe the discomfort and aid the skin to heal and recover.

The risk of skin cancer

An increasingly frequent sequel to excessive exposure to the sun is skin cancer, and the reductions in the earth's ozone layer make this likely to become dramatically more common in future years, even in countries some distance away from the Equator.

The sun has an ageing effect on the skin, so enjoy it but use good suntan and aftersun moisturizing creams and keep out of the midday sun. Sunbeds can damage skin. They do not protect against sunburn; you still need to be careful when out in hot sunshine.

Below *Take sensible precautions to minimize exposure to sunlight, such as covering up when you are out and about and staying out of the sun during the hottest part of the day.*

Compress

For a mild case of sunburn, start by cooling areas of red skin, as for minor burns. Applying a chilled infusion of chamomile (*Chamaemelum nobile*), elderflower (*Sambucus nigra*) or lavender (*Lavandula* spp) flowers, as a compress, is very soothing. Cooled distilled witch hazel (*Hamamelis virginiana*) also makes a good compress.

Poultice

Strawberries and yogurt both take the heat out of sunburnt skin. Mash them up together (make sure you use plain yogurt) and apply directly to the skin as a poultice, keeping it in place with a piece of gauze or cotton fabric.

Essential oils

Lavender essential oil may be used as for burns, directly on the skin; if you are not sure of its purity, dilute it (adding 5 drops to a small bowl of water) and carefully dab it on to the skin. Chamomile essential oil, also diluted, may be similarly used, but only on unbroken skin.

Either of these oils could also be added to the bath (5–8 drops); make sure the water is no more than tepid, as a hot bath would make the problem worse.

Marigold skin salve (see Skin Irritations) is a useful all-purpose cream to apply to sun-reddened skin, after first cooling it with a herbal infusion.

Below right *Rose and chamomile are good essential oils to use on sun-damaged skin. Put a few drops in bath water.*

Routine after-sun care

Essential oils of rose, chamomile, lavender or sandalwood make excellent aftercare for leathery, sun-damaged skin. Dilute any one of these in a base oil, such as sweet almond, (adding 2–3 drops to 5ml/1 tsp base oil) and massage in gently twice a day. Rose oil, although it is expensive, is probably the best one to choose: it is safe to use on sensitive skins, provided it is a pure essential oil and not synthetic.

After-sun treatment

- For a refreshing spray to use after exposure to the sun, mix 8 drops rose oil in 25ml/5 tsp water and apply with an atomizer.
- For a soothing and cooling oil for sunburnt skin mix 5 drops each of rose essential oil and chamomile essential oil together with 45ml/3 tbsp each grapeseed oil and virgin olive oil and 15ml/1 tbsp wheatgerm oil. Combine all the oils in a bowl. Massage gently into the sun-reddened area.

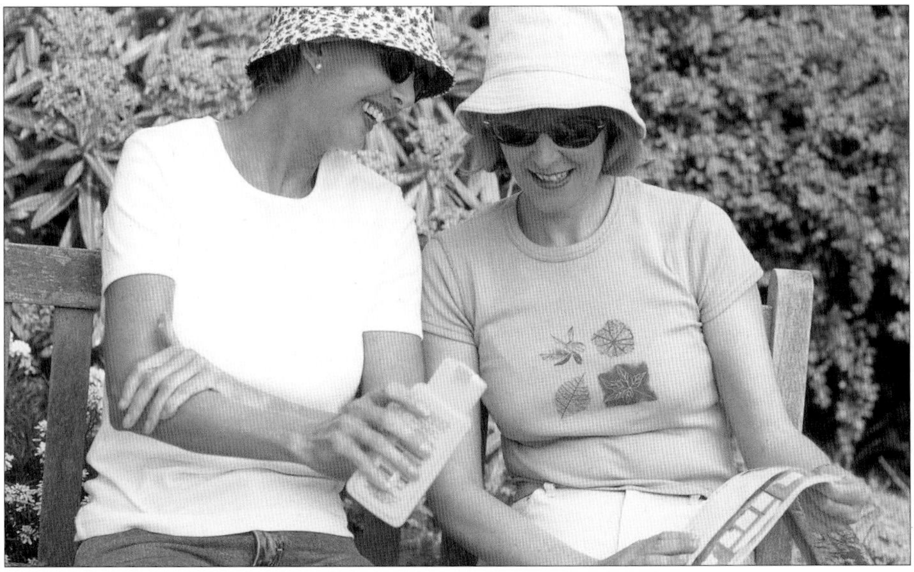

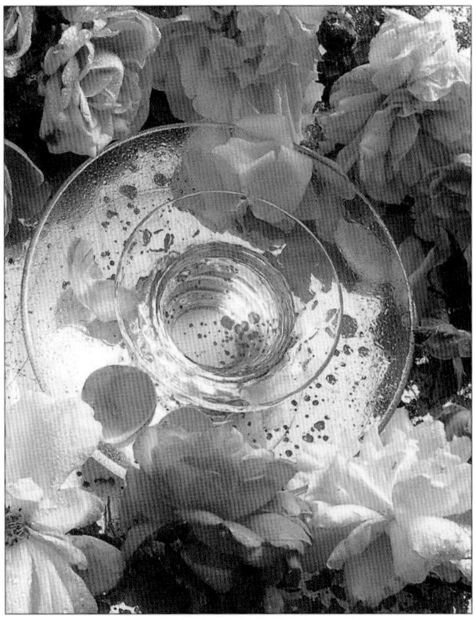

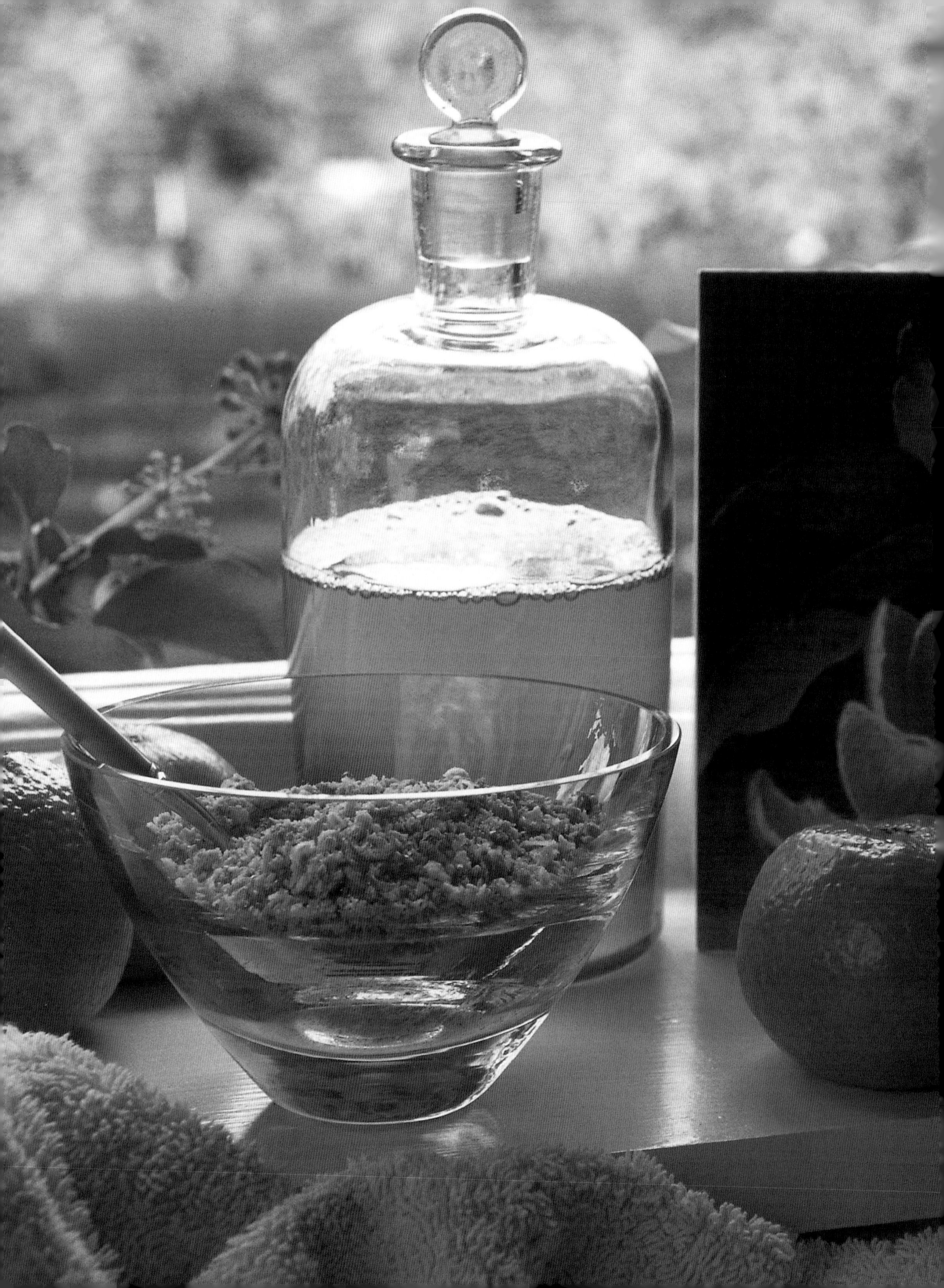

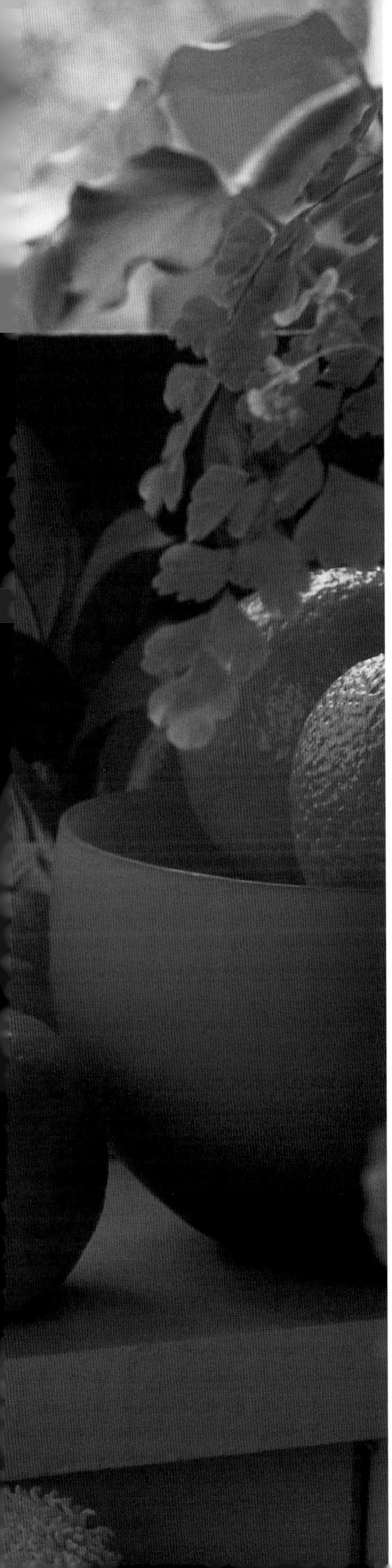

Herbal Beauty Treatments

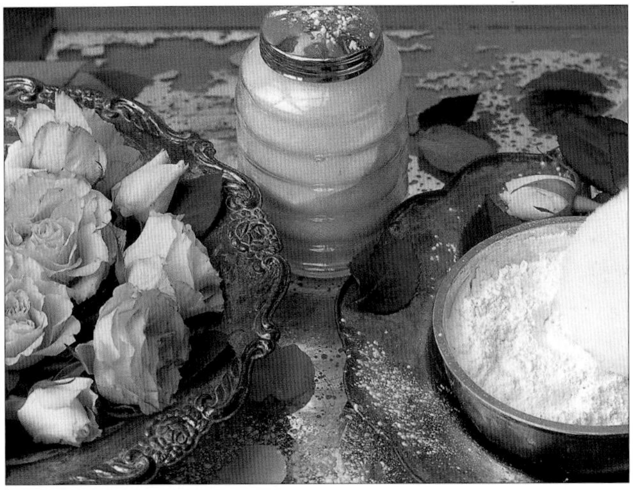

Using simple beauty treatments made with herbs, flowers and basic natural ingredients contributes greatly to general health and well-being. Many commercial beauty products contain parabens and other chemicals, which studies have found could have an injurious effect on the system, so it makes sense to find alternatives where practicable.The recipes in this chapter show how to make your own hair products and face creams, body lotions, dusting powders and many other items for daily hygiene and general beauty care. They are easy to follow and the products take little time to prepare. It is important to follow guidelines on how to store them and how long they should be kept.

Above *Fragrant dusting powder scented with herbal flowers is a luxurious beauty treat with which to pamper yourself.*

Left *Beauty preparations can be made with a variety of natural ingredients.*

Healthy Hair

Modern hair care products can make your hair look good, but many of them contain potentially harmful chemicals that you may prefer to avoid. Using the same ones consistently can also lead to build-up on hair and scalp, so it makes sense to give your hair a rest by using herbal treatments and natural ingredients, which have been tried and tested and provide a simpler way to keep hair in top condition.

Herbal shampoo

This is the most difficult hair-care item to produce in "natural" form. All commercial shampoos contain some form of detergent, which may strip the hair of its natural oils, but also have an effective cleansing action.

The easiest way to make a "herbal" shampoo that will leave your hair clean and shiny is to add 2–3 drops essential oil to 15ml/1 tbsp ready-made organic shampoo base (available from specialist suppliers); or you could mix the shampoo base with an equal quantity of a strong herbal infusion. A mild, fragrance-free, pH-balanced shampoo can be used as a base.

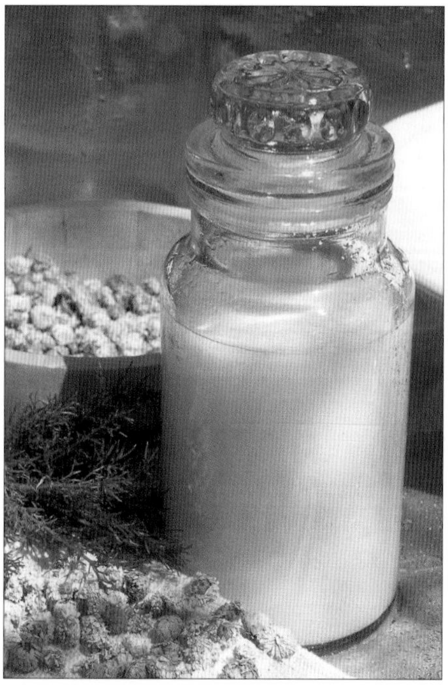

Above *Herbal shampoo has a gentle, less abrasive action than commercial shampoo.*

HAIR RESCUER

This rich, nourishing formula helps to improve the condition of dry and damaged hair.

Ingredients

Makes enough for 1 treatment

30ml/2 tbsp olive oil
30ml/2 tbsp light sesame oil
2 eggs
30ml/2 tbsp coconut milk
30ml/2 tbsp runny honey
5ml/1 tsp coconut oil

1 Combine all the ingredients together in a blender or food processor, until smooth.

2 Transfer to a bottle. Keep refrigerated and use within 3 days.

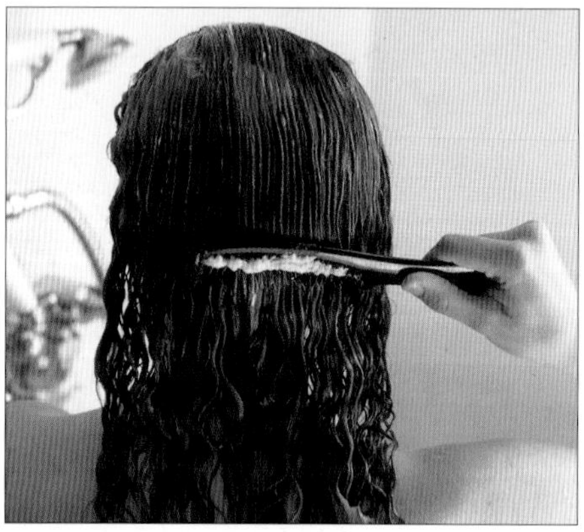

3 Comb the mixture through your hair after shampooing, leave for 5 minutes.

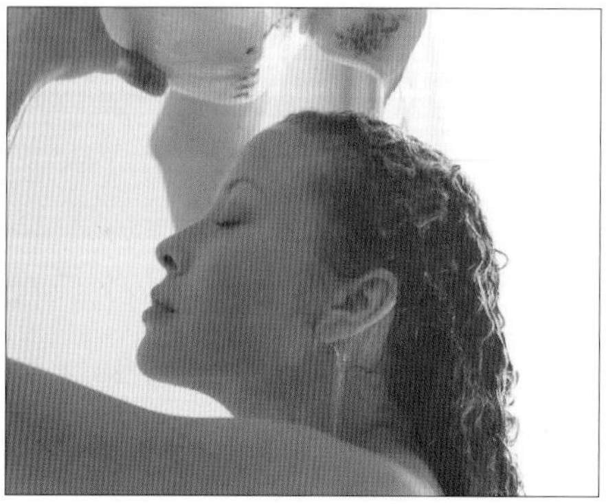

4 Rinse the hair with warm water and gently rub dry with a towel.

Conditioners and herbal rinses

The best way to keep hair looking glossy is to use a natural conditioner followed by a herbal rinse. Oil-based preparations need to be used before shampooing; lighter ones made of natural ingredients can be used after a shampoo and washed out with warm water and a herbal rinse. For dry to normal hair try a mixture of avocado and egg, for oily hair yogurt makes a good conditioner.

To revive dry or sun-damaged hair, an oil-based treatment, rich in essential oils, works best.

NETTLE RINSE FOR DANDRUFF

This herbal rinse helps to keep the hair shiny and in good condition. Make it freshly the evening before you wash your hair.

Ingredients

25g/1oz fresh nettle leaves (*Urtica dioica*)
25g/1oz nasturtium flowers and leaves
1 litre/1¾ pints/4 cups water
30ml/2 tbsp cider vinegar
30ml/2 tbsp distilled witch hazel

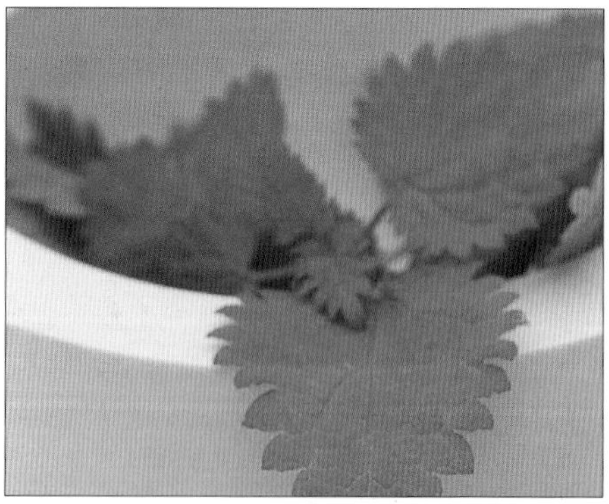

1 Put the nettles and nasturtium flowers and leaves in a heatproof bowl. Boil the water and pour it over the nettles and nasturtiums. (Nettles lose their sting in boiling water.)

2 Leave to stand overnight. Strain off the herbs and add the vinegar and witch hazel.

3 Hold your head over a portable bowl as you pour the rinse through your hair. Keep pouring the rinse from the bowl back into the pitcher and re-apply at six times.

CHAMOMILE RINSE FOR FAIR HAIR

Combined with cider vinegar, chamomile and rosemary have been used in hair rinses for hundreds of years. The herbs enhance hair colour and the vinegar is a wonderful scalp conditioner. Chamomile has long been favoured by blondes for their fair hair; although it does not bleach, it enhances the hair's natural colour.

Ingredients

Makes enough for 3 treatments

50g/2oz dried chamomile (*Chamaemelum nobile*) flowers
900ml/1 1/2 pints boiling water
50ml/2fl oz cider vinegar
5 drops chamomile essential oil

1 Put the chamomile flowers into a wide-necked jar and pour the water on top.

2 Seal the jar and leave to stand overnight. Strain the infusion repeatedly through muslin (cheesecloth) or paper coffee filters, until it is clear.

3 Add the cider vinegar and essential oil. Store in a stoppered glass bottle in the refrigerator and use within a week, as a final rinse when washing your hair.

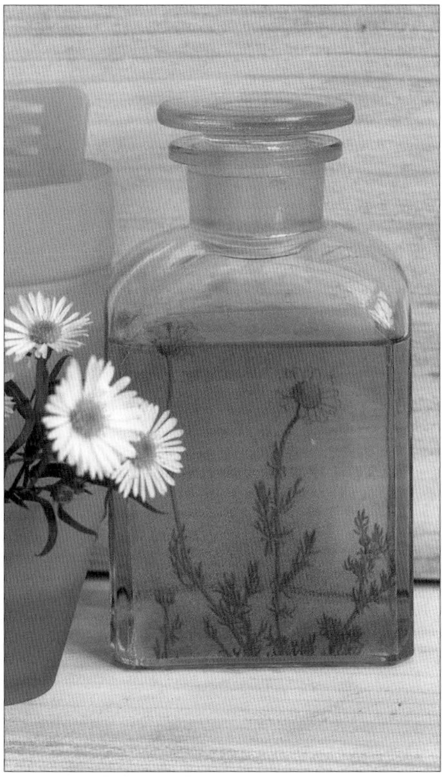

ROSEMARY RINSE FOR DARK HAIR

Fresh rosemary has a high essential oil content and is also beneficial for dry hair.

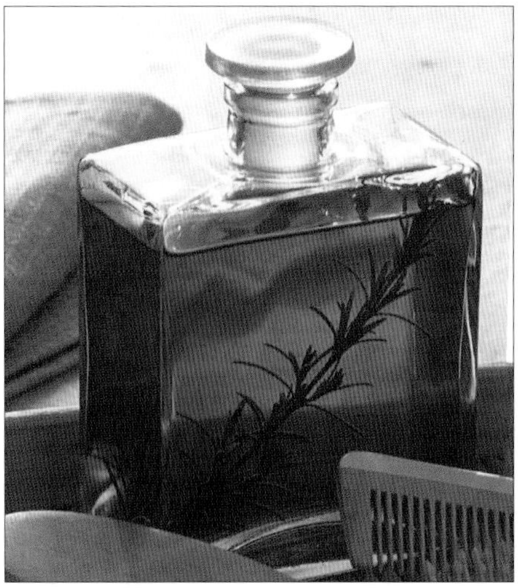

Ingredients

40g/1 1/2oz fresh rosemary (*Rosmarinus officinalis*)
1 litre/1 3/4 pints/4 cups boiling water
50ml/2fl oz cider vinegar

Make as for the chamomile rinse. Use frequently for shiny hair.

Below *Herbal rinses add gloss and shine.*

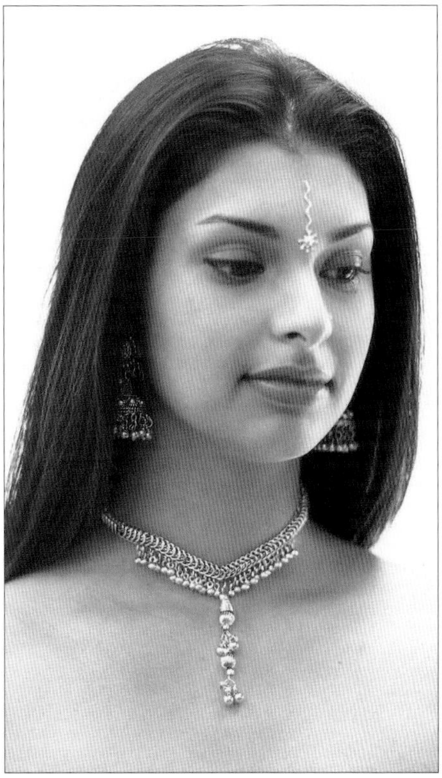

WARM OIL HAIR TREATMENT

Use this treatment once a month to improve the hair texture and to condition the scalp.

Ingredients

Makes enough for 5 treatments

90ml/6 tbsp coconut oil
3 drops rosemary essential oil
2 drops tea tree essential oil
2 drops lavender essential oil

1 Gently warm the coconut oil in a bowl over hot water until it melts, then mix in the rest of the ingredients.

2 Apply sparingly, while still warm, to dry hair; the head should not be saturated. Massage it in before covering your head with a hot towel for 20 minutes.

3 Shampoo as normal. Reheat the remaining oil for subsequent uses.

Below *The regular use of herbal conditioners gives hair a healthy gleam.*

Below far left *A chamomile rinse adds a sheen to fair hair. Herbal hair care is gentler on the scalp and will not cause the chemical build-up associated with commercial products.*

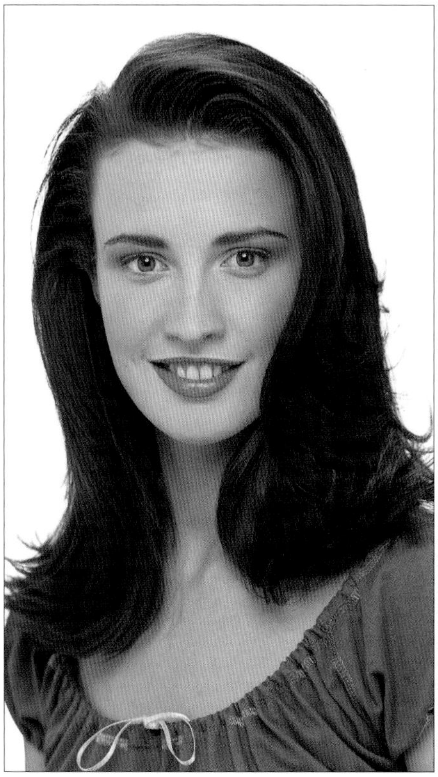

Facial Care

The most delicate skin on the body's surface is on the face, and caring for it will pay dividends in maintaining a fresh, clear complexion and slowing down the skin's ageing process. A healthy lifestyle and a nutritious diet are essential for good skin. Smoking, a bad diet, and too much sun are the skin's worst enemies. Otherwise, the old mantra of "cleanse, tone and moisturize" holds good, preferably using natural products based on herbs and flowers.

Cleansing

On a daily basis a gentle wash with mild soap and water is enough, with a fragrance-free cream to remove make-up, but for an occasional deep cleansing treatment, rosewater mixed with natural ingredients makes an effective cream or face mask.

Toning

Infusions of flowers and herbs make excellent skin toners. Apply with cotton wool (cotton balls) after removing a face mask or make-up, or use at any time to freshen the skin. These natural toners must be kept chilled and used up within a few days as they soon deteriorate.

Moisturizing

This is the most essential step for keeping skin young and healthy looking. A light cream that will not drag the skin is best.

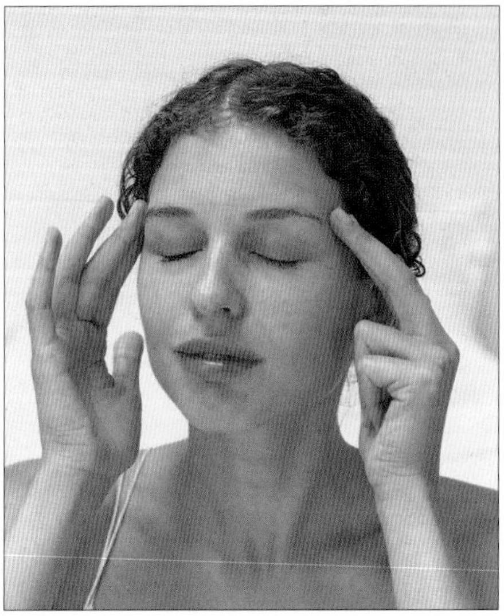

ROSE CREAM CLEANSER AND FACE MASK

A simple cleanser, with both soothing and cooling properties, can be made from rosewater and cream. The addition of honey and oatmeal transforms it into a nourishing face mask or an exfoliating scrub. The face mask is suitable for dry skin, but gentle enough for sensitive faces. Both the cleanser and the mask should be made in small quantities, kept in the refrigerator and used within 2 days.

Ingredients

For the cleanser
105ml/7tbsp triple-distilled rose water
45ml/3 tbsp double (heavy) cream

For the face mask
30ml/2 tbsp pure unblended clear honey
5ml/1tsp triple-distilled rosewater
45ml/3 tbsp double (heavy) cream
30ml/2 tbsp fine ground oatmeal

1 To make the cleanser, stir the rosewater and the double cream together until the mixture is well blended. Apply to the face on cotton wool (cotton balls).

2 To make the face mask, gently warm the honey, then mix in the rosewater and double cream. Add the oatmeal, stir well and leave for 10 minutes.

3 Smooth over the face and neck and leave on for 10 minutes before washing off very thoroughly. As with all masks, this is most effective if used while relaxing in a bath.

4 To use the mixture as a facial scrub, smooth it over the skin and then massage gently before washing off thoroughly.

Left *Simple preparations made with fresh flowers and used every day keep skin looking its best.*

Right *Dark red roses are best for colour. The toner on the left is made from fragrant "Ena Harkness", with elderflower tonic on the right.*

ROSE PETAL TONER FOR SENSITIVE SKIN

Any fragrant roses are suitable for this recipe, as long as they have not been sprayed with pesticide. Pink or red ones are best. Pick the flowers when they are fully open but have not started to fade, preferably in the morning.

Ingredients

40g/1½oz fresh rose petals
600ml/1 pint/2½ cups boiling water
15ml/1 tbsp cider vinegar

1 Put the rose petals in a bowl, pour over the boiling water and add the vinegar. Cover and leave to stand for 2 hours, then strain into a clean bottle.

2 Keep in the refrigerator or a cool place and use up within 2 days.

ELDERFLOWER TONER FOR DRY SKIN

This has a gentle non-astringent action suited to dry skin. Pick the flowers as soon as they open, and use them fresh or dried.

Ingredients

25g/1oz elderflowers
600ml/1 pint/2½ cups boiling water
15ml/1 tbsp cider vinegar

Make as for rose petal toner above.

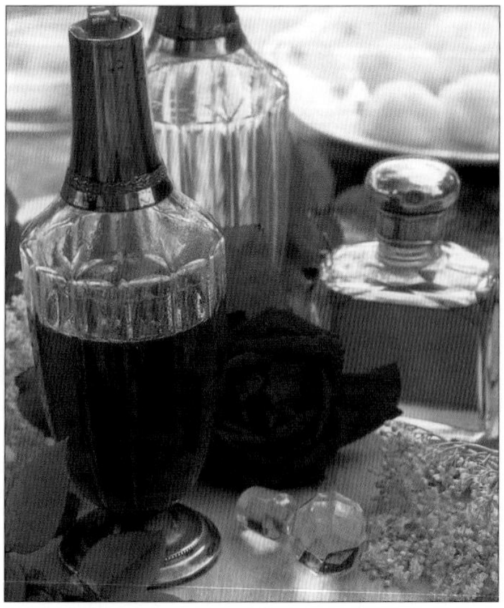

MARIGOLD TONING MILK FOR INFLAMED SKIN AND THREAD VEINS

Pot marigold flowers are soothing and healing. Thread veins are not going to disappear if you use this preparation, but its cooling action does help. Remember that sun, extremes of temperature and too much alcohol all make the condition worse.

Ingredients

6–8 fresh pot marigold (*Calendula officinalis*) flowers
300ml/½ pint/1¼ cups milk
3 drops tincture of benzoin
5ml/1 tsp infused calendula oil (not an essential oil)

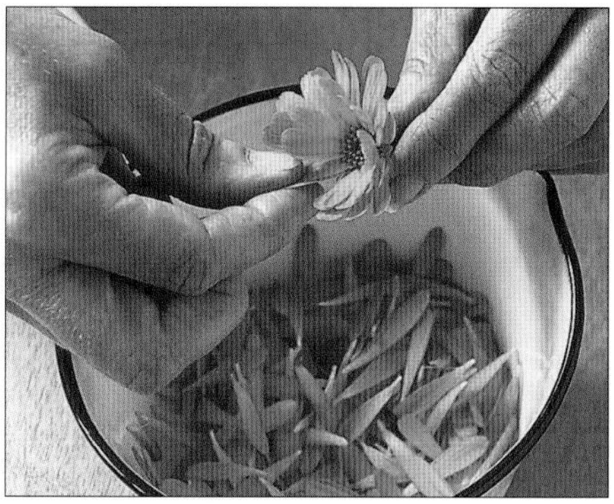

1 Pull the petals off the marigold flowerheads and put them in an enamel pan. Pour in the milk, cover and simmer gently for about 30 minutes.

2 Remove the pan from the heat and stir in the tincture of benzoin and the calendula oil. Leave until cool, then strain the mixture into a jug (pitcher).

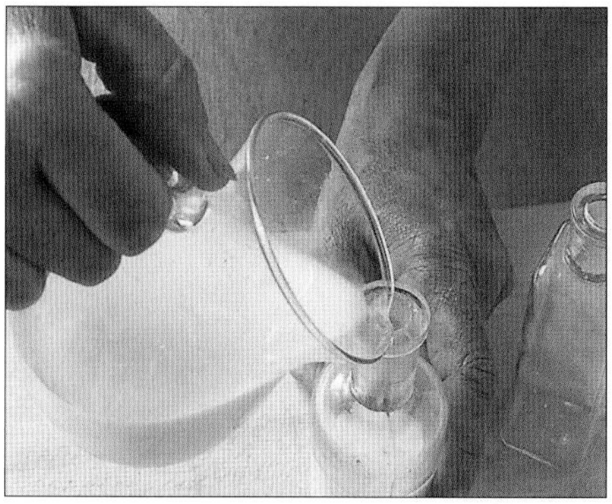

3 Pour the marigold milk into a glass bottle. Keep the lotion chilled and use within 3 days to soothe the skin.

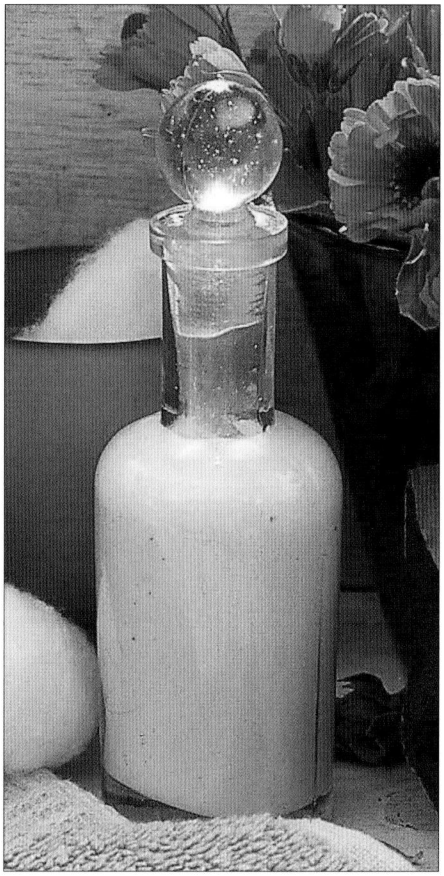

Above *Apply soothing marigold milk to the face with cotton wool (cotton balls).*

ELDERFLOWER MOISTURIZER

A moisturizing cream is a must to prevent dry skin. It will help to keep wrinkles at bay and protect the skin from wind and weather. Making your own moisturizer ensures the use of simple ingredients and herbs that will be gentle on your skin. This recipe includes elderflowers, which have a long-standing reputation for lightening the skin.

Ingredients

15g/½ oz dried elderflowers (*Sambucus nigra*)
600ml/1 pint/2½ cups boiling water
30ml/2 tbsp emulsifying ointment
5ml/1 tsp beeswax
30ml/2 tbsp almond oil
2.5ml/½ tsp borax

Right *Elderflower moisturizer is a must for keeping skin soft and wrinkles at bay. The flowers are musk-scented and abundant in early summer.*

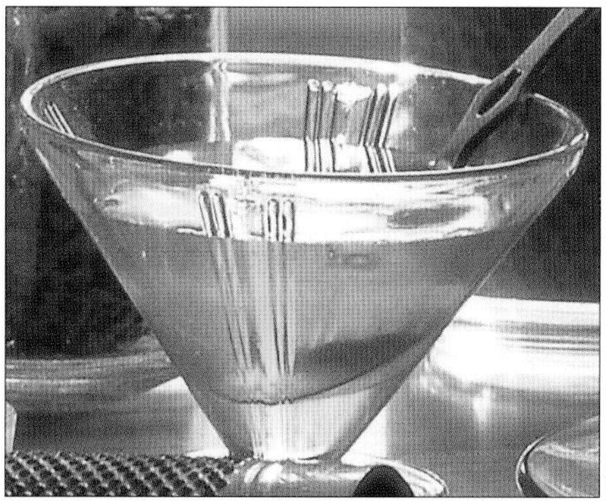

1 Make the elderflower infusion by pouring the boiling water over the elderflowers. Leave to stand for 30 minutes, then strain. You will need 120ml/4fl oz/½ cup.

2 Put the emulsifying ointment, beeswax and almond oil into a bowl, and the elderflower infusion and borax into another. Set both over hot water and stir until the oils are melted and the borax is dissolved.

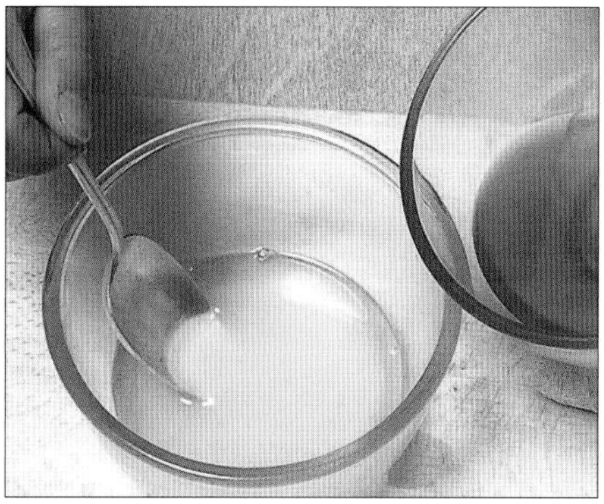

3 Mix the liquids together. Leave to cool, stirring at intervals, until it starts to set. Pour into a jar and keep for up to 2 months.

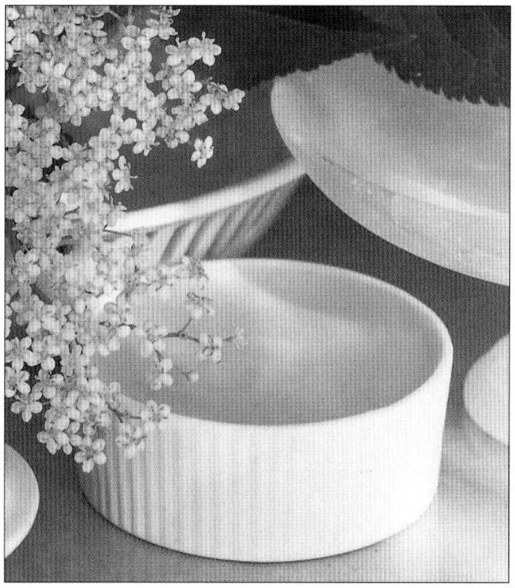

Eyes and Lips

The skin around the eyes is the most delicate on the face and the first to show signs of tiredness or stress. Eye creams can make matters worse, especially if their texture is too heavy; there is also a tendency to drag the skin when applying them. Simple herbal compresses are the best way to revive and revitalize tired eyes, and the relaxation involved in lying down with the eyes closed and gently covered is a bonus.

CHAMOMILE COMPRESS

This is a tried and tested treatment for tired eyes. Although it can be done using herbal teabags, if you have time it is worth making the compresses from muslin (cheesecloth) and whole chamomile flowers rather than the more powdery mix that often goes into teabags. Whether you are using cloth bags or teabags, cover them with boiling water, leave them to cool, then put them in the refrigerator to get cold. Lie down for 20 minutes with the compresses over the eyes.

Ingredients

5g/⅕oz chamomile (*Chamaemelum nobile*) flowers
2 x 15cm/6in square unbleached muslin
20cm/8in fine ribbon or string.

Place a handful of chamomile flowers in the centre of each muslin square. Gather the muslin into a bundle and tie it with ribbon or string.

Below *A compress made with chamomile flowers is restful for tired eyes.*

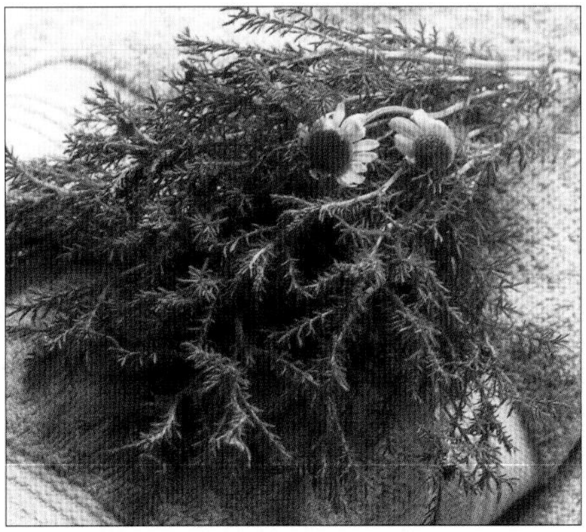

LAVENDER LIP BALM

It is quite simple to make your own soothing cream for lips chapped by weather or illness. Beeswax and cocoa butter are rich emollients; wheatgerm oil, with its high vitamin E content, is a powerful antioxidant and lavender essential oil is well known for its healing ability. You can also apply a simple mixture of honey and rosewater as a salve for sore or chapped lips.

Ingredients

5ml/1 tsp beeswax
5ml/1 tsp cocoa butter
5ml/1 tsp wheatgerm oil
5ml/1 tsp almond oil
3 drops lavender essential oil

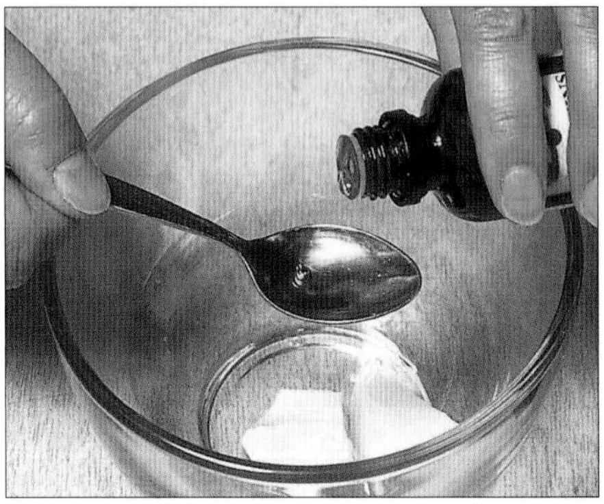

1 Put the beeswax into a small bowl and add the cocoa butter, wheatgerm oil and almond oil. Set the bowl over a pan of simmering water.

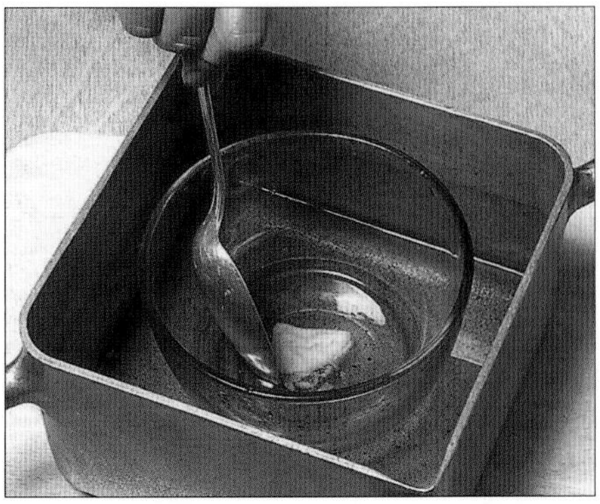

2 Stir the mixture constantly until the beeswax has melted.

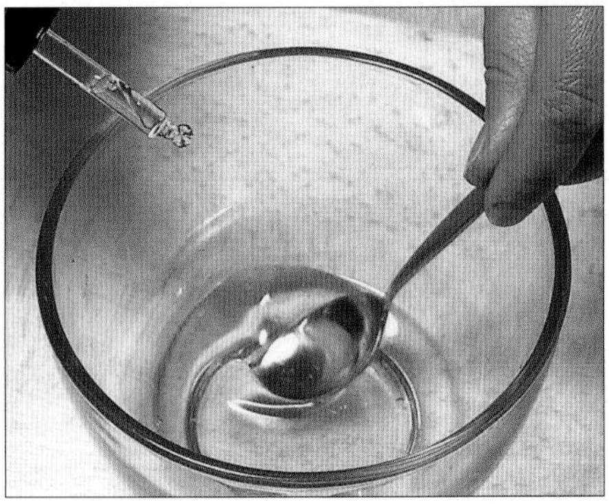

3 Remove the bowl from the heat and allow the mixture to cool for a few minutes before mixing in the lavender oil. Pour into a small jar and leave to set.

Below *Lavender lip balm is rich and soothing with a pleasant scent.*

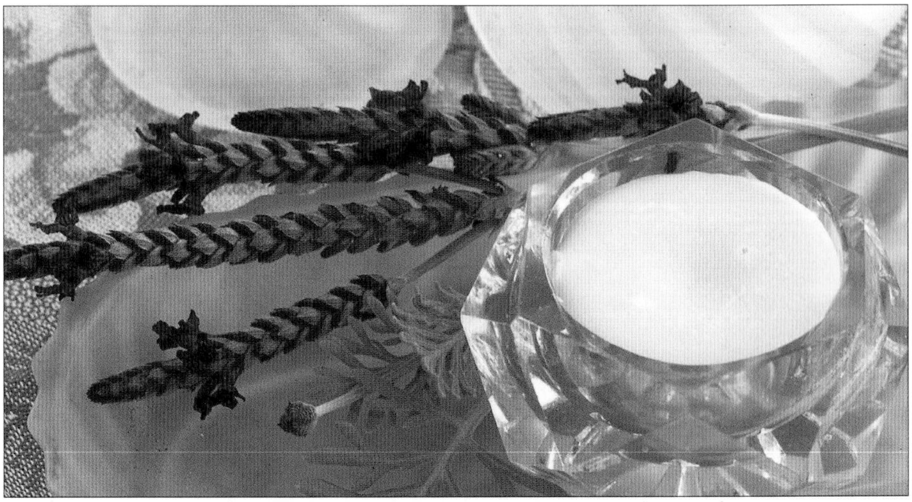

Teeth and Fresh Breath

Herbs can be used in many ways to keep the breath fresh and the teeth clean. Although you may not wish to use a herbal tooth powder all the time, it does provide a viable, natural alternative to manufactured products, which may contain a long list of synthetic chemical ingredients.

Simple teeth cleansers

- **Sage** (*Salvia officinalis*) – Rub teeth with fresh sage leaves.
- **Lemon peel** – Pare the peel off the fruit and rub over the teeth to remove stains.

Simple breath fresheners

- **Parsley, watercress, mint** – Chew the fresh leaves after eating a garlicky meal.
- **Whole spices** – Suck or chew fennel seeds, star anise, angelica, caraway, calamus root, cinnamon stick, or cloves after a meal.
- **Rosewater** – Dilute half-and-half with water for rinsing the mouth.
- **Lavender infusion** – Infuse 15ml/1 tbsp dried lavender (*Lavandula*) in 300ml/½ pint/1¼ cups water and use as an oral rinse.

Below *Keep the teeth clean and the breath fresh with natural cleansers and rinses.*

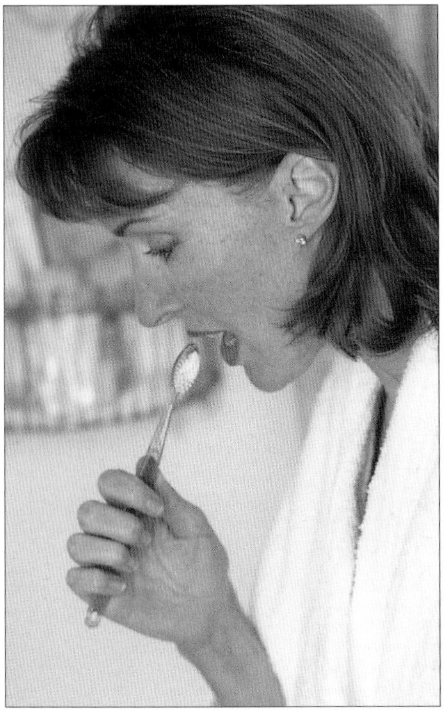

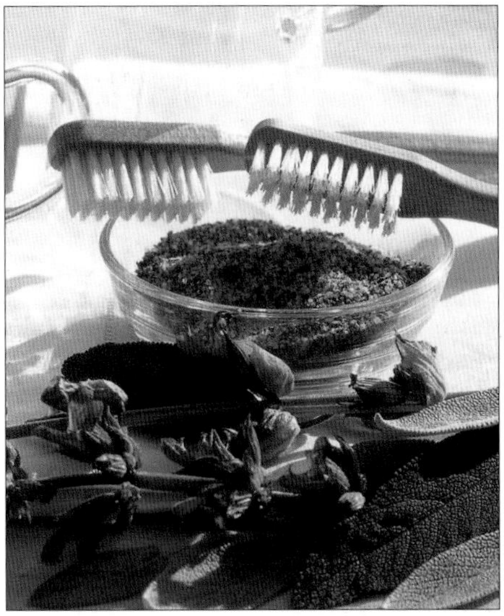

Above *Powdered sage and salt make a traditional mixture for cleaning the teeth.*

SAGE AND SALT TOOTH POWDER

The cleansing action of sage and salt will make your mouth tingle. Rinse your mouth well with plenty of fresh water after using this tooth powder. For a milder effect, substitute 15ml/1 tbsp orris root powder for the salt.

Ingredients

25g/1oz fresh sage (*Salvia officinalis*) leaves
60ml/4 tbsp sea salt

1 With a pair of scissors, snip the sage leaves into an ovenproof dish.

2 Mix in the salt, grinding it into the leaves with a wooden spoon or pestle. Bake the mixture in a very low oven for about 1 hour, until the sage is dry and crisp.

3 Pound the mixture again until it is reduced to a powder. Keep in a jar in the bathroom and use on a dampened toothbrush instead of toothpaste.

Right *Consider incorporating herbal ingredients into a chemical-free range of toiletries. Such products are now more widely available in health food stores and larger supermarkets.*

SPICED LEMON VERBENA MOUTHWASH

Commercial antiseptic mouthwashes can upset the natural acid balance of the mouth. A herbal mouthwash is gentler and this one – which is made with tangy lemon verbena – is particularly pleasant to use.

Ingredients

5ml/1 tsp each ground nutmeg (*Myristica fragrans*), ground cloves, cardamom pods and caraway seeds
small handful fresh lemon verbena leaves (*Aloysia triphylla*) or 15g/½oz dried lemon verbena
600ml/1 pint/2½ cups purified water
30ml/2 tbsp sweet sherry

1 Put the spices and lemon verbena into a pan with the water. Bring to the boil and simmer for 30 minutes.

2 Strain through a sieve lined with kitchen paper, then add the sherry and pour into a clean bottle.

3 To use, dilute 15–30ml/1–2 tbsp in a tumbler of water.

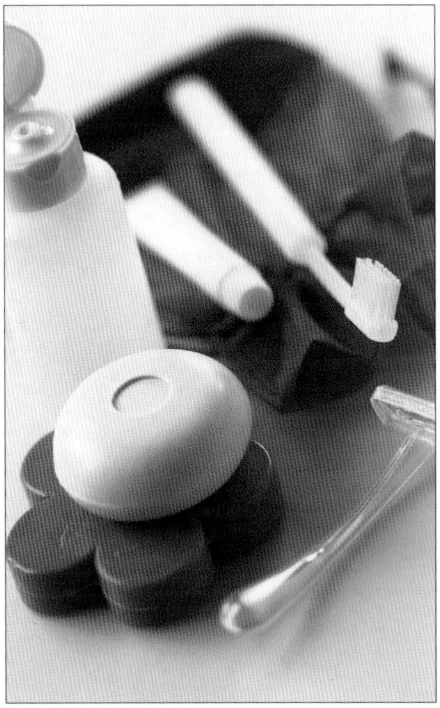

Hands and Nails

The demands of daily living, from gardening to home maintenance and domestic chores, can all take their toll on the hands and nails. Exposure to cold wind and weather is also hard on the hands. To keep them looking their best, a weekly manicure incorporating a toning hand mask and gentle massage will make all the difference: lightly press and squeeze the base of each hand with the other one, and pull and stretch the fingers.

Use a herbal hand cream regularly to keep the skin soft. When making the rose hand cream you can leave out the lanolin if you are likely to have an allergic reaction to it. Roses are ideal ingredients for their fragrance and gentle action.

ROSE GERANIUM NAIL OIL

Massaging the base of your nails every day will encourage healthy growth. You can also use this oil as part of a manicure.

Ingredients

50ml/2fl oz/¼ cup almond oil
10ml/2 tsp apricot kernel oil
5 drops geranium essential oil
2 drops rose essential oil

1 Mix all the ingredients together in a small bowl.

2 Clean the nails thoroughly then soak them for at least 10 minutes in the solution. Massage the cuticles at the same time.

ROSE HAND MASK

This is a good way to restore the tone and texture of the skin – and using it also forces you to relax for 15 minutes. Smooth on some rose hand cream afterwards.

Ingredients

45ml/3 tbsp medium or fine oatmeal
30ml/2 tbsp rose infusion or triple-distilled rosewater
5ml/1 tsp almond oil
5ml/1 tsp lemon juice
5ml/1 tsp glycerine

1 Mix all the ingredients together to form a soft paste. You may need to add a little extra rose infusion or rosewater if the mixture seems too stiff.

2 Spread the mask all over the backs of the hands and the fingers. Leave it in place for 15 minutes.

3 Rinse off the hand mask in warm water to leave hands feeling soft and smooth. (Oatmeal has a mildly exfoliating action.)

Below *An infusion of rose petals makes a fragrant addition to a hand mask.*

Below left *Keep nails in tip top condition with a herbal essential oil treatment.*

Below right *This fragrant cream is nourishing.*

ROSE HAND CREAM

This fragrant hand cream is rich in nourishing oils and waxes. Two bowls of thin clear liquids, when combined together, miraculously produce a rich, thick mixture that has the consistency of cream cheese.

Ingredients

50ml/2fl oz/¼ cup rosewater
45ml/3 tbsp distilled witch hazel
2.5ml/½ tsp glycerine
1.5ml/¼ tsp borax
30ml/2 tbsp emulsifying ointment or beeswax
5ml/1 tsp lanolin
30ml/2 tbsp almond oil
2 drops rose essential oil

1 Gently heat the rosewater, witch hazel, glycerine and borax in a small pan until the borax has dissolved. In a double boiler melt the wax, lanolin and almond oil over a gentle heat.

2 Slowly add the rosewater mixture to the oil mixture, stirring constantly as you do so. It will quickly turn milky and thicken.

3 Remove from the heat and continue to stir while it cools, then add the rose essential oil.

4 Pour the cream into china or glass pots and store in a cool place. It will keep for up to two months if carefully stored.

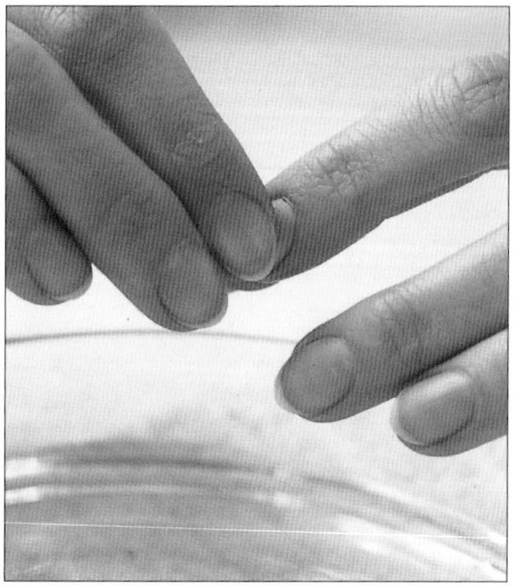

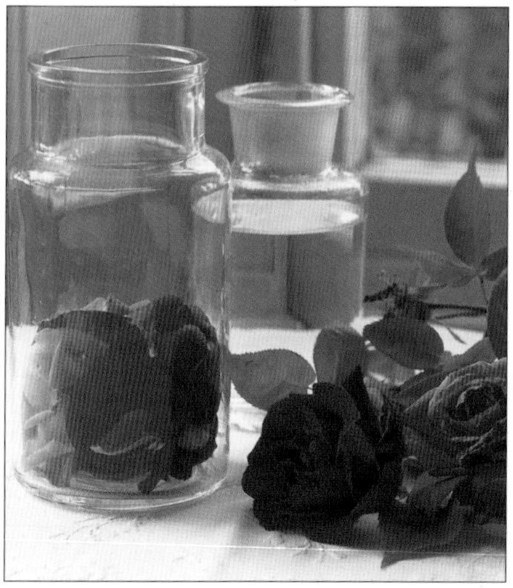

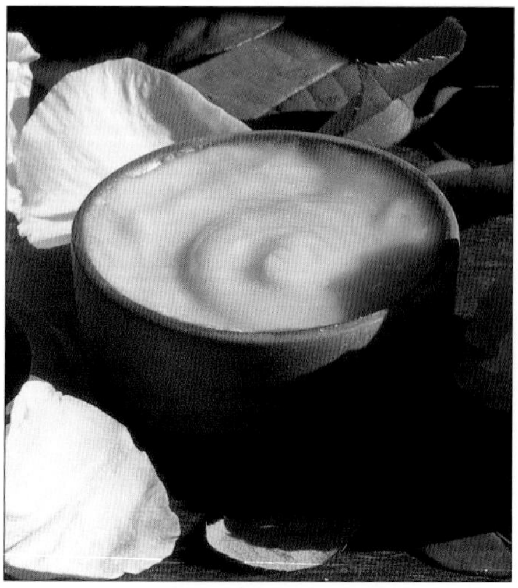

Foot Treatments

While the hands tend to suffer from damage caused by overuse and daily chores, the feet are more likely to suffer from general neglect. We take them completely for granted (until they let us down) and seldom pamper and look after them the way we do the rest of the body. But if your feet feel good, it will be reflected in the whole of your face and body, so time spent caring for them will be amply rewarded.

LEMON VERBENA AND LAVENDER FOOT BATH

This fragrant foot bath is ideal for tired, aching feet. Use it before you go to bed to help you unwind and relax.

Ingredients

15g/½ oz dried lemon verbena (*Aloysia triphylla*)
30ml/2 tbsp dried lavender (*Lavandula* spp)
5 drops lavender essential oil
30ml/2 tbsp cider vinegar

1 Put the lemon verbena and lavender in a basin and pour in enough hot water to cover the feet.

2 Allow to cool, then add the lavender oil and cider vinegar. Soak the feet for 10–15 minutes, then dry them thoroughly.

Below *Massage the feet regularly with plenty of nourishing cream to keep the skin supple.*

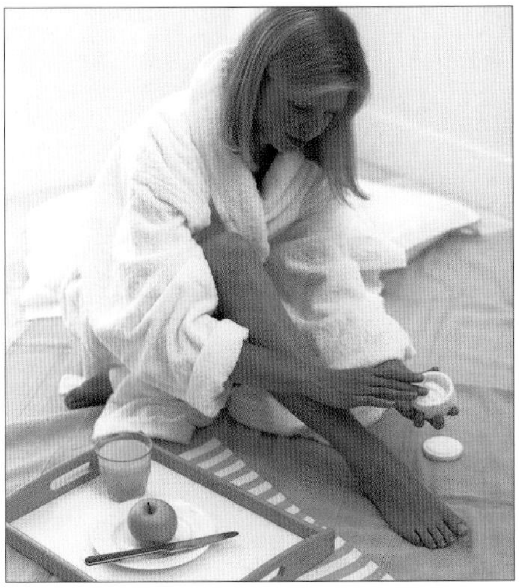

HERBAL FOOT BATH FOR ACHING FEET

There is nothing like a fragrant foot bath for refreshing tired feet. At the same time, it revitalizes the whole being, its warmth relaxes the body and the scent of the herbs calms the mind. Foot baths are comforting if you have a cold and, with the right herbs, they can help fight fungal infection.

Ingredients

50g/2oz mixed fresh herbs: peppermint (*Mentha x piperita*), yarrow (*Achillea millefolium*), pine needles, chamomile (*Chamaemelum nobile*) flowers, rosemary (*Rosmarinus officinalis*), houseleek (*Sempervivum tectorum*)
1 litre/1¾ pints/4 cups boiling water
15ml/1 tbsp borax
15ml/1 tbsp Epsom salts

1 Roughly chop the herbs, put them in a large bowl and pour in the boiling water. Leave to stand for 1 hour.

2 Strain, and add the liquid to a basin containing about 1.75 litre/3 pints/7½ cups hot water – the final temperature of the foot bath should be comfortably warm.

3 Stir in the borax and Epsom salts. Immerse the feet and soak for 15–20 minutes. Pat dry and rub in some foot cream.

Below *A foot bath revitalizes the whole body.*

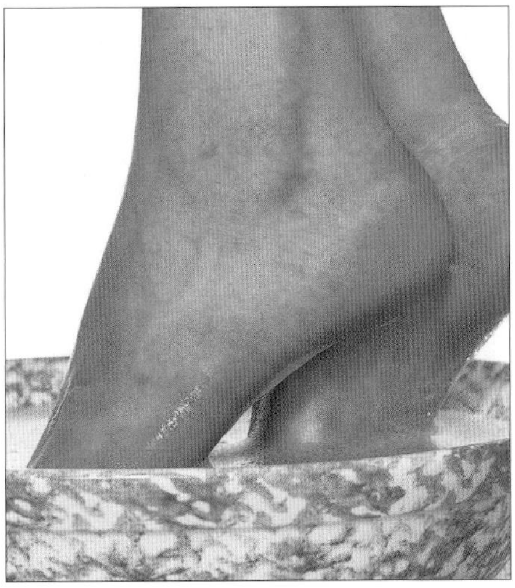

TEA TREE FOOT CREAM

One of the best essential oils to incorporate in a foot cream is tea tree. It has healing, antiseptic properties and also has a fungicidal action, which will protect the feet from the various unpleasant foot complaints that can be picked up at the pool or gym.

Although most creams and lotions are best stored in glass or ceramic containers, in this case it is sensible and practical to keep the lotion in a pump-action plastic bottle, which makes it much easier to use.

Ingredients

120ml/4fl oz unscented hand cream
15 drops tea tree essential oil

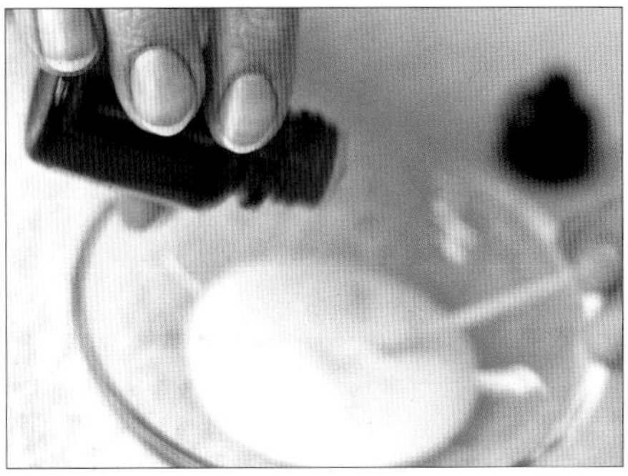

Put the hand cream in a bowl. Stir in the essential oil. Massage the cream into clean, dry feet.

Below *Tea tree oil has antiseptic properties to help keep feet free from infections.*

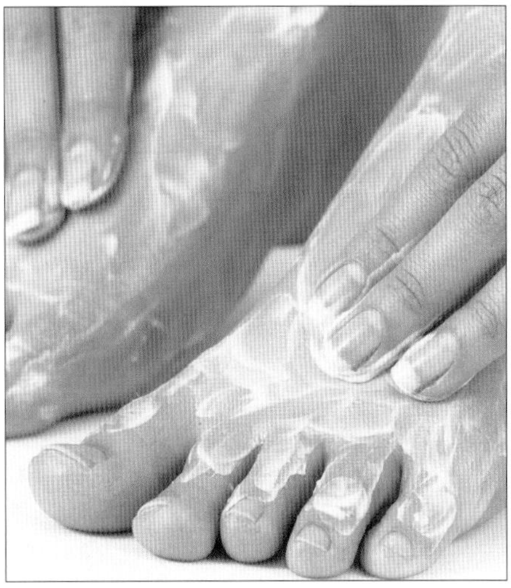

Skin Treatments

The lavish use of a body lotion after a daily bath or shower will help prevent skin drying out and losing its elasticity. Making your own is not difficult and the simple ingredients, flower waters and floral essential oils are nourishing and revitalizing. Both the recipes given here make lotions that will keep for up to 2 months if stored in sealed jars in a cool, dark place.

COCONUT AND ORANGEFLOWER BODY LOTION

This creamy preparation is wonderfully nourishing for dry skin. It is solid at room temperature but melts when lukewarm.

Ingredients

50g/2oz coconut oil
60ml/4 tbsp sunflower oil
10ml/2 tsp wheatgerm oil
10 drops orangeflower essence

1 Put the coconut oil in a bowl over a pan of gently simmering water. Once it has melted, stir in the sunflower and wheatgerm oils.

2 Leave to cool, then add the orangeflower essence and pour into a jar. It will solidify after several hours.

Below *Wheatgerm oil is rich in vitamin E, which protects skin cells against premature aging. Coconut oil is rich and moisturizing.*

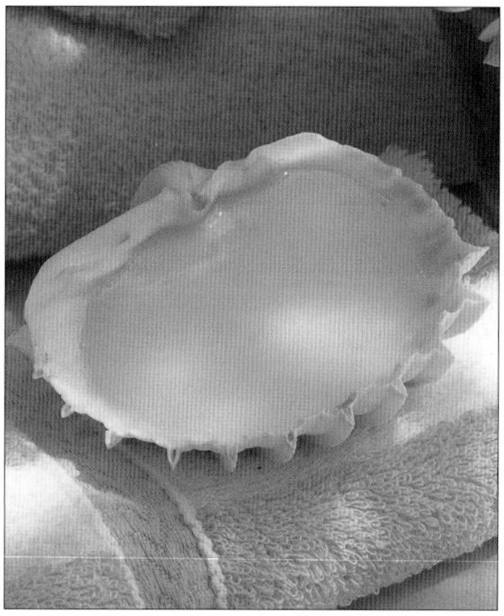

ROSE BODY LOTION

This recipe gives a rich, creamy lotion. If you prefer a runnier, more liquid texture, increase the amount of water in the mixture by 30ml/2 tbsp.

Ingredients

45ml/3 tbsp hot, recently boiled water
2.5ml/½ tsp borax
5ml/1 tsp beeswax
30ml/2 tbsp emulsifying ointment
25ml/5 tsp apricot kernel oil
20ml/4 tsp cold-pressed sunflower oil
10 drops rose essential oil

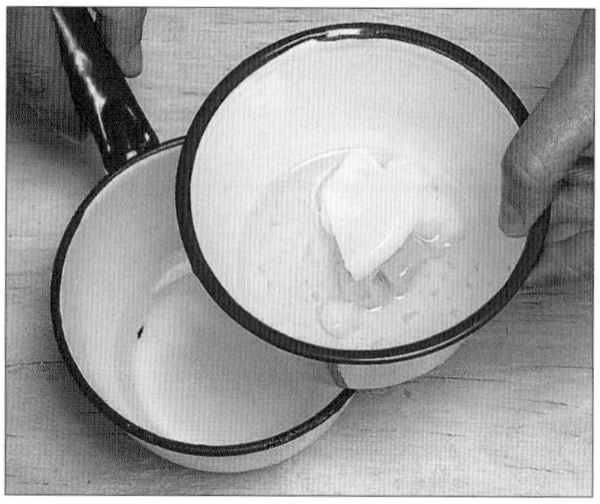

1 Dissolve the borax in the boiled water. Melt the beeswax and emulsifying ointment with the apricot kernel and sunflower oils in a double boiler (or in a bowl set over a pan of simmering water). Remove from the heat once the wax has melted and stir well.

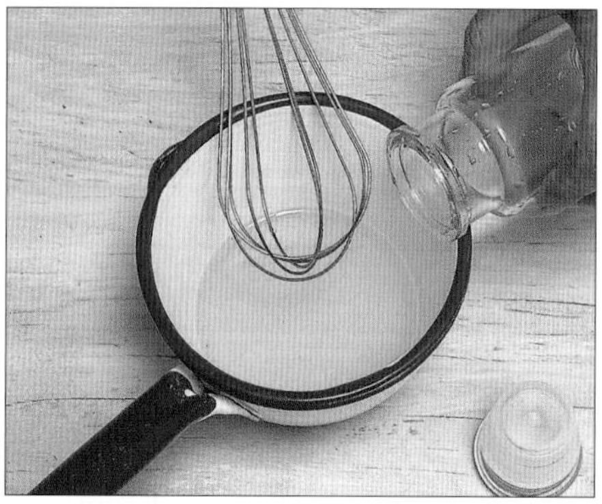

2 Add the borax solution, whisking as you do so. Keep whisking until it cools, then add the rose oil. Pour the lotion into a tinted glass jar, seal and store in a cool place.

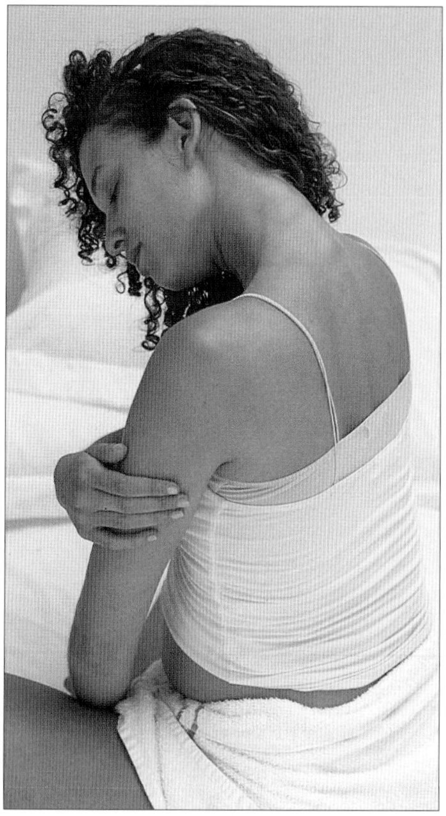

Above *Smoothing on body lotion after a bath or shower moisturizes dry skin and softens rough patches.*

Below *A rose-scented body lotion is ideal for sensitive skins. Make a double quantity, keeping some for yourself to use regularly and some to give away.*

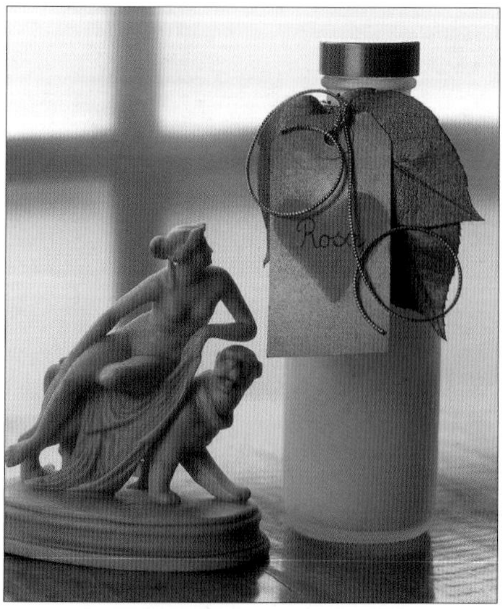

Dusting powder

There is a tendency to think of dusting powders as being the province of bathed babies and elderly ladies, but this needn't be so. A talcum powder, dusted all over the body, is a wonderful way to coat the body with fragrance.

Dusting powders can be made from scratch or you can use unscented talc as a base. Either way you will be able to formulate a scented powder quite different from commercial talcum powders. Dusting powders look wonderful in shallow bowls on a dressing table accompanied by a pretty powder puff.

Single fragrance dusting powders

These dusting powders are the simplest of all to make, especially if your base is ready-made unscented talcum powder. For each 75ml/5 tbsp talc you will need 15ml/1 tbsp cornflour (cornstarch), scented with 5 drops of your favourite essential oil. Fragrance is so personal that you will need to decide for yourself the properties of the different oils, but it is generally accepted that jasmine sets the scene for seduction, roses are romantic and peppermint or lemon are good to use after vigorous exercise at the gym.

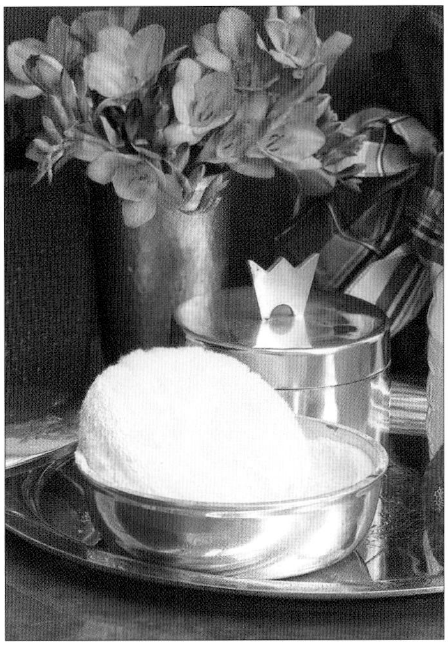

Left *Fragrant dusting powder makes the skin feel wonderfully soft and smooth.*

LUSCIOUS LAVENDER BODY POWDER

A soft blend of lavender, coriander and geranium, with a hint of fresh lemon, gives this body powder a delightful fragrance. Use it after your evening bath or shower or when you've been to the gym. The fragrance is better absorbed when the skin is slightly damp and the pores are open. Apply with a powder puff or cotton wool (cotton balls).

Ingredients

60ml/4 tbsp white kaolin clay (available from pharmacies) mixed with 60ml/4 tbsp arrowroot and 60ml/4 tbsp cornflour (cornstarch) or 180ml/12tbsp unscented talc
15ml/1 tbsp cornflour
3 drops lavender essential oil
3 drops coriander essential oil
3 drops lemon essential oil
3 drops geranium essential oil

1 Mix together the kaolin clay, arrowroot and cornflour (cornstarch) in a deep bowl, or put the unscented talc in the bowl.

2 Put the 15ml/1 tbsp of cornflour into a separate bowl and add the essential oils. Stir thoroughly.

3 Add the scented cornflour to the larger bowl and mix together thoroughly. Decant into a container.

Below *Lavender body powder has a delicious, light fragrance.*

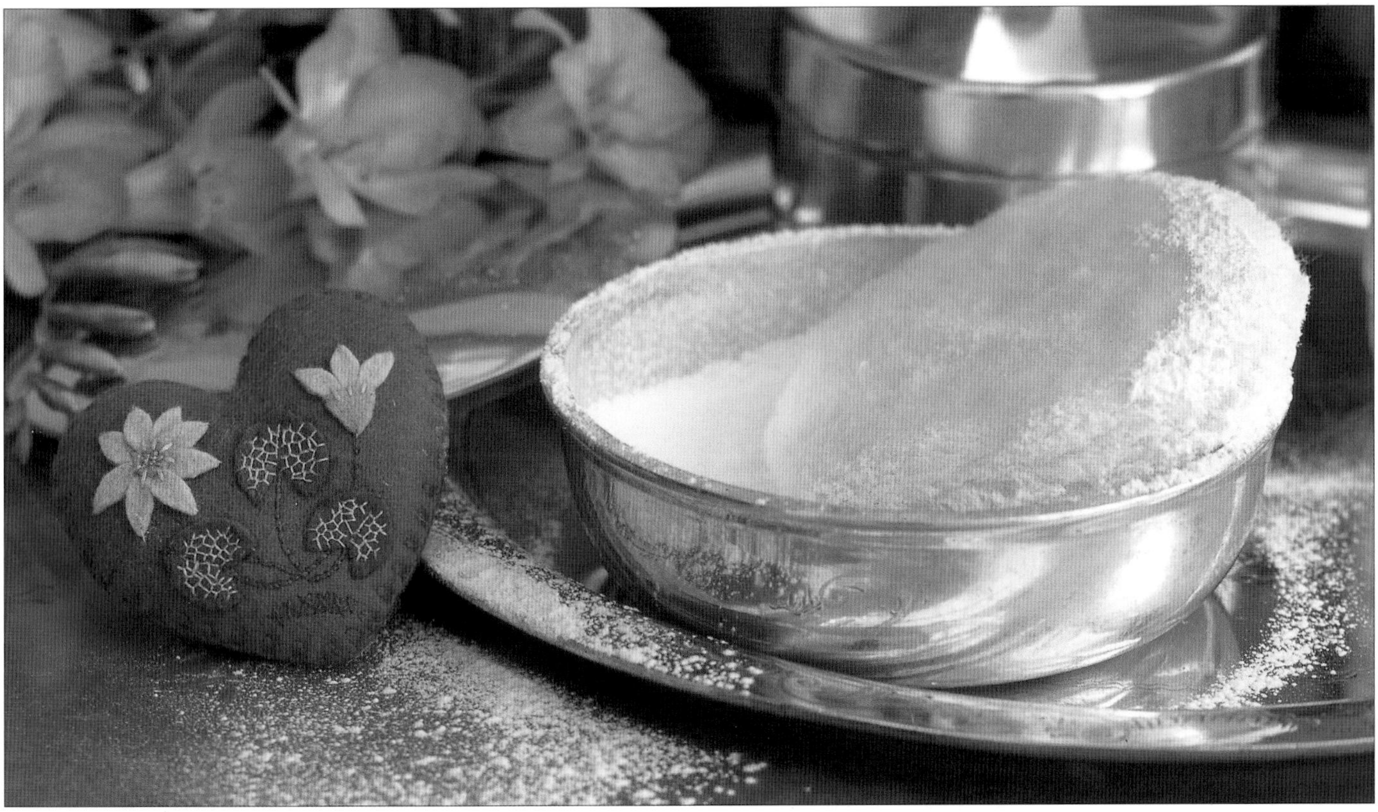

Bathing

Herbal baths provide the ideal way to relax the mind and body, to revive and restore the system. Instead of putting fresh herbs into bath bags, essential oils can be added directly to the water. The occasional use of an exfoliating body scrub will leave skin revitalized and a milk and honey bath oil restores vital nourishment. As a final touch, making your own soap provides the opportunity to incorporate ingredients to suit individual likes and needs.

Below *Taking time out to relax in a warm bath is beneficial for mind and body.*

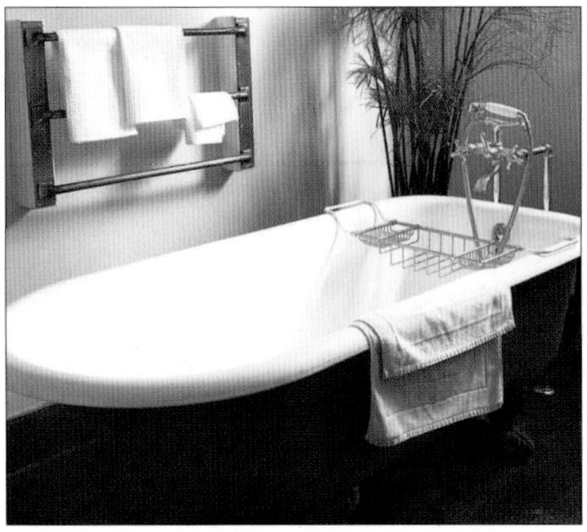

MILK AND HONEY BATH OIL WITH ROSEMARY

Milk is well known for its cleansing and lubricating qualities when applied to the skin. The addition of a little shampoo makes this a dispersing oil, so it does not leave a greasy rim around the bath.

Ingredients

2 eggs
45ml/3 tbsp rosemary herb oil
10ml/2 tsp honey
10ml/2 tsp baby shampoo
15ml/1 tbsp vodka
150ml/¼ pint/⅔ cup milk

1 Beat the eggs and oil together, then add the other ingredients and mix thoroughly. Pour into a clean glass bottle.

2 Add 30–45ml/2–3 tbsp to the bath and keep the rest chilled. Use within 2 days.

Essential oils in the bath

Add 5–6 drops essential oil straight from the bottle directly into a full bath. Do not add while the water is still running as the oil will evaporate too quickly and be wasted. Alternatively, mix two or three essential oils together in a base of sweet almond oil or jojoba oil. Then add 20 drops of the mixed oil to the bath. The quantities given are for a 50ml bottle of base oil.

- **Anti-stress mix**: 10 drops each marjoram, lavender and sandalwood.
- **Invigorating mix**: 5 drops rosemary, 5 drops camphor, 10 drops peppermint.

Stimulating scrubs

Face and body scrubs are increasingly popular as part of a beauty regime. The slightly rough texture of the scrub will efficiently exfoliate and stimulate the skin, leaving it clean and soft and ready for moisturizing. It is also a good idea to exfoliate before applying tanning lotion. Used at any time of the year but especially in the dark, cold months when the body never sees the sun, a scrub will remove dead skin and tone the skin, leaving it looking revitalized, but it should not be used too often, especially on sensitive skins.

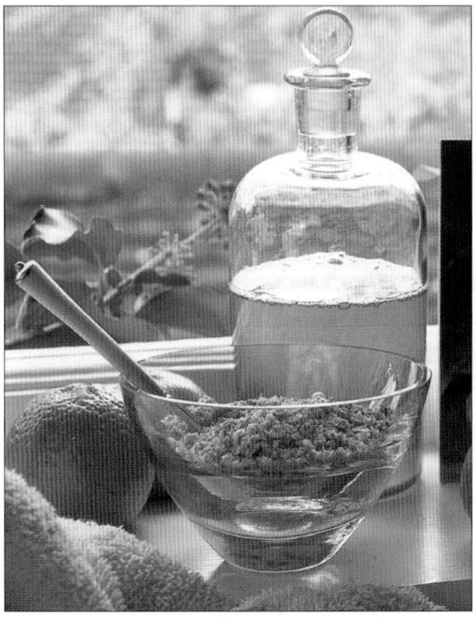

Above *Regular use of a rough-textured body scrub invigorates and smooths the skin.*

CITRUS BODY SCRUB

The slightly gritty texture of this exfoliating scrub provided by ground sunflower seeds, oatmeal, sea salt and orange peel helps to remove dead skin cells and stimulates the blood supply to the skin, leaving you tingling and toned. The combination of the aromatic orange peel and the grapefruit oil gives it a fresh scent.

Ingredients

Makes enough for 5 treatments
45ml/3 tbsp freshly ground sunflower seeds
45ml/3 tbsp medium oatmeal
45ml/3 tbsp flaked sea salt
45ml/3 tbsp finely grated orange peel
3 drops grapefruit essential oil
almond oil, to mix

1 Thoroughly mix all the ingredients except the almond oil and store in a sealed glass jar.

2 Mix to a paste with almond oil before using. Rub over the body, paying particular attention to areas of hard, dry skin such as the elbows, knees and ankles.

3 Remove the residue before showering or bathing.

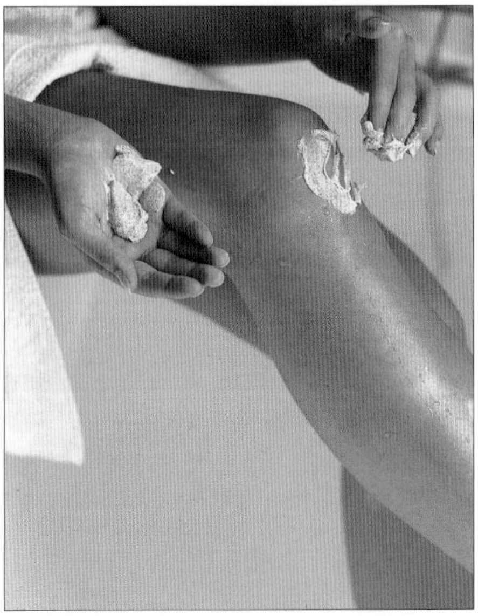

Above *Knees and elbows are prone to dryness so use this body scrub to treat those areas.*

LEMONGRASS SOAP

The toning and antiseptic qualities of lemongrass not only help relieve oily skin and acne, but can also help tighten up post-pregnancy or post-diet skin. Use the soap within a month.

Ingredients

Makes 2 bars

150g/5oz unscented soap (preferably made with vegetable oils)

12 drops lemon grass essential oil

1 Using the finest side of a cheese grater, grate the soap into a bowl.

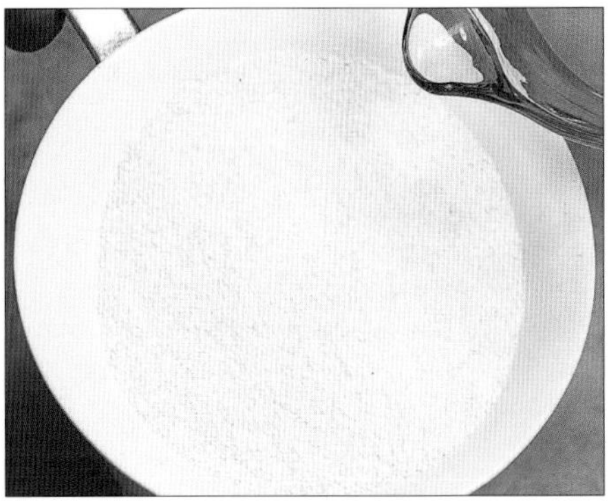

2 Add water to the bowl in the proportion of one part water to two parts soap.

3 Put the bowl over a pan of simmering water and heat the mixture gently, stirring continuously, until it coalesces. You will see this happening slowly and the soap will become thicker, gradually getting harder to stir. Remove the pan from the heat.

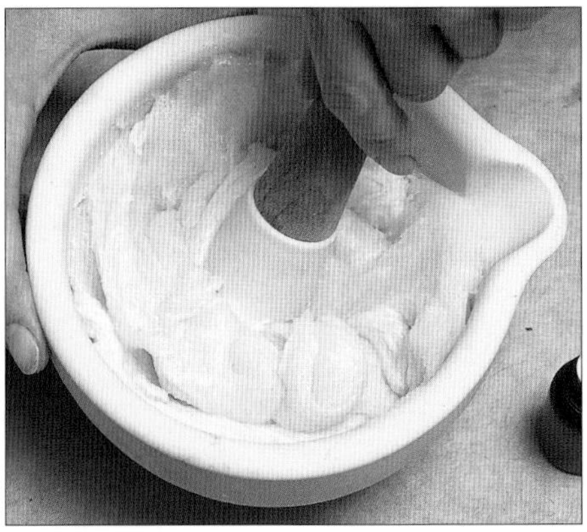

4 Tip the soap into a pestle and mortar and add the lemongrass oil. Mix well to distribute the oil.

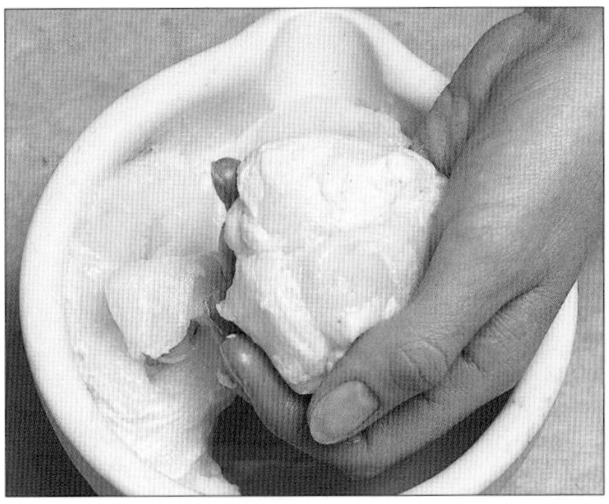

5 With wet hands, take about half the soap and work into a bar.

6 Repeat to make another bar. Leave on a wooden board to dry out and set hard. This may take a couple of days.

Below *For a calming bath, add a handful of neroli-scented calming milk bath mixture and wash with soaps made with pure vegetable oils because they are the kindest to the skin. Lemon grass root is toning and antiseptic in action.*

CALMING MILK BATH MIXTURE

Chamomile and neroli both have many valuable properties, essentially to soothe and calm. Chamomile is a wonderfully gentle herb, used to settle upset stomachs and to treat insomnia; it is also used in beauty preparations to pacify sensitive skin. Neroli oil comes from the flowers of the Seville orange tree and is known to relieve depression, anxiety and insomnia. Add this soothing mixture to a running bath and allow a traditional remedy to soak away the cares of everyday life.

Ingredients

120ml/4fl oz/½ cup fine sea salt

240ml/8fl oz/1 cup powdered milk

6 drops chamomile essential oil

12 drops neroli essential oil

Mix the sea salt, powdered milk and essential oils well. Place in a covered container and leave for 3 weeks for the oils to permeate the ingredients before adding to the bath.

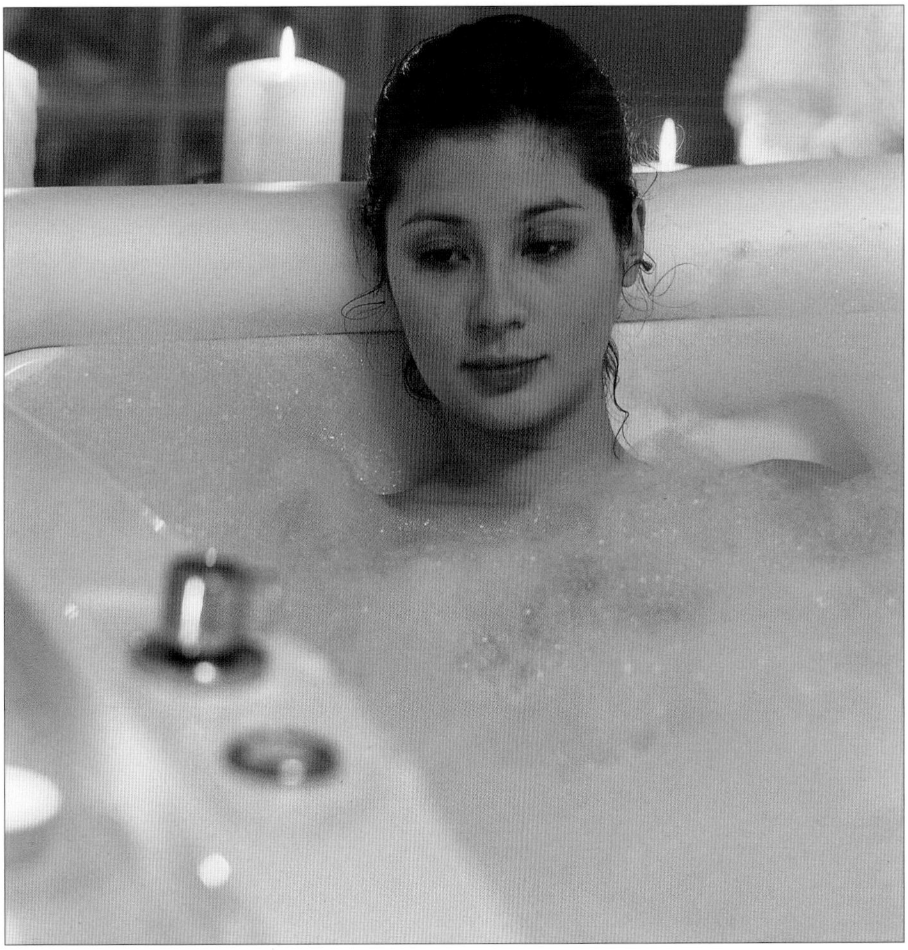

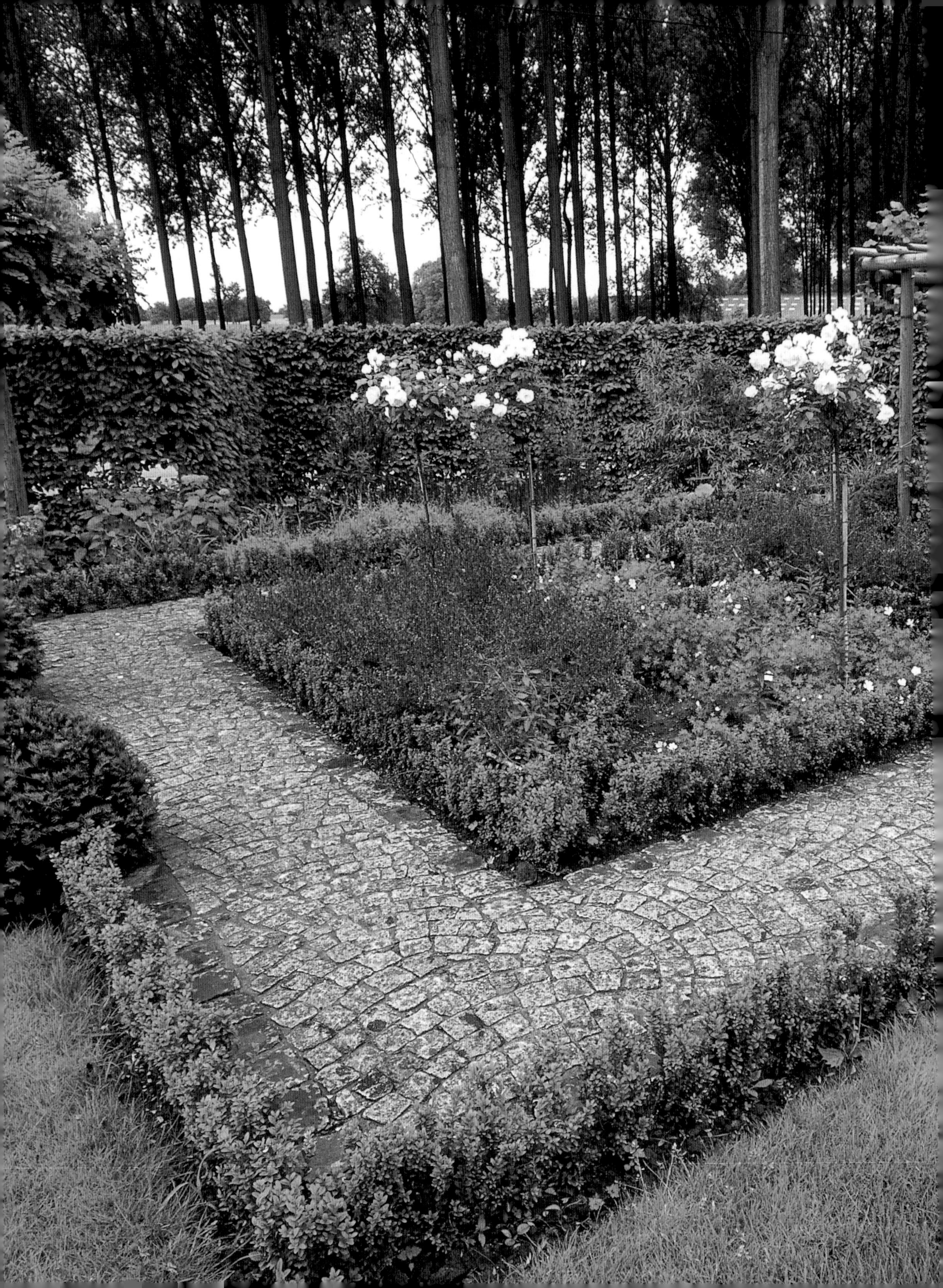

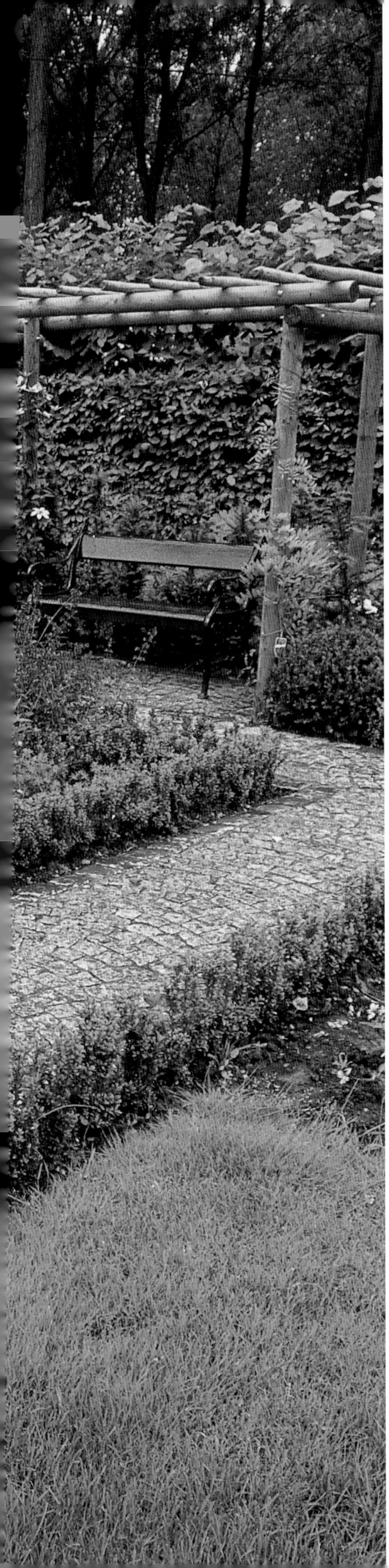

Directory of Herbs

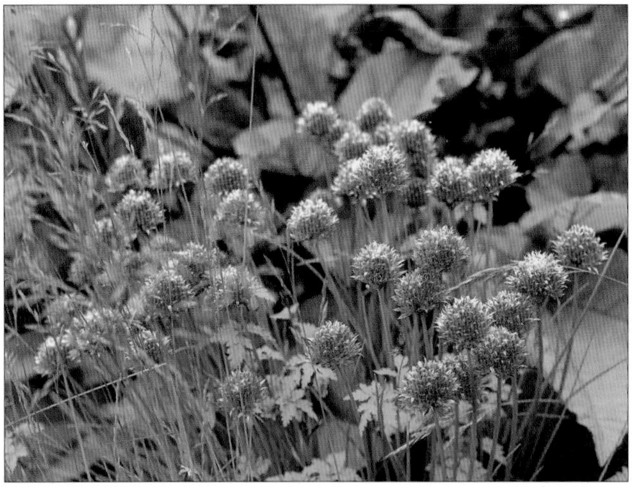

This section describes 235 herbs in alphabetical Latin name order, with a photograph of each one to aid identificiation. Each entry gives a brief history of the herb, including traditional associations and folklore, followed by a description of its characteristcs, habit, growth and cultivation. The principal uses, including medicinal, culinary, household and commercial, are also outlined. Medicinal uses in this section are for reference only and should not be taken as practical recommendations. Many herbs can be toxic if taken to excess, especially in the form of essential oils, and some may cause adverse reactions in certain people. If in doubt as to its suitability, consult a qualified practitioner before using any of these herbs medicinally.

Above *Chives (*Allium schoenoprasum*) with Herb Robert.*

Left *A wide range of herbs have an attractive shape and form and can easily be incorporated into a design for a small garden.*

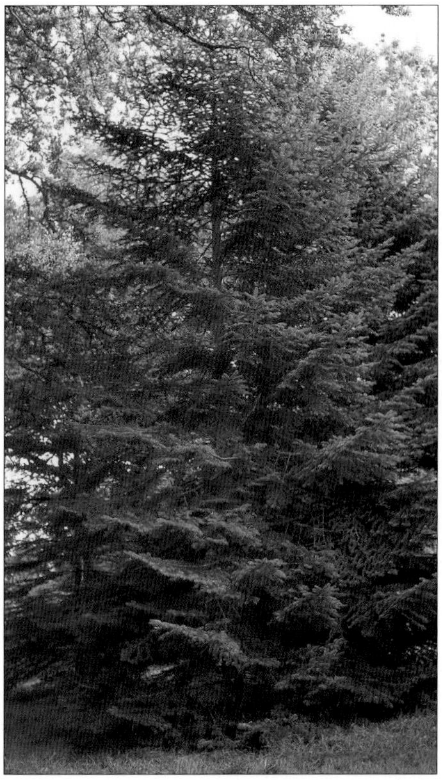

PINACEAE

Abies alba

Silver fir

History and traditions The silver fir was the source of "Strasbourg Turpentine", as described by the French doctor and botanist Pierre Belon in *De Arboribus Coniferis*, 1553, and listed in the London *Pharmacopoeia* until 1788. Its manufacture is covered in the famous work on distillation techniques, *Liber De Arte Distillandi* by the Strasbourg physician Hieronymus Braunschweig, 1450–1534. Turpentine is now more usually made from a selection of several different species of pine, but both *Abies alba* and *A. balsamea* still have a place in many herbal medicines and modern pharmaceutical preparations.
Description It grows from 25–45m/80–150ft and has glossy, dark green needles, silver underneath. It is monoecious – that is, the small male cones and much larger female cones, which are reddish brown when ripe and up to 15cm/6in long, are produced on the same tree.
Related species *A. balsamea* has smooth grey bark, studded with resin blisters, and is strongly scented with balsam.
Habitat/distribution Native to mountainous regions of central and southern Europe, also found in North and Central America.
Growth Prefers moist but well-drained, slightly acid soil and does not flourish in polluted air. It may be propagated from seed, sown in late autumn or winter, with a period of stratification to aid germination.
Parts used *A. alba,* leaves, resin tapped from mature trees. *A. balsamea,* leaves, oleo-resin collected from blisters on the trunk. Essential oil from resin of both species.

USES Medicinal *A. alba* and *A. balsamea* have aromatic, antiseptic properties, stimulate circulation and increase blood flow and are expectorant and diuretic in action. They are common ingredients of proprietary remedies for coughs and colds, bath preparations, liniments and rubs for rheumatism and neuralgia. Oleo-resin from *A. balsamea* is used in North American traditional medicine for chest infections, cuts, burns, skin eruptions and venereal disease.
Cosmetic The essential oil is an ingredient of cosmetics, perfumes and soaps.

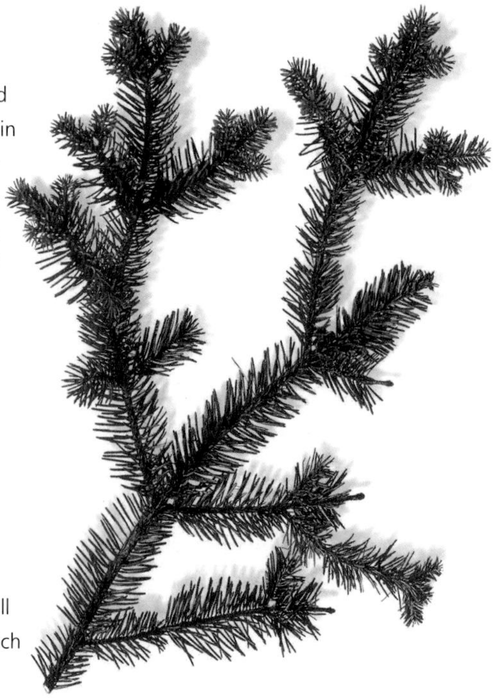

Above *The leaves of a silver fir are fine and needle-like.*

CAUTION Silver fir is an irritant, which can cause skin reaction in sensitive subjects.

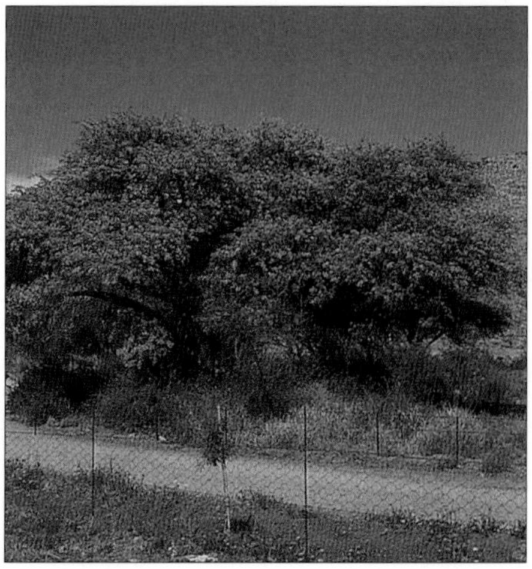

LEGUMINOSAE/MIMOSACEAE

Acacia senegal

Gum Arabic

History and traditions The ancient Egyptians imported what appears to be acacia gum, and it was referred to in the writings of the Greek physician, Theophrastus, in the 4th century BC. Gum arabic is mentioned in many old herbals as an ingredient of pomanders and medicines.
Description *A. senegal*, which produces gum arabic, reaches 6m/19ft tall, has grey bark, pale green pinnate leaves and small pale yellow balls of flowers. There are over 1,000 species in the *Acacia* genus, often called wattles, many of which produce gums for commerce. *A. nilotica* (above) is the source of an inferior gum arabic.
Habitat/distribution The genus is found in dry areas in tropical to warm-temperate zones of Africa, Asia, Australia, Central and South America.
Growth *A. senegal* is tender, requiring a minimum temperature about 15°C/60°F. It needs a slightly acid, well-drained soil and full sun and is propagated by seed, germinated at 21°C/70°F.
Parts used Resin of *A. senegal* (it dissolves in water to form a mucilage which makes a bonding agent).

USES Medicinal Gum arabic is a demulcent, soothes inflamed tissues and is used in pastilles, lotions and pharmaceutical preparations.
Culinary Although it has no place in the domestic kitchen it is used in the food industry in a wide range of products, including confectionery and chewing gum.

CAUTION There are statutory restrictions on the cultivation of wattles in some places.

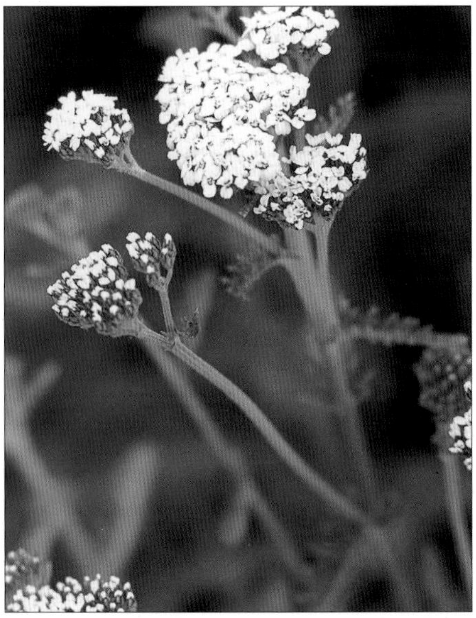

COMPOSITAE/ASTERACEAE

Achillea millefolium

Yarrow

History and traditions The Latin name honours the legendary Achilles, whose soldiers are said to have staunched their wounds with this plant in the Trojan War, and it has a long tradition as a wound herb. *Millefolium* refers to the many segments of the finely divided leaves. This herb has attracted a wealth of folklore over the centuries, as its common names reveal.
Description A pungent perennial with flat, creamy-white to pinkish flower heads rising on tough stalks 15–30cm/6–12in above a mat of greyish-green, finely-divided leaves. With its creeping roots and efficient self-seeding it is extremely invasive.
Related species There are many ornamental cultivars of *A. millefolium* including 'Moonshine', with light yellow flowers, and the rich crimson 'Fire King'. *A. ageratum* (formerly *A. decolorans*), English mace, is a little-known culinary herb with a mildly spicy flavour, used to flavour chicken dishes, soups, stews and sauces.
Habitat/distribution Widespread in temperate zones, found in grasslands, waste ground and by roadsides. Native of Europe and western Asia, naturalized in North America, Australia and New Zealand.
Growth Propagated by division of roots. The wild species is invasive and when grown as a garden plant it is advisable to keep it in a container or to restrict the roots by surrounding with tiles pushed into the soil.
Parts used The whole plant, fresh or dried.

Yarrow folklore

As "devil's nettle" or "devil's plaything", yarrow was thought to be dedicated to Satan and widely used in charms and spells. It had a place in Druid ceremonies and was made into herbal amulets or strewn on the threshold of houses against witches and evil forces. A bunch hung on the door, and tied to the baby's cradle for good measure on Midsummer's Eve, was hoped to ensure an illness-free year ahead.

Several claims are made for yarrow's supernatural powers in the 15th-century "Book of Secrets", attributed to Albertus Magnus. If put to the nose it will protect "from all feare and fatansye or vysion" and rather more wildly, if the juice is smeared on the hands, when plunged into water they will act as magnets for fish.

Yarrow features in many traditional rhymes connected with finding true love:

Yarrow, yarrow, long and narrow,
Tell unto me by tomorrow,
Who my husband is to be.

Another rhyme, attributed to the county of Suffolk in England and to eastern Europe, refers to yarrow's propensity to cause a nosebleed:

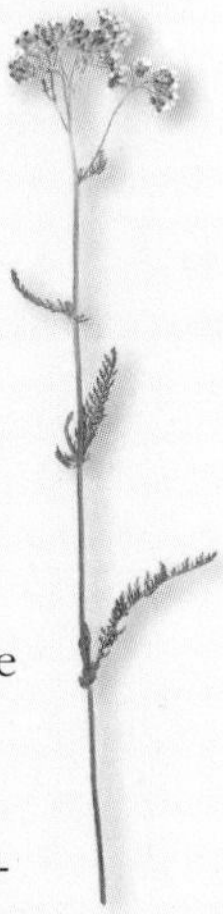

Green 'arrow, green
'arrow, you bears a
white blow,
If my love loves me my
nose will bleed now.

And if eaten at the wedding feast, it was claimed that bride and groom would remain in love for seven years.

As well as its role as a wound herb, reflected in the names soldier's woundwort, herb militaris and carpenter's weed, it was credited with both stopping a nosebleed or bringing one on (a supposed way of relieving migraine), as occasion demanded. It has a pungent smell and, as "old man's pepper", was made into snuff.

USES Medicinal The essential oil contains azulene, which has anti-inflammatory properties. It increases perspiration and is taken internally, as a tea, for colds and feverish conditions, and applied externally for wounds, ulcers and nosebleeds. It is still used today in contemporary herbalism as a uterine tonic and to reduce heavy menstrual bleeding. It is also thought to lower blood pressure and to relieve indigestion.
Cosmetic A weak infusion of the flowering tops in distilled water makes a cleanser or refreshing toner for oily skins.
Other names Soldier's woundwort, herb militaris, carpenter's weed, old man's pepper, nose bleed, devil's nettle, milfoil and also thousand leaf.

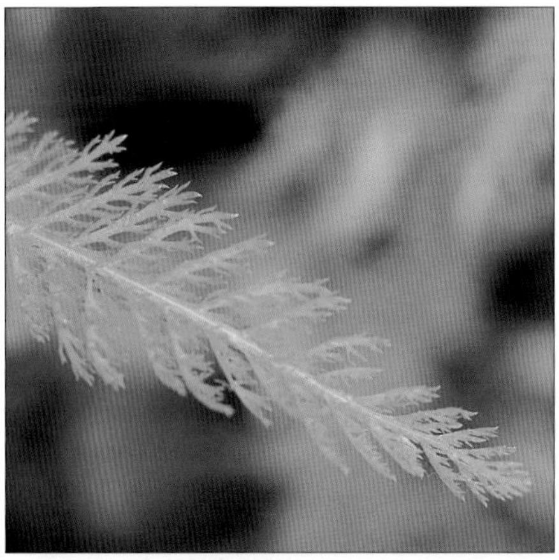

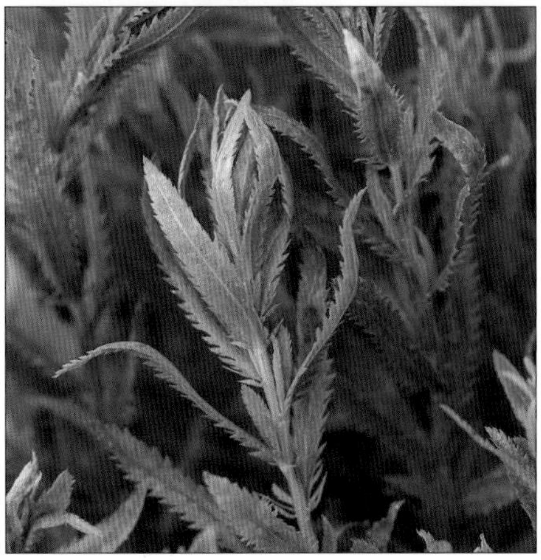

Above right *The divided leaves of* Achillea millefolium, *also known as thousand leaf.*

Right Achillea ageratum, *English mace.*

CAUTION Large does can cause headaches. Allergic rashes and skin sensitivity to sunlight may result from prolonged use.

RANUNCULACEAE

Aconitum napellus

Aconite

History and traditions The generic name is from the Greek for a dart (*akontion*) in recognition of its erstwhile use as an arrow poison, but the species name, *napellus*, meaning "little turnip", is supposedly for the shape of the roots, and gives no hint of the deadly nature of this plant. The popular name, monkshood, describes the curious shape of the flowers, while the common name for *A. lycoctonum,* wolf's bane, is a reference to its ability to despatch this once much-feared animal by sprinkling the juice over raw meat as bait. Stories of the dangers of aconite abound in herbals through the ages, such as Gerard's account of the "ignorant persons" of Antwerp who were taken with "most cruel symptoms and so died" when served the leaves in a salad as a "lamentable experiment".

Description The helmet-shaped, inky-blue flowers give this hardy herbaceous perennial a slightly sinister appearance appropriate to its properties. It has tuberous roots and delphinium-like foliage from which the flowering stems rise to a height of 1.5m/5ft.

Related species There are about 100 species, all of which are highly poisonous. *A. lycoctonum* has yellow, sometimes purple, flowers and *A. carmichaelii,* syn. *A. fischeri*, is sometimes used in Chinese medicine as a painkiller.

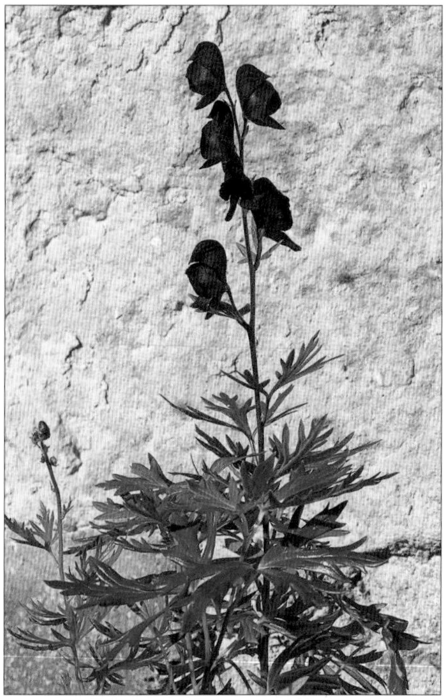

Habitat/distribution Widespread in Europe and in northern temperate regions, in damp woodlands, meadows and mountainous areas.

Growth Plant in moist, fertile soil and part-shade. Propagation is by division of roots in the autumn for flowering in the second year. Seeds sown in spring will not flower for 2–3 years.

Parts used Dried root tubers.

Other name Monkshood.

USES Medicinal The alkaloid, aconite, gives it toxicity. As a strong sedative and painkiller, it should be used only by qualified practitioners. A very small dose causes numbness of lips, tongue and extremeties and can lead to vomiting, coma and death.

CAUTION The whole plant is highly toxic and if ingested can kill. Contact with skin may cause allergic reactions – always handle with gloves. Subject to legal restrictions in some countries.

ACORACEAE

Acorus calamus

Calamus

History and traditions The first specimens to reach Europe were imported from Asia by the botanical garden in Vienna in the 16th century. Calamus, which means "reed" in Greek, then became popular as a scented strewing herb. Cardinal Wolsey used it extensively for this purpose in Hampton Court Palace. This was yet another example of his extravagance in the eyes of his contemporaries, due to its comparative rarity – at the time calamus was grown only on the Norfolk Broads some distance away. It was also one of the ingredients in Moses's instructions to make "an ointment compound after the art of the apothecary" as a holy anointing oil (Exodus 30:25).

Description A pleasantly aromatic perennial with a thick much-branched rhizome, it has similar-shaped leaves to the irises, although is not botanically related to them. The flower head is a spadix, emerging from the side of the leaf, but it is not usually fertile in Europe and cool northern climates, owing to lack of appropriate insects for pollination.

Related species *A. gramineus*, native to the Far East, is a miniature species, used in Chinese medicine. Its compact size makes it suitable for growing in ornamental ponds.

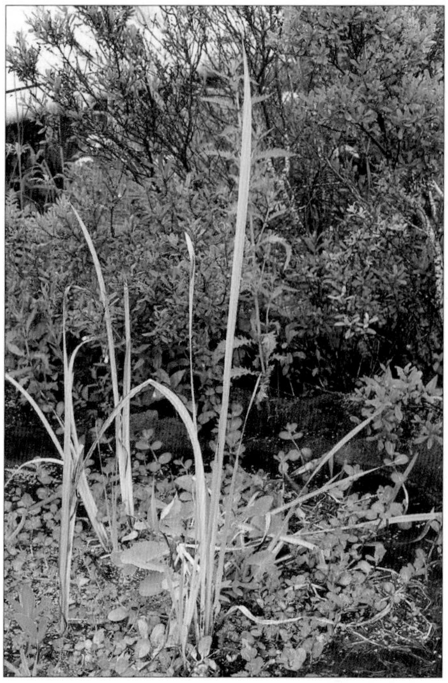

Habitat/distribution *A. calamus* (above) is indigenous to central Asia and eastern Europe, and is now widespread in marshy areas and by shallow waterways of northern temperate zones.

Growth Vigorous and easy to propagate, it must have moist soil and plenty of water. Grows best by water margins. Propagate in spring or autumn by cutting rhizomes in small pieces, each with 2–3 buds, and planting in muddy ground.

Parts used Rhizomes, essential oil.

USES Medicinal Used for digestive problems and to dispel intestinal worms. It is slightly sedative to the central nervous system and is traditionally used in Ayurvedic medicine following strokes, and also for bronchial complaints. Externally it is used as an alcohol rub for aching muscles.

Aromatic The essential oil, separated by steam distillation, is a perfumery ingredient. Herbalists of old called it "*calamus aromaticus*", and the ground root was added to potpourris, scented sachets, tooth and hair powders.

Household In Asia it is sometimes used as an insecticide powder to deter ants.

Other names Sweet flag, sweet rush and myrtle grass.

CAUTION Excessive doses can cause adverse reactions, including vomiting.

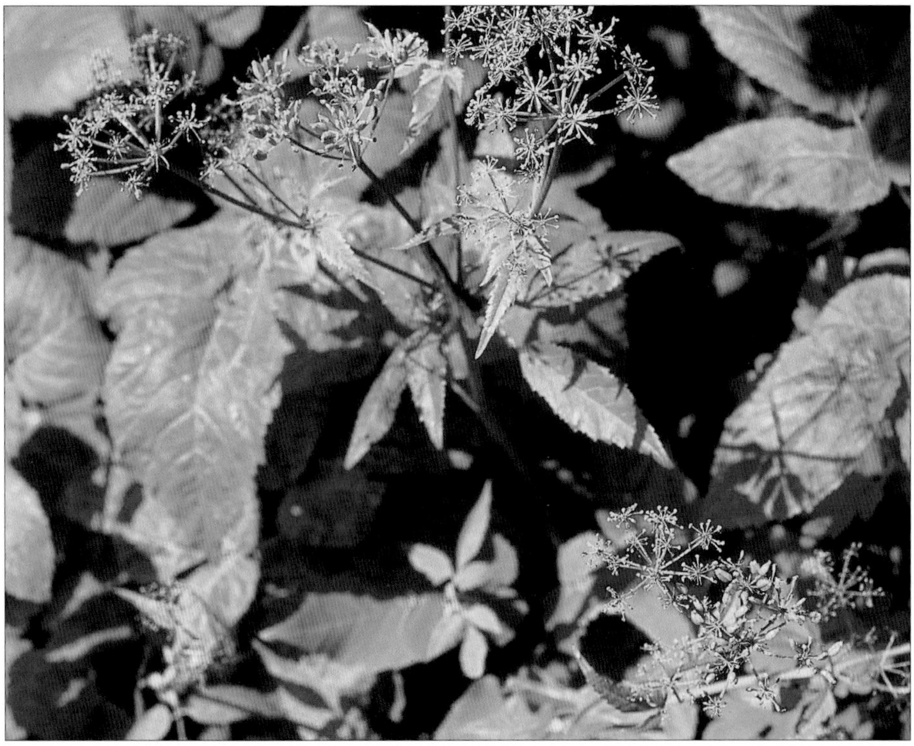

UMBELLIFERAE/APIACEAE

Aegopodium podagraria

Ground elder

History and traditions The specific name comes from the Latin word for gout, *podagra*, and it was grown in monastery gardens in medieval times as a cure for that disease. The name bishops' weed could be a reference to an episcopal tendency to gout, due to high living and a rich diet of meat and alcohol, or to the plant's prevalence around ecclesiastical sites. It is dedicated to St Gerard, the patron saint of gout sufferers.

Description A herbaceous perennial with a creeping root system, it spreads rapidly, smothering other plants and self-seeds. Umbels of white flowers rise on long stems to 90cm/36in above the leaves in summer.

Related species *A. podagraria* 'Variegatum' is a variegated cultivar with cream patterning at the leaf margins. It is not as invasive as the common variety and makes a pretty border, especially when grown with white lilies or tulips.

Habitat/distribution Native to Europe, naturalized in North America; found in woodlands and wasteground.

Growth Ground elder is a rampant weed that grows in any soil and is almost impossible to eradicate once established. This plant is definitely not suitable for cultivation as it will take over.

Parts used Leaves, stems.

USES Medicinal An anti-inflammatory herb with astringent properties, it has a long tradition as a treatment for gout, sciatica and rheumatism. It can be taken internally as an infusion, and is applied externally for stings and burns.

Culinary Though fairly unpleasant in taste, the young leaves and shoots can be added to salads, or cooked like spinach.

Other names Goutweed, bishops' weed and herb Gerard.

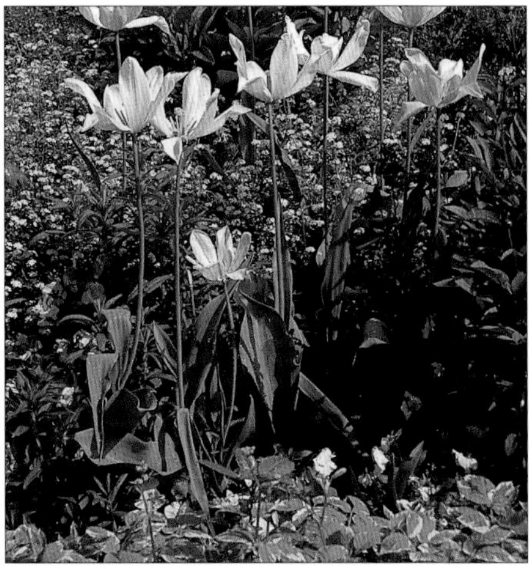

Above Aegopodium podagraria *'Variegatum' (Variegated ground elder) in the foreground with white, lily-flowered tulips.*

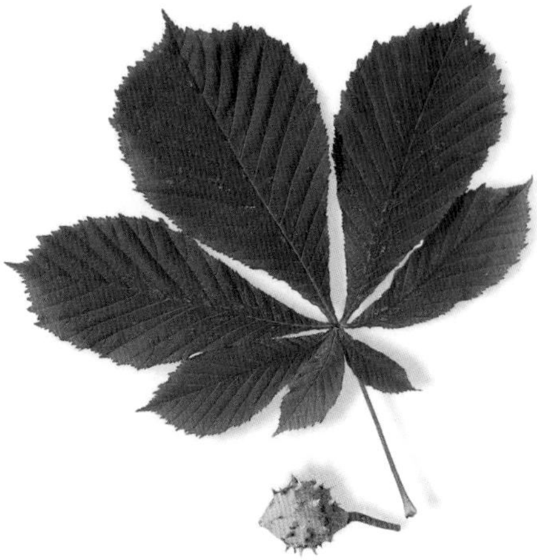

HIPPOCASTANACEAE

Aesculus hippocastanum

Horse chestnut

History and traditions This spectacular tree was introduced to western Europe in the mid-16th century, when it was grown in Vienna from seeds brought from Istanbul by the botanist Clusius (Charles de L'Ecluse), although it does not seem to have been widely used for medicinal purposes until the late 19th century. The origins of the name are confused, but are all tied to the use of this tree as animal fodder. *Hippocastanum* is the Latin for "horse chestnut", which the Romans supposedly fed to their livestock.

Description A stately, deciduous tree, 30–40m/98–130ft in height, it has palmate leaves, sticky resinous buds and candelabras of white or pink-tinged flowers in spring. The spiny, globular, green fruit contains glossy reddish-brown seeds (conkers, also called chestnuts).

Habitat/distribution Occurs in eastern Europe, eastern Asia and North America, introduced to Britain and western Europe.

Growth Propagate by seeds, sown in autumn. Often self-seeds and grows rapidly in any soil.

Parts used Bark, seeds.

USES Medicinal Effective in the treatment of oedema and varicose veins. The plant may be used internally and externally and has the following actions: venotonic, anti-inflammatory, antieccymotic (against bruises). Use as a cream to help varicose veins.

CAUTION The whole fruit is mildly toxic and should never be eaten. Only for use by qualified practitioners. Should not be applied to broken skin because saponins in the plant could be an irritant.

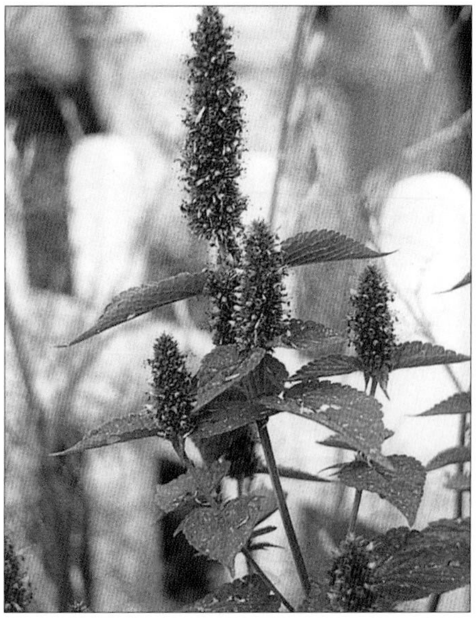

LABIATAE/LAMIACEAE

Agastache foeniculum

Anise hyssop

History and traditions A traditional medicinal herb of Native Americans, it became popular with colonists as a bee plant for the distinctive aniseed flavour it gave to honey.

Description A hardy, short-lived perennial with soft, ovate leaves, strongly scented with aniseed. Bold purple flower spikes last all summer. Clumps are 60–90cm/24–36in in height.

Related species *A. rugosa*, known as Korean mint, or wrinkled giant hyssop, is also a hardy perennial, 1m/3ft high, with pointed, mint-scented leaves and mauve flower spikes.

Habitat/distribution *A. foeniculum* is native to North and Central America, and *A. rugosa* comes from eastern Asia.

Growth Grows best in rich moist soil in full sun. Although reasonably hardy, *A. foeniculum* will not stand prolonged frost or temperatures below -6°C/20°F. Propagate by division or softwood cuttings in spring.

Parts used Leaves, flowers – fresh or dried.

USES Medicinal The leaves have antibacterial properties and are taken as an infusion to alleviate coughs and colds, or as a digestive.

Culinary The leaves of both *A. foeniculum* and *A. rugosa* make refreshing tea with a minty flavour. They can be floated in soft drinks and fruit cups to add piquancy. Add a few leaves to a salad to boost flavour and goodness. The dried or fresh leaves may be added to cooked meat dishes and go well with pork.

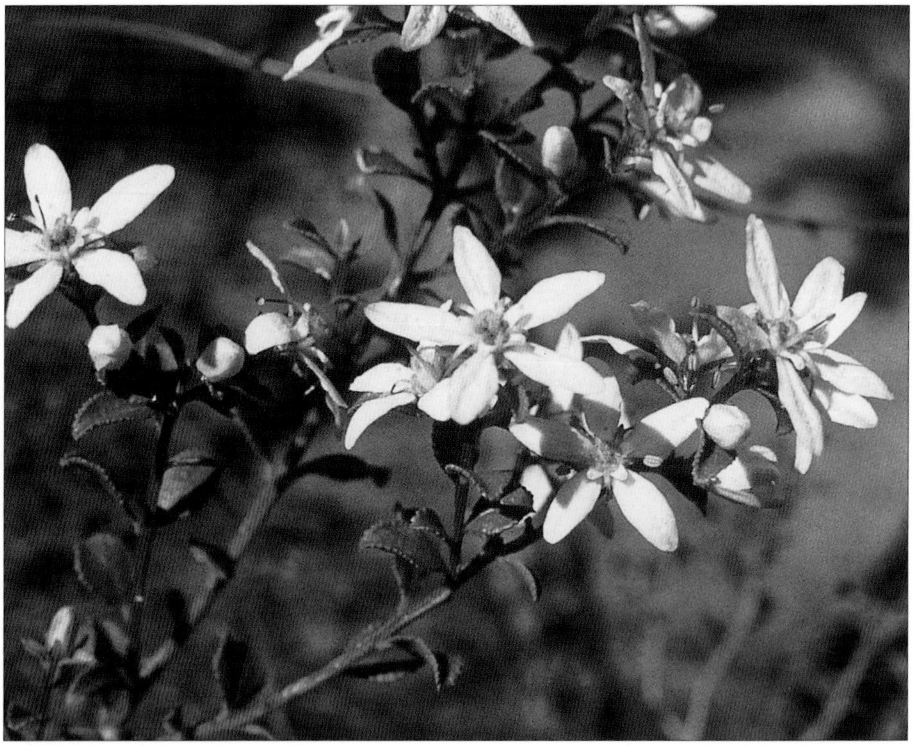

RUTACEAE

Agathosma betulina

Buchu

History and traditions A prized medicinal plant of the indigenous people of South Africa, its virtues were discovered by colonists of the Cape who introduced it to Europe at the end of the 18th century. In the 1820s the dried leaves were exported in some quantity to Britain and thence to North America, to be included in proprietary medicines and used to flavour cordials. John Lindley in his *Flora Medica*, 1838, records that several species of *Agathosma*, collected as 'bucku', were "found to be an excellent aromatic stomachic and very efficacious as a diuretic. The infusion is much praised as a remedy in chronic inflammations of the bladder and urethra and in chronic rheumatism." All of these uses remain valid in herbal medicine today.

Description A tender, evergreen shrub, 1–2m/3–6ft in height, it has glossy, yellowish-green leaves, which are leathery in texture and studded with oil glands which smell of blackcurrants. White flowers appear in spring. A member of the rue family, it is highly aromatic, scenting the air wherever it grows in quantity.

Related species Several species are used, all indiscriminately termed buchu, or "buka", meaning powder in the local language. *A. betulina* is held to be the most effective for medicinal purposes, *A. crenulata,* oval buchu, has ovate leaves and *A. serratifolia*, long buchu, serrated, lance-shaped foliage. These plants were once classified as "barosma" and the term "barosma powder" for buchu is still sometimes used.

Habitat/distribution Dry hillsides of Cape Province, South Africa.

Growth Grown as a conservatory plant in temperate zones, a minimum temperature of 5°C/41°F is required. Pot in ericaceous (lime-free) compost. It must not be overwatered, which can lead to rot, and should be cut back hard in spring to keep it in shape and control size. It grows outside in warm, frost-free regions, and needs well-drained, acid soil and full sun.

Parts used Leaves, which are harvested when the plant is in flower, and dried.

USES Medicinal A strong urinary antiseptic. Used internally to treat urinary infections, especially cystitis, coughs and colds, rheumatism, arthritis and digestive disorders. Applied externally for bruises and sprains.

Culinary Gives a blackcurrant taste to soft drinks and cordials and is used to flavour a local liquor "buchu brandy".

Household Made into a powder to deter ants and other insects.

Other name Round buchu.

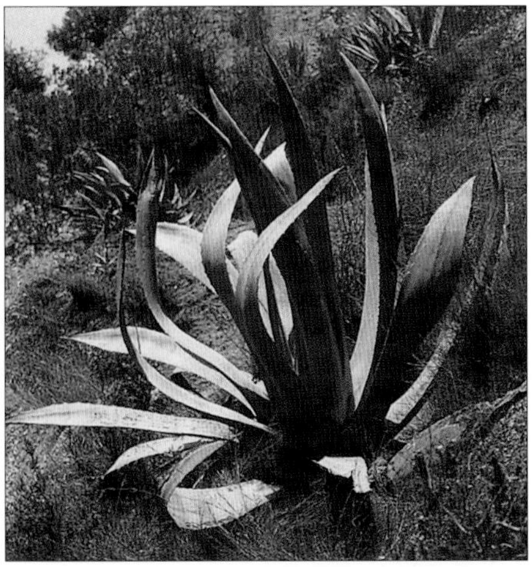

AGAVACEAE

Agave americana

Agave

History and traditions Agave comes from the Greek for admirable. It gained the name "century plant" from the mistaken belief that it flowers only after a hundred years – but most bloom after ten years.

Description A tender succulent whose rosettes of spiky grey-green leaves are 1–2m/3–6ft high with a spread of 2–3m/6–10ft. The tall bell-shaped flower spikes, resembling small trees, rise to 8m/26ft. Agaves should not be confused with aloes, and are not botanically related.

Related species *A. americana* 'Variegata' is a cultivar with yellow margins to the leaves.

Habitat/distribution Originally from tropical zones of the Americas, especially Mexico, this plant is now naturalized in southern Europe, India, and Central and South Africa.

Growth Needs well-drained soil, full sun and a minimum temperature of 5°C/41°F. Propagate by offsets. In cool climates it can be grown as a conservatory plant but takes up a lot of space.

Parts used Leaves, roots, sap.

USES Medicinal The sap has anti-inflammatory properties, and is applied externally for burns, bites and stings, by breaking open a leaf.

General The root has cleansing properties and is used for washing clothes and in commercial soap production. Fibres are woven into rope. The powdered leaf makes snuff and the whole plant is much employed as a stock-proof fence.

CAUTION Can provoke a reaction in those with a history of skin problems.

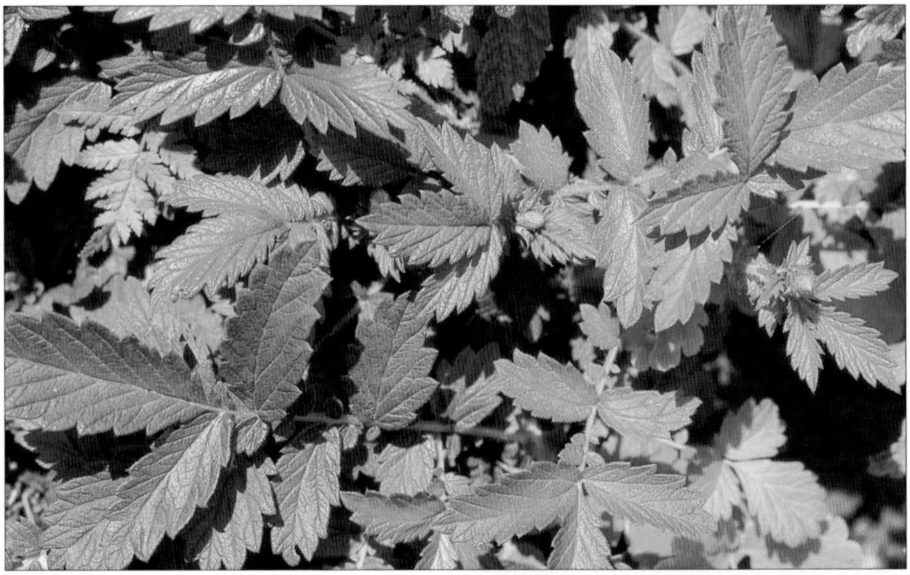

ROSACEAE

Agrimonia eupatoria

Agrimony

History and traditions The species name is from Mithradates Eupator, King of Pontus, who died in 64BC. He practised magic, was a great believer in herbal potions and was thought to have rendered himself immune to injury by saturating his body with lethal poisons.

The Anglo-Saxons attributed magical powers to agrimony, including it in charms and dubious preparations of blood and pounded frogs.

A sprig under the pillow supposedly brought oblivion, until removed. It was also credited with healing wounds, internal haemorrhages, snake bites, charming away warts and mending bad backs. Retaining its reputation through the centuries, it became the principal ingredient of *eau d'arquebusade*, a lotion for treating the wounds inflicted by the arquebus, a 16th-century firearm and forerunner of the musket. It was an essential ingredient of a springtime drink, still taken by country folk into the early years of this century as a "blood purifier".

Description A perennial with compound pointed leaves, covered in soft hairs. In summer and autumn it has small yellow flower spikes with a hint of an apricot scent. It grows to a height of 30–60cm/1–2ft.

Habitat/distribution Found on waste grounds and roadsides throughout Europe, Asia and North America.

Growth A wild plant which tolerates poor, dry soil, it can be propagated by seed sown in spring or by root division in autumn.

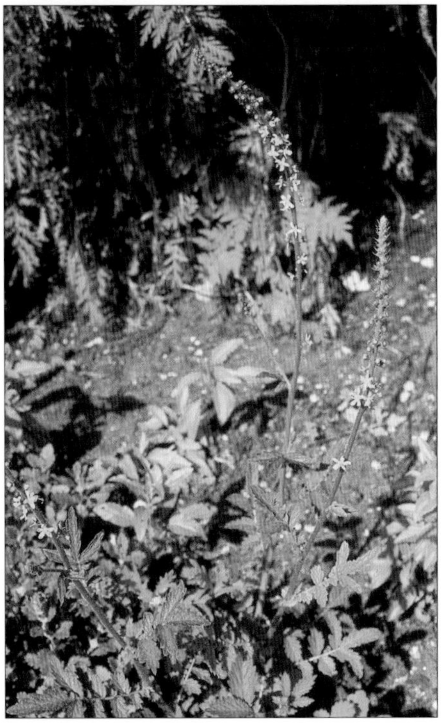

Above *Agrimony in flower.*

Parts used Dried flowering plant.

USES Medicinal Has anti-inflammatory, anti-bacterial and astringent properties and is taken internally for sore throats, catarrh, diarrhoea, cystitis and urinary infections. It has been documented as a traditional medicine to treat type 2 diabetes. Applied externally as a lotion for wounds.

Household Yields a yellow dye.

Other names Church steeples, sticklewort and cockleburr.

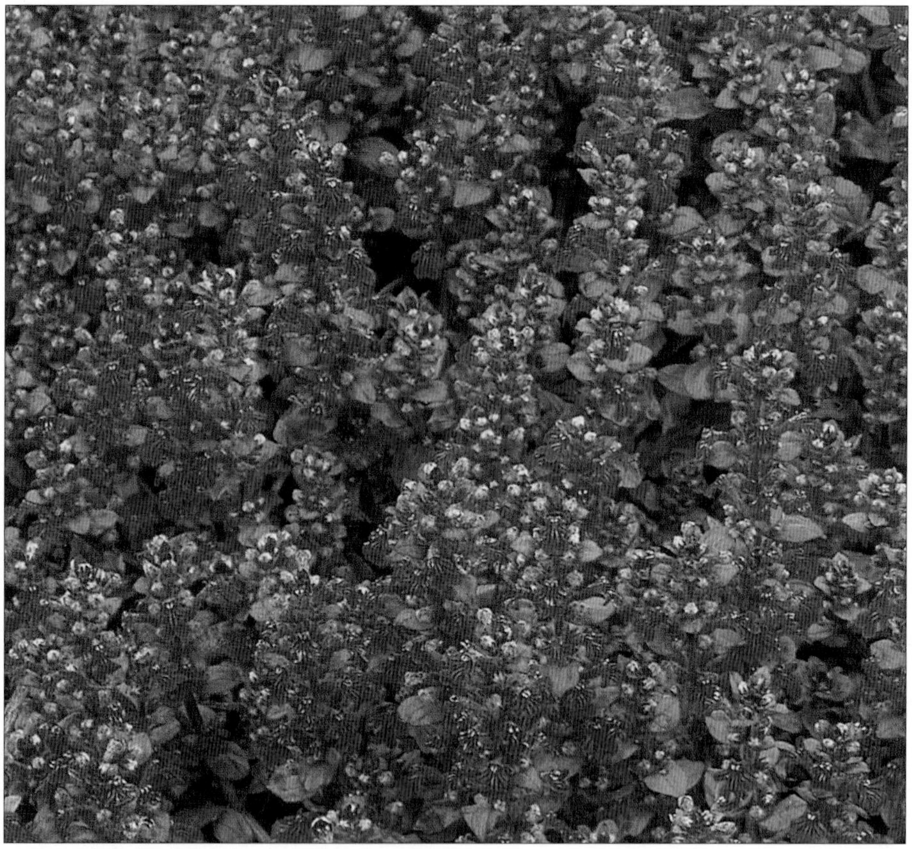

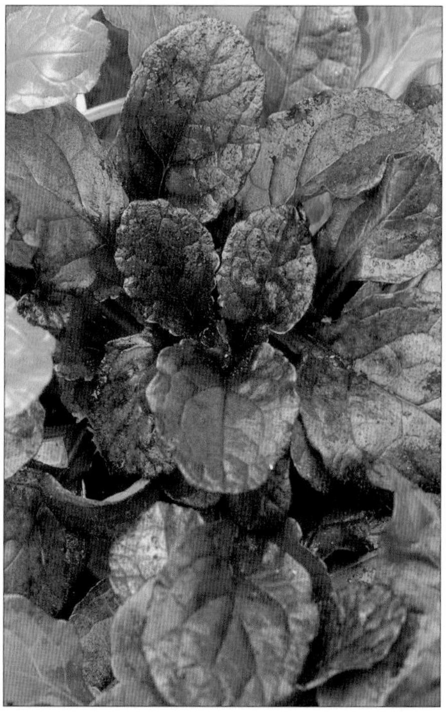

Above Aguja reptans *'Atropurpurea'.*

Below Aguja reptans *'Multicolor'.*

LABIATAE/LAMIACEAE

Ajuga reptans
Bugle

History and traditions The apothecaries knew it as "bugula" and along with self-heal, *Prunella vulgaris,* it was valued for many centuries as a wound herb. Culpeper thought highly of it: "If the virtues of it make you fall in love with it (as they will if you be wise) keep a syrup of it to take inwardly, and an ointment and plaster of it to use outwardly, always by you". He recommended it for all kinds of sores, gangrene and fistulas. Gerard, who found many specimens growing "in a moist ground upon Black Heath, near London", backs him up, expressing the view that it is common knowledge in France "how he needs neither physician nor surgeon that hath Bugle and Sanicle".

Description A hardy perennial, 10–30cm/ 4–12in high, growing on a creeping rootstock, it has attractive blue flower spikes in spring or early summer, growing from rosettes of basal leaves. White or pink-flowered mutants occasionally occur.

Related species Cultivars with richly coloured foliage make rewarding subjects for the herb garden. *A. r.* 'Atropurpurea' has purple-bronze leaves, *A. r.* 'Multicolor' has colourful variegated foliage of pink, crimson and cream with a hint of green, and *A. r.* 'Variegata' has greyish-green leaves with creamy margins.

Habitat/distribution In damp ground in woodlands and meadows. Native to Europe and introduced elsewhere, it is also found in northern Africa and parts of the Middle East.

Growth Ajugas make excellent ground cover and are easy to propagate by separating and replanting the leafy runners at any time of the year, but preferably in spring or autumn when sufficient moisture can be provided. They do need a moist soil to flourish well, and sun or partial shade.

Parts used Whole plant.

USES Medicinal Its reputation, sadly, has not stood the test of time and bugle is no longer widely used in herbal medicine today. But it is said to be mildly astringent and is sometimes still recommended, in the form of a lotion or ointment, for treating cuts and bruises.

Other names Carpenter's herb and sicklewort.

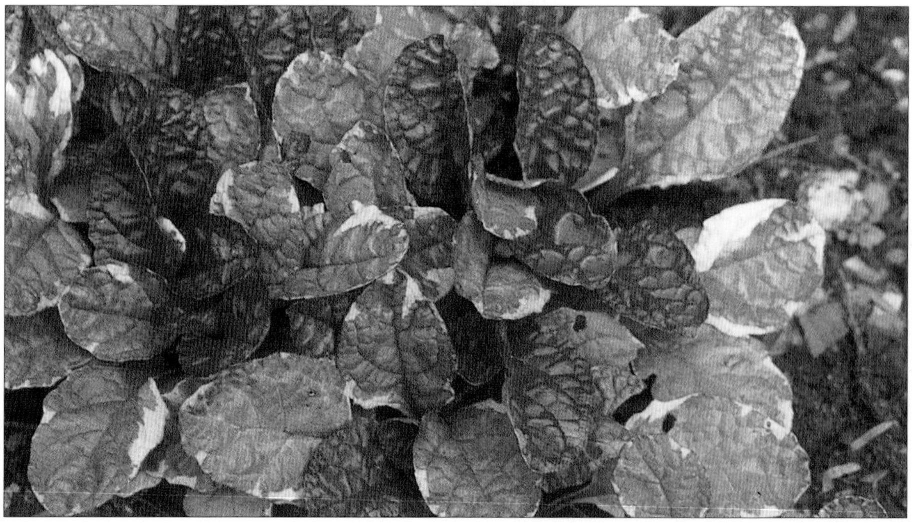

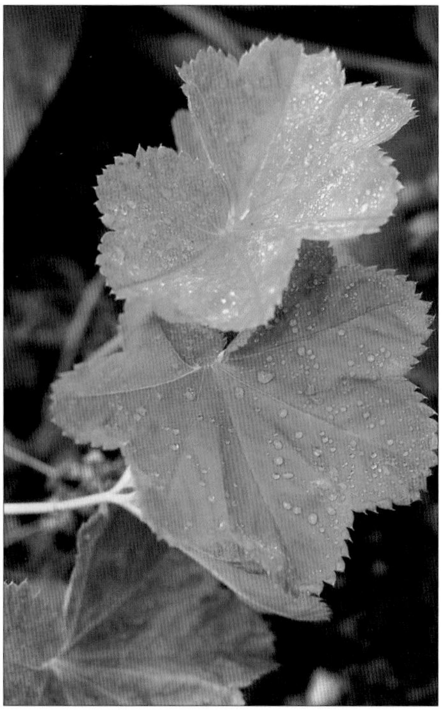

ROSACEAE

Alchemilla vulgaris

Lady's mantle

History and traditions This herb was unknown to the writers of the ancient classical world, but was a popular "magic" plant in northern Europe from earliest times, rising to prominence during the Middle Ages for its connections with alchemy. It was also sometimes associated with the Virgin Mary and dubbed Our Lady's mantle, subsequently shortened to lady's mantle, the scalloped leaves supposedly resembling a sculptured cloak. It was traditionally prescribed for infertility and "women's troubles" and was said to regulate the menstrual cycle and ease menopausal symptoms – as it still is prescribed by herbalists today.

Description A perennial 40–50cm/16–20in, it has hairy, branched stems and deeply lobed leaves (seven or nine lobes) with serrated edges and a froth of yellowish-green flowers in late spring and throughout summer.

Related species *A. alpina*, another medicinal species, is lower-growing at 10–20cm/4–8in, with star-shaped leaves. *A. mollis,* from the Carpathian mountains and known as "the garden variety", is the most attractive of the three with paler green, scalloped leaves and a more luxurious show of greeny-yellow flowers. It is widely grown in herb gardens, but has less medicinal value.

Habitat/distribution Found in mountainous areas, meadows, pasture lands and on rock ledges in Europe and throughout northern temperate regions.

Growth Grows in any soil in sun or partial shade. Self-seeds prolifically but germination of seed sown artificially is erratic. The easiest way to propagate is by division in spring or autumn. Species planted together hybridize readily.

Parts used Leaves.

USES Medicinal A herb traditionally used in gynaecology to treat menstrual irregularities and some symptoms of menopausal change. Applied externally for vaginal itching, as a lotion for sores and skin irritation, or as a mouthwash.

Culinary The leaves are edible and sometimes shredded and added to salads, but their slightly bitter, undistinguished taste hardly warrants this treatment.

Other names Lion's foot, bear's foot and leontopodium (in French, it is called Pied-de-Lion and in German, Frauenmantle).

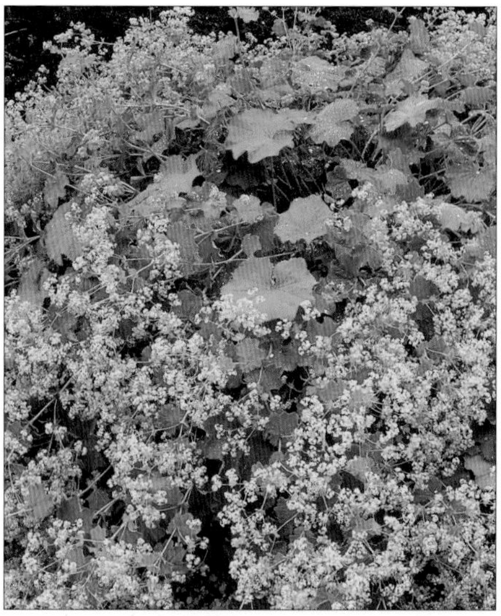

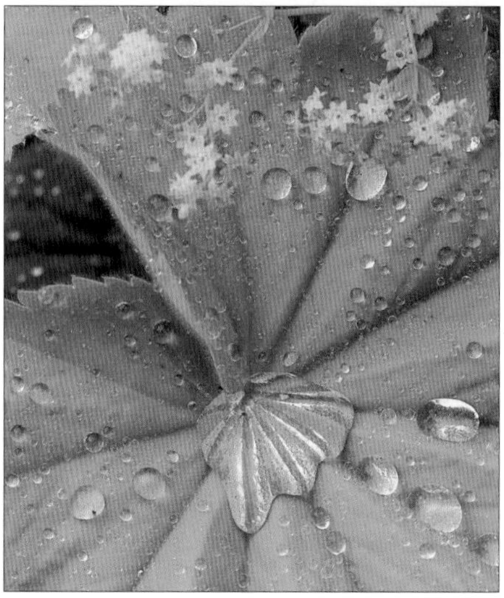

Above right Alchemilla mollis *has a froth of greeny-yellow flowers throughout summer.*

Right *The concave shape of* Alchemilla xanthochlora *and* A. mollis *leaves forms a dip where drops of moisture collect.*

The alchemy connection

The magic of lady's mantle lies in its ability to hold moisture drops, often dew, trapped in the central dips of the leaves and by their waxy surface. Dew was a much-prized ingredient in the recipes of the alchemists of old and here was an accessible source. So the herb was named "Alchemilla" – the little alchemist.

In its narrowest and best-known sense, the primary concern of alchemy was the transformation of base metal into gold, but its wider significance is that it marked the beginnings of systematic chemistry. Leading alchemists of the 13th century were Albertus Magnus, Roger Bacon and Arnold de Villeneuve, who wrote widely on the subject. Although they believed in the "philosopher's stone" (the instrument capable of transmuting metals into gold), they were also pre-occupied with the discovery of a divine water, or elixir of life, capable of healing all maladies – with the purest dew as a necessary component.

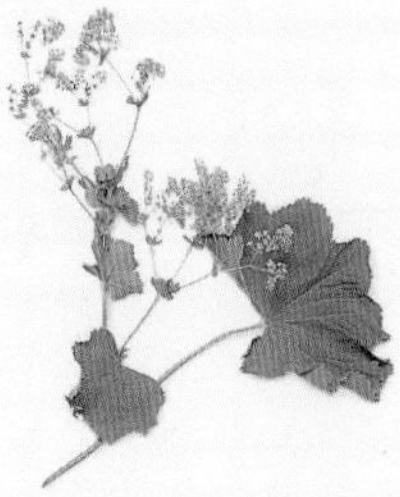

In the 16th century, the Swiss physician, Paracelsus, took up some of the tenets of alchemy, including the concept of the "prima materia" and the "quinta essentia", the primary essence of a substance, but gave it a new direction. The chief objective was the making of medicines, dependent on a study of the properties of plants and their effects on the body.

LILIACEAE/ALLIACEAE

Allium

The onion genus provides us with some of the most useful medicinal and culinary herbs. The characteristic strong smell is a result of the sulphur compounds contained within, which are beneficial to the circulatory and respiratory systems and have antibacterial properties. It also makes them among the most popular and powerful flavouring agents in worldwide cuisine.

History and traditions The use of onions and garlic can be traced back to the ancient civilizations of Babylonia, Egypt, Greece and Rome. One variety of onion was accorded divine honours in Egypt, and the pyramid builders are said to have been sustained by doses of garlic.

Many of the old writers on herbs, from Pliny onwards, refer to the medicinal properties of garlic, but not everybody was unanimous in its praise. Horace made the outrageous claim that it is "more poisonous than hemlock", when he was ill following a meal containing garlic. And, in 16th-century Britain, the herbalist Gerard remained doubtful of its virtues. In this he was unusual, as the pungent smell of both onions and garlic ensured a widespread belief that their juice protected from infection and in times of plague they were much in demand. One old recipe book gives water distilled from onions as a treatment for the bites of a rabid dog. The smell of garlic is particularly lingering and all-pervasive and may well be responsible for superstitions about its capacity to ward off vampires and the devil.

Avoiding garlic breath

Chewing fresh parsley helps to disguise the smell of garlic on the breath. If you do not like the taste of garlic, but want to benefit from its healthy attributes, it can be taken in capsule form (available from good health stores or pharmacies).

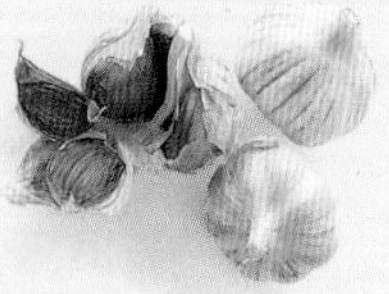

Right Allium cepa *Proliferum Group produces bulbs on its stems.*

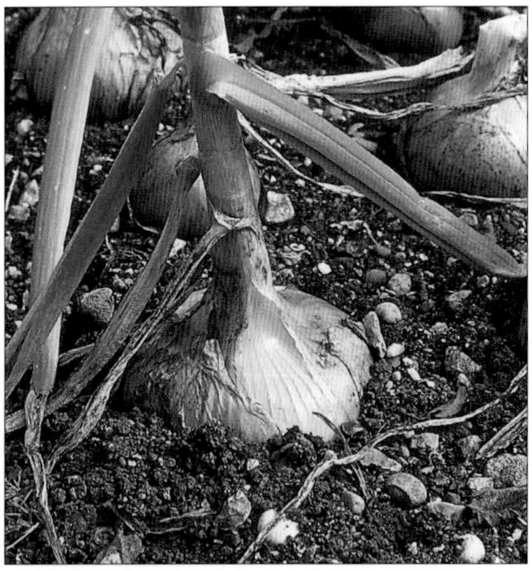

Allium cepa
Onion

Description Single bulbs at the base of each stem form the familiar culinary onion.
Related species There are numerous cultivars. *Allium cepa* Proliferum Group is the attractive tree onion, whose flowers produce large bulbils with leaves attached.
Habitat/distribution Origins unknown but probably originated in Central Asia, now grown worldwide.
Growth Propagate from sets in early summer or seed sown in spring or autumn. Plant in well-drained soil, rich in nutrients. Bend over tops in late summer to speed ripening, and dry bulbs before storing.
Parts used Fresh bulb.

USES Medicinal See box opposite.
Culinary Popular vegetable and flavouring agent.

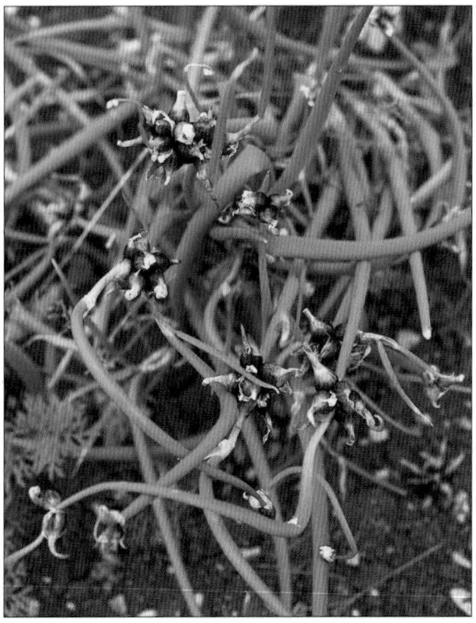

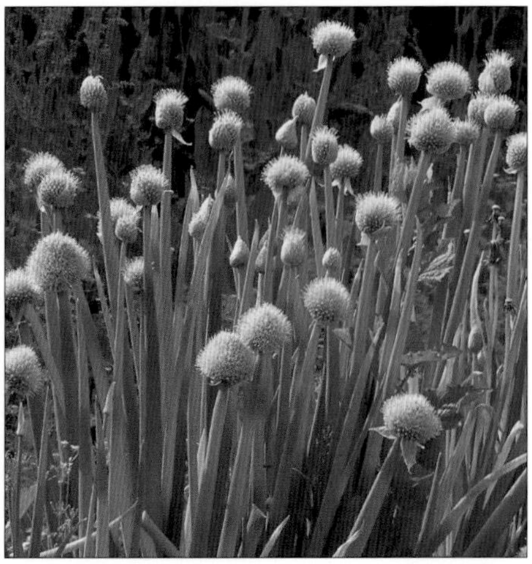

Allium fistulosum
Welsh onion

Description Evergreen hardy perennial 60–90cm/2–3ft tall, with hollow stems and leaves. Tightly packed greenish-white globes form the flowers in spring.
Habitat/distribution Native of Siberia, China and Japan. Widely grown elsewhere.
Growth Grow in well-drained, reasonably rich soil and divide clumps every three years. Seeds can be sown directly into the ground after frost.
Parts used Leaves, bulbs.

USES Medicinal The Welsh onion shares the decongestant, antibacterial properties of garlic and onions, but it is thought to be less concentrated and efficacious.
Culinary Pull the whole plant to make use of the bulb at the root, or cut the leaves and snip into salads and stir-fries.

Garlic bread

2–3 garlic cloves, peeled
25g/1oz/2 tbsp butter
1 tsp fresh parsley, finely chopped
1 tsp lemon juice
4 slices of bread, cut from a baguette

Using a garlic press, crush the garlic cloves into a small bowl. Beat the crushed garlic with the butter, parsley and lemon juice until softened and evenly combined. Spread it evenly over the slices of bread. Toast under a hot grill, or put on a baking tray in a hot oven, until browned.

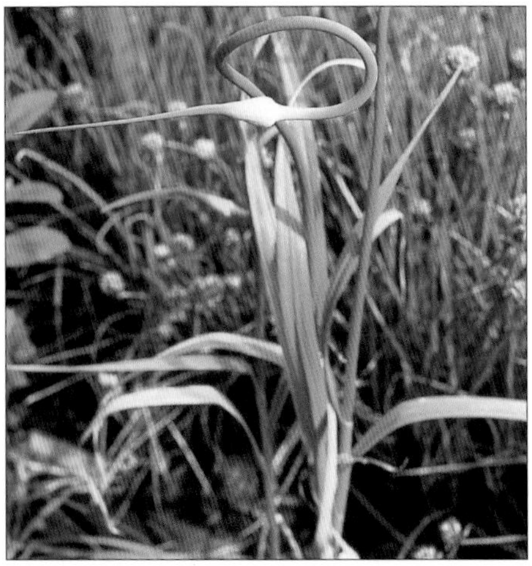

Allium sativum
Garlic

Description A hardy perennial, it is often cultivated as an annual. Bulbs are made up of cloves, or bulblets, in a papery, white, or pinkish-white casing. The clump of flat leaves grows to 60cm/2ft. Flowers are greenish white.
Habitat/distribution Originally from India or Central Asia, now grown worldwide, but does not flourish in cold, northern climates.
Growth Plant bulbs in autumn or winter in rich soil and a sunny position. Lift in late summer and dry in the sun before storing. Increase by dividing bulbs and replanting.
Parts used Bulbs, separated into cloves.

USES Medicinal See box below.
Culinary Popular flavouring agent.

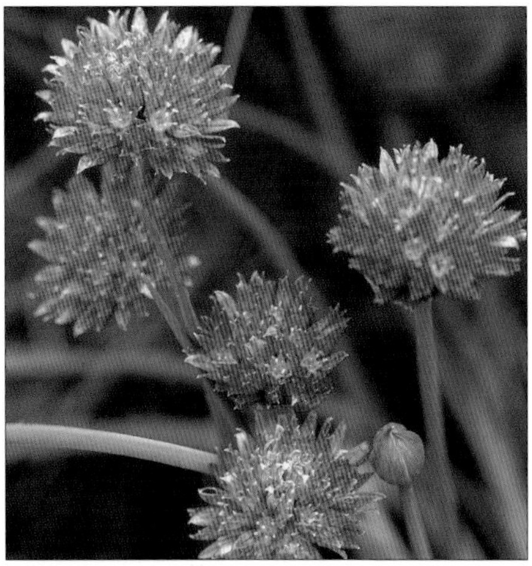

Allium schoenoprasum
Chives

Description A hardy perennial with clumps of cylindrical leaves growing from small bulblets to 30cm/12in. The leaves do not withstand very cold winters. Purple flower globes appear in early summer. There are both fine and broad-leafed cultivars.
Habitat/distribution Native to cool regions of Europe, naturalized in North America. Found in dry and damp, rocky areas, grasslands and woods.
Parts used Leaves, flowers.

USES Culinary A prime culinary herb, with no medical applications, it has a milder flavour than its onion cousin, *Allium cepa*. Snip leaves into salads, sauces and soups. Flowers can be used as a garnish.

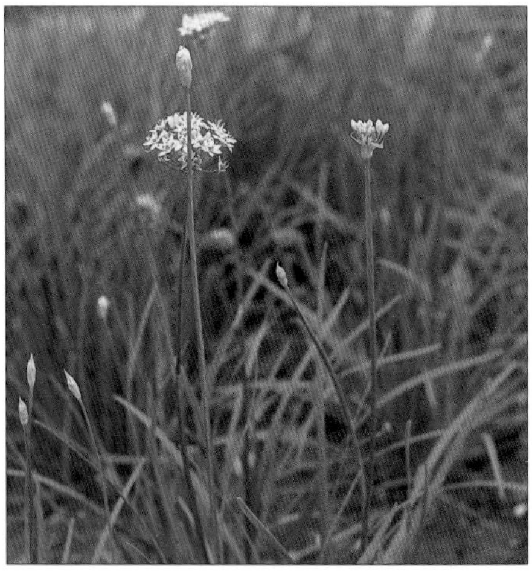

Allium tuberosum
Garlic chives

Description A perennial with sheaths of coarse, flattened leaves growing from a rhizome (modified stem) to a height of 50cm/20in. Star-shaped white flowers appear in late summer.
Parts used Fresh leaves.

USES Culinary Use as chives.

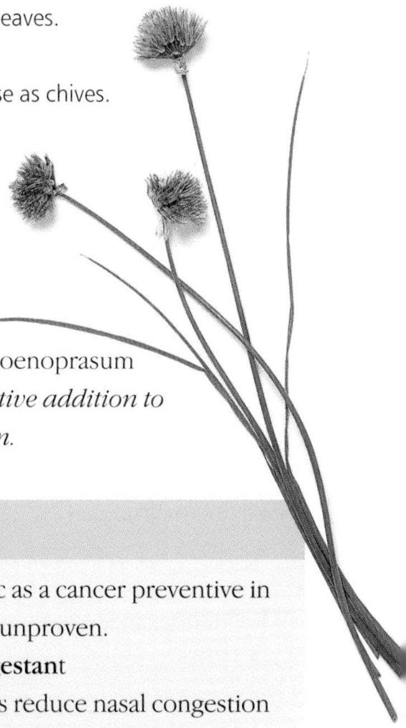

Right Allium schoenoprasum *makes an attractive addition to the flower garden.*

Medicinal use of garlic and onions

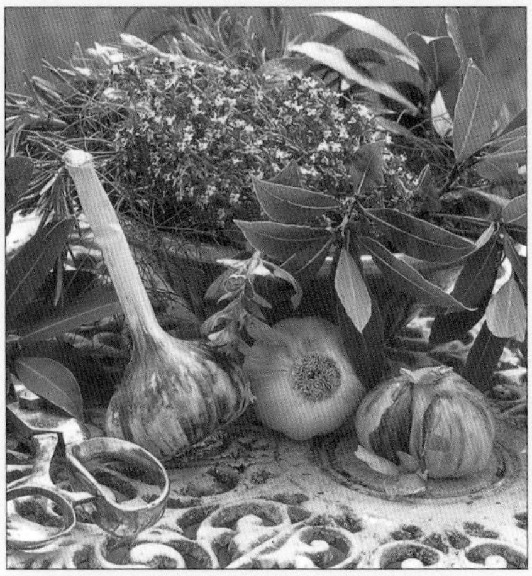

Above *Regularly eating garlic helps to keep your heart healthy.*

Helps lower blood pressure and blood cholesterol
Both garlic and onions may help to lower blood pressure and blood cholesterol. They are also thought to raise levels of beneficial high-density lipoproteins in the blood – these are molecules which play a part in clearing cholesterol from body tissues.
Helps prevent blood clotting
Research studies have also found that eating onions and garlic inhibits blood clotting and helps prevent circulatory diseases such as coronary heart disease, thrombosis and strokes. Studies using animals revealed that a garlic compound, allyl disulphide, helped prevent growth of malignant tumours – but the case for garlic as a cancer preventive in humans is as yet unproven.
Acts as a decongestant
Garlic and onions reduce nasal congestion and ease cold symptoms, especially when eaten raw, as volatile components are lost in cooking.
Has antiviral and antibacterial properties
The juice of a freshly-cut onion is a useful first-aid measure to relieve insect bites, bee stings and the itching of chilblains.

CAUTION Garlic can interact with anti-coagulant drugs such as warfarin.

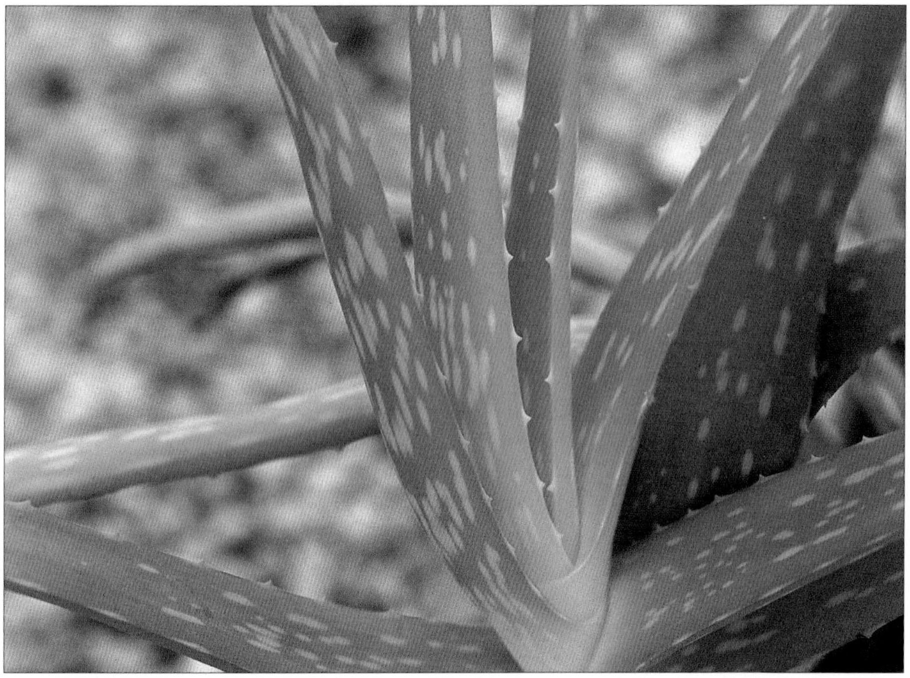

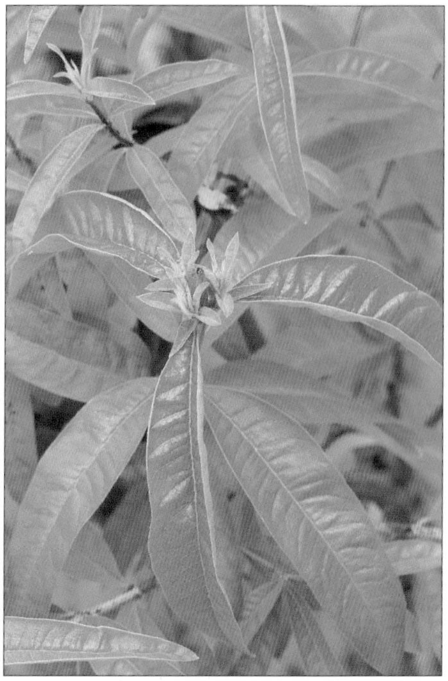

ALOEACEAE

Aloe vera syn. *A. barbadensis*

Aloe vera

History and traditions The medicinal value of this plant was recognized by the Egyptians and used as an embalming ingredient. One story goes that Aristotle tried to persuade Alexander the Great to conquer the Indian Ocean island of Socotra (near the Gulf of Aden), for its aloes, being the only known place where they grew at the time. The plant was introduced to Europe in the 10th century and became established over the centuries as an important ingredient in proprietary medicines.

Description A tender succulent, 60–40cm/2–3ft tall, with clusters of elongated, very fleshy, greeny-grey leaves, spiked at the edges, and tubular yellow flowers.

Related species Of the 300 species of aloes only a few have medicinal properties, including *A. perryi* and the South African *A. ferox,* which has red spikes at the leaf edges. *A. vera* is the most potent.

Habitat/distribution Origins are uncertain, but it is widespread in tropical and subtropical regions in dry, sunny areas.

Growth It needs a well-drained soil, full sun and a minimum temperature of 5°C/41°F. In cold climates it can be successfully grown as a conservatory or house plant. Pot up in gritty compost (soil mix), do not overwater, and allow to dry out completely between waterings.

Parts used Leaves, sap. The leaves are cut and the sap is used fresh, preserved and bottled or dried to a brown crystalline solid for use in creams, lotions and medicinal preparations.

USES Medicinal It is the mix of constituents in this plant that gives it exceptional healing properties. Aloe gel and resin may be used. Aloe resin has laxative and anti-inflammatory activity. The gel is immune-enhancing, anti-viral, anti-inflammatory, demulcent and emollient. It contains minerals; antioxidant vitamins C, E, B_{12}, beta-carotene and lignin. *A. vera* gel from the leaf is applied externally to promote healing of wounds, burns, sunburn, eczema and skin irritations. It is taken internally for digestive tract problems and there is also some evidence that it may help conditions where the immune system is not functioning well. It has laxative properties and "bitter aloes" is the name for the strong, purgative medicine that is made from the leaves.

Cosmetic It is an ingredient of many commercial cosmetic products.

Other names Aloes, Barbados aloe, Cape aloe and Curaçao aloe.

CAUTION Only to be taken internally with professional healthcare advice. Not to be taken internally if pregnant or in large doses. Subject to legal restrictions in some countries.

VERBENACEAE

Aloysia triphylla syn. *Aloysia citriodora*

Lemon verbena

History and traditions This lemon-scented shrub from South America was introduced to Europe in the 1790s. It is said to be named after Maria Louisa, wife of Carlos IV of Spain, Aloysia being a corruption of Louisa. The Victorians liked it for its long-lasting lemon fragrance, calling it "the lemon plant", and dried it for use in scented sachets.

Description Frost- to half-hardy deciduous shrub with rough-textured, strongly lemon-scented, spear-shaped leaves, dotted on the underside with oil glands. Racemes of tiny mauve-white flowers appear in late summer. In warm climates, where no frost occurs, it grows to 4.5m/15ft, but in cooler regions it is unlikely to grow to more than 1.5m/5ft. It is closely related to the *Lippia* genus, with which it was once classified.

Habitat/distribution Native to Chile and Argentina, it is widely grown in tropical and subtropical zones of the world, in Australia, New Zealand and temperate regions of Europe.

Growth It will usually survive a minimum temperature of -5°C/23°F, provided it is grown in a sheltered, south-facing site in well-drained soil. It will not tolerate prolonged cold and frost, especially if grown in a heavy soil. May be grown as a pot plant if given winter protection.

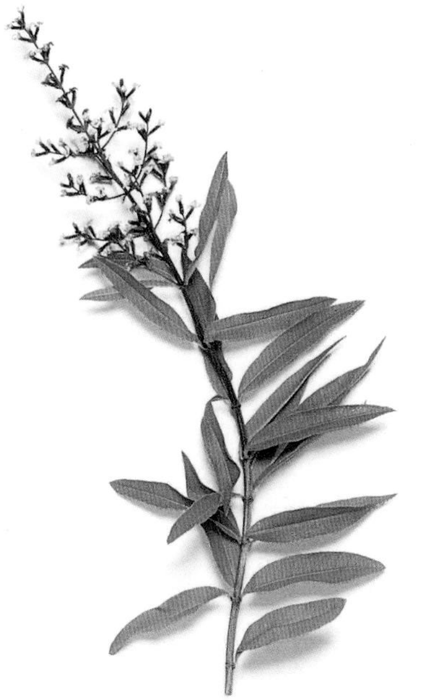

Above *Lemon verbena has a strong sherbert lemon scent.*

Right *Lemon verbena in flower – it keeps its scent well when dried.*

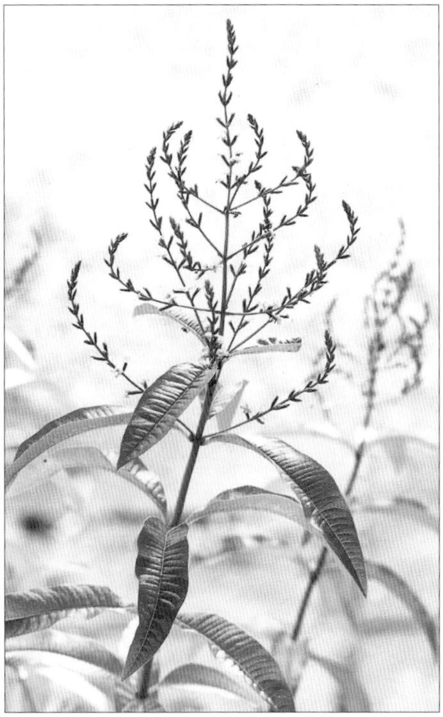

New leaves do not appear until late spring or early summer. Cut back hard in spring, when it will regenerate from old wood. It is propagated from cuttings, taken in late summer, but needs heat to produce roots and during development of the seedlings.
Parts used Leaves, essential oil.

USES Medicinal Has been traditionally used to treat various diseases, including bronchitis, insomnia, anxiety, digestive and heart problems.
Culinary The leaves (fresh or dry) make a refreshing tea. If used with great discretion, as the taste is strong, they can be included in savoury stuffings and sauces, or used to flavour cakes and ice cream.
Aromatic The benefit of this herb is that the leaves retain their lemon scent, when dried, for several years. They help to deter insects and are ideal for sachets and making potpourri. The essential oil was widely used in perfumery, but has been discovered to sensitize the skin to sunlight.

Lemon verbena potpourri

dried peel of 1 lemon
2 cups dried lemon verbena leaves
1 cup dried chamomile flowers
15cm/6in cinnamon stick, crushed
1 cup dried pot marigold petals
5ml/1 tsp orris root powder
2–3 drops essential oil of lemon verbena (optional)

To dry the lemon peel, scrape it off the fruit with a vegetable peeler, spread on paper and put in a warm place (such as an airing cupboard) for about two weeks, until crisp.

Mix the dried lemon peel, dried lemon verbena leaves, dried chamomile flowers, crushed cinnamon, dried pot marigold petals, orris root powder and oils together. Seal in a tin and put in a warm place for 2–3 weeks, shaking occasionally. Put in a bowl to scent the room, covering when not in use to retain the scent, or in drawstring sachets to hang in a wardrobe.

Lemon verbena essential oil will give the potpourri a stronger fragrance. It is also useful for adding zest to the mixture at a later date, as it will lose strength when constantly exposed to light and air.

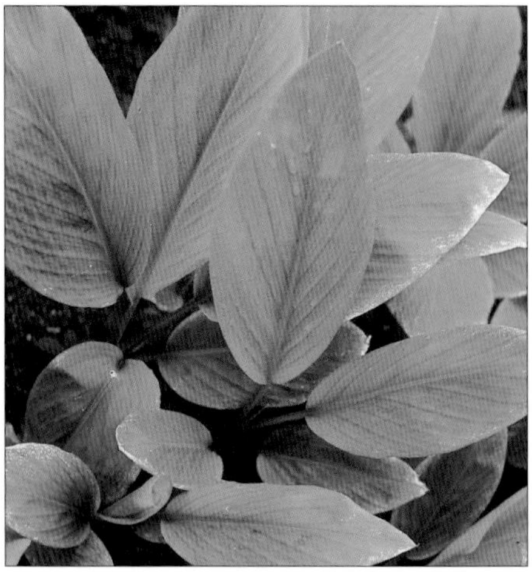

ZINGIBERACEAE

Alpinia officinarum

Galangal

History and traditions Very similar to ginger, this plant has a long history as a spice and medicinal plant and has been used in Ayurvedic and Chinese medicine since ancient times. 'Galangal' comes from the Arabic word *Khalanjan*, which could in turn be derived from a Chinese word meaning "mild ginger". Known in Europe since the 9th century, it was probably introduced by Arab or Greek physicians.
Description A tropical evergreen with tall clumps of ovate to lanceolate leaves growing from ginger-scented rhizomes to a height of 1.2m/4ft. Flowers are pale green and white. *A. officinarum*, lesser galangal, is the more important species for both medicinal and culinary purposes.
Related species *A. galanga*, greater galangal, is a larger plant, growing to 2m/6ft, and has a less marked ginger aroma.
Habitat/distribution Found in tropical rainforest and grassland areas of southeast Asia and Australia.
Growth It can be grown only in climates with high humidity and minimum temperatures of 15–18°C/59–64°F. Needs well-drained soil and partial shade. Propagated by division of the rhizomes when new shoots appear.
Parts used Rhizome, oil.

USES Medicinal A good digestive aid. It has antibacterial and antifungal properties, is used for feverish illnesses and fungal infections. *A. galanga* is considered less effective medicinally.
Culinary Both species are used as a ginger-like flavouring in Thai and southeast Asian cookery.

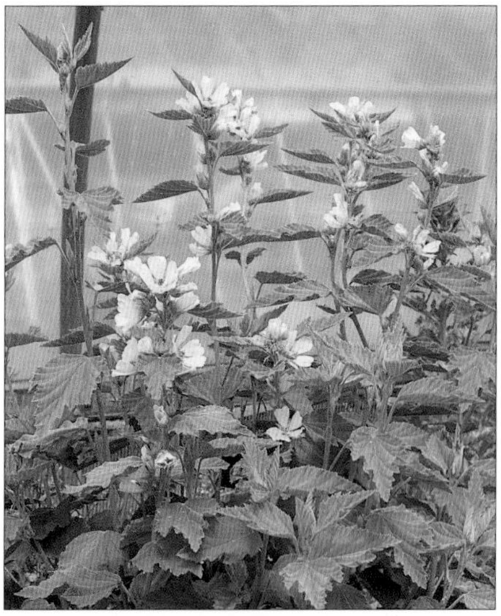

MALVACEAE

Althaea officinalis

Marshmallow

History and traditions The generic name comes from the Greek, *altho*, meaning "to cure". The family name, Malvaceae, is also of Greek derivation, from *malake*, meaning soft, indicating the emollient, healing properties of this plant, which have long been recognized. Pliny remarked: "Whosoever shall take a spoonful of Mallows shall that day be free from all diseases that may come to him." Early recorded uses include poultices to reduce inflammation and spongy lozenges to soothe coughs and sore throats. It is from this the modern confectionery is descended, though it no longer contains any of the herb. Marshmallow root was eaten as a vegetable by the Romans and in many Middle Eastern and European countries was a standby in times of famine when food was scarce. In more recent times it was a springtime country tradition to eat the young shoots, or make them into a syrup, to "purify the blood".

Description A hardy perennial with soft, downy leaves and pale pink flowers in summer, it reaches 1–1.2m/3–4ft in height. It has large, fleshy taproots.

Habitat/distribution Found in salt marshes, near sea coasts and in moist inland areas, throughout Europe, in temperate regions of Asia, North America and Australia.

Growth Prefers moist to wet soil and a sunny situation. Propagated by division in autumn or by seed sown in late summer, though germination is often erratic.

Parts used Leaves, roots, flowers.

USES Medicinal The herb contains a demulcent mucilage and is anti-inflammatory in action. *Althaea* is used primarily to calm digestive complaints such as constipation, diarrhoea, irritable bowel syndrome and heartburn, It is also used to influence the pulmonary systems. It may also be applied locally to ulcers, boils, inflammation of the skin and insect bites.

Culinary At one time the young roots and leaves were boiled, then fried with onions as a spring vegetable, or added to salads – but neither is very palatable.

> **CAUTION** Marshmallow may delay the absorption of other drugs.

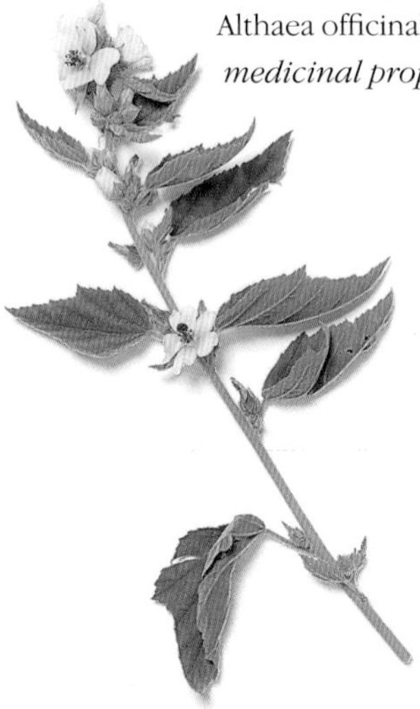

Below *All parts of* Althaea officinalis *have medicinal properties.*

Below left and right Alcea rosea, *the garden hollyhock, has racemes of single blooms in pink, purple and white. There are also many cultivars with double flowers.*

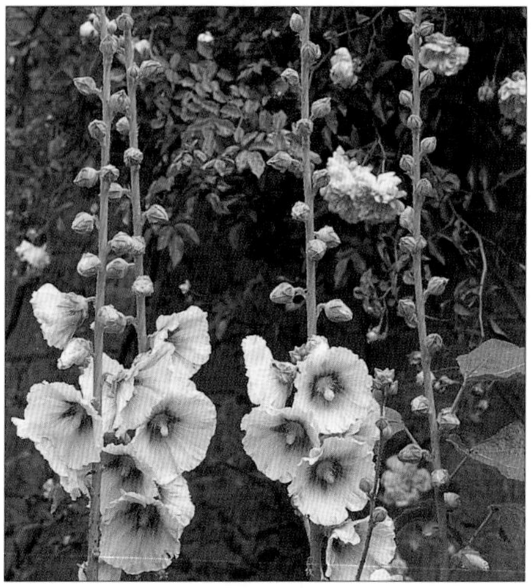

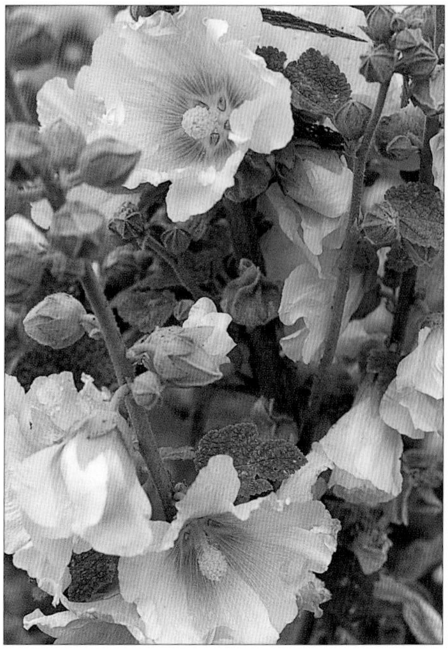

Related species

MALVACEAE

Alcea rosea formerly *Althaea rosea*

Hollyhock

This spectacular biennial, which first came to Europe from China in the 16th century, is closely related to *Althaea officinalis* and used to be classified in the same genus. It too has soothing properties and the flowers were once used to make cough syrups and to treat chest complaints, but the medicinal properties of its less showy relative are now considered superior. It is still worth its place in the herb garden for its old-fashioned grace and large colourful blooms (pink, purple, yellow or white) on towering spikes. It is easy to grow in well-drained soil and a sunny position from seeds sown *in situ* in spring or late summer.

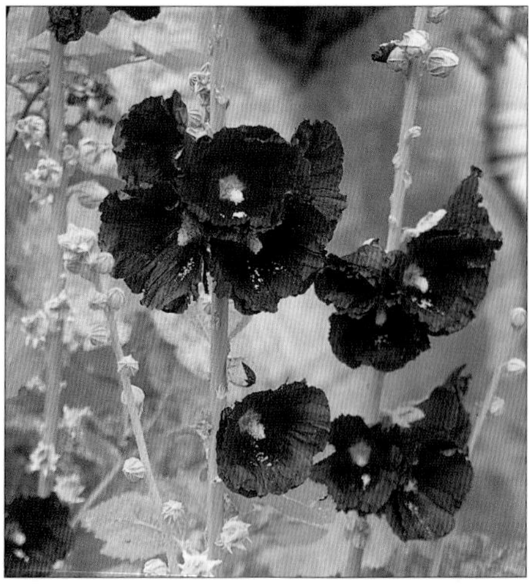

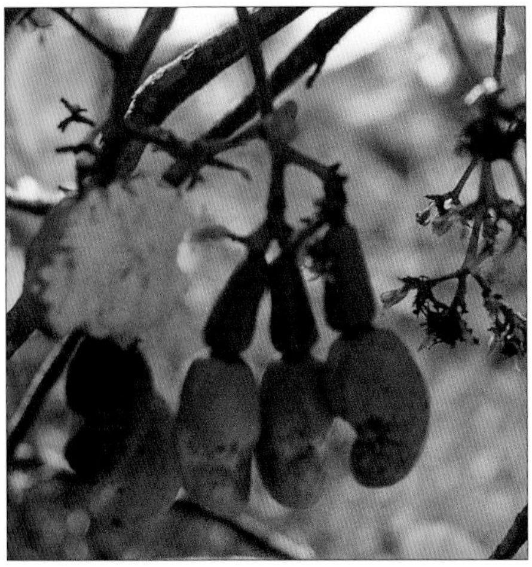

ANACARDIACEAE

Anacardium occidentale

Cashew nut

History and traditions A native of South and Central America and the Caribbean islands, this well-known nut tree was introduced to India from Brazil by Portuguese colonists in the 16th century, who originally planted it to prevent soil erosion on hillsides in Goa.
Description An evergreen tree, reaching 12m/40ft, it has dark green, rounded, oval leaves. Panicles of pinkish-green flowers are followed by the fleshy fruit, known as the cashew apple, each of which has a kidney-shaped nut suspended from its base, containing a white seed.
Habitat/distribution Naturalized and cultivated in tropical zones worldwide.
Growth Tender trees which need well-drained, sandy soil, periodic high rainfall and a minimum temperature of 18°C/64°F.
Parts used Leaves, bark, fruits, seeds.

USES Medicinal The bark and leaves are used in traditional herbal medicine in Africa to treat malaria.
Culinary The nut, or kernel, is a good source of fibre and protein. It is rich in minerals and mono-unsaturated fat, making it a healthy choice of snack when eaten in moderation. Juice from the fruit is made into soft drinks and distilled to produce spirits.
Other The outer shell of the nut produces a thick, tarry black oil used in engineering, and as a timber preservative to protect against insects.

CAUTION Oil from the cashew nut shell is an irritant and can cause painful skin blistering.

UMBELLIFERAE/APIACEAE

Anethum graveolens

Dill

History and traditions An ancient herb known in biblical times and described both by Pliny, AD23–79, and by the Greek physician Dioscorides, AD40–90, in *De Materia Medica*. It appears in the 10th-century writings of Alfric, Archbishop of Canterbury, and was a favourite herb in Anglo-Saxon charms against witchcraft, at which time it was also burned "to disperse thunder clouds and sulphurous air". The common name is likely to have come from the Saxon word *dillan*, to lull, for its ability to soothe colicky babies and for the ancient Greek tradition of covering the head with dill leaves to induce sleep. The culinary connection with cucumber goes back a long way. Charles I's cook, Joseph Cooper, records a recipe for pickling cucumbers in dill in his book of 1640. It has a long tradition of use in India and Eastern countries as a medicinal and culinary herb.
Description An aromatic annual, 1m/3ft tall, with a single stem and feathery leaves. It has terminal umbels of tiny yellow flowers in midsummer and elliptic, flattened fruits. Resembles fennel, but is shorter and has a subtler, less strongly aniseed flavour.

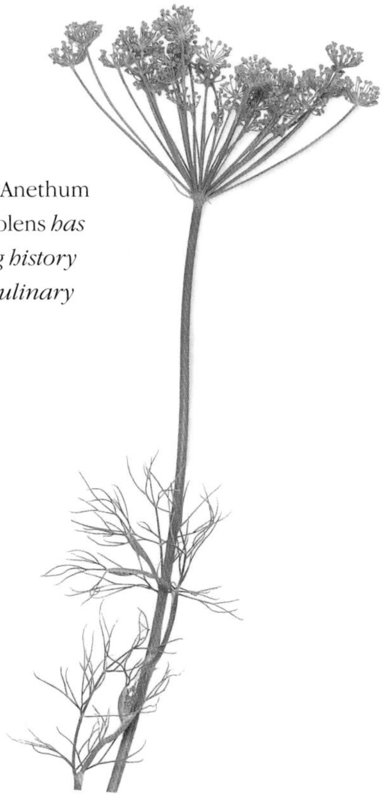

Right Anethum graveolens *has a long history as a culinary herb.*

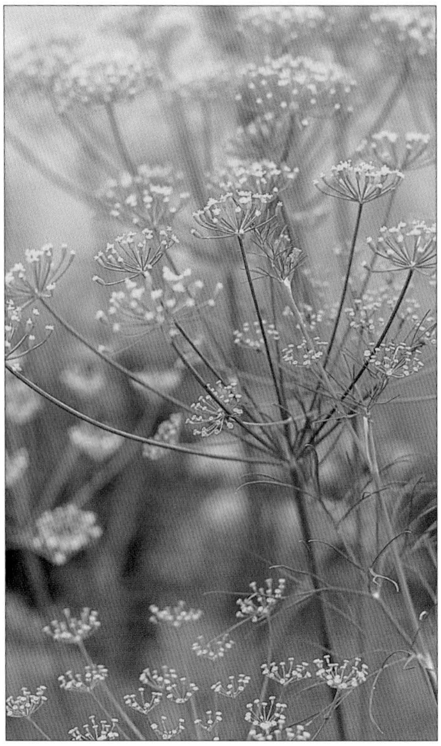

Related species Indian dill is known as sowa. It is usually classified as *A. sowa,* but this is either a subspecies of *A. graveolens* or very closely related.
Habitat/distribution Originated in southern Europe and Asia, now widely grown in herb gardens worldwide.
Growth Plant dill in well-drained but nutrient-rich soil, in full sun. Requires adequate moisture as it bolts (runs quickly to seed) in poor, dry soil. Best propagated from seed sown in spring, straight into the ground where it is to grow, as it does not take well to being transplanted. Should not be grown near fennel as the two plants crosspollinate.
Parts used Leaves, seeds.

USES Medicinal A cooling, soothing herb which aids digestion, prevents constipation and is an ingredient of "gripe water" given to babies for indigestion. In Indian herbal medicine dill and fenugreek seeds are included in preparations for diarrhoea and dysentery. Poultices of the leaves are applied to boils and to reduce swelling and joint pains. Seeds are chewed to cure bad breath.
Culinary Leaves and seeds add a caraway-like flavour to fish, seafood and egg dishes and go well with bland-tasting vegetables, especially cucumber and potatoes. Widely used in Scandinavian cuisine. In Indian cookery, it is added to curries, rice dishes, soups, pickles and chutneys.

UMBELLIFERAE/APIACEAE

Angelica archangelica

Angelica

History and traditions According to legend, this herb took its name from the angel who revealed its virtues to a monk during a plague epidemic. It was thought to give protection from infection. It is also variously connected with the archangel Gabriel who is said to have appeared to the Virgin Mary at the Annunciation, and the archangel Michael, whose feast day is in May. In all northern European folklore it has an ancient reputation for its powers against witchcraft and evil spirits. In Lapland poets wore crowns of angelica, supposedly to gain inspiration from its scent. John Parkinson in his *Theatre of Plants*, 1640, wrote of it: "The whole plante, both leafe, roote and seede, is of an excellent comfortable scent, savour and taste."

Description Angelica is a statuesque biennial, though it often lives for three years. The whole plant is subtly aromatic. Standing 1.2–2.4m/4–8ft high, it has hollow stems, large, deeply divided pale green leaves and globular umbels of green flowers in early summer, followed by flat, oval seeds.

Related species *A. atropurpurea*, American angelica, has red stems. *A. sylvestris* is the wild European angelica.

Habitat/distribution Native to Europe and parts of Asia. Introduced in other parts of the world.

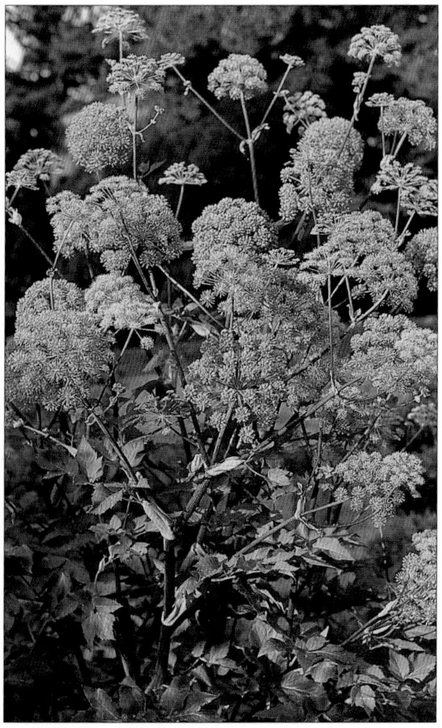

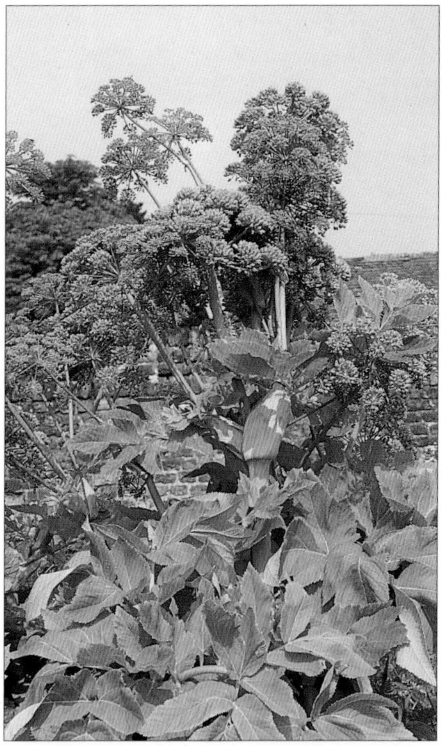

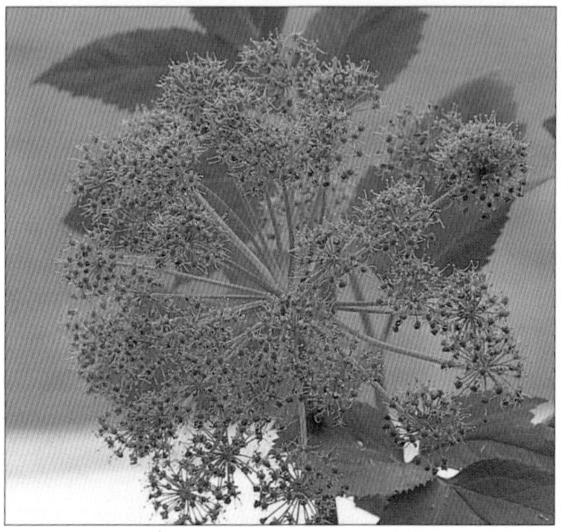

Growth Prefers a rich, damp soil but tolerates most conditions, provided it is not too dry. Plant in sun or partial shade. Self-seeds freely. Propagate by seed sown in autumn, in situ or in pots; seed remains viable for 6–12 months.

Parts used Leaves, stems, roots, seeds.

USES Medicinal Has anti-inflammatory properties, lowers fevers and acts as an expectorant. Infusions of the root are used to aid digestive disorders and bowel complaints. Furocoumarin content increases skin photosensitivity and may cause skin irritation in susceptible people.

Culinary In Europe young stems are candied, cooked with rhubarb, tart fruits and berries to reduce acidity. It can be added to jams or marmalade (ginger and angelica make a good combination), seeds are added to biscuits (cookies). Seeds and roots are constituents of Benedictine, Chartreuse and other liqueurs.

CAUTION Not to be taken in pregnancy, during heavy menstrual flow, or if taking anti-coagulant medication, such as aspirin. May increase skin photosensitivity. Caution with inflammatory gastrointestinal tract conditions such as active peptic ulcers and gastritis.

Far left Angelica atropurpurea *is a North American species with red stems.*
Left *A seed head of angelica.*

Culinary angelica

Angelica and rhubarb

Angelica has a pleasantly aromatic, slightly sweet taste, which enhances the flavour of rhubarb and reduces its acidity, so that less sugar is necessary. Only the very young leaf stems should be used, as older ones are coarse and stringy. Allow two or three 15cm/6in pieces for each 450g/1lb of rhubarb sticks. Cut them into small pieces and add to your favourite rhubarb pie or crumble recipe. Angelica is also excellent puréed with rhubarb to make a fool.

Candied angelica

Old recipe books contain instructions for candying leaves and roots, as well as stems of angelica.

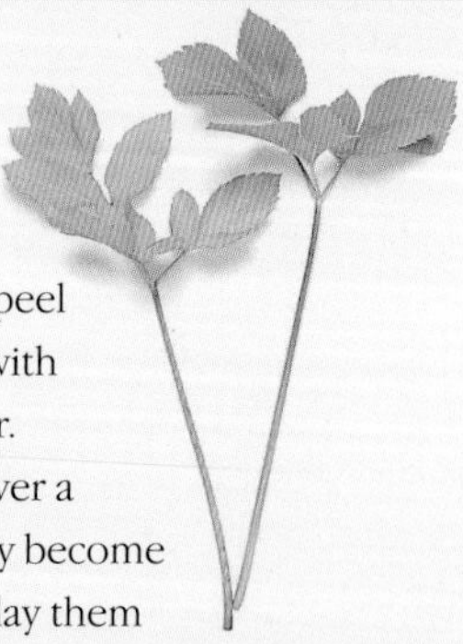

"Boil the stalks of Angelica in water till they are tender; then peel them and cover with other warm water. Let them stand over a gentle fire till they become very green; then lay them on a cloth to dry; take their weight in fine sugar with a little Rose-water and boil it to a Candy height. Then put in your Angelica and boil them up quick; then take them out and dry them for use."

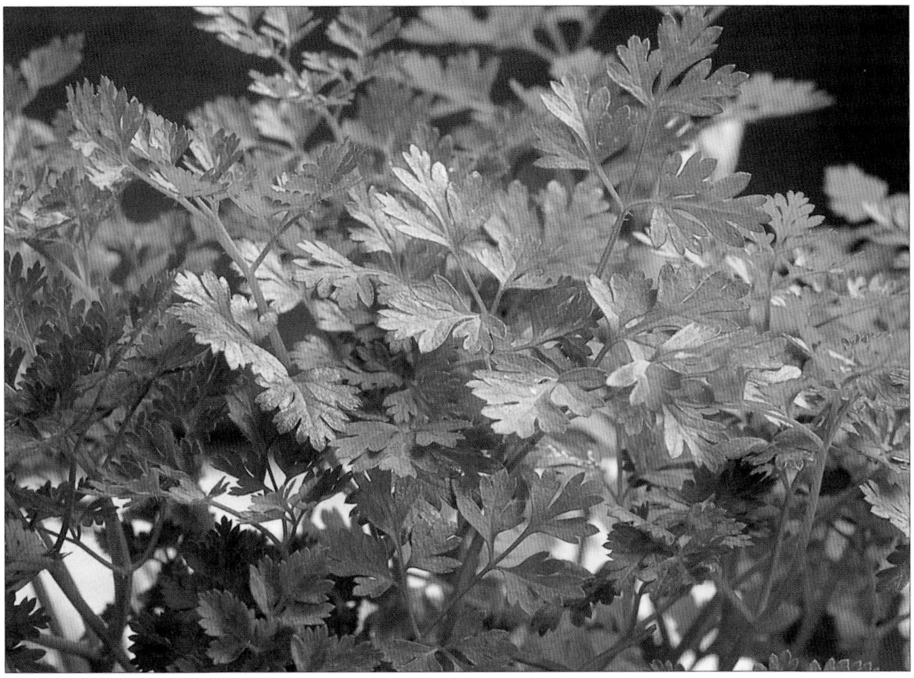

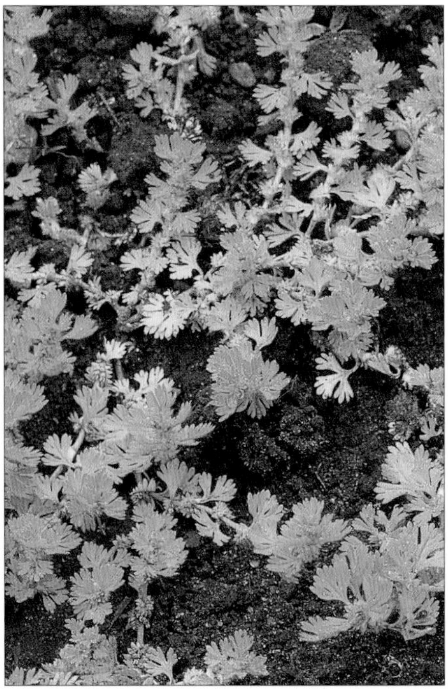

UMBELLIFERAE/APIACEAE

Anthriscus cerefolium

Chervil

History and traditions The Romans were very fond of chervil and it is listed in 15th-century manuscripts as an essential kitchen herb. Confusion sometimes arises, however, as at that time both *A. cerefolium* and sweet cicely, *Myrrhis odorata*, were known as "chervil", sometimes distinguished as "sweet chervil" and "common chervil". John Parkinson, who wrote during the 17th-century in England, indicates: "Common chervil is much used of the French and Dutch people to bee boiled or stewed in a pipkin either by itself or with other herbs, whereof they make a Loblolly and so eate it. Sweete chervil gathered while it is young and put among other herbs for a sallet addeth a marvellous good relish to all the reste."

Description A hardy annual, 30–60cm/1–2ft high, with bright green, finely divided feathery leaves and flat umbels of small white flowers in early summer.

Habitat/distribution Native to the Middle East and southern Russia. Widely cultivated elsewhere in warm and temperate climates.

Growth Chervil prefers light, moist soil and a sunny situation. Propagate from seed sown successionally for a continuous supply. It does not transplant well and runs to seed quickly, but can be sown where it is to grow, or cropped straight from the seed tray.

Parts used Leaves, preferably fresh, cut just before flowering.

USES Medicinal Although it has mild digestive properties, and is sometimes taken as a tea for this purpose, its chief use is culinary.

Culinary The delicate taste, which is more distinctive than parsley, complements most dishes. It brings out the flavour of other herbs and is an essential ingredient, along with parsley, tarragon and chives, of the classic French combination, *fines herbes*. It is best used raw or in a very short cooking process, if the subtle flavour is to be retained.

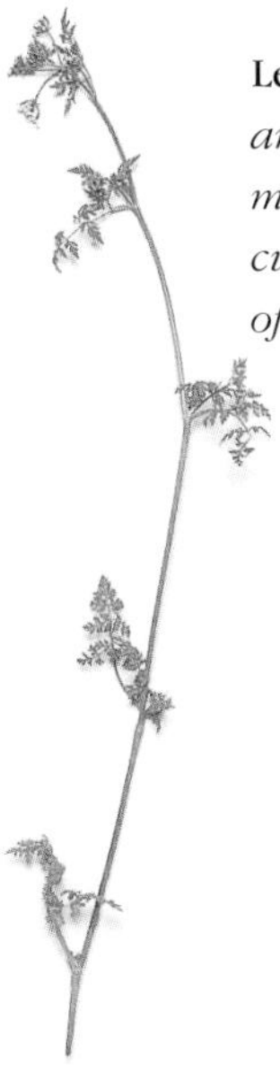

Left *Chervil's light aniseed flavour makes it a culinary herb of distinction.*

ROSACEAE

Aphanes arvensis

Parsley piert

History and traditions The common name comes from this herb's vague resemblance to parsley and from the French name for it, *perce-pierre*, meaning to pierce or break a stone. Breakstone is an alternative country name in English also and refers to its traditional use in treating kidney stones. Culpeper lists as its chief use that "it provokes urine, and breaks the stone", and it is still used for the treatment of kidney stones in herbal medicine today.

Description A prostrate annual with small fan-shaped leaves and inconspicuous green flowers in summer.

Habitat/distribution Found in dry places and wastelands, it is native to Britain and widely distributed throughout the world.

Growth As a wild plant, it grows best in well-drained soil, in sun or partial shade, and tolerates gravelly, stony soils. Propagated by seed sown in spring.

Parts used Leaves.

USES Medicinal A diuretic which also soothes irritated and inflamed tissues. It is used to ease painful urination and in the treatment of kidney and bladder stones.

Culinary It was a popular salad herb during the 16th century, but the taste is uninteresting and it is seldom eaten today.

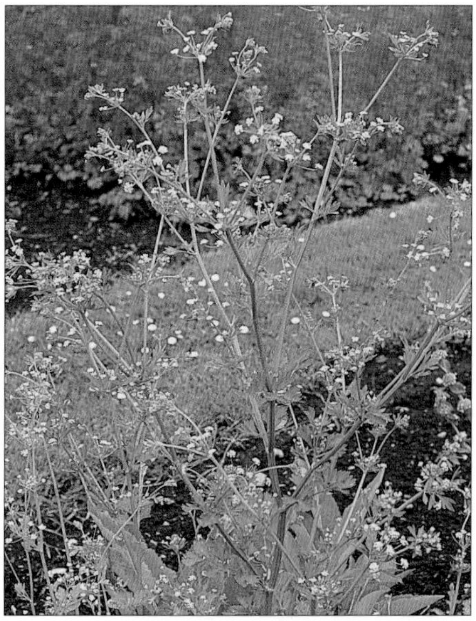

UMBELLIFERAE/APIACEAE

Apium graveolens

Wild celery

History and traditions Although rather bitter in flavour, it was the only celery known until the 17th century, when the cultivated variety we enjoy today, *A. g.* var. *dulce,* was developed.
Description An aromatic biennial with a bulbous, fleshy root. Grooved stems grow from 30–90cm/1–3ft high in the second year. It has pointed, divided leaves (similar in shape to cultivated celery) and umbels of sparse, greenish-white flowers in late summer, followed by small, ridged seeds.
Habitat/distribution Found in marshy, often salty ground in Europe, Asia, northern Africa, North and South America.
Growth It prefers rich, damp soil, sun or partial shade and tolerates saline conditions. Does best in a sheltered position, and bears flowers for seed production in warm climates. It is propagated by seed sown in spring, but needs a temperature of 13–16°C/55–61°F to germinate.
Parts used Roots, stems, leaves, seeds.

USES Medicinal Used in the treatment of arthritis and rheumatism and in Ayurvedic medicine as a nerve tonic.
Culinary The plant is toxic in large quantities. A few seeds may be used for flavouring.

CAUTION Seeds should not be taken if pregnant, or where there is kidney disease or damage. May cause allergic reactions.

COMPOSITAE/ASTERACEAE

Arctium lappa

Greater burdock

History and traditions This plant's names relate to the clinging nature of the burs which follow the flowers. *Arctium* comes from *arktos*, Greek for a bear (supposed to indicate the plant's roughness), and *lappa* from a word meaning to seize, though some authorities also connect the species name with the Celtic word for hand, *llap*. The English common name is a little more obvious in derivation, "bur" referring to the prickles and "dock" to the shape of the large leaves. Culpeper lists its popular names as "Personata", "Happy-Major" and "Clot-bur".
Description A biennial, or short-lived perennial, which grows to 1.5m/5ft tall. It has long, ovate leaves covered in down and thick, hairy stems. Purple thistle-like flowers appear in mid to late summer, followed by fruits (seed heads) made up of hooked spines or burs.
Related species *A. minus,* lesser burdock, has similar properties. *A. lappa* 'Gobo' is a culinary cultivar grown in Japan.
Habitat/distribution Greater burdock is native to temperate regions of Asia and widely distributed throughout Europe and North America, found on roadsides, waste ground and in nitrogen-rich soil.
Growth It is usually collected from the wild, but a cultivated species is grown in Japan. Prefers a moist soil, sun or partial shade and it self-seeds quite freely.
Parts used Roots, stems, seeds, leaves (rarely).

CAUTION Contact dermatitis is possible in those who are sensitive. May increase severity of existing symptoms. Only to be taken on the advice of a herbal or medical practitioner.

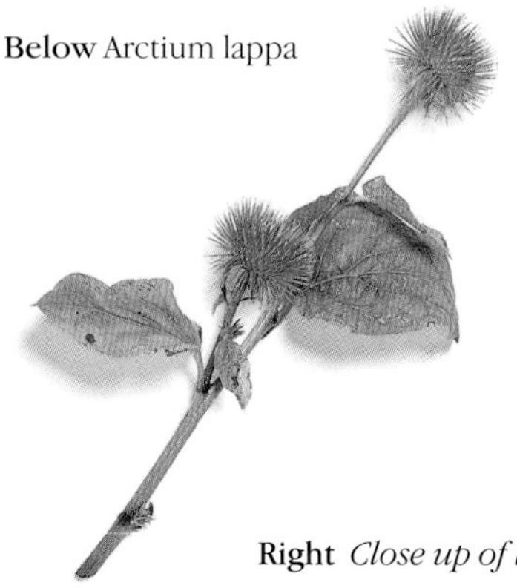

Below Arctium lappa

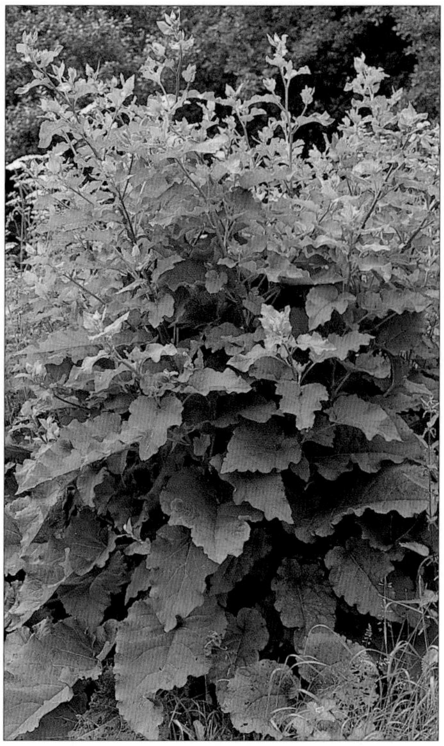

USES Medicinal It has antibacterial and fungicidal properties and is used as a decoction or poultice for inflamed skin, sores, boils and disorders such as eczema and psoriasis. It is also taken for gastric ulcers and is said to increase resistance to infection. Used in traditional Chinese medicine.
Culinary It is cultivated in Japan for the roots, which are eaten as a vegetable. The stalks, before flowering, can be chopped and added to salads, or cooked as a celery-like vegetable. In the past, they were sometimes candied, in the same way as angelica.
Cosmetic An infusion of the leaves, or decoction of the roots, makes a tonic skin freshener or hair rinse for dandruff.
Other names Lappa and beggar's buttons.

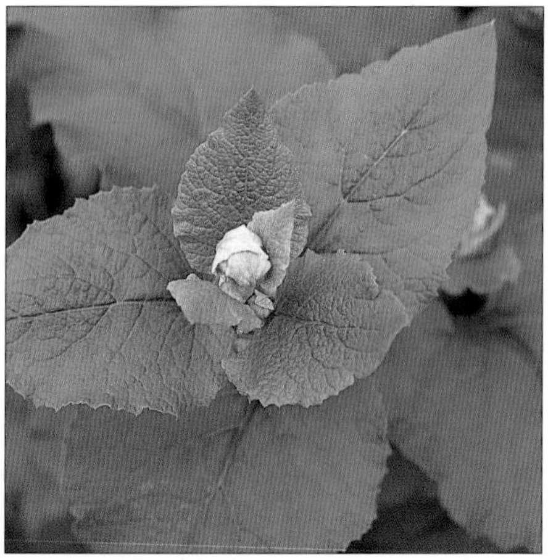

Right *Close up of leaf*

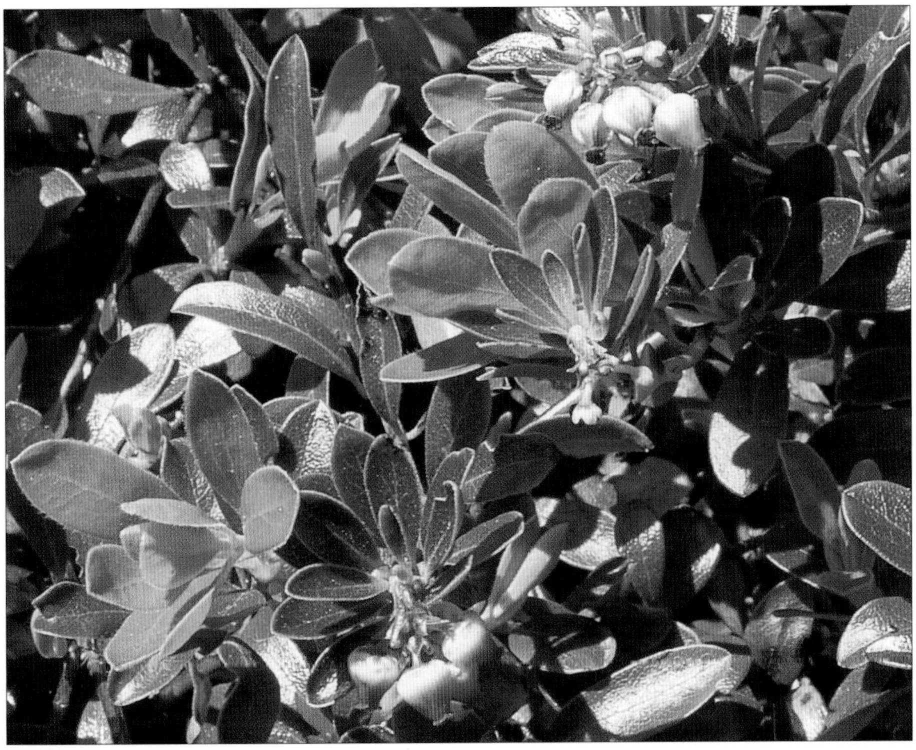

ERICACEAE

Arctostaphylos uva-ursi

Bearberry

History and traditions The generic name from the Greek, *arcton staphyle*, and the specific, *uva-ursi,* from the Latin, both mean "bear's grapes", perhaps because bears enjoyed the fruit, or maybe the sour taste of this plant was only thought fit for consumption by bears? It is listed in 13th-century herbal manuscripts and was described in detail by the 16th-century Dutch botanist Clusius (Charles de L'Ecluse). In the 17th century John Josslyn discovered this herb growing in North America, where many of the Native American tribes made use of its medicinal properties and added it to smoking mixtures. He found it to be highly effective against scurvy. It was considered medicinally important in 18th-century Europe, and remained so into the 20th century, appearing in the British *Pharmacopoeia*.

Description A creeping, evergreen shrub, growing to 15cm/6in, with dark green, leathery, small, oval leaves. Terminal clusters of tiny, white or pink, bell-shaped flowers appear in summer, followed by red fruit.

Habitat/distribution Found in rocky moorland and woodland, in northern Europe, Scandinavia and Russia, northern Asia, Japan, North America and cool, northern hemisphere regions.

Growth Needs moist, sandy or peaty soil. Ericaceous compost (soil mix) must be used if container-grown and for propagating, which can be done from seed, by layering in spring or from cuttings, taken with a heel, in summer.

Parts used Leaves – usually dried.

For commercial use they are collected from the wild, mostly in Scandinavia and Russia, field cultivation having proved too costly.

USES Culinary Although the berries are edible, they taste extremely sharp, and are more suitable as "grouse feed", (a use given in one herbal). The leaves were at one time a popular tea in Russia.

Medicinal Constituents include arbutin and methylarbutin, which have been established as effectively antibacterial, especially against urinary infections, such as cystitis. Avoid long-term use due to high tannin content.

General The leaves have a high tannin content and have been used in the past in leather tanning and to produce a dark grey dye.

Other names Mountain box and uva-ursi.

CAUTION Bearberry should not be taken by women during pregnancy, by children, or where there is kidney disease.

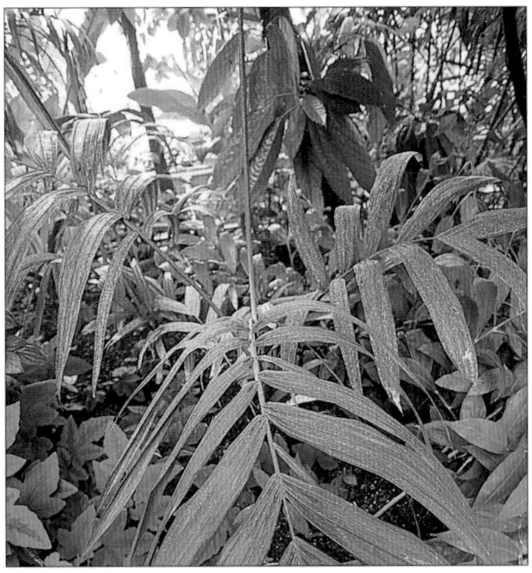

PALMAE/ARECACEAE

Areca catechu

Betel nut

History and traditions The Chinese discovered the medicinal properties of this tree by 140BC, when they brought it back from their conquests of the Malayan archipelago. It is the main ingredient of paan or "betel nut", a mixture of areca nut, lime and spices, wrapped in betel leaf, *Piper betle*, and it is widely chewed throughout the Middle East and Asia. It induces mild euphoria and is supposed to increase sexual virility.

Description A tall palm, reaching 20m/65ft in height, with numerous feathery leaflets making up its 2m/6ft long leaves. The pale yellow flowers appear when the tree is about 6–8 years old, followed by bunches of up to 100 round, orange fruits.

Habitat/distribution A native of Malaysia, and found throughout India, the Far East and eastern Africa, usually on coastal sites. Introduced in American tropical zones.

Parts used Fruit, rind, seeds.

USES Medicinal Stimulates the flow of saliva, and accelerates heart and perspiration rates. Chewed to sweeten breath, strengthen gums, improve digestion, and suppress intestinal worms – but permanently stains teeth red. Research is being carried out in America on this tree as a source of a potential anti-cancer drug. However, excessive chewing can lead to cancer of the mouth.

CAUTION Toxic in large doses, excess causes vomiting and stupor. Legal restrictions are in force in some countries.

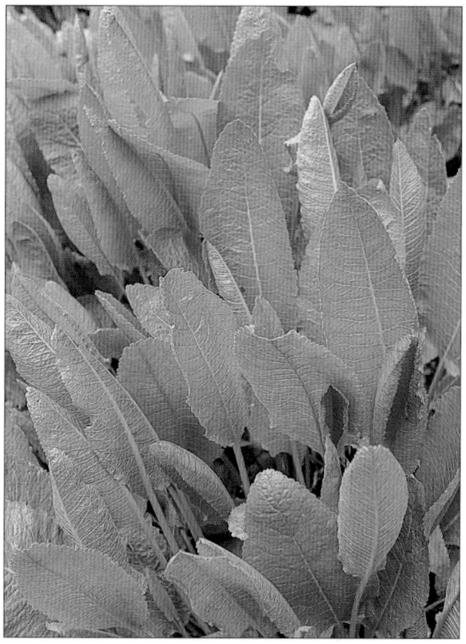

CRUCIFERAE/BRASSICACEAE

Armoracia rusticana

Horseradish

History and traditions Horseradish was valued in the Middle Ages for the medicinal properties of both leaves and root. The great English botanist and herbalist William Turner, writing in 1548, referred to it as 'Red Cole', and it was not commonly called horseradish until so named in England, in Gerard's Herbal of 1597. At that time it was used in Germany and Scandinavia to make the hot and spicy condiment we know today, but this did not become popular in Britain until well into the 17th century. John Parkinson, in 1640, describes its use as a sauce in Germany, adding, "and in our own land also", but he considered it "too strong for tender and gentle stomaches". In 1657, William Coles reiterated that it was the practice in Germany for "the root, sliced thin and mixed with vinegar (to be) eaten as a sauce with meat".

Description A perennial, with a deep, fleshy taproot and large bright green, oblong to ovate leaves, with serrated margins, sprouting from the base to a height of 60cm/2ft. Racemes of tiny, white flowers on drooping stems, up to 1.2m/4ft long, appear in summer.

Habitat/distribution In the wild it is found in dampish soils in Europe and western Asia. Now naturalized in many parts of the world.

Growth In theory it prefers a moist soil, but in practice flourishes in most conditions. It can be propagated by seed in spring, or by root cuttings in spring or autumn. It grows vigorously and, once established, is nearly impossible to eradicate as it regenerates from the tiniest scrap of root left in the soil.

Parts used Leaves, roots.

USES Medicinal The root may be taken in the form of a syrup for bronchial infections, catarrh and coughs and as a general tonic for debility. Horseradish is known as a "central" or "circulatory" stimulant (meaning it increases activity) for the heart and circulation.

Culinary The young, fresh leaves have a milder flavour than the pungent root and can be added to salads or chopped into smoked-fish pâtés. The fresh root is shredded to make a strong-flavoured, creamy-textured horseradish sauce, traditionally served with beef, but also excellent as an accompaniment to cold, especially smoked, meat and fish, hard-boiled eggs and stuffed aubergines (eggplants). For a milder flavour, grated apple, sprinkled with lemon juice and vinegar, can be mixed with horseradish.

To make horseradish sauce

2–3 pieces of fresh horseradish root
10ml/2 tbsp cider vinegar
115g/4oz fromage frais (farmers' cheese)
salt, pepper and a pinch of sugar
10ml/2 tsp fresh, chopped dill

Scrub the horseradish root, grate it finely, and cover with the vinegar. Or, for a smoother texture, mix the horseradish and vinegar in an electric blender till pulped. Mix in the fromage frais, seasonwith salt, pepper, sugar and chopped dill.

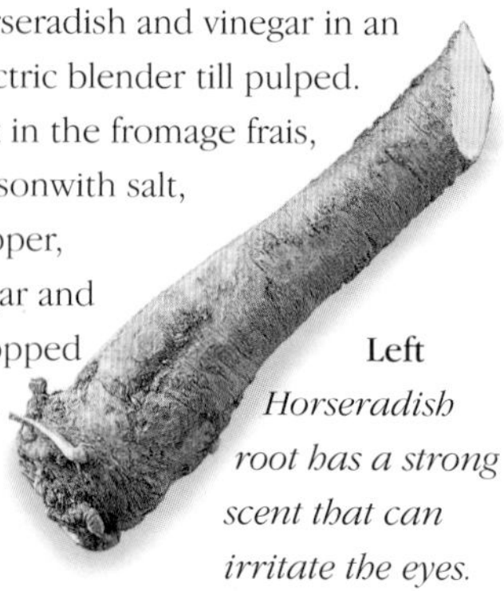

Left *Horseradish root has a strong scent that can irritate the eyes.*

CAUTION May provoke allergic reactions. Large internal doses may cause vomiting. Should not be taken if suffering from stomach ulcers or thyroid problems.

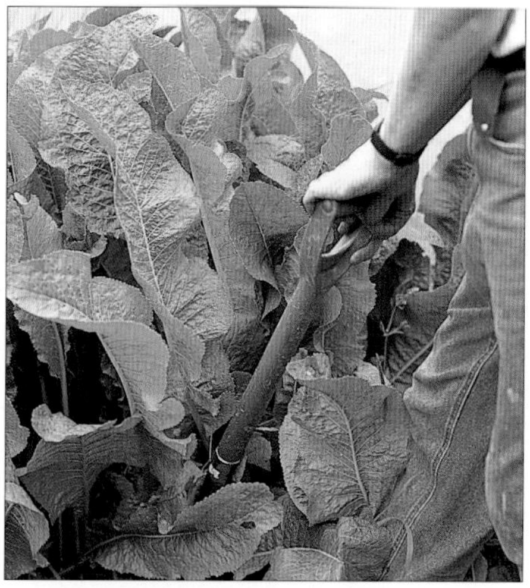

Above *Digging up roots of established plants to make horseradish sauce.*

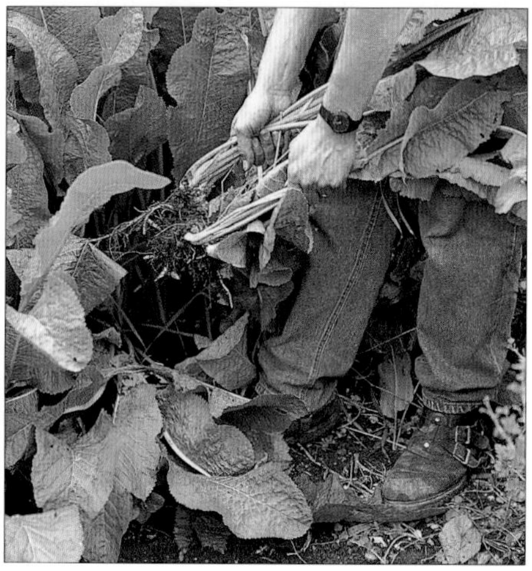

Above *Leaving some behind will ensure an ongoing supply of material.*

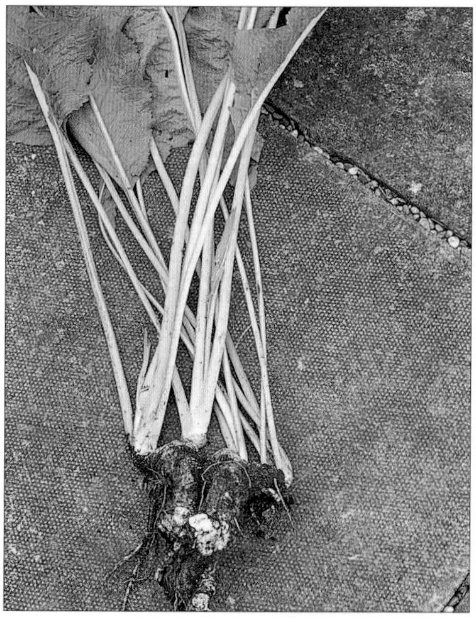

Above *Home-grown horseradish roots make a pungent sauce.*

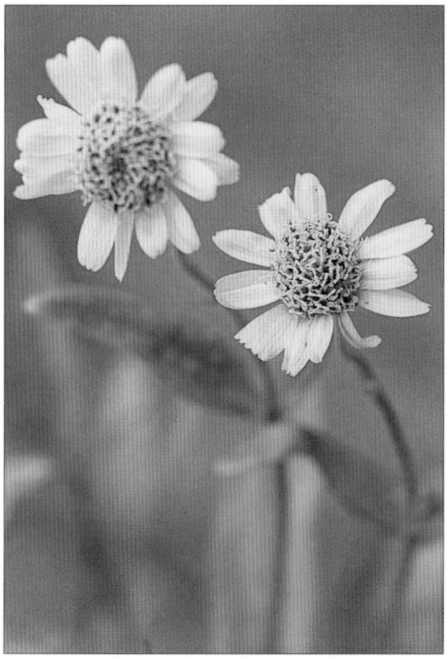

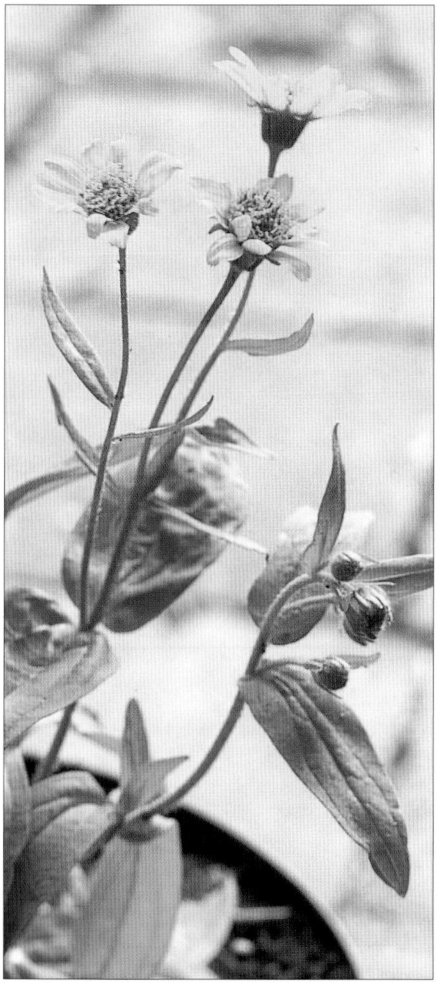

Above *Flowers of* Arnica montana.

Right *Golden arnica flowers and pink* Mimulus lewisii *cover a hillside in bloom in Glacier National Park, United States.*

COMPOSITAE/ASTERACEAE

Arnica montana
Arnica

History and traditions Pier Andrea Mattioli, a household name in herbs in the 16th century, and physician at the Court of the Holy Roman Emperor Ferdinand I, in Prague, rated arnica highly. It became fashionable when he wrote about it in his standard work, *Commentarii*, a version of which appeared in Venice in 1544. It was widely used in the folk medicine of other European countries, principally Germany and Austria, where it has remained an important medicinal herb to this day. Arnica was used by Native Americans to treat muscular injury and back pain.

Description An alpine perennial with a creeping rootstock, it has a basal rosette of small, ovate, downy leaves and flowering stems growing to 30–60cm/1–2ft. The daisy-like flowers are golden yellow and borne in midsummer.

Related species *A. fulgens* is a North American species said to be even more medically powerful.

Habitat/distribution Found in mountainous regions of central and northern Europe and North America. *A. montana* is becoming rare in the wild and is protected in many countries.

Growth It prefers a sandy soil, enriched with humus, and a sunny position. As an alpine plant it needs a cool climate, and does not thrive in wet, waterlogged soil – grow arnica in containers or raised beds if necessary.

Parts used Flowers – dried, for use in pharmaceutical preparations.

USES Medicinal Recent research has established both the therapeutic value of this herb and its toxicity. It has a stimulating effect on the heart muscle and the circulatory system, but effects are rapid and correct doses crucial, with a high risk of overdose. It has antiseptic, anti-inflammatory properites when applied externally and is available as a pharmaceutical ointment for bruises. It is also used in homeopathy, for a range of conditions, including sprains, aching muscles, sore throats and sea sickness. In Britain it is legal only for external use and in the United States it is considered unsafe.

Other names Leopard's bane, mountain arnica, mountain daisy and mountain tobacco.

CAUTION Highly toxic and should not be taken internally, except in homeopathic remedies when the dosage is very small. It may cause dermatitis when used externally – do not apply to broken skin. Legally restricted in some countries. Use with advice from qualified medical practitioners.

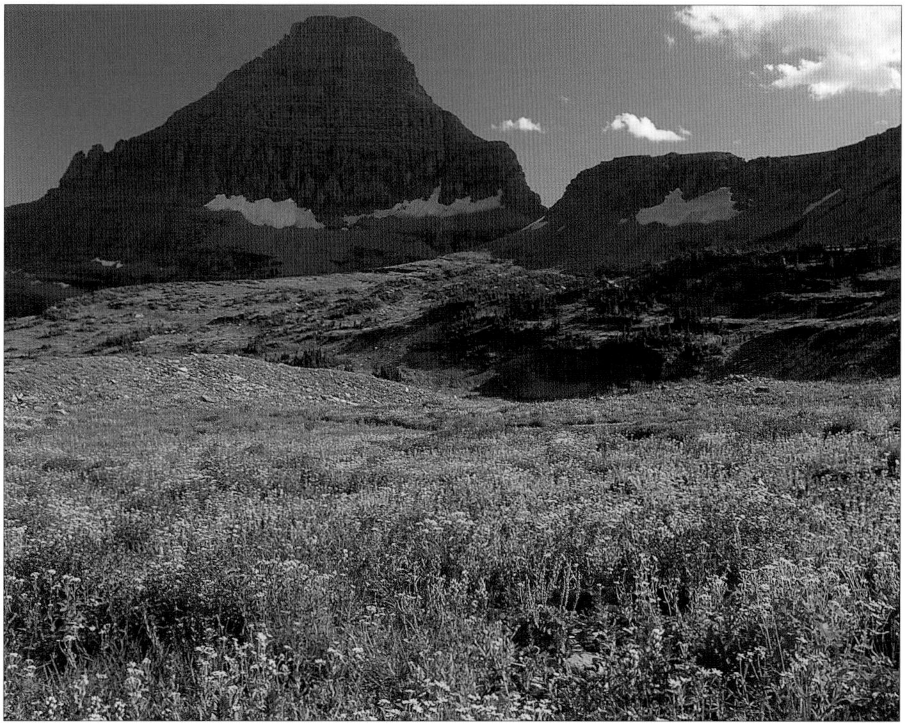

COMPOSITAE/ASTERACEAE

Artemisia

This genus of some 300 species, containing many garden ornamentals, supplies four of the best-known herbs. These include one of the most popular culinary herbs, tarragon, which is the exception of the four in character and uses.

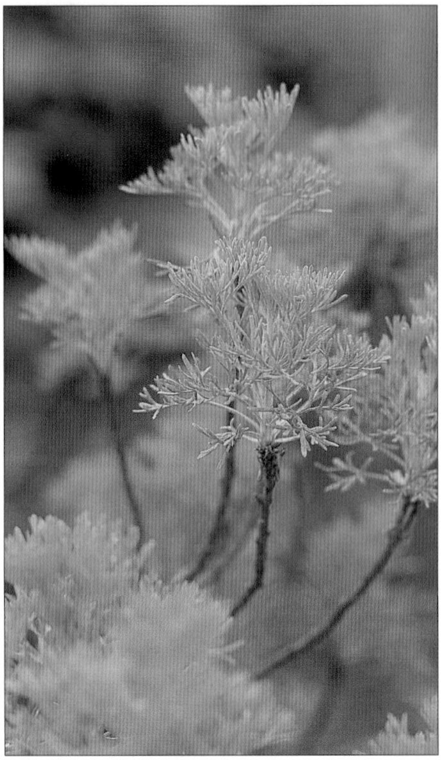

Artemisia abrotanum
Southernwood

History and traditions A native of southern Europe, southernwood was introduced to Britain in about 1548, where the popular name, southernwood, directly described its origins as a woody plant from the south. It soon became established as a cottage garden favourite, attracting new names and associations. 'Lad's love' and 'old man' came about because smearing its ashes in an ointment base was supposed to make pimply youths sprout virile beards and bring new growth to bald heads. Other authorities claim that boys in love wore it in their hats, or gave sprigs as love tokens to the objects of their affections. The French name "*garde-robe*" refers to the habit of including this herb in sachets to protect clothes from insect infestation. It was also thought to protect from infection and was included in nosegays carried for the purpose.

Description A shrubby semi-evergreen (it loses foliage in winter in cold climates and as the plants age), it grows to 1m/3ft tall and has feathery, grey-green leaves with a clean, lemony scent. It seldom flowers in northern climates, but in warmer southern regions small yellow flowers appear in summer.

Habitat/distribution Southernwood is native to southern Europe and parts of Asia, introduced and widespread in temperate zones and naturalized in North America.

Growth Prefers a light soil, full sun and tolerates drought. It is easy to propagate from softwood cuttings throughout summer, or heeled cuttings from old wood in autumn. Needs clipping back hard in late spring to prevent straggly, woody growth. Plants are best replaced after 6–8 years.

Parts used Leaves.

USES Medicinal Southernwood tea is said to stimulate the appetite and digestion. It is also prescribed for menstrual problems. At one time it was given to children to rid them of their threadworms.

Culinary Although there is some evidence of its use in southern European cookery, it is really far too bitter for the purpose.

Aromatic Its insect repellent properties and pleasant smell when dried make it a first choice herb for sachets to keep moths and insects at bay, or to include in potpourri.

Other names Lad's love and old man.

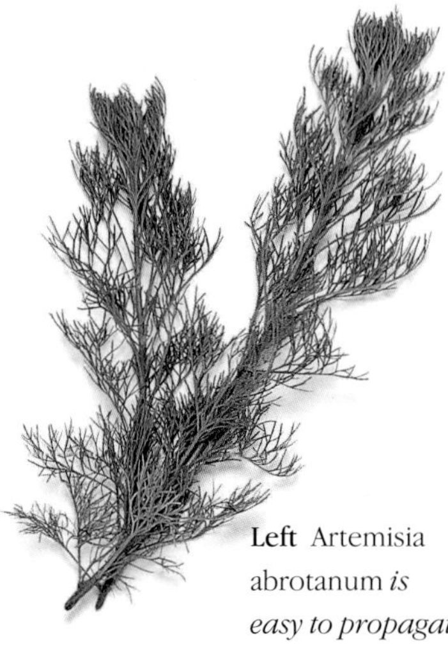

Left Artemisia abrotanum *is easy to propagate from cuttings.*

CAUTION Taken internally, southernwood stimulates the uterus and should never be given to pregnant women.

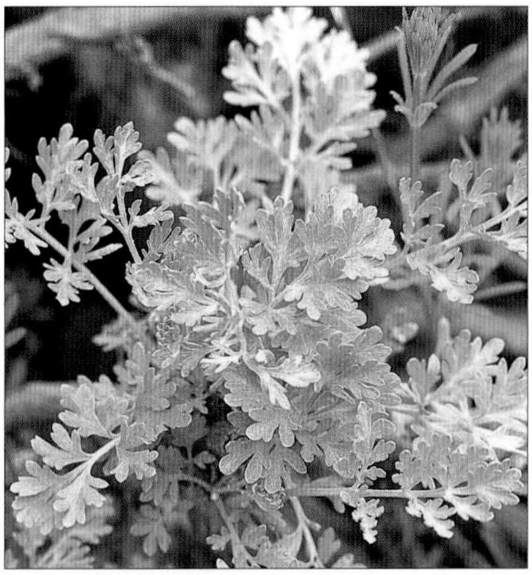

Artemisia absinthium
Wormwood

History and traditions This bitter herb was once highly valued medicinally, with a reputation for overcoming bodily weakness. As a 15th-century manuscript declares: "Water of wormwood is gode – Grete Lords among the Saracens usen to drinke hitt." And Sir John Hill, in his *Virtues of British Herbs* (1772), alleging that the Germans have a tendency to overeat, says this is made possible by a habit of washing down each mouthful with a decoction of wormwood.

Description A perennial subshrub, 1m/3ft in height, leaves are silvery grey, downy and finely divided. Flowers are yellowish green, tiny and ball-shaped, borne on bracts in late summer.

Habitat/distribution Found wild in temperate regions of Europe, North and South America, Asia and South Africa. Widely introduced as a garden plant.

Parts used Leaves, flowering tops.

USES Medicinal A strong herb with some toxicity. Has anti-inflammatory properties, expels intestinal worms and stimulates the uterus. Sometimes recommended for digestive problems, poor appetite and general debility. Best taken on professional advice.

Aromatic Strongly insect-repellent, it is dried for inclusion in sachets against moths, fleas and other insects, or made into tinctures and infusions to deter them.

CAUTION It should not be given to children, pregnant or breast-feeding women. Taken habitually, or in excess, it can cause vomiting, convulsions, delirium and hyperacidity.

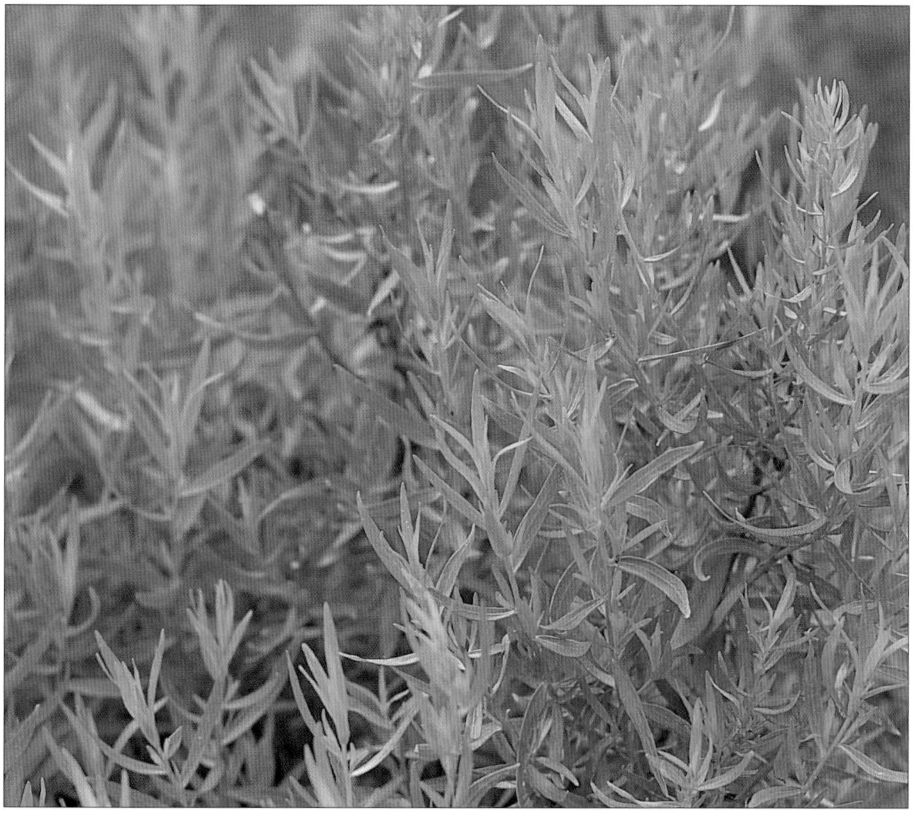

Artemisia dracunculus
French tarragon

History and traditions The species' name, *dracunculus*, is from the Latin meaning "a little dragon" after its supposed ability to cure the bites of serpents and mad dogs. A native of southern Europe, it was first introduced to the royal gardens of Britain in Tudor times. John Evelyn in his *Acetaria* (1699) recommended it as "highly cordial and friendly to the head, heart, and liver" and advised that it "must never be excluded from sallets".
Description A perennial 1m/3ft high, with branched erect stems, and slim, pointed leaves. Flowers are inconspicuous and greyish green but appear only on some plants grown in warm climates – it does not flower at all in cool northern climates. Not to be confused with the subspecies, known as Russian tarragon, a larger, more vigorous plant, with coarser leaves and practically no discernible aroma.
Habitat/distribution A native of southern Europe and Asia, widely distributed in temperate zones worldwide.
Growth It prefers a fairly moist, but well-drained soil and full sun. Tarragon needs protection in winter in colder climates, especially in areas where frost is prolonged or where the ground becomes waterlogged. Propagate by division of roots in spring or autumn. It cannot be propagated from seed.
Parts used Fresh or dried leaf.

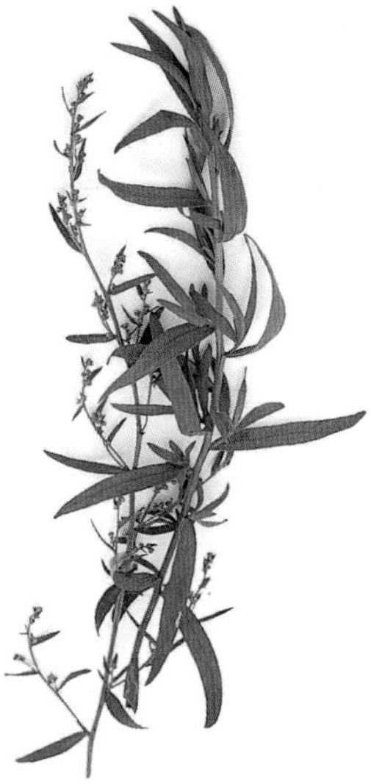

Right *French tarragon is a superbly flavoured culinary herb.*

USES Culinary One of the top culinary herbs for distinction of flavour, it is used in salads, savoury pâté, cooked meat, fish and egg dishes.
Well known for its affinity with chicken, it also enhances the flavour of root vegetables such as carrots and parsnips. Vinegar flavoured with tarragon is a classic condiment and it is a main ingredient of sauces and stuffings.

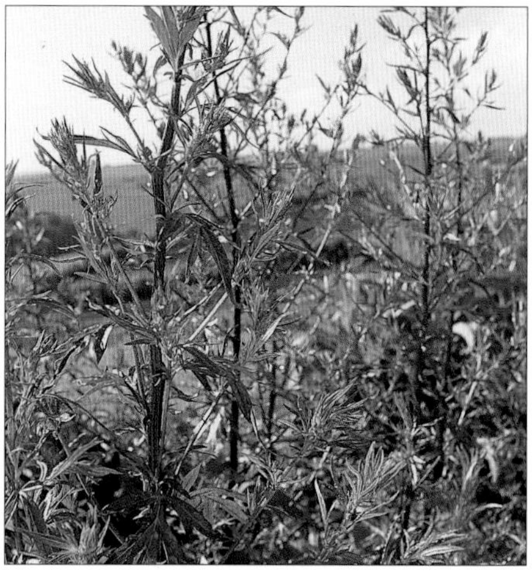

Artemisia vulgaris
Mugwort

History and traditions Ascribed magical properties by cultures in Europe, China and Asia. It was one of the nine herbs in the Anglo-Saxon charm against flying venom and evil spirits, when it was held to be "Mighty against loathed ones / That through the land rove" (Anglo-Saxon Ms, Harleian Collection). Roman soldiers are said to have put it in their shoes to prevent aching feet on long marches. Mugwort has a rich history in magic and protection, and is known to help sift stagnant energy and focus a restless mind. It is renowned for helping to access lucid dreaming states and is used in meditation.
Description A straggly perennial, 1–1.5m/3–5ft tall. Leaves are grey green with white undersides and slightly downy. In the summer panicles of inconspicuous grey-green flowers appear.
Habitat/distribution A wild plant growing by streams and rivers, in wastelands, hedgerows, field margins in Europe, Asia and North America.
Parts used Leaves.

USES Medicinal As with some of the other artemisias, it is said to have digestive properties, stimulates the appetite and acts as a nerve tonic. It is a diuretic and used in regulating menstruation. In Traditional Chinese Medicine a different species, *Artemisia argyi* is used in moxibustion.
Culinary At one time it was included in stuffings and sauces but the slightly bitter, unpalatable taste makes it hardly recommendable.
Aromatic Has insect-repellent properties.

CAUTION Only to be taken on professional advice.

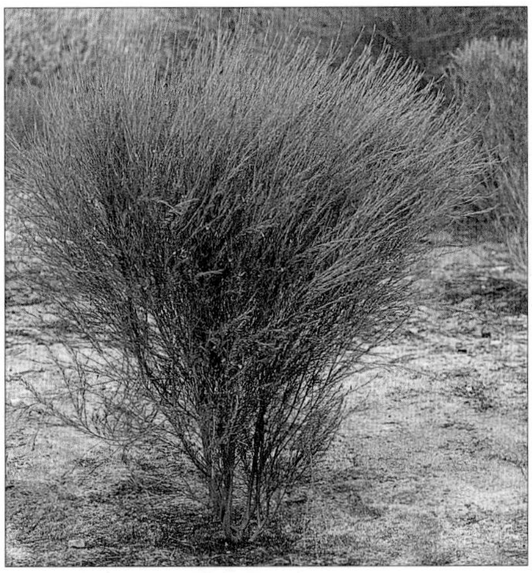

LEGUMINOSAE/PAPILIONACEAE

Aspalathus linearis

Rooibos

History and traditions A traditional tea plant of native South Africans of the Cape, it was adopted by European travellers and colonists in the late 18th century. It has gained popularity in the 20th century for its soothing, medicinal properties and its antioxidant content. It makes a pleasant-tasting tea with a refreshing flavour.
Description A small shrub up to 2m/6ft in height, with bright green, thin, linear leaves, bearing short, leafy shoots in their axils. Small yellow pea flowers are followed by long pods. The leaves turn a reddish brown during processing, which gives the tea its name.
Habitat/distribution Native to dry, mountainous areas of Cape Province, South Africa.
Growth A frost-hardy bush – it cannot tolerate temperatures below –5°C/23°F, or prolonged severe weather. Requires dry, sandy soil and full sun. Propagated by seed sown in spring. Pinch out shoots, as it grows, to encourage bushiness. Commercially cultivated in South Africa.
Parts used Leaves and shoots – sun-dried and fermented to make tea.

USES Medicinal High in vitamin C and mineral salts, it is taken internally for digestive disorders and to relieve allergies and eczema and applied externally for skin irritations.
Culinary Pleasant as an alternative to tea with a low caffeine and tannin level. It is sometimes used as a flavouring herb in sauces and soft drinks and as an ingredient of a local alcoholic liquor.
Other name Red bush tea.

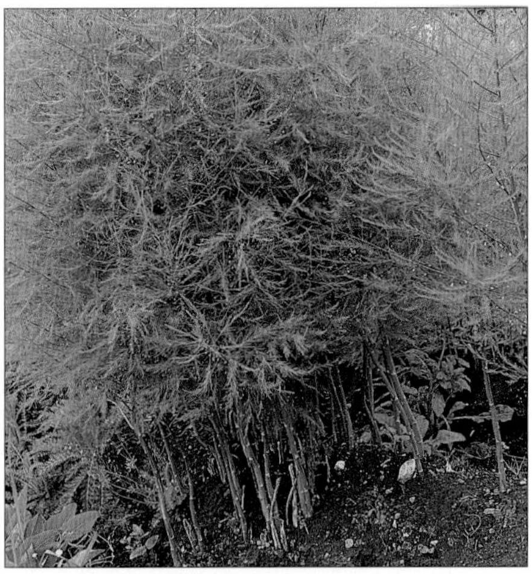

ASPARAGACEAE/LILIACEAE

Asparagus officinalis

Asparagus

History and traditions Appreciated as a delicacy by the ancient Greeks and Romans and mentioned by Pliny in his *Natural History*. The name is originally from a Greek word, the medieval Latin for which was "sparagus", leading to the popular derivation of sparrow-grass. This was once so widely used that a commentator remarked in 1791, "The corruption of the word into *sparrow-grass* is so general that *asparagus* has an air of stiffness and pedantry about it." Gerard recommended its culinary virtues and Culpeper stressed the medicinal properties. His assertion that it clears the sight and eases toothache no longer holds sway, but he also recommended it for sciatica, as do herbalists today.
Description A perennial whose fleshy shoots are eaten as a delicacy. If left uncut it develops feathery leaves to a height of 1–1.5m/3–5ft with small greeny-white flowers followed by red berries.
Habitat/distribution Native to coastal, sandy areas and woodlands of Europe and Asia, now widely cultivated throughout the world.
Growth It requires rich, well-drained loam and a sunny position. Plants may be propagated from seed, but beds are usually established from bought one-year-old crowns. It takes three years to produce the vegetable, but beds then last 10–12 years.
Parts used Young shoots.

USES Medicinal Asparagus has cleansing, restorative properties, combats acidity and is taken for rheumatism, sciatica and gout, as either a food or an infusion. It also has diuretic and laxative properties, and is taken for urinary infections, but it should be avoided where there is kidney disease. An important medicinal herb in India traditionally used in cases of impotence, though no research has been undertaken that supports this.
Culinary High in vitamins A and C and minerals, including calcium, phosphorus and iron. Young shoots, lightly steamed, are served as a vegetable with melted butter or a vinaigrette sauce, or puréed to make soup.
Other name Sparrow-grass.

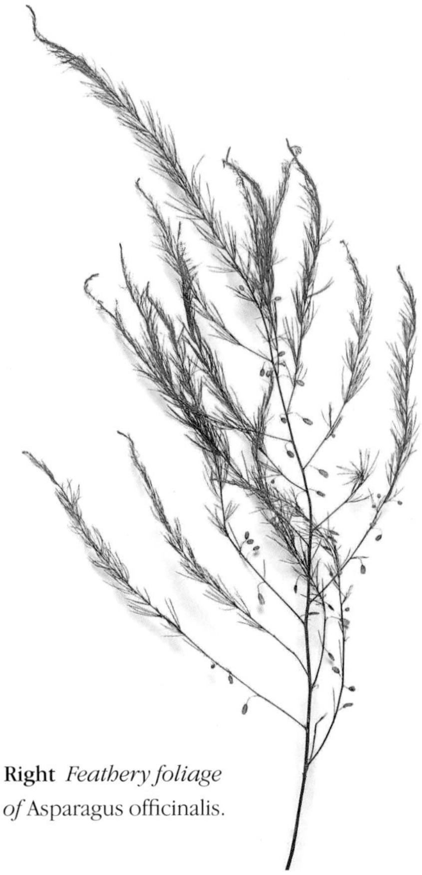

Right *Feathery foliage of* Asparagus officinalis.

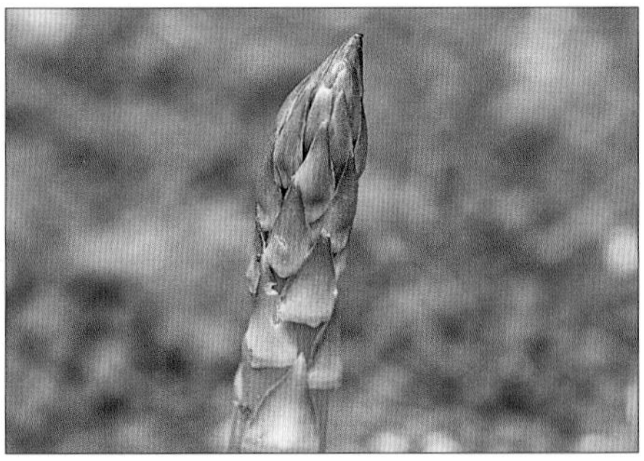

Above *Asparagus emerging from the soil.*

CAUTION Only to be taken medicinally on professional advice.

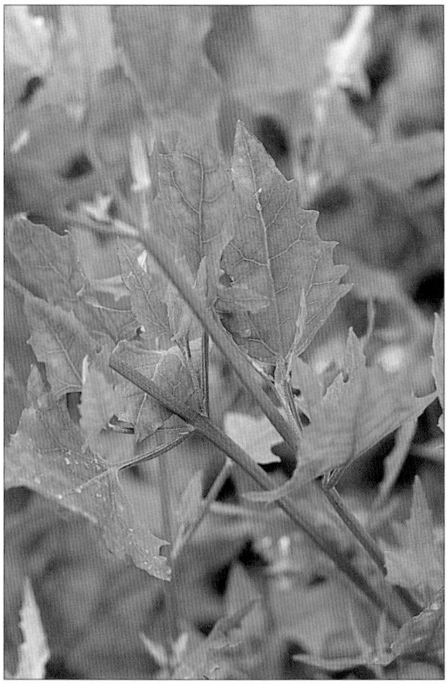

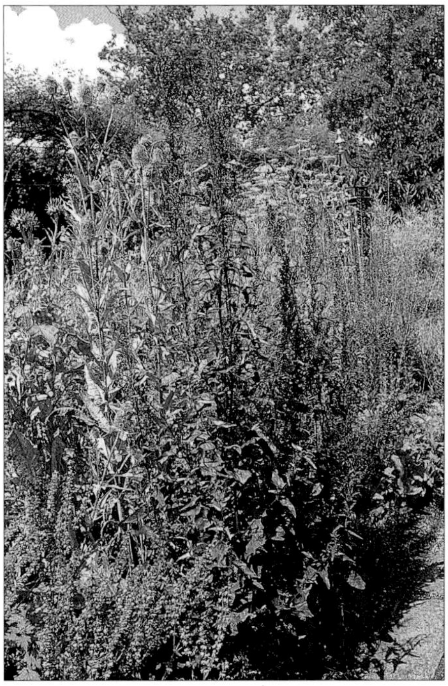

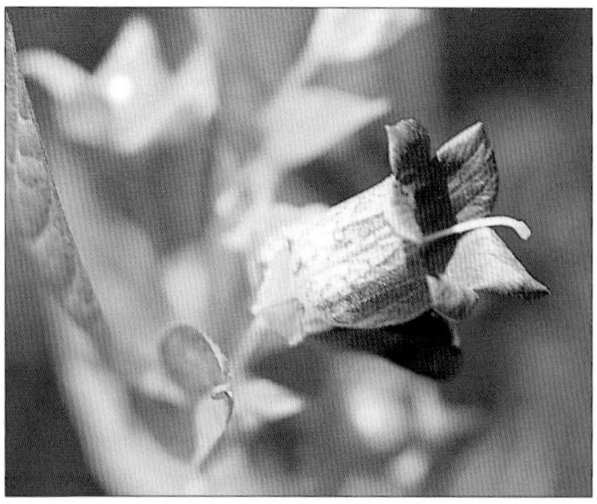

CHENOPODIACEAE

Atriplex hortensis

Orache

History and traditions This herb was eaten as a spinach-like vegetable by Native American tribes, and introduced to Britain in 1548. Sixteenth-century herbalists considered it to be effective against gout when applied as a poultice with honey, vinegar and salt. John Evelyn in his *Acetaria* (1719) refers to its "cooling properties" and recommends it as a salad herb or vegetable, advising that, like lettuce, it should be boiled in its own moisture. Culpeper agreed that it could be eaten as a salad but thought its real virtue lay in the seeds, which he claimed made an effective laxative in the form of an alcohol tincture.

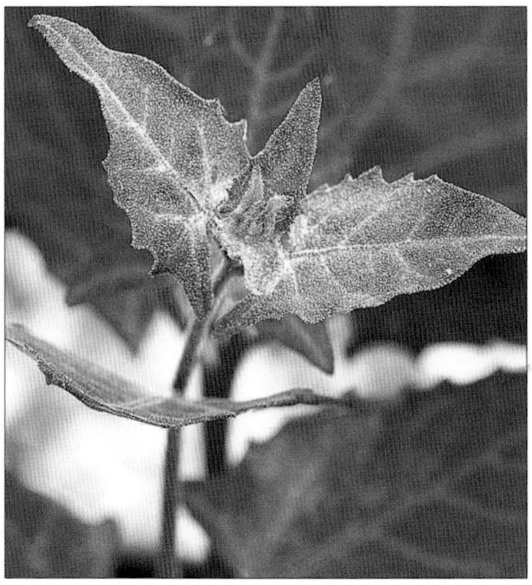

Above Atriplex hortensis *var.* rubra, *red orache, makes a spectacular plant in the border, and the leaves add colour to salads.*

Description An upright annual, growing to 1.2m/4ft, it has spear-shaped green to purple leaves, slightly downy when young, and a mass of yellow-green, sorrel-like flowers, borne on tall spikes, in summer.
Related species *A. hortensis* var. *rubra*, or red orache (above) is a more attractive cultivar, with purple-red foliage and flowers, followed by spectacular seed heads sought after by flower arrangers.
Habitat/distribution Occurs in Asia, North America and Europe, often in coastal areas. It is widely cultivated in temperate and warm regions worldwide.
Growth Flourishes in any soil, tolerates dry conditions but growth is more luxuriant in moister, more fertile soil. Prefers an open, sunny position. Propagated by seed sown *in situ* in spring. Self-seeds prolifically.
Parts used Leaves.

USES Culinary Leaves of red orache add colour and interest to salads, but, despite some recommendations, neither red nor green make very succulent spinach substitutes when cooked as vegetables.
Other name Mountain spinach.

Left *Leaves of* Atriplex hortensis *var.* rubra.

SOLANACEAE

Atropa belladonna

Deadly nightshade

History and traditions In 16th-century Venice this plant was known as *herba bella donna*, and used to dilate the pupils of their eyes by women who sought to beautify themselves. Its potential to cause fatalities was well understood at the time, the apothecaries' name for it being *solatrum mortale*, which translates as "deadly nightshade". Writing at the end of the 16th century, Gerard pontificates on its dangers, advising that a plant "so furious and deadly" should be banished from "your gardens".
Description A bushy perennial, 1–1.5m/3–5ft tall, it has ovate, dull green leaves, bearing single, purple-brown, bell-shaped flowers in the axils in summer, followed by shiny black berries.
Related species Not to be confused with the *Solanum* genus, many of which are poisonous also and include other nightshades – as well as potatoes, aubergines (eggplant) and climbers.
Habitat/distribution Native to Europe and Asia, introduced and naturalized elsewhere.
Growth Grown as a commercial crop (for the pharmaceutical industry) in well-drained, moist soil and full sun – warm, dry conditions increase the alkaloid content.
Parts used Whole plant – dried and processed.

USES Medicinal It contains the alkaloid, atropine, which dilates the pupils of the eye and gives the plant its toxic, sedative properties. A constituent of pharmaceutical drugs, used as pre-medication before surgery and in eyedrops for ophthalmic treatment.

CAUTION Highly poisonous. Do not use internally. Use under professional supervision only.

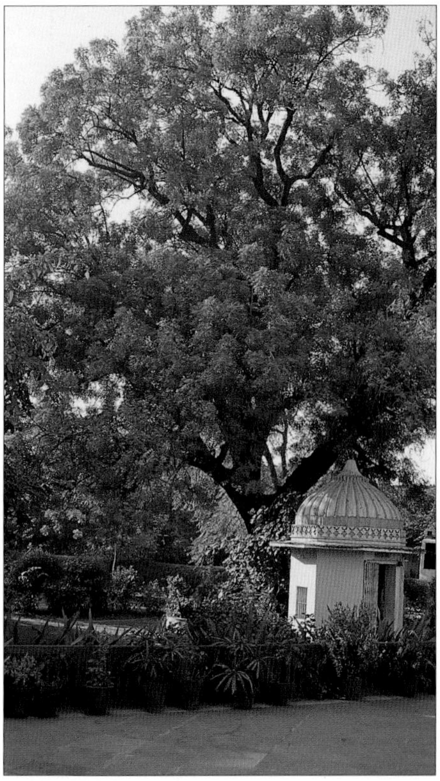

MELIACEAE

Azadirachta indica

Neem tree

History and traditions A common tree of southern Asia, it has played an important role in Ayurvedic medicine, and in agriculture and domestic life as an insect repellent since earliest times. The first part of the botanical name is from a Persian word meaning "noble tree", reflecting its many useful properties, which remain valid to this day. The Neem Foundation, Bombay, dedicated to its study, was established in 1993 and the tree's potential as a source of a low-cost, environmentally-friendly pesticide for field crops in developing countries is currently being investigated.

Description A large, evergreen tree, 12–15m/40–50ft tall, it has dense pinnate leaves. Clusters of small white flowers appear in spring to be followed by long greeny-yellow fruits each containing a seed. The wood secretes resin, and *margosa* or *neem* oil is made from the seeds.

Habitat/distribution Occurs in India, Sri Lanka, Myanmar, southeast Asia and tropical regions of Australia and Africa. Widely planted as shade trees to line the roads.

Growth It will not grow in temperatures below 15°C/59°F. It requires sun and tolerates poor, dry soil.

Parts used Leaves, bark, seeds, oil, resin.

USES Medicinal Neem has anti-inflammatory and insecticidal properties, reduces fever, and acts as a tonic and detoxicant, increasing vitality. Traditionally in Indian herbal medicine, it has been used to treat malaria and leprosy. Also used externally for skin disorders and irritations, especially boils and ulcers, and in eye and ear complaints. Twigs can be used to clean teeth, prevent breath odour and protect from infection.

Cosmetic Reputed to prevent hair loss if a decoction of the leaves is applied as a rinse. The oil is used in hair and skin lotions, toothpaste and soap.

General Makes an effective mosquito and insect repellent, and insecticide for crops. In its countries of origin the dried leaves are used to protect stored clothes or books from insect damage. Although it has been found to be safe and efficient as a sheep dip, this use has not been developed commercially.

Other name Margosa.

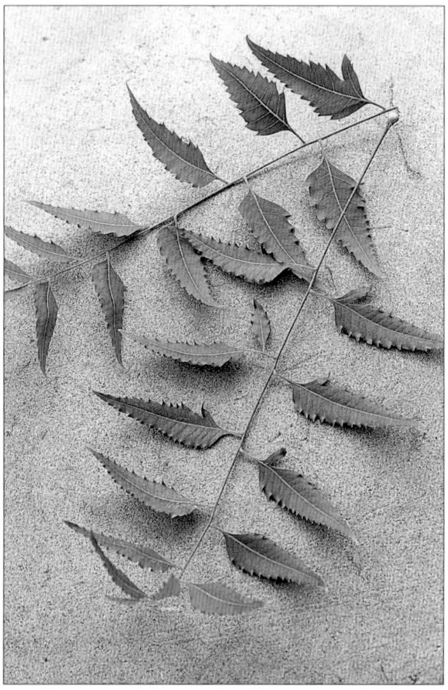

Above *Neem leaves have excellent insecticidal properties.*

CAUTION Seek medical advice before taking internally. Can interact with pharmaceutical drugs. Not to be taken if pregnant, while breast-feeding or on fertility treatment. Not to be taken long term or in high doses.

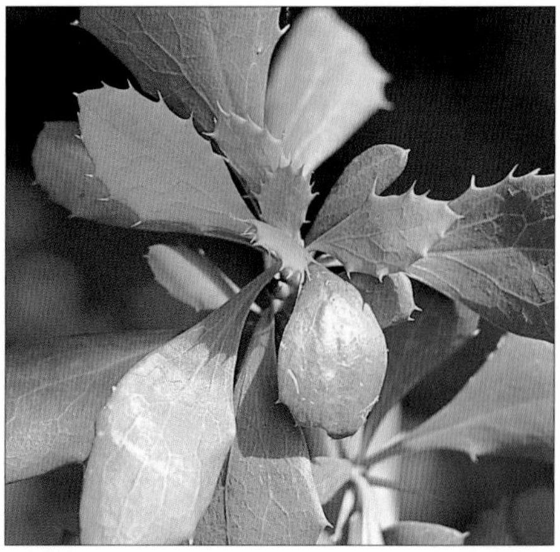

BERBERIDACEAE

Berberis vulgaris

Barberry

History and traditions Barberry has been grown since medieval times for medicinal and culinary use and as a dye plant, producing a yellow colour. It was said to be excellent for "hot agues" and all manner of burnings and scaldings. It had a reputation for blighting wheat, now justified, as it is a known host of the disease, wheat rust.

Description A shrub which grows to 2m/6ft, with sharp spines on the stems and small oval leaves. Clusters of yellow flowers in late spring are followed by the shiny red fruits (berries).

Habitat/distribution Found in hedges and woodland in Europe, also in Asia, the Americas and northern Africa.

Growth A wild plant, it grows on any soil in sun or partial shade. It is propagated by layering or by taking cuttings in early autumn and can also be grown from seed.

Parts used Leaves, bark, roots, fruit.

USES Medicinal Barberry can have a strong effect on the liver causing an increase in bile production and a mild to moderate laxative effect. It has a bitter tonic effect and reduces nausea.

Culinary The berries are very bitter, but high in vitamin C. At one time they were made into jams, jellies, preserves and tarts.

CAUTION Only to be taken on the advice of a qualified herbalist or medical practitioner. Not to be taken if pregnant or when breast-feeding.

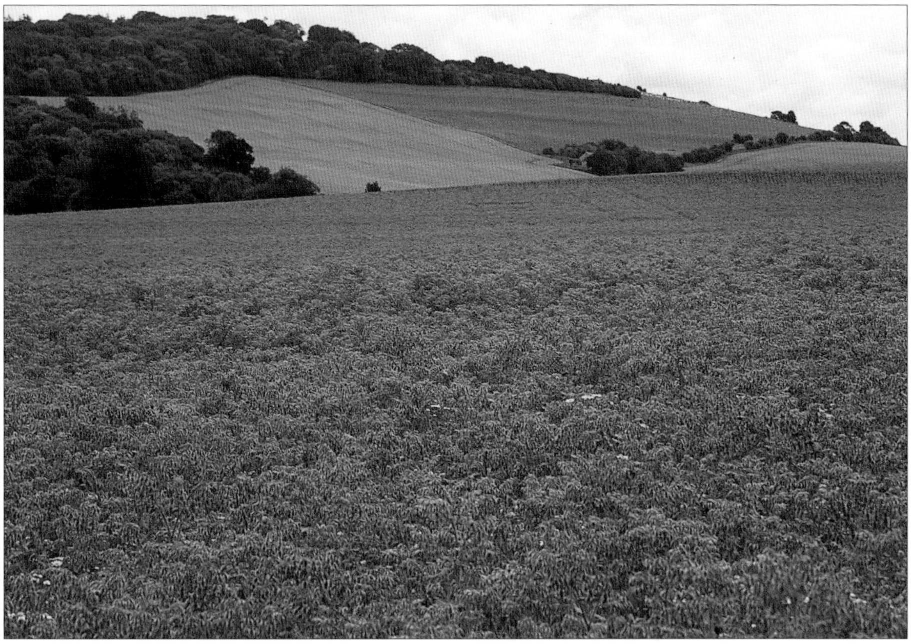

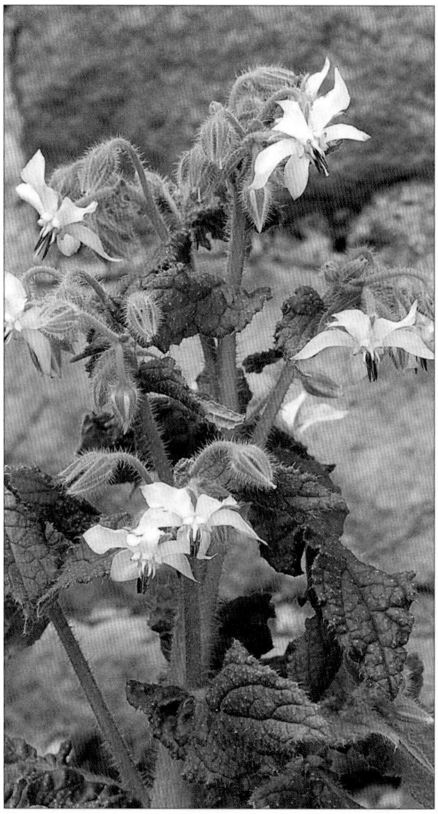

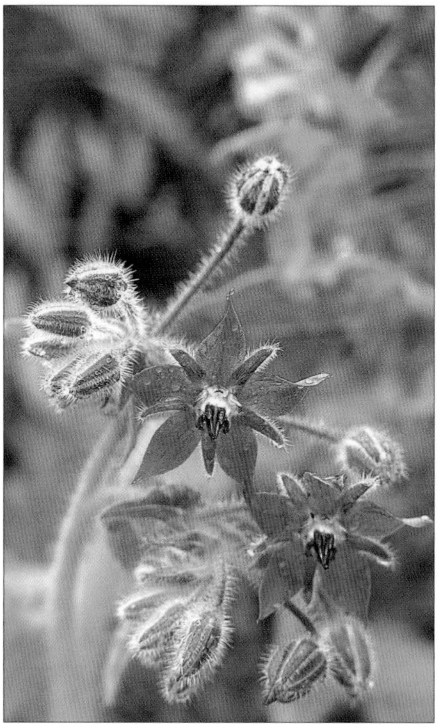

BORAGINACEAE

Borago officinalis

Borage

History and traditions There are various historical references to the ability of this herb to bring comfort and cheer. Gerard mentions references to it in this context by Pliny and Dioscorides, along with the Latin tag: "*Ego Borago, gaudia semper ago*", which he translates as "I, Borage, bring alwaies courage". He goes on to advise adding the flowers to salads to "exhilerate and make the mind glad", the leaves to wine to "drive away all sadnesse, dulnesse and melancholy", making a syrup of the flowers to calm a "phrenticke or lunaticke person" or, for even greater force and effect, candying them with sugar. According to John Parkinson, the 16th-century English herbalist, their attractive colour and form made the flowers a favourite motif in needlework.

Description A short-lived hardy annual, 60–90cm/2–3ft high, with a sprawling habit of growth, hollow, hairy stems, downy leaves and blue (sometimes pink) star-shaped flowers with black centres. It is very attractive to bees.

Related species *B. officinalis* 'Alba' is a white-flowered variety.

Habitat/distribution Native to the Mediterranean region from Spain to Turkey. Now naturalized in most of Europe and in many other parts of the world.

Growth Grows in any soil, even if poor and dry, but it makes a lusher, healthier plant, less prone to mildew, given better soil and more moisture. Prefers a sunny position. It is easy to propagate from seed sown in spring or autumn, and despite common advice to the contrary, the seedlings may be successfully transplanted when young, if they are well watered until established. It also self-seeds.

Parts used Leaves, flowers, oil from the seeds.

USES Medicinal A cooling, anti-inflammatory herb with diuretic properties. It is also said to be mildly antidepressant. Used externally to soothe inflamed skin and in mouthwashes and gargles. The seeds contain gamma-linolenic acid, and oil extracted from them is used as an alternative to evening primrose oil for hormonal problems and skin complaints. Borage is grown as a commercial crop for its oil, which is used in pharmaceutical drugs and cosmetic products.

Culinary The leaves have a faint flavour of cucumbers and are added to soft drinks and wine cups. The flowers make a pretty garnish for salads, and are candied or dried as decorations for sweet dishes and cakes.

CAUTION Borage may cause allergic reactions in some people. The leaves, but not the oil, have been found to contain very small amounts of an alkaloid that may cause liver disease. The plant, but not oil extracted from the seeds, is legally restricted in some countries. Use with advice from qualified medical practitioners.

Top left *Borage is grown as a commercial crop for the pharmaceutical and cosmetic industries.*

Top Borago officinalis *'Alba'.*

Above *Borage flowers make a pretty garnish for salads and drinks.*

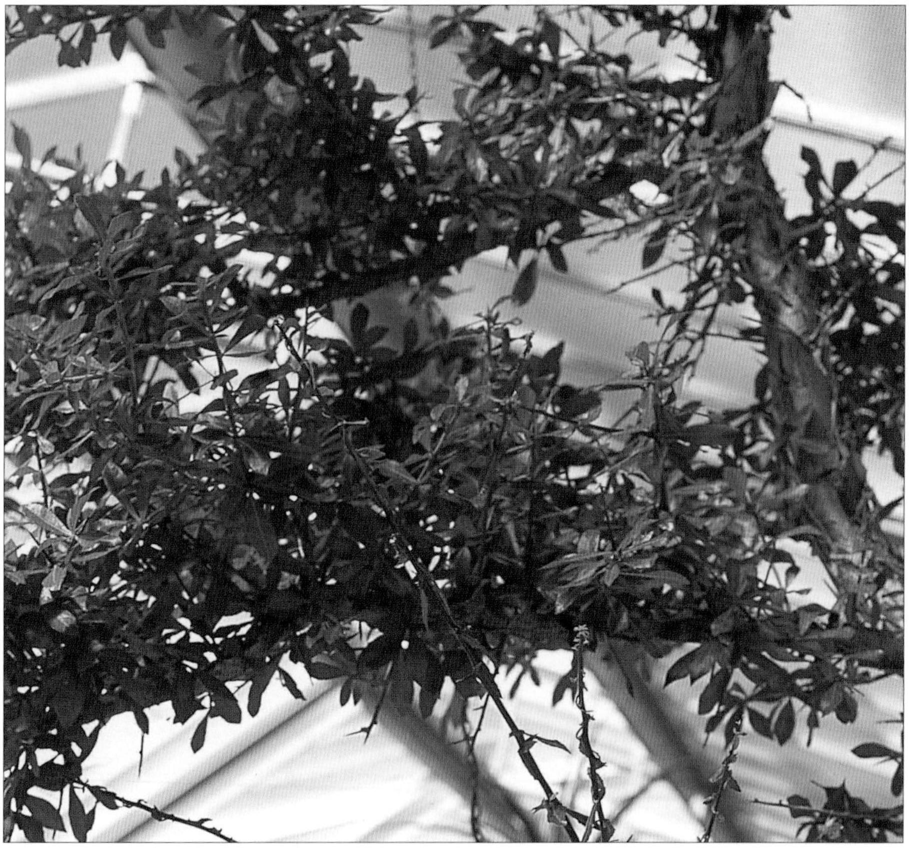

BURSERACEAE

Boswellia sacra syn. *B. carteri*

Frankincense

History and traditions Since ancient times, frankincense has been an ingredient of incense, used in the religious ceremonies of the Egyptians, Babylonians, Assyrians, Hebrews, Greeks and Romans, and is still used in religious ritual to this day. It was highly valued by early civilizations as an item of trade, considered as precious as gold, and was one of the gifts said to have been given to Jesus Christ at his birth by the wise men from the east (Matt. 2:11). It is also thought to have been used by Cleopatra as a cosmetic for smoothing skin. In charred form it made *kohl*, the black eyeliner worn by eastern women. Ancient medicinal uses include Pliny's claim that it provided an antidote to hemlock poisoning and Avicenna's recommendations that it should be prescribed for tumours, ulcers, vomiting, dysentery and fevers. There is also some evidence that at one time it was used in China for leprosy.
Description A small deciduous tree, 2–5m/6–16ft in height, with papery bark, pinnate leaves and racemes of small greenish-white flowers. The gum is secreted in the wood.
Related species Several species of *Boswellia* produce frankincense – formerly it was mostly derived from *B. sacra* and *B. papyrifera*. Today, *B. carteri* and *B. frereana* are usual sources. *B. serrata* (from India) is grown for timber.
Habitat/distribution *B. sacra* comes from Somalia and southern Arabia, *B. papyrifera* from Nigeria and Ethiopia, *B. carteri* and *B. frereana* from Somalia across to eastern Africa, found in desert scrubland. Many *Boswellia* species are threatened with extinction in the wild, due to over-exploitation and over-grazing.
Growth Grows wild, in shallow, rocky soil.
Parts used Gum resin – obtained by incising the trunk to produce a milky sap, which hardens into yellowish globules. Available in the form of grains or powder.

USES Medicinal Frankincense has anti-inflammatory and anti-arthritic properties. The resin has antiseptic properties and is used in Chinese and Ayurvedic medicine. The essential oil is used in aromatherapy to counteract anxiety.
Aromatic Its chief use is as an ingredient of incenses and fragrant preparations. Also added to commercial cosmetics and is a constituent of an anti-wrinkle face cream.
Other name Olibanum.

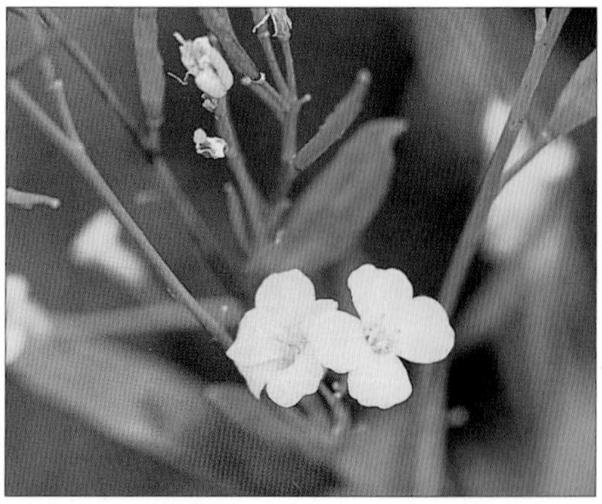

BRASSICACEAE

Brassica nigra

Mustard

History and traditions Mustard has a long history both as a medicinal and as a flavouring herb. The ancient Greeks thought highly of it and Hippocrates recommended that it be taken internally, or as a poultice, for a variety of ailments. It probably came to Britain with the Romans, who mixed the seeds with wine as a condiment and ate the leaves as a vegetable. Gerard describes pounding the seeds with vinegar to make an "excellent sauce" for serving with meat as a digestive and appetite stimulant.
Description An erect annual, 1–1.2m/3–4ft high, with narrow, lobed leaves and racemes of bright yellow flowers, followed by pods containing reddish-brown seeds.
Related species *B. juncea,* or brown mustard, being easier to harvest mechanically, though less pungent, has largely replaced the medicinal *B. nigra.* White mustard (*Synapsis alba,* syn. *Brassica alba)* is grown for commercial production. It is used to make American mustard and is the species sown with cress as a salad.
Growth Requires rich, well-dressed soil and full sun and is propagated by seed sown in spring.
Parts used Leaves, seeds – seedpods are picked before they are fully ripe and dried.

USES Medicinal Mustard has warming and antibiotic properties and is applied externally in poultices, baths or footbaths for rheumatism, aching muscles and chilblains. A mustard foot-bath is a traditional British remedy for colds.
Culinary The ground seeds, mixed into a paste, make the familiar "hot-flavoured" condiment to serve with a range of dishes. The whole seeds are added to curries, soups, stews, pickles and sauces. Young leaves are eaten with cress, or added to salads.

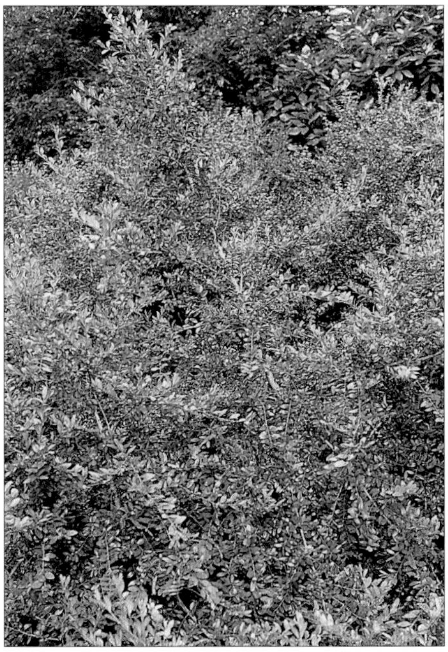

BUXACEAE

Buxus sempervirens

Box

History and traditions The gardens of ancient Rome featured formally clipped box hedges and topiary, a fashion which was enthusiastically revived in Renaissance Europe, when knot gardens and elaborate parterres dominated designs for gardens. Box foliage has been used to decorate the house for American Thanksgiving and at Christmas time in Europe, when it was made into "kissing boughs" or "Advent crowns" (depending on inclination and piety) – sprigs were tied on to frames and decorated with ribbons, candles and shiny red apples. Sometimes known as "boxwood" for its fine-grained, durable wood, traditionally used to make engraving blocks, wooden tools, musical instruments and fine furniture.

Description Common box is an evergreen shrub, or small tree, growing to about 4.5m/14ft, with glossy green, ovate leaves and a strange, rather acrid scent.

Related species There are over 70 species, ranging from tender to hardy. *B. sempervirens* 'Suffruticosa' is a dwarf form – for edging and low hedges: *B. sempervirens* 'Elegantissima' is slow growing with variegated cream and silver-green foliage; *B. sempervirens* 'Latifolia Maculata' has gold leaves; and *B. microphylla* makes low-growing mounds of dark green.

Habitat/distribution Occurs in Europe, Asia, Africa, North and Central America.

Growth Requires well-drained, but not poor, soil, sun or shade. Although hardy, *B. sempervirens* does not thrive in very cold winters and new growth is damaged by frosts – clip after frosts to avoid encouraging vulnerable new shoots. Propagated by semi-ripe cuttings, in late summer.

Parts used Leaves, bark, wood.

USES Medicinal Said to be effective against malaria, but contains toxic alkaloids, and is little used in herbal medicine today. It is currently being researched for its potential as treatments for cancer, HIV and AIDS.

CAUTION Poisonous, can be fatal if taken internally. May cause skin irritations.

Above Buxus sempervirens, *common box.*

Below left to right *Clipped dwarf box,* Buxus sempervirens *'Suffruticosa', the variegated leaves of* B. sempervirens *'Elegantissima' and the compact and very hardy* B. microphylla *var.* koreana.

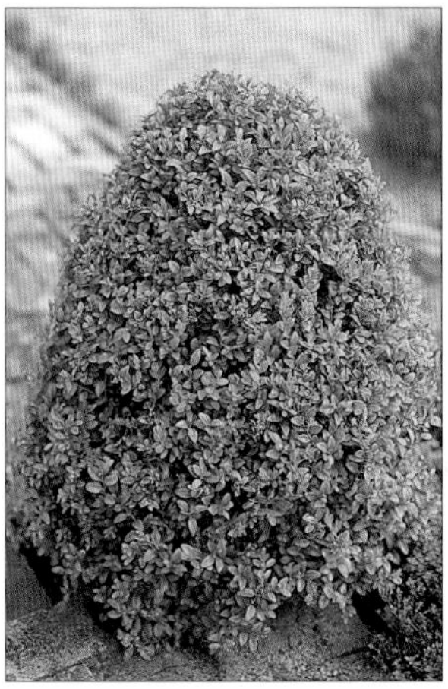

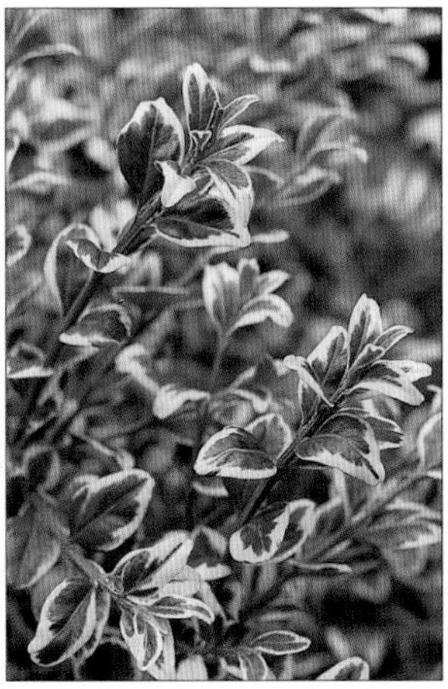

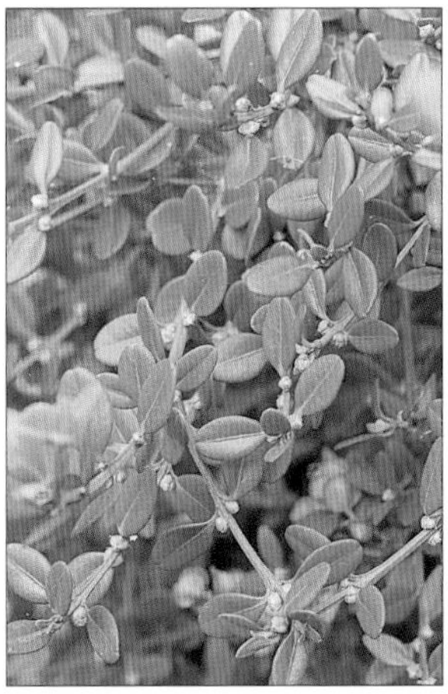

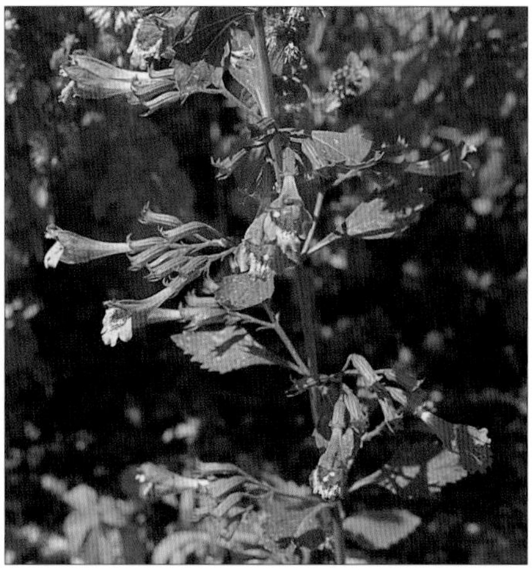

LAMIACEAE

Calamintha nepeta

Calamint

History and traditions Now regarded as an ornamental, calamint was once an important medicinal herb, considered to be effective for "hysterical complaints" and "afflictions of the brain", as well as for a range of ailments from leprosy to indigestion. It had a reputation for hindering conception and inducing abortion.

Description A small, bushy perennial, 30–60cm/1–2ft high, it has small, ovate leaves and a mass of tubular pinky-mauve flowers in summer.

Related species The medicinal calamint of the apothecaries was *C. officinalis,* now classified as *C. sylvatica*, but *C. nepeta* seems to have been used interchangeably. *C. grandiflora* has larger flowers and *C. grandiflora* 'Variegata' is a cultivar with cream and green variegated foliage.

Habitat/distribution Native to Europe, found in grassland, woodland and chalky uplands of central Asia and northern temperate zones.

Growth Prefers well-drained, not-too-rich soil and a sunny position. The easiest method of propagation is by division in spring.

Parts used Leaves or flowering tops.

USES Medicinal It is taken as a tonic, or for indigestion, in the form of an infusion.

Culinary The young leaves and flowers, fresh or dried, may be infused to make a lightly mint-scented tea or added to salads.

CAUTION Not to be taken during pregnancy, as one of its constituents is pulegone (also found in pennyroyal, *Mentha pulegium),* which stimulates the uterus.

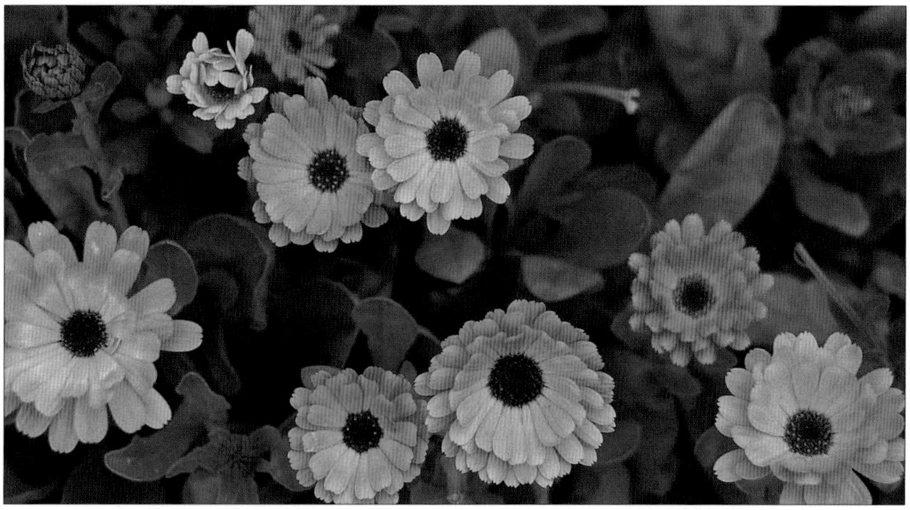

ASTERACEAE

Calendula officinalis

Pot marigold

History and traditions This cheerful, familiar flower was valued for its medicinal, culinary and cosmetic properties in early civilizations of both east and west. Calendula is the diminutive of the Latin *calendulae* and thus "a little calendar or little clock" (*Oxford English Dictionary).* This ties in neatly with its habit of closing its petals when there is no sun as described by Shakespeare in *A Winter's Tale*:

The Marigold that goes to bed wi' the sun
And with him rises weeping.

In medieval England the usual name was simply "golds" – Chaucer refers to a garland of "yellow golds" as an emblem for jealousy and it was only later dubbed "marigold" in honour of the Virgin Mary. Its brightness inspired claims of exceptional virtues from an ability to draw "wicked humours" out of the head (*Macer's Herbal,* 15th century), which makes some sense of a fantastical tale in the *Book of Secrets of Albertus Magnus (*1560) of how an amulet of marigold petals, a bay leaf and a wolf's tooth will ensure that only words of peace will be spoken to the wearer. In Tudor times the petals were dried in huge quantities and sold in grocers' shops to flavour winter stews. They were made into conserves and syrups and also added to salads.

Description A low-growing annual – to 50cm/20in – with hairy, slightly sticky leaves and large orange-yellow daisy-like flowers throughout summer into early autumn.

Related species There are a number of hybrids and ornamental cultivars that do not necessarily have the same medicinal value, but may be used for culinary and cosmetic purposes and to add to potpourri. The *Tagetes* genus of marigolds are not related. Many are toxic and should not be used for the same purposes as *Calendula.*

Growth Easy to grow in any soil. Propagate from seed sown in autumn or spring. Regular dead-heading ensures a good supply of blooms over a long period. Self-seeds prolifically.

Parts used Flowers – petals can be used fresh or dried.

USES Medicinal Pot marigold has anti-inflammatory, antiseptic properties and is also antibacterial and antifungal. Used to help with PMS to reduce bloating and bring on menstrual bleeding. It makes an excellent ointment for soothing irritated, chapped skin, eczema, insect bites and sunburn. It may also be made into an infused oil, for the same purpose, by steeping petals in warm vegetable oil. It is an uplifting, "sunshine" herb, finding light in dark places.

Culinary Once known as "poor man's saffron", the fresh or dried petals add rich colour to rice dishes and salads and may be sprinkled over sweet dishes or baked in buns and biscuits.

Cosmetic Petals are added to beauty creams, or made into an infusion as a lotion for oily skins.

Aromatic Whole dried flowers, or petals, lend colour to a fragrant potpourri.

CAUTION Not to be confused with inedible marigold (*Tagetes*). Occasionally causes allergic reactions.

Pot marigold salad with curried eggs

This dressing has a mild, creamy curry flavour. Serve this salad with baked ham and thick wholemeal (whole-wheat) bread.

Serves 4
4 medium eggs
5ml/1 tsp mild curry powder or paste
75ml/5 tbsp single (light) cream
15ml/1 tbsp chopped parsley
1 bag of mixed salad leaves with light and dark red lettuce
1 pot marigold head, using the petals only

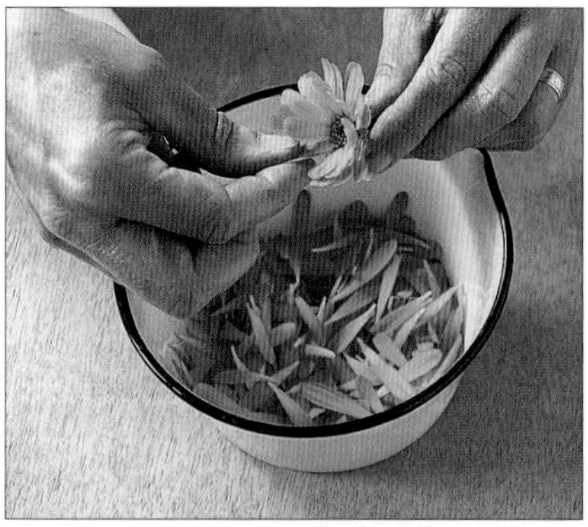

1 Boil the eggs in a saucepan of boiling water for 4 minutes. Allow to cool. Shell and cut into quarters. Stir together the curry powder or paste, mayonnaise and cream in a mixing bowl.

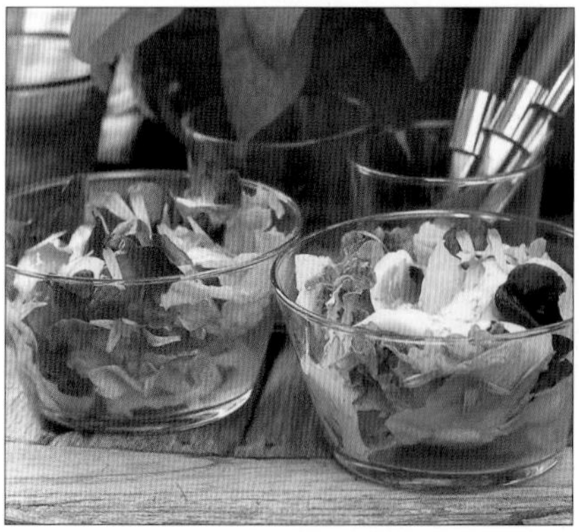

2 Put the chopped parsley and salad leaves in individual bowls. Add one egg to each bowl, then pour over the curried cream sauce. Add the marigold petals.

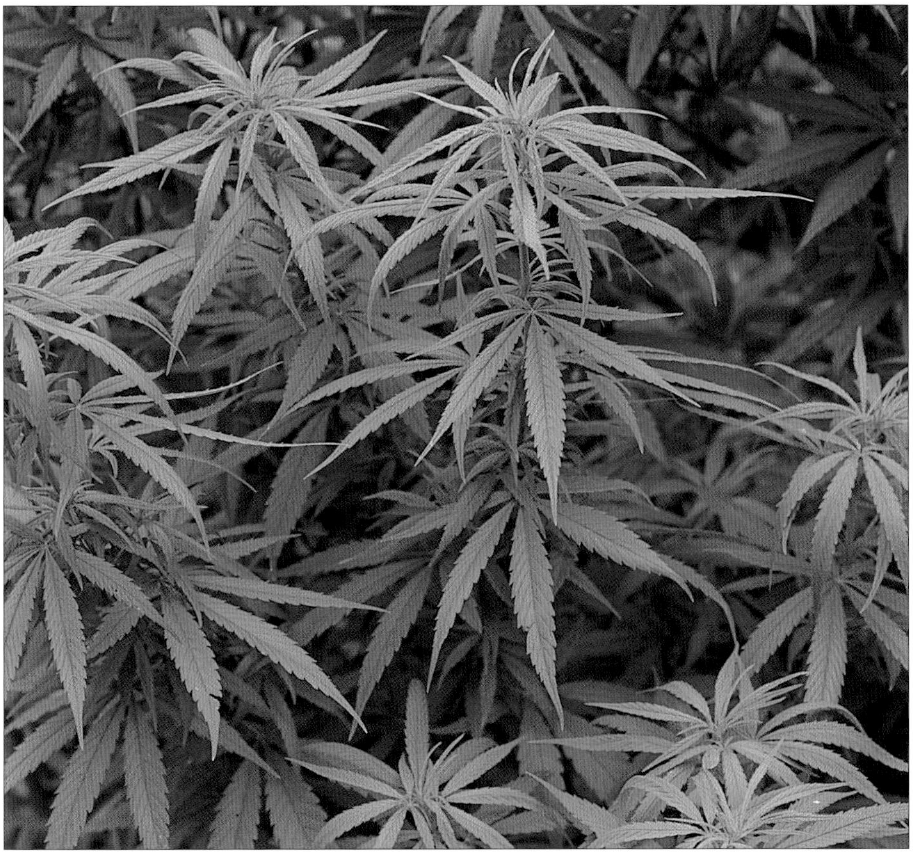

CANNABACEAE

Cannabis sativa

Cannabis

History and traditions Cannabis has a long history as a medicinal plant, being mentioned in ancient Chinese and Indian texts dating from the 10th century BC. Herodotus reports that the Scythians (nomadic people of Iranian origin, living between the 7th and 2nd centuries BC) "crept into their huts and threw the seeds onto hot stones". Pliny thought very highly of this plant's medicinal values. Hildegarde of Bingen in AD1150 refers to it as a relief for headaches, and it is mentioned in all the great Renaissance herbals – though its narcotic effects were well understood and it was known as "The Leaf of Delusion".

As hemp, it has been grown for its fibre since ancient times, and it provided rope for the hangman in 16th-century Britain (old names are "gallowgrass" and "neckeweed").

Description An annual which grows to 5m/16ft in height, on erect stems with narrow, toothed leaves and panicles of inconspicuous green flowers.

Habitat/distribution Cannabis is native to northern India, southern Siberia, western and central Asia; it can be grown throughout temperate and tropical regions.

Parts used Leaves, flowering tops – processed in various forms, under various names, such as "marijuana", "pot", "dagga", "kif", "ganja", "charas" or "churras", and "bhang".

USES Medicinal Cannabis is widely used as an illegal narcotic drug. It can be addictive, and is weakening and harmful in excess, but there is some evidence of its therapeutic value for diseases such as cancer, multiple sclerosis, cerebral palsy and glaucoma. There is also a growing body of clinical research for its therapeutic value in treating anxiety, depression and PTSD (post-traumatic stress disorder). Its anti-inflammatory properties show potential for conditions such as inflammatory bowel disease and rheumatoid arthritis.

General Rope is made from the fibre. Seeds are the source of hempseed oil used in varnishes, foods and cosmetics. Hemp *per se* does not contain appreciable amounts of THC (tetrahydrocannabinol carboxyli). It is legal in some places.

Other name Hemp.

CAUTION It is illegal in most countries.

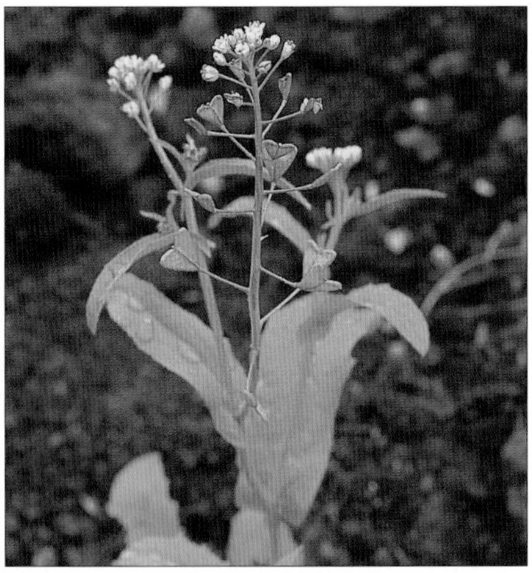

CRUCIFERAE/BRASSICACEAE

Capsella bursa-pastoris

Shepherd's purse

History and traditions Most of its names in English, Latin and other European languages refer to the resemblance of the seeds to purses or little pouches. It is of ancient origin, seeds were found at Catal Huyuk, a site dating from 5950BC, and in the stomach of Tollund Man. Following a visit to America, John Josselyn listed it in his herbal in 1672 as one of the plants unknown to the New World before the Pilgrim Fathers went there. Despite being a common weed, it has proved a valid medicinal plant in this century – extracts were used during World War I to treat wounds.

Description An annual, or more usually biennial, plant with a flower stem rising to 50cm/20in from a basal rosette of oval, dentate leaves. It has tiny white flowers, followed by triangular seedpods.

Habitat/distribution Grows worldwide in temperate zones in fields and waysides on gravelly, sandy and nitrogen-rich soils.

Growth A wild plant, it tolerates poor soil. It can be propagated from seed. Self-seeds freely.

Parts used Leaves – fresh, or dried for use in infusions and extracts.

USES Medicinal Contains a glycoside, diosmin, which has blood-clotting effects and is reputed to stop internal haemorrhages and reduce heavy menstruation when taken as an infusion of the dried leaf. Also taken for cystitis and applied externally for eczema and skin complaints.

Culinary The leaves are rich in vitamins A, B and C and, although not very tasty, make a healthy addition to salads.

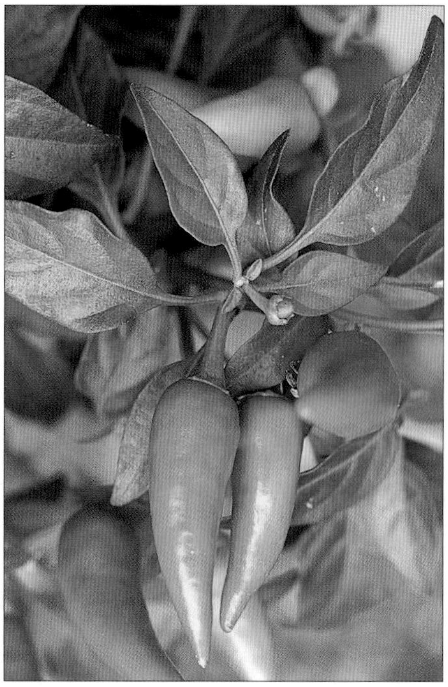

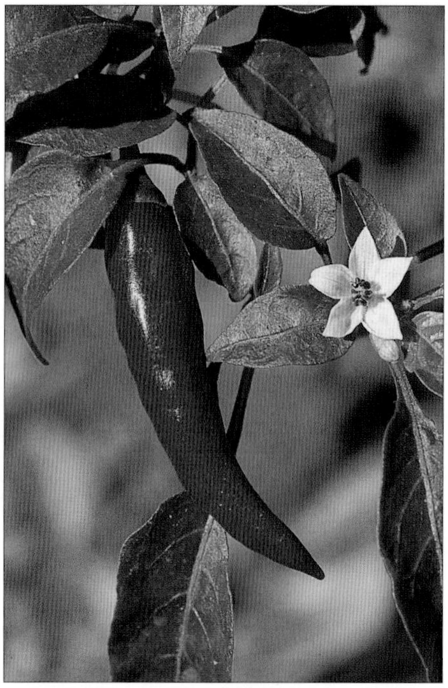

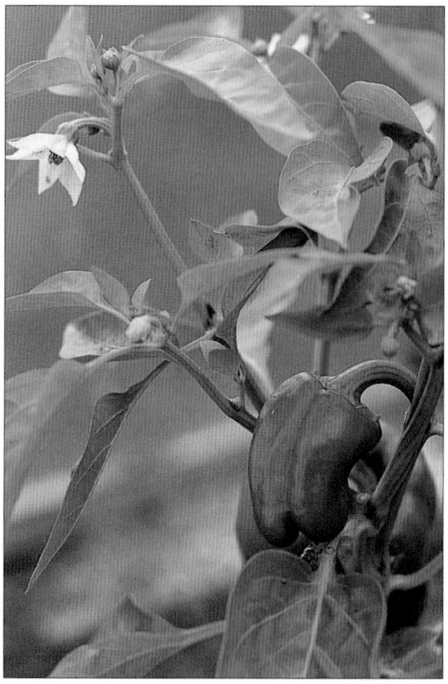

SOLANACEAE

Capsicum

History and traditions Capsicums were first brought to Europe and the West from Mexico following Columbus's voyage of 1492, when the doctor who accompanied him noted their uses by the Native Americans as pain relievers, toothache remedies and for flavouring food. The Portuguese were responsible for their spread to India and Africa.

Habitat/distribution They are now grown in tropical and subtropical regions worldwide, and under glass in temperate zones. They can be grown outdoors in many areas of North America and in the southern states are a major commercial crop.

Description *Capsicum annuum* var. *annuum* are annuals, sometimes short-lived perennials, and most grow into small bushy plants 60–90cm/2–3ft high; a few may reach 1.5m/5ft. They have glossy lance-shaped to ovate leaves and small white flowers followed by conical, or spherical, green, ripening to red, fruits.

Species Most cultivated peppers are of the species *C. annuum* var. *annuum*. There are over 1,000 cultivars grown across the world, with fruit in a wide range of shapes, sizes and degrees of pungency, divided into five main groups:

1. **Cerasiforme Group (cherry peppers)** – with small, very pungent fruits.
2. **Conoides Group (cone peppers)** – with erect, conical fruits.
3. **Fasciculatum Group (red cone peppers)** – slender, red, very pungent fruits.
4. **Grossum Group (bell peppers, sweet peppers, pimento)** – these have large, sweet, bell-shaped fruit, green, then ripening to red or yellow. Rich in vitamin C, they lack the medicinal properties of the hot, pungent peppers.
5. **Longum Group (cayenne peppers, chilli peppers)** – fruits are usually drooping, very pungent and the source of chilli powder, cayenne pepper and hot paprika. *C. frutescens* is a name often used for varieties of *C. annuum* whose fruits are used in Tabasco sauce.

Growth Frost-tender plants, which must be grown under glass in cool temperate climates. Plant in loam-based (John Innes) growing medium (soil mix), water freely, feed with a liquid fertilizer once a week and mist flowers with water daily to ensure that fruit sets. Propagation is from seed, at a temperature of 21°C/70°F in early spring. Outside, they are grown in well-drained, nutrient-rich soil.

Parts used Fruits – eaten ripe or unripe; or dried (ripe only) for powders.

USES Medicinal It is the bitter alkaloid, capsaicin, which gives peppers their hot taste and has been established by modern research as an effective painkiller – it works by depleting the nerve cells of the chemical neurotransmitter which sends pain messages to the brain. Peppers are antibacterial and also contain vitamins A, C, and mineral salts. Pungent varieties increase blood flow, encourage sweating, stimulate the appetite and help digestion. In tropical countries they are useful food preservatives and help prevent gastric upsets. Taken internally or used as gargles (infusions of the powder) for colds, fevers and sore throats; applied externally (in massage oil or compresses) for rheumatism, arthritis, aching joints and muscles. A pharmaceutical analgesic cream, with capsaicin as active ingredient, has recently been developed for reducing rheumatic pain.

Culinary Sweet red or green peppers make delicious cooked vegetables or raw salad ingredients. Hot chilli peppers are added to pickles and chutneys; dried to make cayenne pepper, chilli powder or paprika (from milder-tasting fruits); added to dishes in Indian, Mexican, Thai and other worldwide cuisines.

Other names Peppers and chilli peppers.

Top centre Capsicum frutescens, *a hot chilli pepper.*

Top right Capsicum annuum *var.* annuum, *Grossum Group, a sweet, bell pepper.*

CAUTION Chillies may cause inflammation and irritation to skin and eyes, so wear gloves when handling them. If taken internally to excess, they may cause digestive disorders.

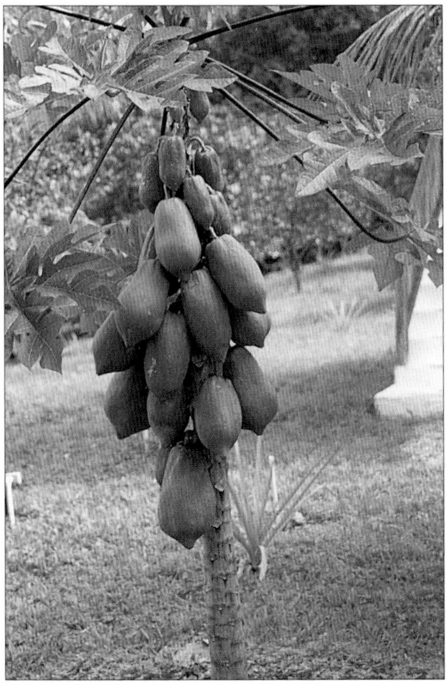

CARICACEAE

Carica papaya

Papaya

History and traditions Originally from South and Central America and the West Indies, this tree with its fragrant, fleshy fruit was unknown in Europe before the end of the 17th century. The Spanish took it to Manila and, with the expansion of trade and travel at the beginning of the 18th century, it made its way to Asia and Africa and is now grown in tropical countries around the globe.
Description A small, evergreen tree, up to 6m/20ft in height with deeply cut, palmate leaves, forming an umbrella-shaped crown. The large, ovoid fruits have dark green, leathery skin, ripening to yellow, containing sweet orange-yellow flesh and numerous tiny black seeds surrounding a central cavity.
Habitat/distribution Native to South and Central America, occurs widely in tropical zones.
Growth A tender, tropical plant, it will not grow in temperatures below 13°C/55°F. Requires rich, moist soil, and a sunny, humid climate.
Parts used Fruit, seeds, leaves – fresh. Sap, known as "papain", is extracted from the unripe fruits by scarification, and produced in dried or liquid form.

USES Medicinal The fruit is one of the best natural digestives, containing enzymes similar to pepsin. Juice is applied externally to destroy warts and for skin eruptions and irritations. Seeds and papain are used in preparations to expel intestinal worms.
Culinary Fruit is high in vitamin C and minerals, and is eaten fresh, canned or made into ice creams, desserts and soft drinks. Papain is used commercially as a meat tenderizer, and, on a domestic level, the inside of the skin of the fruit and leaves are wrapped round meat for the same purpose. Seeds have a pungent flavour and are sometimes eaten, or used as food flavouring, in countries where it is grown.
Cosmetic Juice smooths skin, removes freckles and reduces sun damage. Papain is included in commercial cosmetic products.
General Papain is used as an insecticide against termites, as an ingredient of chewing gum, to reduce cloudiness in beer and to make woollen and silk fabrics shrinkproof.

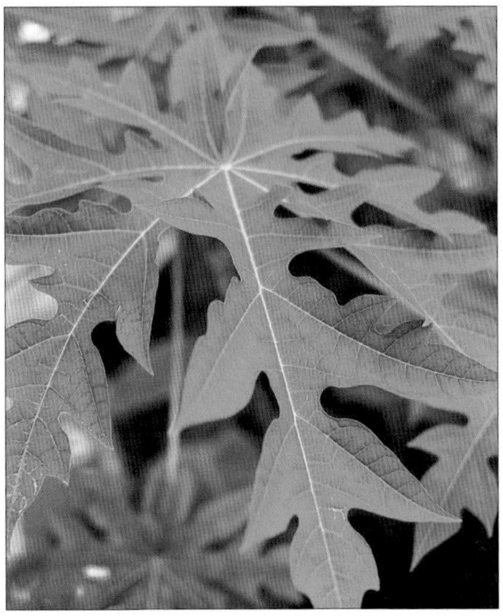

Above *Papaya leaves are used to tenderize meat.*

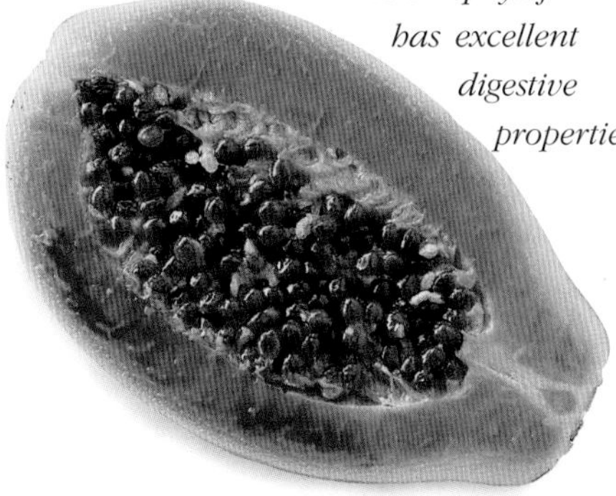

Left *Papaya fruit has excellent digestive properties.*

CAUTION Do not take in large quantities or as a concentrated extract during pregnancy.

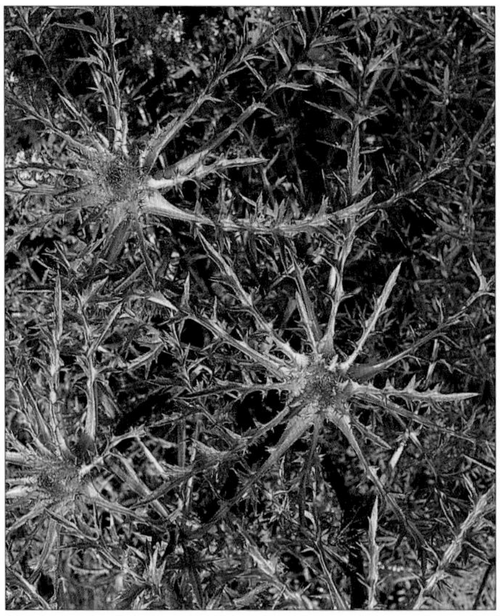

COMPOSITAE/ASTERACEAE

Carlina acaulis

Carline thistle

History and traditions In medieval times this thistle was thought to be an antidote to poison and the root was sometimes chewed to relieve toothache. It is said to be named after the Emperor Charlemagne, following a dream that it would cure the plague.
Description A low-growing, short-lived perennial, 5–10cm/2–4in high, with a deep tap root, it has basal rosettes of spiny leaves and large stemless flowers with silvery-white bracts surrounding a brown disc-shaped centre.
Habitat/distribution Native to Europe and Asia, it is found in fields, grasslands and waste ground on poor dry soils in sunny positions.
Growth It grows best in a poor, dry soil. If kept too wet it will rot, and if the soil is too rich it becomes lax, overgrown and loses its neat, stemless habit. Propagated from seed sown in autumn and overwintered in a cold frame.
Parts used Roots – dried for use in decoctions, liquid extracts and tinctures.

USES Medicinal It has antibacterial and diuretic properties. A decoction of the roots is used as a gargle for sore throats, for skin complaints and to clean wounds. It is taken internally for urine retention.
Culinary Claims have been made for the flower centres as substitute artichoke hearts.

CAUTION Large doses taken internally are purgative and emetic.

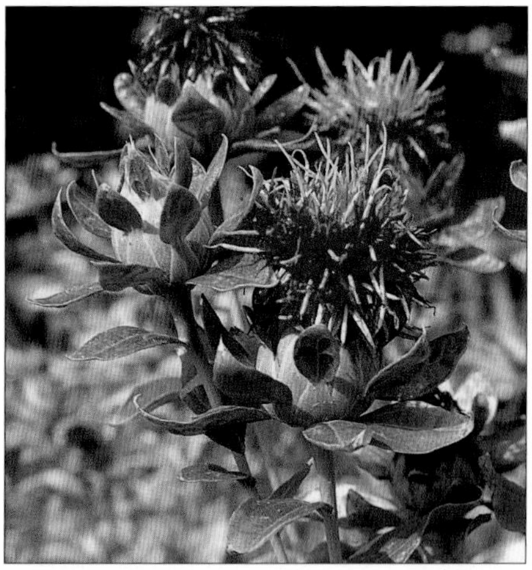

COMPOSITAE/ASTERACEAE

Carthamus tinctorius

Safflower

History and traditions Cultivated in Egypt, China and India since ancient times, safflower was a valued dye plant – producing a pink dye, used for the original "red tape" of Indian bureaucracy. It was introduced to Europe from the Middle East during the mid-16th century for its medicinal properties, and is now cultivated for the oil extracted from the seeds.
Description A hardy annual, growing to 1m/3ft high, with finely toothed, long, ovate leaves and shaggy, thistle-like, yellow flower heads set in spiny bracts.
Habitat/distribution Native to Asia and Mediterranean regions, widely cultivated for its seeds in many countries, including Asia, India, Africa and Australia.
Growth Grows in any light, well-drained soil and tolerates dry conditions. Propagated by seed, sown in spring.
Parts used Flowers, seeds, oil.

USES Medicinal The oil contains 75 per cent linoleum acid and is a useful source of essential fatty acids. Tea, infused from fresh or dry flowers, is taken to reduce fevers and is mildly laxative. Infusions are applied externally for bruises, skin irritations and inflammations.
Culinary Oil extracted from the seeds is low in cholesterol and has a delicate flavour. The flower petals, which are slightly bitter, have been used as a substitute for saffron in colouring food.
Household Flowers produce a yellow dye with water and red dye with alcohol. They are dried for adding to potpourri and as "everlasting" flowers for dried arrangements.

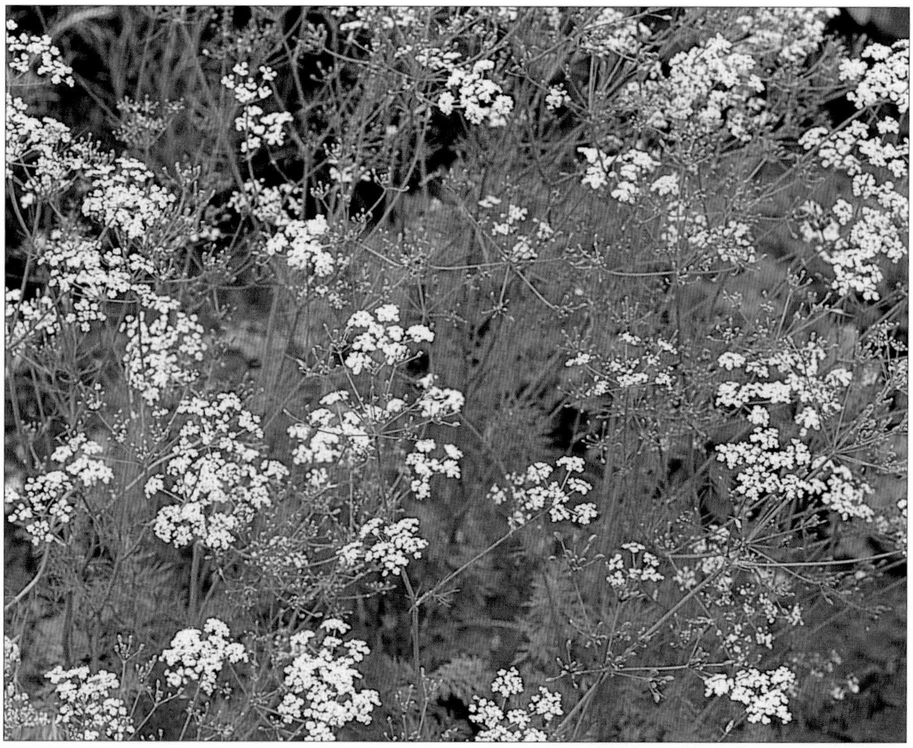

UMBELLIFERAE/APIACEAE

Carum carvi

Caraway

History and traditions Caraway seeds have been found during archaeological excavations at Neolithic sites in Europe and the plant was well known to the Egyptians, Greeks and Romans. The seeds were a popular culinary flavouring in Tudor England, cooked with fruit and baked in bread and cakes. They were made into sugared "comfits", and frequently served as a side dish with baked apples, as in Shakespeare's *Henry IV* when Falstaff is invited to take "a pippin [apple] and a dish of carraways". This custom is said to have continued into the early 20th century at formal dinners of London livery companies. There is also an old superstition that caraway has retentive powers, and, if sprinkled about, is capable of preventing people and personal belongings from straying.
Description A biennial 45–60cm/18in–2ft tall, it has feathery leaves, with umbels of white flowers appearing in its second year, followed by ridged fruits (popularly known as seeds).
Habitat/distribution Native to Asia and central Europe in meadowlands and waste grounds. Introduced and cultivated elsewhere.
Growth Prefers well-drained soil and a sunny position. Propagated from seed sown in spring, preferably *in situ* as it does not transplant well.

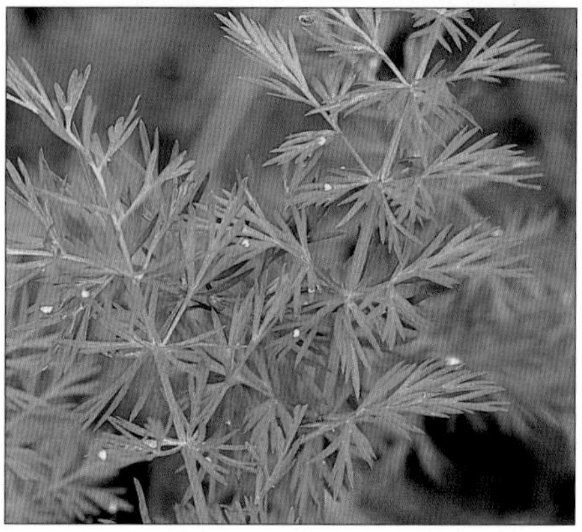

Above *Young, tender caraway leaves add flavour to salads.*

Parts used Leaves, seeds, essential oil from the seeds.

USES Medicinal Caraway has carminative properties (combats flatulence). A few seeds chewed after a meal or an infusion of the seeds may relieve bloating and excessive wind.
Culinary Seeds are used to flavour cakes, biscuits, bread, cheese, stewed fruit, baked apples, cabbage and meat dishes. Also as a pickling spice and to flavour the liqueur, Kümmel. Young leaves make a garnish and are added to salads.
Aromatic Essential oil (containing over 50% carvone, which gives it its aromatic scent) is used as a flavouring in the food industry and in perfumes and cosmetics.

FAGACEAE

Castanea sativa

Sweet chestnut

History and traditions Sweet chestnut trees were grown in ancient Greece and Rome. The Greek physician, Theophrastus, wrote of their medicinal virtues and the Romans enjoyed eating them. They were probably introduced to Britain by the Romans and there are records of chestnuts grown in the Forest of Dean being paid as tithes, during the reign of Henry II, 1154–1189. Writing in the mid-17th century, Culpeper considered the "inner skin" of the chestnut would "stop any flux whatsoever" and that the ground, dried leaves made into an electuary (medicinal paste) with honey made "an admirable remedy for the cough and spitting of blood". Their culinary diversity was praised by the 17th-century diarist and gourmet, John Evelyn, as "delicacies for princes and a lusty and masculine food for rusticks", while he regretted that all too often they were mere animal fodder.

Description A deciduous tree, growing to 15m/50ft with dark grey, furrowed bark, and narrow, glossy, serrated-edged leaves. The small white flowers, appearing in spring, are followed by clusters of prickly green spherical fruits, containing 1–3 edible brown nuts. Trees grown in cool, northerly regions do not produce the same quality of large, succulent fruits as those grown in warmer, Mediterranean climates.

Habitat/distribution Occurs in woodlands of southern Europe, Asia, North America and northern Africa.

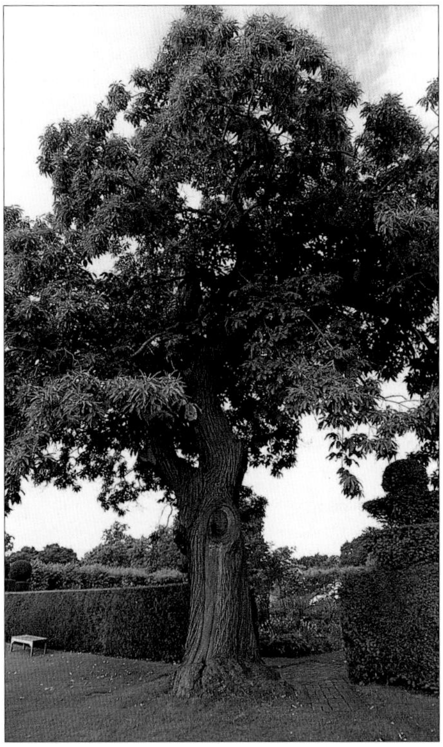

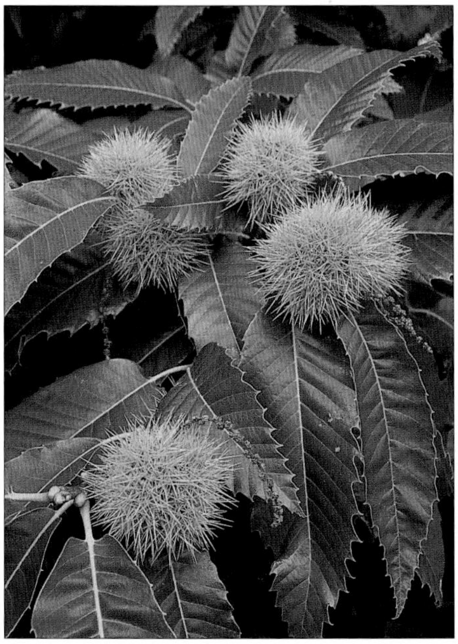

Growth Grows best in well-drained loam in sun or partial shade. Propagated by seed sown in autumn.

Parts used Leaves, seeds (nuts).

USES Medicinal Infusions of the leaves are taken for coughs and colds and used as a gargle for sore throats. Also said to be helpful for rheumatism.

Culinary Chestnuts are equally suited to savoury and sweet dishes. They are the classic stuffing ingredient for turkey, other poultry and game, and make excellent soups, pâtés, and accompaniments to vegetable and meat dishes. Sweetened purée forms the basis of desserts, especially in France, where chestnuts are also crystallized as "marrons glacés".

Other name Spanish chestnut.

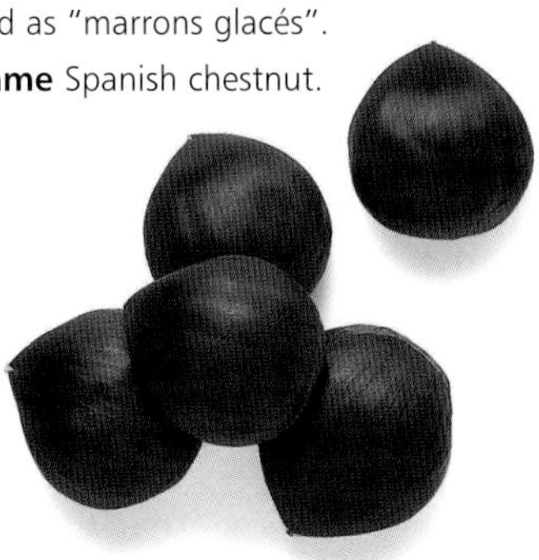

Above *Sweet chestnuts.*

Left *Spiky fruits contain the edible nuts.*

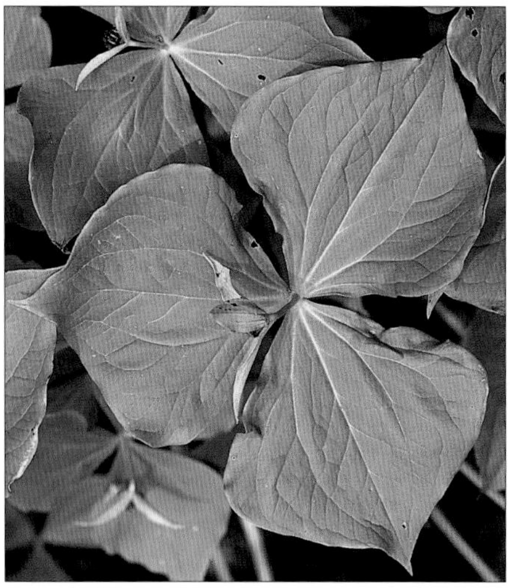

BERBERIDACEAE

Caulophyllum thalictroides

Blue cohosh

History and traditions A herb used in the traditional medicine of the Native Americans to facilitate childbirth. Its value being appreciated by the wider population, it was listed at the end of the 19th century as an official medicinal herb in the United States pharmacopoeia. The name "cohosh" is from a local tribal language.

Description A perennial which grows on a rhizomatous rootstock. The palmate leaves develop with, or just after, the yellow-brown flowers. Fruits split open to reveal spherical seeds, which turn from green to deep blue as they ripen.

Habitat/distribution Occurs in moist woodlands in North America.

Growth Requires moist, rich soil, in partial or deep shade. Divide plants in spring. Propagation from seed is slow and germination may often be erratic.

Parts used Rhizomes and roots are dried for inclusion in powders, liquid extracts and other medicinal preparations.

USES Medicinal Do not use in pregnancy unless used under the guidance of a herbalist or other qualified health professional. A herb with a long traditional use in gynaecology. Do not use if you are trying to conceive, during early pregnancy or lactation.

Other names Squaw root and papoose root.

CAUTION Not to be used without the advice of a qualified medical practitioner.

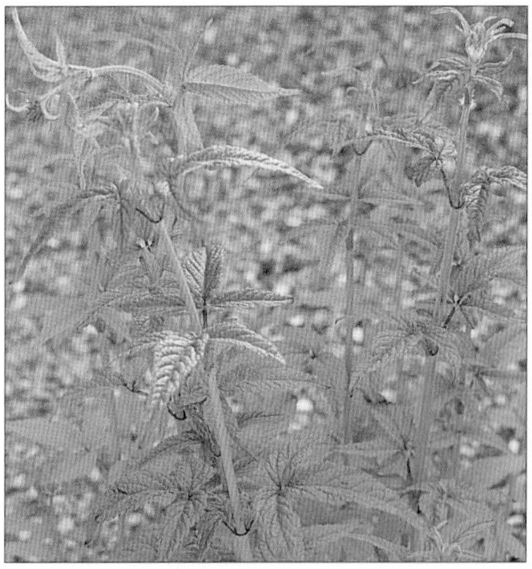

LABIATAE/LAMIACEAE

Cedronella canariensis syn *C. triphylla*

Balm of Gilead

History and traditions This upstart from the Canary Islands is something of a fraud, sniffily dismissed by Mrs Grieve, in *A Modern Herbal* (1931) as being "called Balm of Gilead for no better reason than that its leaves are fragrant". But it has largely taken over from ancient, more worthy contenders for the name, because it has a similar musky, balsam scent, though not, apparently, any worthwhile medicinal uses. The original Balm of Gilead is usually taken to be *Commiphora opobalsamum,* a rare and protected desert shrub, once valued for its balsam-scented resin. Another source of Balm of Gilead is the balsam poplar, *Populus balsamifera.*
Description A half-hardy shrubby perennial, up to 1m/3ft in height, it has lightly serrated, trifoliate leaves and pink flower clusters, made up of tubular, two-lipped florets.
Habitat/distribution A native of the Canary Islands, where it is found on sunny, rocky slopes. Introduced elsewhere.
Growth Requires well-drained soil and full sun. It does not withstand frost and although it may be grown outside in a sheltered position, in cool climates it needs winter protection. Propagation is easiest from softwood cuttings taken in late spring. Germination from seed is erratic and requires heat.
Parts used Leaves, flowers.

USES Culinary Fresh or dry leaves may be infused to make an invigorating tea.
Aromatic Leaves and flowers are dried for adding to potpourri.

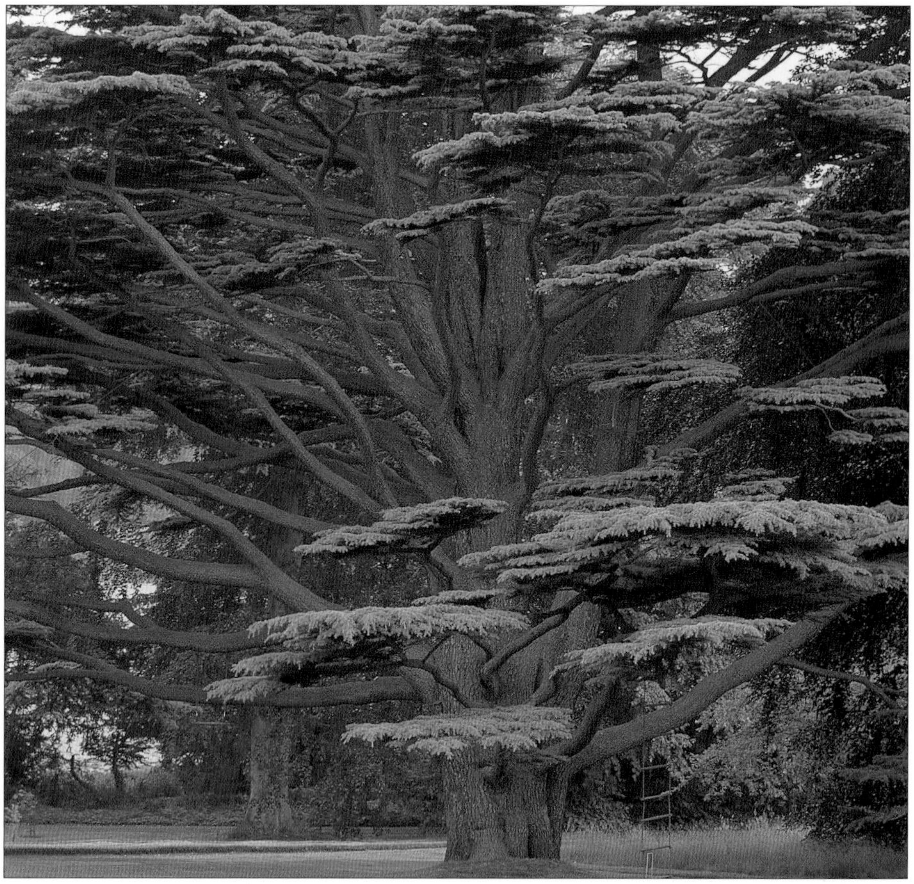

PINACEAE

Cedrus libani

Cedar of Lebanon

History and traditions The ancient Egyptians used oil of cedar for embalming and in their religious rituals. These beautiful, wide-spreading trees, with their head-clearing pine scent, were much prized in biblical times and celebrated in the Song of Solomon ("His countenance is as Lebanon, excellent as the cedars"). And in the Canticles, that evocative Hebrew love poem, also attributed to Solomon, the beloved is compared to many plant fragrances, and told, "The smell of thy garments is like the smell of Lebanon." King Solomon is also alleged to have denuded Lebanon of its cedars to build his massive temple.
Description A tall, 30–40m/100–130ft coniferous tree, with a dark brown or grey, deeply ridged trunk and wide branches bearing whorls of needle-like leaves. It carries both male and female cones, the latter being the larger. They are green at first, turning brown as they ripen over a two-year period, when they break up to release the seeds. Cedars often reach a great age, living for several hundred years.
Related species There are only four species of conifers which are true cedars, all rich in aromatic essential oil. As well as *C. libani,* there is *C. atlantica* (Atlas cedar) and *C. brevifolia* (Cyprus cedar), both classified by some authorities as subspecies of *C. libani,* and *C. deodara,* the Indian cedar.
Habitat/distribution Native to forests of the Mediterranean region from Lebanon to Turkey (*C. libani),* the Atlas Mountains in North Africa (*C. atlantica),* Cyprus (*C. brevifolia)* and the western Himalayas (*C. deodara).*
Growth Fully hardy trees, they grow in any well-drained soil and a sunny position.
Parts used Wood, essential oil.

USES Medicinal The essential oil has antiseptic, fungicide and insect-repellent properties. It is used as a steam inhalation for bronchial and respiratory complaints, to soothe skin irritations, for alopecia, dandruff and other scalp problems. It also has a calming effect for states of anxiety.
Aromatic The oil is added to perfumery, soaps and cosmetics. The wood is used to make furniture and storage chests which, due to its aromatic properties, helps to deter moths and insects.

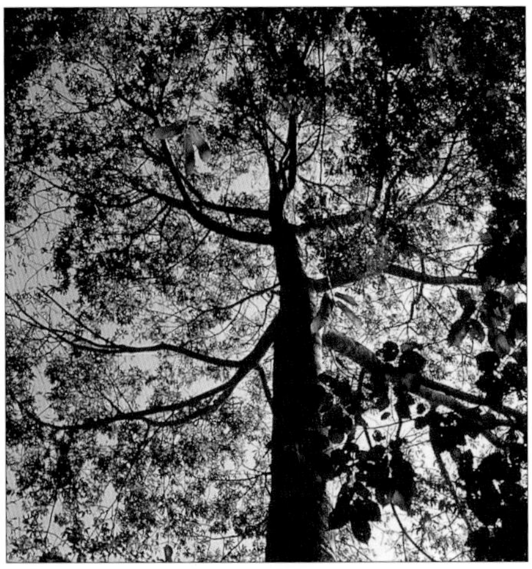

BOMBACACEAE

Ceiba pentandra

Cotton tree

History and traditions The Ceiba is the national tree of Guatemala and was held sacred by the ancient Mayans of Central America. They believed it grew through the centre of the universe, with its roots in the nine levels of the underworld, its trunk in the thirteen levels of the upperworld and its branches in heaven. The myth still prevails in the area, that this graceful tree is the home of the temptress, Ixtobai, recognizable by her backward-facing feet, who lures unfaithful husbands to disappear with her into the underworld through the trunk.
Description A deciduous, or semi-evergreen, tree growing to 40m/130ft with wide-spreading branches and palmate leaves. The flowers are followed by large pods, containing seeds protected by white, fluffy, silky-textured padding, collected to make kapok.
Habitat/distribution Occurs in rainforests and other damp, wooded areas in tropical North, South and Central America, Africa and Asia.
Growth Requires a temperature of 15°C/59°F. Grown in fertile, moist, but well-drained soil and full sun. Usually propagated by cuttings.
Parts used Leaves, bark, seeds, seed-pod fibre.

USES Medicinal The bark and leaves are made into decoctions, taken internally, for bronchial and respiratory infections, or applied externally in the form of baths. The leaves are boiled in sugar to make cough syrup and applied as a compress for headaches, fevers and sprains.
Culinary The seeds are toxic, but an edible, non-toxic oil is extracted from them which is used locally for cooking.

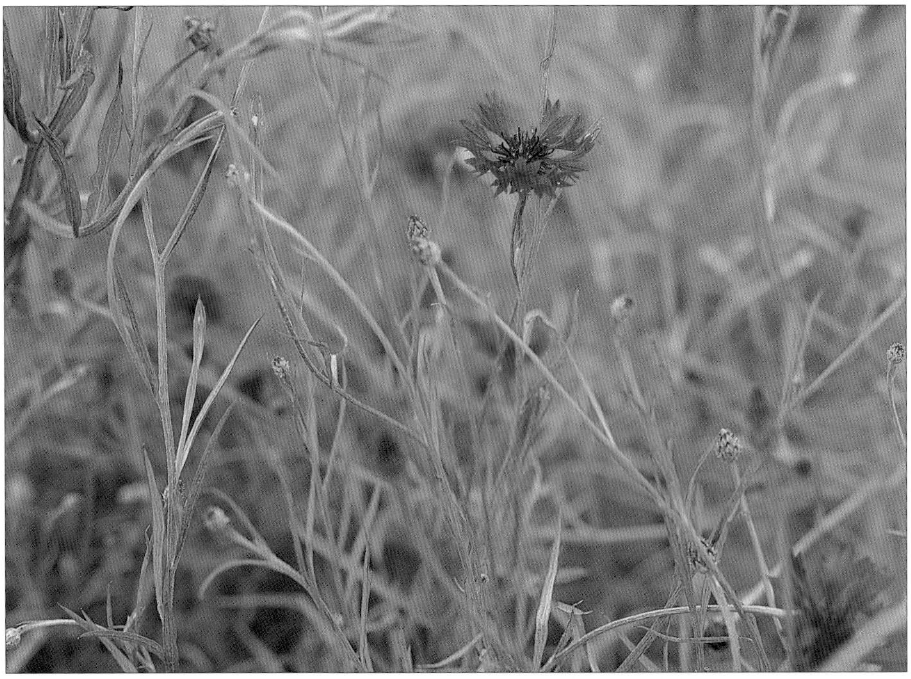

COMPOSITAE/ASTERACEAE

Centaurea cyanus

Cornflower

History and traditions These pretty blue flowers were once a common sight in cornfields, as their name suggests, but have largely been ousted by the techniques of modern agriculture. In his *Herbal* of 1597, Gerard reports that the Italian name for the cornflower is a reference to blunting sickles, "because it hindereth and annoyeth the reapers, dulling and turning the edges of their sickles" and he includes "hurt-sickle" among its English names of blew-bottle, blew-blow and corne-floure. Although Culpeper found many uses for these flowers, Gerard's view was that there is "no use of them in physic", although they are recommended by some for inflammation of the eye.
Description An annual which grows from 20–80cm/8–32in tall, with grey-green lanceolate leaves and bright blue shaggy flower heads. Cultivated kinds also have pink, purple or white flowers.
Related species *C. montana* is a perennial species, found mainly in mountainous areas of Europe. The wild plant, *C. scabiosa,* is often called knapweed.
Habitat/distribution Native to Europe and the Mediterranean region, naturalized in North America, also found in Asia and Australia. Becoming less common in the wild, widely cultivated and grown in gardens.

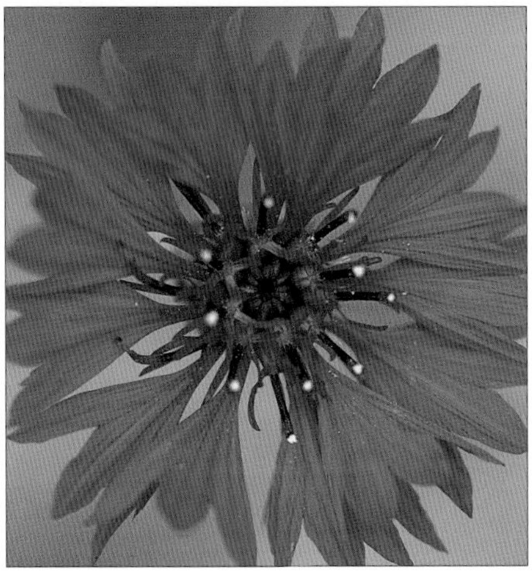

Above *Cornflowers, once a common weed, are frequently cultivated in gardens for their striking colour and form.*

Growth A hardy annual, it is easy to grow from seed sown in spring *in situ*, as it resents being transplanted. May be given an early start by sowing in autumn or very early spring, in plugs, or biodegradable pots, to minimize root disturbance. Plant in well-drained soil and a sunny position.
Parts used Flowers.

USES Medicinal Traditionally used in the past to make eyewashes for tired or strained eyes, but seems to have little place in herbal medicine as practised today.
Aromatic Flowers are dried for potpourris.
Other name Bluebottle.

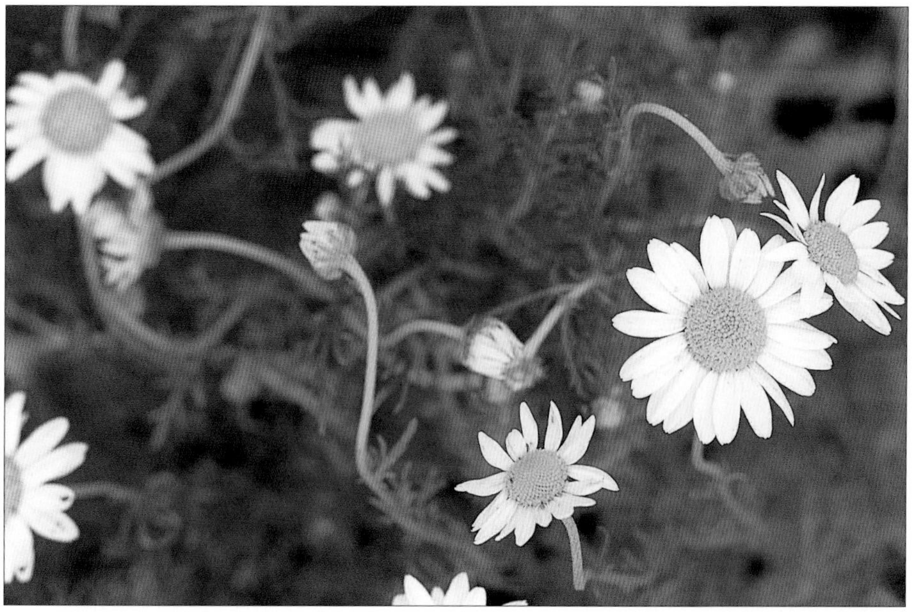

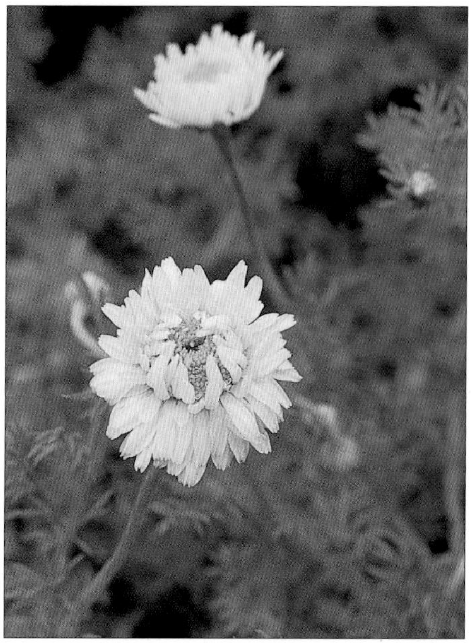

COMPOSITAE/ASTERACEAE

Chamaemelum nobile

Chamomile

History and traditions "Thys herbe was consecrated by the wyse men of Egypt unto the Sonne and was rekened to be the only remedy for all agues", says William Turner in his *Newe Herball,* 1551, in reference to the veneration of chamomile by the ancient Egyptians. The Greeks called it "earth apple", from which its generic name is derived (*kamai*, meaning "on the ground" and *melon*, apple), and in modern Spanish chamomile is called *"manzanilla",* meaning "little apple". It does indeed have an apple-like fragrance, especially noticeable after rain or when the plant is lightly crushed. To the Anglo-Saxons it was *"maythen"* and was one of the sacred herbs of Woden. It was featured in the Nine Herbs Lay, a charm against the effects of "flying venom" and "loathed things that over land rove" from the *Lacnunga* in the Harleian manuscript collection, British Museum. Over the centuries chamomile has been celebrated for its soothing properties, and its fragrance heads the list in an anti-stress prescription from *Ram's Little Dodoen,* 1606: "To comfort the braine smel to camomill, eate sage … wash measurably, sleep reasonably, delight to heare melody and singing".

Description An evergreen perennial with finely divided, feathery leaves growing to 15cm/6in. The white daisy-like flowers, with yellow disc centres, are borne singly on long stems rising to 30cm/1ft.

Related species *C. nobile* 'Flore Pleno' is a cultivar with creamy-coloured double flowers. The whole plant is more compact than the species, about 10cm/4in tall including flower stems, and makes a good edging plant. *C. nobile* 'Treneague' is a non-flowering cultivar which forms a dense carpet useful for lawns and seats and grows to about 6cm/2$^1/_2$in.

Habitat/distribution Indigenous to Europe, it is widely grown in North America and many other countries. It is found in the wild on sandy soils in grasslands and waste ground.

Growth Prefers light, sandy soil and a sunny position. It is possible to propagate *C. nobile* from seed sown in spring, but the easier and more usual method is by division of runners or "offsets". *C. n.* 'Flore Pleno' and *C. n.* 'Treneague' must be vegetatively propagated.

Parts used Flowers, essential oil.

USES Medicinal Chamomile has an antiseptic, anti-inflammatory action and is soothing and a relaxant. It is taken as a tea for nausea and indigestion and to help promote sound sleep, and may also be helpful in relieving painful menstruation. It is made into ointments or lotions for skin irritations and insect bites. The true essential oil is very expensive and contains azulene, which gives it a deep blue colour. It is frequently used for skin complaints and eczema (diluted in witch hazel or a pure, mild vegetable oil) and as a steam inhalation for asthma, sinusitis or catarrh.

Cosmetic An infusion of the flowers makes a rinse to give a shine to fair hair, or a skin freshener for sensitive skins. Essential oil or infusions are added to face or hand creams and fresh flowers floated in hot water make a deep-cleansing facial steam treatment.

Aromatic The dried flowers are added to sleep pillows and sachets or put into potpourri.

Other name Roman chamomile.

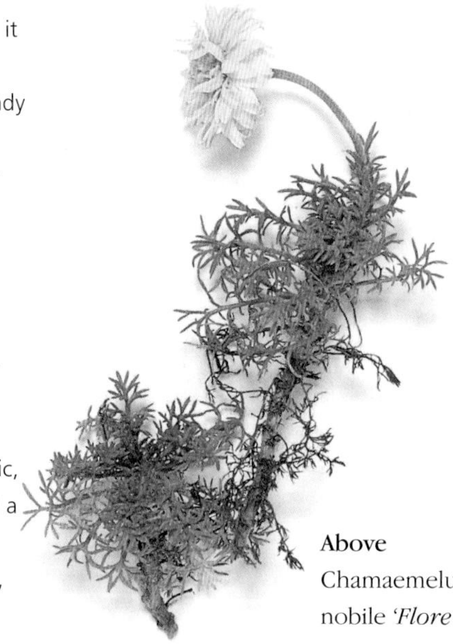

Above Chamaemelum nobile *'Flore Pleno'.*

Top *The double flowers of the dwarf edging plant* C. nobile 'Flore Pleno'.

CAUTION Despite being such a benevolent herb (when recommended doses and guidelines are followed), if taken internally to excess it may cause vomiting and vertigo. The plant may cause contact dermatitis.

Related species

COMPOSITAE/ASTERACEAE

Matricaria chamomilla syn. *Matricaria recutita*

Wild/German chamomile

History and traditions The name *matricaria* comes from its early gynaecological uses in herbal medicine.

Description *M. chamomilla* syn. *M. recutita* is a tall hardy annual which grows to 60cm/2ft. Although from a different genus (due to botanical differences), flowers, feathery foliage and scent are similar in appearance to that of *Chamaemelum nobile*. Not to be confused with the scentless mayweeds, or false chamomiles *Matricaria inodora* and *Tripleurosperum maritimum*, or the almost scentless corn chamomile (*Anthemis arvensis*).

Habitat/distribution Occurs all over Europe, Western Asia and India.

Growth Propagated from seed, sown *in situ* in early spring, it grows easily in any dry, light soil.

Parts used Flowers – they have similar properties to those of *Chamaemelum nobile*.

USES As for *C. nobile*.

Other names Scented mayweed.

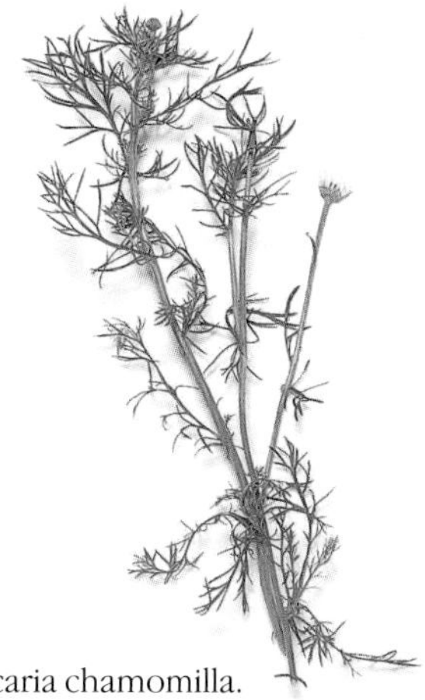

Above Matricaria chamomilla.

To make oyle of chamomile

Take oyle a pint and halfe, and three ounces of camomile flowers dryed one day after they be gathered. Then put the oyle and the flowers in a glasse and stop the mouth close and set it into the sun by the space of forty days.

The Good Housewife's Handbook, 1588

A chamomile lawn

Chamomile has been popular since medieval times for scented lawns, paths or places to sit, all of which still make delightful features in the herb garden.

A chamomile lawn requires regular hand weeding to keep it looking good and does not take heavy wear. The trick is to think small – grow it as a scaled-down version of a lawn, plant it round a fountain or sundial, or as a mini lawn between paving.

- Use rooted cuttings or offsets of non-flowering *Chamaemelum nobile* 'Treneague', edged (or for a "flowery-mead" effect, interspersed) with *C. n.* 'Flore Pleno'.
- Choose an area with light, preferably sandy soil, prepare it well, eliminating weeds and removing stones. Rake in a little peat to hold water and help the plants settle in quickly.

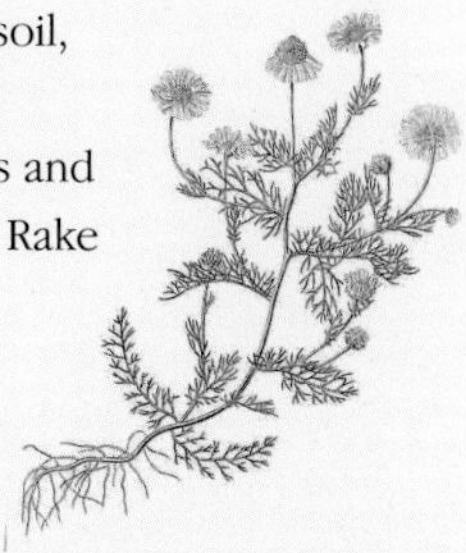

- Set plants 10cm/4in apart, water them in and keep lightly moist until established.
- To maintain the lawn, weed regularly and fill in any gaps that appear with new plants.

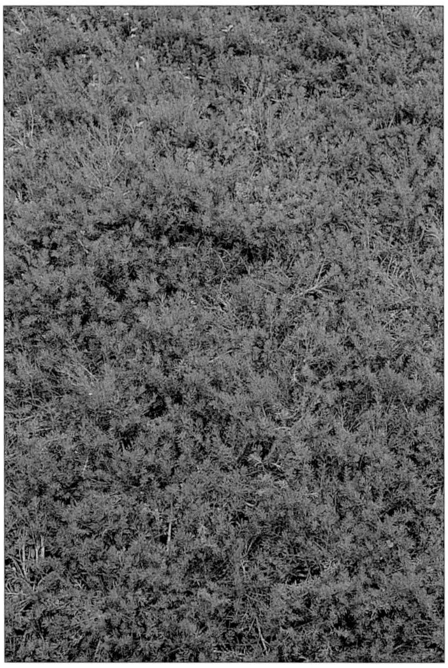

Above *A lawn of* C. n. *'Treneague'.*

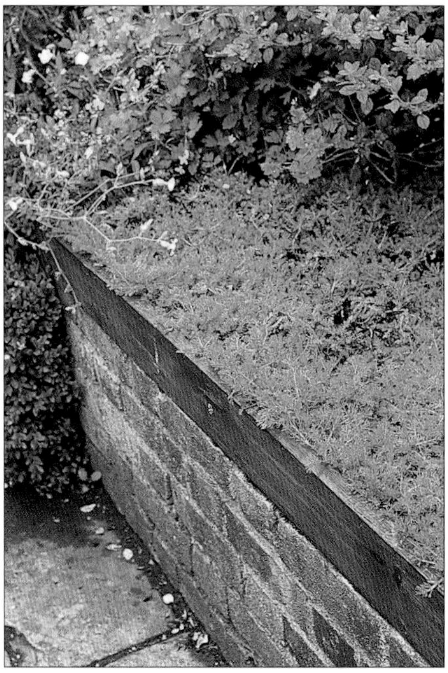

Above *A brick-built chamomile seat.*

A chamomile seat

These are always attractive and have the added advantage that the area of chamomile is small enough to make maintenance simple of the seat. It is also a good way to grow chamomile in a garden with heavy or clay soil, as the seat forms a raised bed to provide a free-draining environment.

- The base of the seat may be constructed with brick, stone or timber, filled with rubble and a very thick layer of topsoil for planting.
- It is best to keep to *C. n.* 'Treneague' only for this, as flowers sticking out of a bench spoil the effect. Plant as for the lawn.
- If back and arm rests are required for the seat, they could be made of the same material as the base. Clipped box also looks very effective.

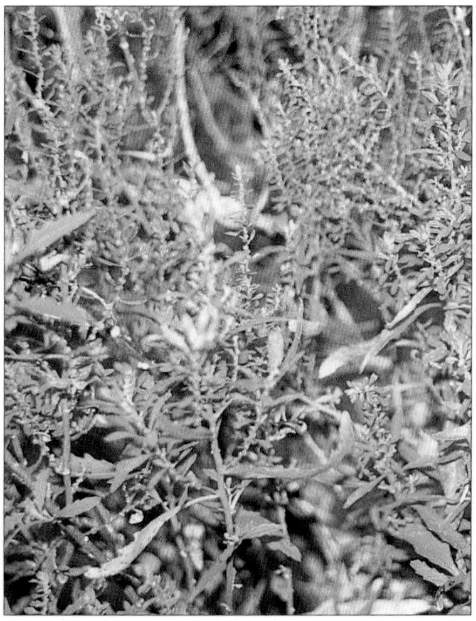

CHENOPODIACEAE

Chenopodium ambrosioides

American wormseed

History and traditions American wormseed was introduced to Europe in the 17th century from Mexico, where it was taken as a tea and used in traditional medicine.

Description An annual, 60cm–1.2m/2–4ft high, it has longer, more lanceolate leaves than those of *C. bonus-henricus* and a strong acrid scent. The tiny, green flowers are followed by small nutlike, one-seeded fruits.

Habitat/distribution Native to tropical Central America, naturalized throughout much of USA and grown in other countries also.

Growth Frost-hardy (to -5°C/23°F), American wormseed grows in any well-drained soil. Propagated by seed sown in spring; in warm climates it often self-seeds freely.

Parts used Flowering stems, essential oil.

USES Medicinal Its chief use has always been to expel intestinal worms. It has also been recommended for nervous disorders, asthma and problems with menstruation. The volatile oil of chenopodium is a powerful insecticide as well as a vermifuge (a medicine that expels intestinal worms), but should never be administered in this concentrated form as it is highly toxic.

CAUTION Poisonous in large doses, it should be taken only under medical supervision and is legally restricted in some countries.

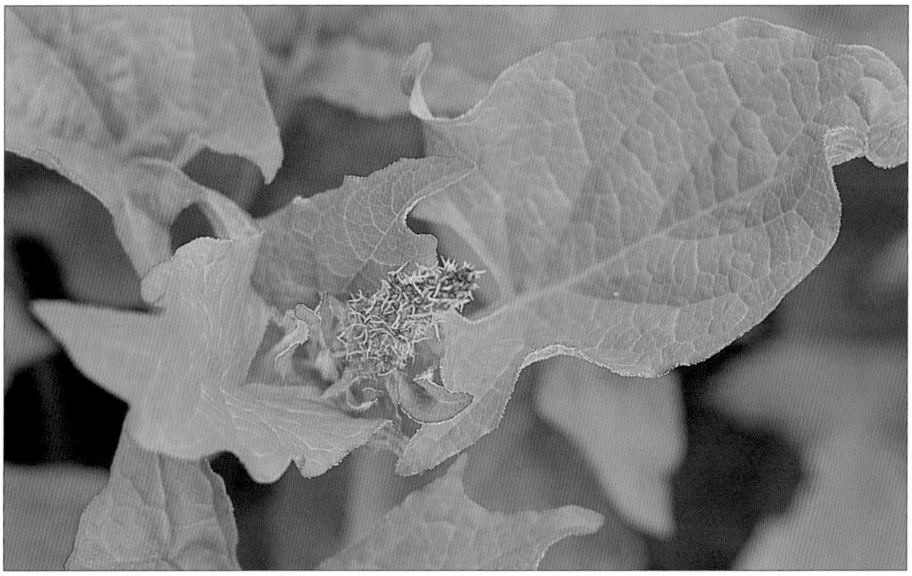

CHENOPODIACEAE

Chenopodium bonus-henricus

Good King Henry

History and traditions According to the 16th-century physician and botanist, Rembert Dodoens, of the Netherlands, this plant was dubbed *bonus henricus,* "good Henry", to distinguish it from a poisonous plant, *malus henricus,* "bad Henry". There is some uncertainty as to who "Henry" was, but one source claims it is a generic term for mischievous elves. "King" appears to have been spin-doctored into the English popular name to give this rather unattractive plant a spurious connection with King Henry VIII, "Good King Hal". The Latin name *Chenopodium* is derived from the Greek for "goose foot", an eloquent reference to the shape of the leaves.

Description A perennial which grows 60cm/2ft tall and spreads indefinitely, it has fleshy, downy stems, dark green, arrow-shaped leaves and greenish-yellow spikes of sorrel-like flowers in early summer.

Related species *Chenopodium album*, White Goosefoot – also known as allgood and fat hen (because it does a good job of fattening poultry) – as well as pigweed, mutton tops and lamb's quarters. It has long been a staple food of both animals and people. The Iron Age Dane, Tollund Man, made a last meal of it before he was hanged, seeds being found in his stomach.

Habitat/distribution Native to Europe but found worldwide on waste ground and previously cultivated land.

Growth This is an invasive plant which needs no cultivation and thrives in any soil. Said to be of "superior quality" if grown in rich soil, but little difference in taste or texture will be noticed. Tough taproots can make it difficult to eradicate if no longer wanted. Easily propagated from seed, or division, in spring.

Parts used Leaves, stems.

USES Medicinal Once made into ointments and poultices for skin complaints (an old name was "smearwort") but has no known medicinal value currently, apart from being mildly laxative.

Culinary Extravagant claims have been made for this plant as being a spinach-like vegetable (leaves) and asparagus substitute (young stems). Although edible if picked when young and tender, the leaves develop a fibrous texture with age which makes them less palatable. John Evelyn (*Acetaria,* 1719) was right when in reference to one of its names, "blite", from the Greek for insipid, he commented that "it is well-named, being insipid enough". It is rich in vitamins C, B^1, iron and calcium – so it may be a case of "eating up your greens" for the sake of your health.

Other names Goosefoot, allgood, fat hen, English mercury and Lincolnshire asparagus.

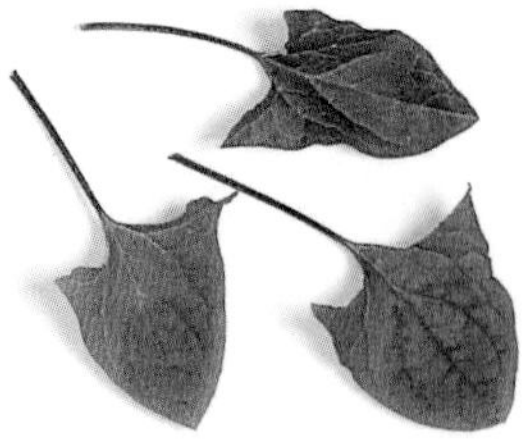

Left *The leaves of* Chenopodium bonus-henricus *were thought to resemble goose feet.*

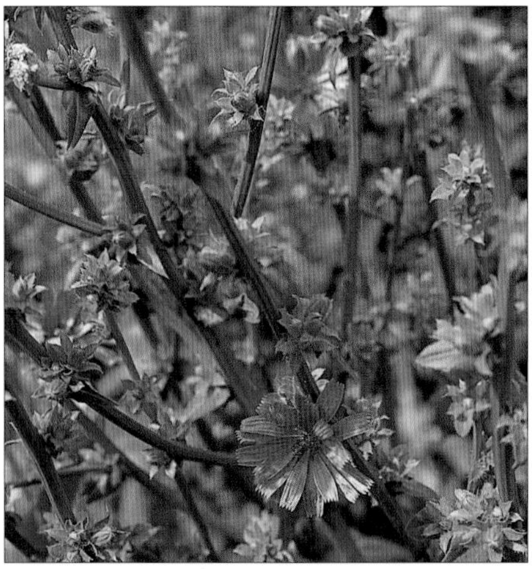

COMPOSITAE/ASTERACEAE

Cichorium intybus

Chicory

History and traditions This herb was cultivated in Egypt over 2,000 years ago, and known to the ancient Greeks and Romans, who used it as a salad ingredient and vegetable. Its use as a coffee substitute is thought to date from 1806 when Napoleon's Continental blockade prevented imports of coffee. It was widely used for the same purpose during the World Wars.

Description A tall, hardy perennial, growing to 1.5m/5ft. It has a deep taproot and thick stem which exudes a milky sap when cut. It has toothed, oval to lanceolate leaves and pale blue flowers appear in summer.

Habitat/distribution Native of the Mediterranean region, western Asia and North Africa, introduced and established worldwide.

Growth For best results grow in rich, but well-drained soil. Propagate from seed sown in spring. Sometimes self-seeds, especially on dry soils.

Parts used Leaves, roots.

USES Medicinal A bitter tonic herb, the dried, crushed root is made into infusions or decoctions for digestive upsets and to improve appetite. It is also a mild stimulant and laxative.

Culinary There are various cultivars whose leaves are added to salads, including red, broad-leafed radicchio types. Blanched heads, or chicons, eaten in salads and cooked as vegetables, are produced by lifting the roots, packing them in boxes in a growing medium, cutting off the leaves and keeping them in complete darkness until white, elongated shoots have sprouted.

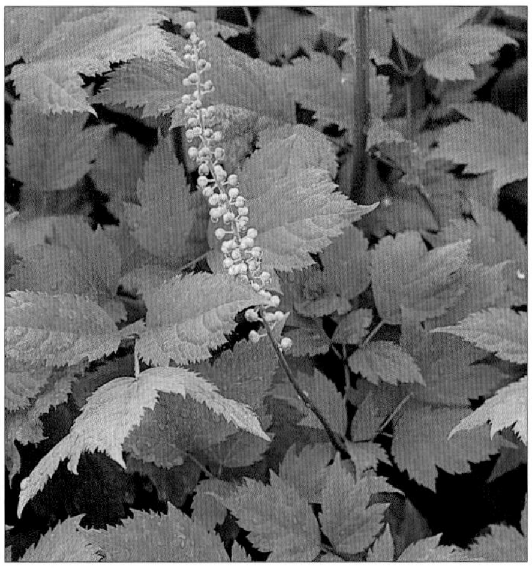

RANUNCULACEAE

Actaea racemosa

Black cohosh

History and traditions The root of this herb was used in the medicine of Native Americans for female complaints and it was thought to be an antidote to poison and to rattlesnake venom. The generic name is from the Latin *cimex,* meaning a bug, and *fugere*, to run, in reference to this plant's insect-repellent properties.

Description A tall, clump-forming, aromatic perennial, with a rather unpleasant smell. It makes an attractive plant for the border with spires of creamy-white, bottle-brush flowers, rising to 1.5m/5ft above the three-lobed basal leaves 40cm/16in high.

Habitat/distribution Native to North America, it is grown in northern temperate regions and occurs in moist grassland or woodland.

Growth Fully hardy, it requires moist, fertile soil with plenty of humus and partial shade. It can be propagated by division of roots or by seed, sown in pots in autumn for overwintering in a cold frame for germination the following spring.

Parts used Rhizomes – dried for use in decoctions, tinctures and extracts.

USES Medicinal For arthritis, rheumatism, menstrual and some menopausal problems.

CAUTION Large doses may cause liver damage or miscarriage. Not to be taken during pregnancy, while breast-feeding, or by anyone with liver disease. Legally restricted in some countries.

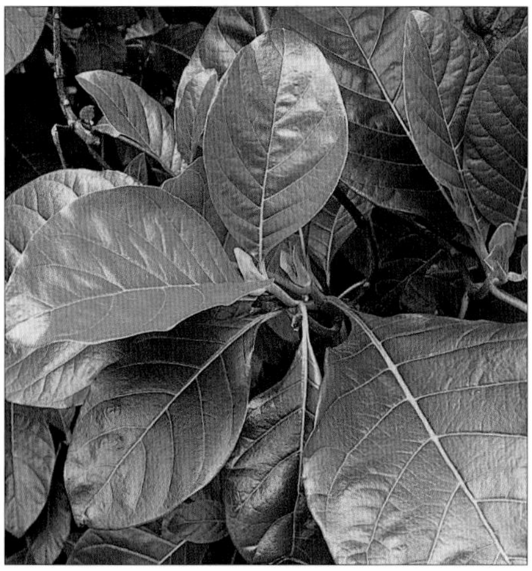

RUBIACEAE

Cinchona officinalis

Cinchona

History and traditions Said to be named after the Countess of Chinchon, wife of the Viceroy of Peru, after she had been cured of a fever (probably malaria) with a cinchona bark medicine in about 1638.

Description Cinchona species are tender, evergreen trees varying in height, according to species and habitat, from 10–25m/30–80ft. The oval leaves are often red-veined and small, crimson flowers are borne in panicles.

Related species There are several species of *Cinchona* of medicinal value, all closely related, including *C. calisaya* and *C. pubescens.*

Habitat/distribution Native to mountainous regions of South America, widely introduced and cultivated in tropical regions worldwide.

Growth In the wild, trees occur in dense, wet forest. Commercial plantations provide well-drained, moist soil and high humidity. Propagated by cuttings.

Parts used Bark – dried and powdered or as a liquid extract.

USES Medicinal Cinchona bark contains the antimalarial alkaloid, quinine, as well as quinidine, which slows the heart rate. It was the major treatment for malaria from the mid-17th century until recently, now largely replaced for this purpose by synthetic drugs. It is still an ingredient of many pharmaceutical preparations for colds and influenza, and of tonic water.

CAUTION For use by medical herbal practitioners only.

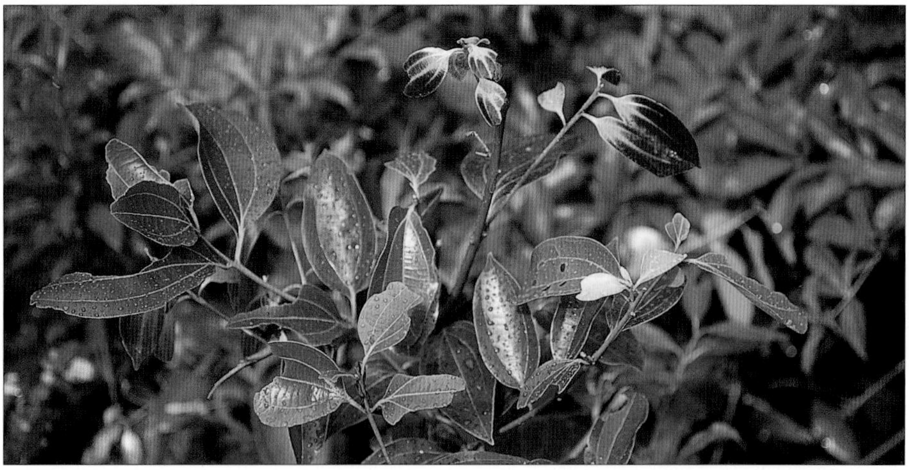

LAURACEAE

Cinnamomum zeylanicum

Cinnamon

History and traditions An important aromatic spice since biblical times, cinnamon was an ingredient of the holy ointment made by Moses. It is also cited as amongst the costly merchandise and luxury items available in Babylon, when the fall of that misguided city is predicted in the biblical book, Revelation. The Portuguese occupied Sri Lanka for its cinnamon in 1536. By the 18th century, cinnamon had become such a valuable commodity in Europe, that the Dutch took control of the island and set up a trading monopoly in the spice.
Description A medium-sized evergreen tree, it grows to about 9m/30ft and has brown, papery bark and ovate, leathery green leaves. Creamy-white flowers are borne in short panicles, followed by olive-shaped dark blue fruits.
Habitat/distribution Native to forest areas of Sri Lanka, southern India and Malaysia and widely cultivated in India, the Seychelles, Brazil, the Caribbean and tropical zones.
Growth Cinnamon grows in sandy soils, and needs plenty of rain, sun and a minimum temperature of 15°C/59°F. Young trees are cut to within 30cm/1ft of the ground, stumps covered in mulch to encourage sprouting for re-harvesting within 2–3 years. It is also propagated by seed.
Parts used Inner bark of young stems – dried and wrapped round thin rods to form quills. Essential oil.
USES Medicinal It has digestive properties, dispels nausea, and is taken for colds, sore throats and rheumatic conditions. The essential oil is antibacterial and antifungal, helps deaden the nerve where there is toothache and is added to steam inhalations for colds and upper respiratory tract infections. It dries up catarrh in productive coughs. Cinnamon is also used to help regulate blood sugar levels in diabetes treatment and to help reduce sugar cravings.
Culinary A popular spice for savoury and sweet dishes. It adds flavour to curries, baked goods, stews and meat dishes, savoury and sweet rice and is a traditional ingredient of Christmas puddings, mince pies, mulled wine and hot spiced drinks.
Aromatic Ingredient of potpourri (powdered or whole pieces) and clove-and-orange pomanders. The essential oil is used in perfumery.

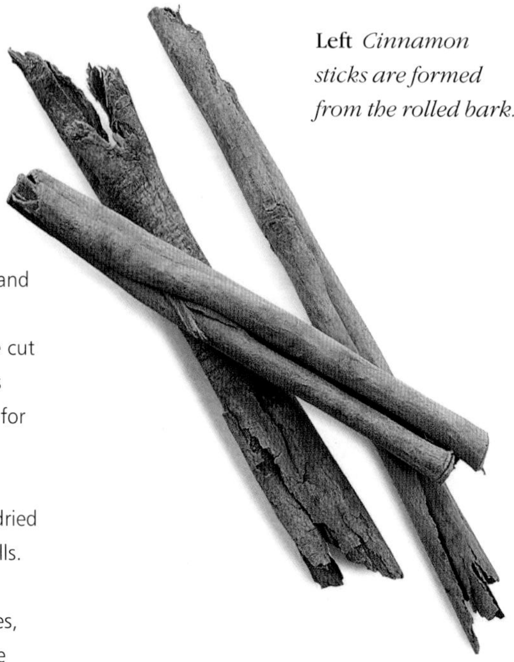

Left *Cinnamon sticks are formed from the rolled bark.*

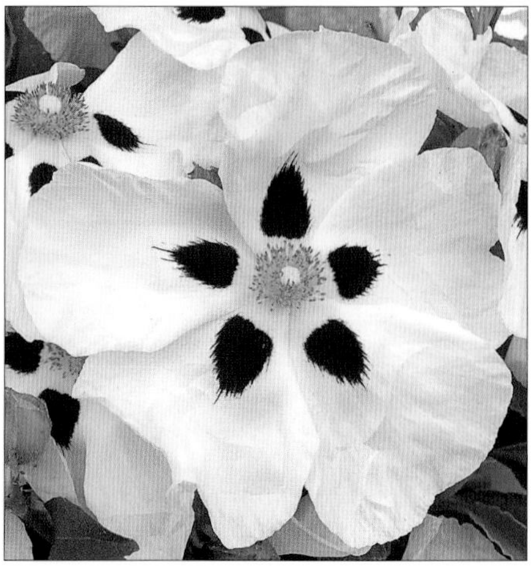

CISTACEAE

Cistus ladanifer

Cistus

History and traditions In his *Relation d'un voyage du Levant,* 1717, French botanist, Pitton de Tournefort, gives an eloquent description of collecting ladanum, a fragrant resin exuded by several species of cistus, by means of dragging a leather-thonged rake (a *ladisteron)* across the plants. He also refers to a method in use since Dioscorides' day, of combing it from the beards of goats allowed to browse on the sticky foliage. It has a perfume reminiscent of ambergris and was one of the main ingredients in the solid, resin-based pomanders popular in the Middle Ages for repelling infection.
Description A hardy evergreen shrub, growing to 2m/6ft, with lanceolate, sticky, dark green leaves. The papery, saucer-shaped white flowers bloom for only one day.
Related species *C. creticus* syn. *C. incanus* subsp. *creticus*, the Cretan rock rose, and also a source of ladanum, is a more compact shrub, growing to 1m/3ft with purplish-pink flowers and yellow stamens.
Habitat/distribution Found in Crete, southern Europe, Turkey, northern Africa and the Canary Islands, on dry, stony soils and sunny hillsides. Introduced and widely grown elsewhere.
Growth Prefers a light, well-drained soil and sheltered site in full sun. It is propagated from seed, sown in containers, in late summer or from softwood cuttings in early summer.
Parts used Dried leaves, oleo-resin – collected from young stems and leaves.

USES Aromatic Used as a fixative in perfumery, and in potpourri and home fragrance products.

RUTACEAE

Citrus

History and traditions The citrus species were unknown to Greek and Roman writers, but they have been cultivated for so long that their origins are hazy. Both oranges and lemons are probably natives of northern India, certainly China, and are thought to have been brought to the West by Arab traders via North Africa, Arabia and Syria, thence to Spain and Sicily. *C. limon,* found in the valleys of Kumaon and Sikkim, in the foothills of the Himalayas, has the Hindustani name *limu* or *nimbu*, which was taken into Arabic as *limun. C. aurantium,* the bitter Seville orange, is the species mentioned in a medicinal context by the Arabian physician, Avicenna, 980–1037, practising at Salerno, and was the orange tree planted in Rome by St Dominic in AD1200. These must also have been the oranges which Edward I's Queen, Eleanor of Castile, is purported to have bought from a Spanish ship which called at Portsmouth in 1290 – sweet oranges were not known in the West before the mid-15th century, introduced from the East by the Portuguese. The custom of wearing orange blossom at weddings is said to have originated with the Saracens, who considered it an emblem of fecundity, and the practice was introduced to Europe by returning Crusaders. Essential oil distilled from the flowers of the bitter orange was said to have an "exquisite fragrance" by the Italian Giambattista Porta in his herbal of 1588. It became known as "oil of Neroli" from 1680, because it was favoured by the wife of the Count of Neroli for perfuming gloves.

Habitat/distribution Originated in Asia, cultivated in the Mediterranean region, in southern parts of North America and other countries.

Growth Orange and lemon trees are tender, and must be protected from frost, but they prefer cool rather than hot conditions. If grown in northern climates, with cold, frosty winters, they should be kept outside in summer and in a temperate conservatory or greenhouse in winter. They need a well-drained, not too acid compost – the correct pH value is crucial, 6–6.5 for lemons and 6.5–7 for oranges. *C. aurantium* and *C. limon* may be grown from seed, or from semi-ripe cuttings – but cultivars do not come true from seed.

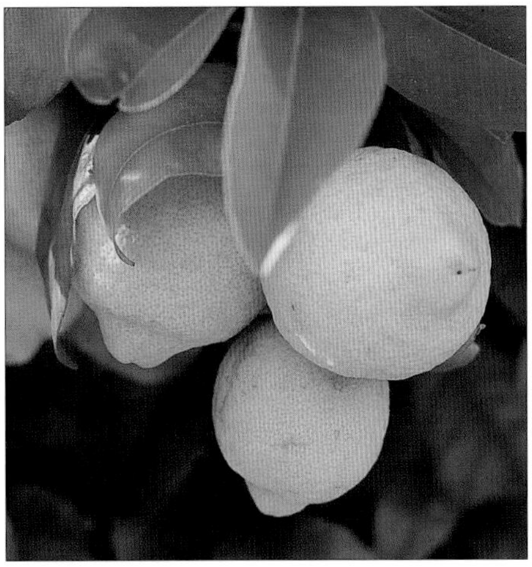

Citrus limon

Lemon

Description A small evergreen tree, 2–6m/6–19ft tall, with light green, oval leaves and thorny stems. Clusters of white flowers, opening from pink-tinted buds, are followed by ovoid, bitter-tasting yellow fruits.

Parts used Fruits, essential oil, expressed from the peel.

USES Medicinal Rich in vitamin C and once used by British seamen to prevent scurvy (limes were also used). Lemons have anti-inflammatory properties and are used in home remedies for colds, frequently in conjunction with honey, which is antiseptic. Applied externally for insect bites and skin irritations.

Culinary The juice and rind are widely used as a flavouring in cooking, and in soft drinks, sauces, pickles, preserves and marinades.

Aromatic The peel is dried for potpourri and home fragrance preparations. The oil is used commercially in perfumery, and to scent soaps and household cleaning products.

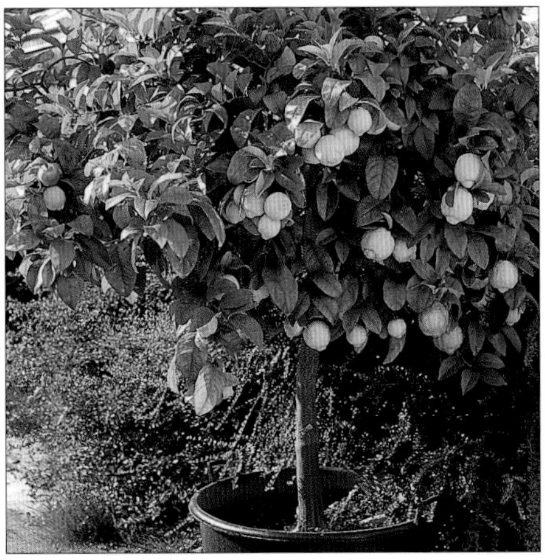

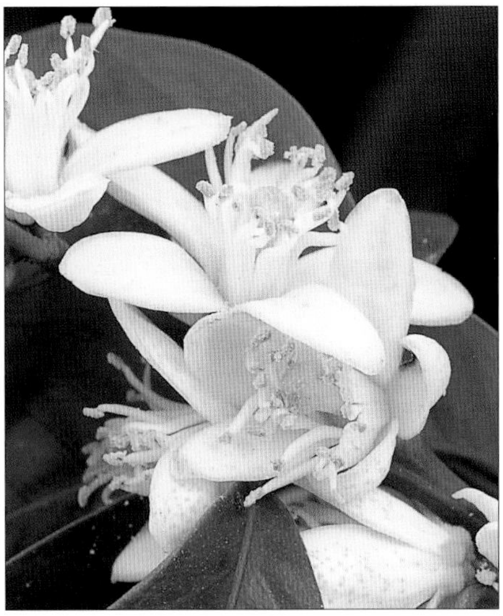

Citrus aurantium

Bitter orange

Description An evergreen tree, growing to 8m/26ft high, with shiny, ovate leaves and fragrant white flowers, followed by bitter, orange fruits.

Parts used Leaves, fruits, flowers. Essential oil of neroli, distilled from flowers; essential oil of petitgrain, distilled from leaves and twigs; distilled orange flower water; oil of orange, expressed from the rind.

USES Medicinal Rich in vitamins A, B and C, and has energizing tonic properties. Infusions of leaves and flowers are used for digestive disorders. The essential oil of neroli is an anti-depressant and calming. It may also be helpful for insomnia.

Culinary The fruits are used to make Seville orange marmalade and a bitter sauce to complement fatty poultry such as duck and goose. Orange flower water has a delicate fragrance, ideal for flavouring sweet dishes. Oil of orange is a flavouring in commercial food products.

Aromatic Essential oils of neroli and petitgrain are used in perfumery.

Cosmetic Orange rind pounded, mixed with rainwater and applied as a poultice is a traditional Indian remedy for acne. Oil of neroli is soothing for dry, sensitive skins as an ingredient of creams and lotions. Also used in many citrus-based cleaning products.

Other name Seville orange.

Left Citrus limon *'Jambhiri'*.

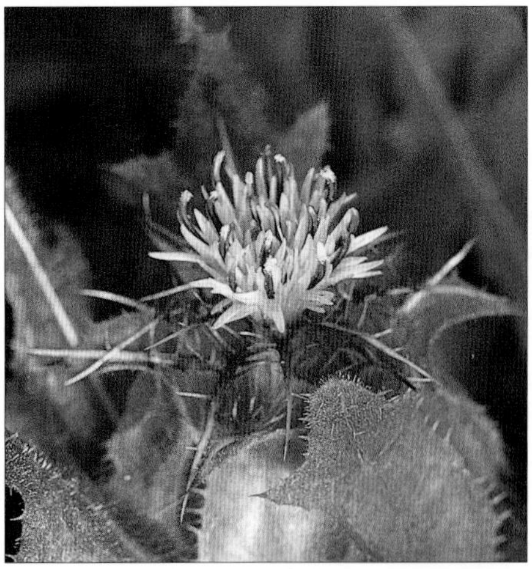

ASTERACEAE

Cnicus benedictus syn. *Carduus benedictus*

Holy thistle

History and traditions It is known as Holy or Blessed Thistle for much the same reasons as the Carline Thistle (*Carlina acaulis*) is named after Charlemagne – it was all down to visions of this plant as a cure for plague. Considering that it does have antiseptic and antibiotic properties, this may not be as far-fetched as it sounds. One writer of a dissertation on treating plague with this thistle said, "I counsell all that have gardens to nourish it, that they may have it always to their own use, and the use of their neighbours that lacke it."

Description The only plant in the *Cnicus* genus, sometimes classified as *Carduus benedictus*. It is an annual with hairy, branched stems, spiny grey-green leaves and solitary yellow flowers set in prickly bracts.

Habitat/distribution A Mediterranean native, it is widely naturalized throughout Europe and North America.

Growth A wild plant, it grows in any ordinary soil, is easily propagated by seed, and self-seeds. Cultivated commercially in Europe for the pharmaceutical industry.

Parts used Whole plant – leaves and flower tops.

USES Medicinal A very bitter herb with antiseptic, antibiotic properties. Taken in the form of an infusion as a tonic and to stimulate the appetite. It was traditionally used for fevers and is said to be helpful for nursing mothers to improve the supply of milk.

Culinary All parts of the plant are edible and have been eaten cooked or in salads.

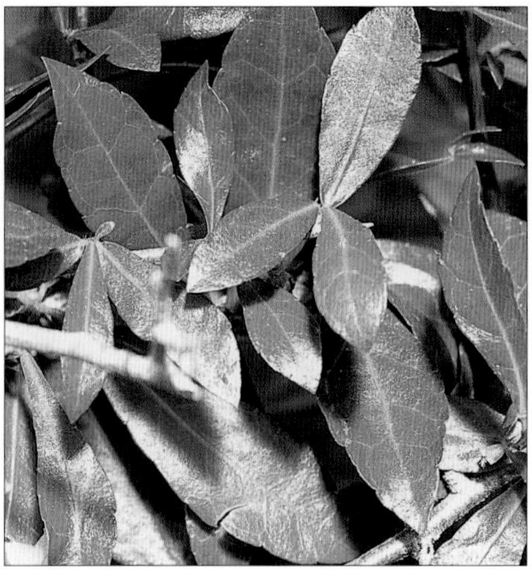

BURSERACEAE

Commiphora myrrha syn. *C. molmol*

Myrrh

History and traditions Myrrh has long been valued for its medicinal properties and as an ingredient of incense, perfumes and ointments. A symbol of suffering, myrrh was used in embalming from the Egyptian period, and the name comes from an ancient Hebrew and Arabic word, *mur,* meaning bitter. It was one of the gifts of the Wise Men to Jesus Christ at his birth and was used, along with aloes and spices, to embalm his body following the crucifixion.

Description A small tree or shrub, growing to about 3m/10ft tall, with spiny branches and sparse trifoliate leaves, made up of small oval leaflets. The gum exudes from the bark naturally, and after incisions have been made, when it flows out as a pale yellow liquid and quickly hardens to a reddish-brown resin.

Habitat/distribution Native to Arabia, Somalia and Ethiopia, where it grows in desert scrub.

Growth Grows wild.

Parts used Oleo-gum resin – known as *bdellium.*

USES Medicinal Myrrh has antiseptic, anti-inflammatory properties and encourages healing when applied to wounds, ulcers, boils and bleeding gums. Sometimes added to tooth powders. A preparation is made from the bark for treating skin diseases. In parts of Africa some species are chewed as a source of moisture and used for cleaning teeth.

Aromatic An ingredient of incense. It has fixative properties when used in perfumery, and is added to potpourri, in granule or powdered form, to "fix" the scent.

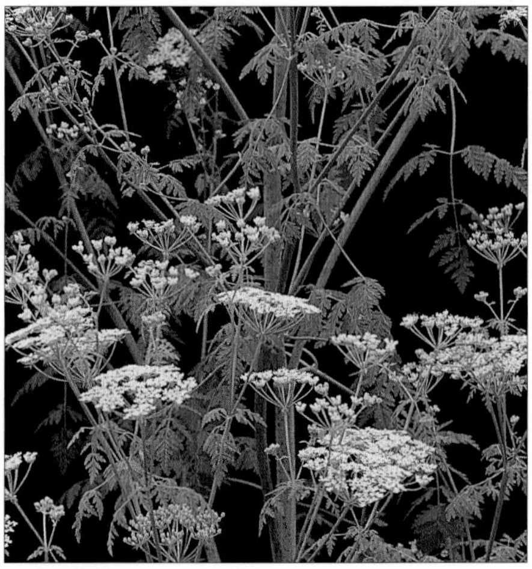

UMBELLIFERAE/APIACEAE

Conium maculatum

Hemlock

History and traditions Poisoning by hemlock was the official method of state execution in ancient Athens. The philosopher Socrates was its best-known victim. It was also used as a medicinal herb in the classical world, mainly for external application. Dioscorides and Pliny, echoed by Avicenna, recommended it for the treatment of skin diseases and cancerous tumours. It appeared in Anglo-Saxon herbals, and an old English myth associated the splotches on the stems with the mark of Cain.

Description A tall, unpleasant-smelling biennial, 1.5–2.4m/5–8ft in height, with purplish-red speckles towards the base of the stems, finely divided, feathery leaves and large umbels of white flowers in midsummer.

Habitat/distribution Indigenous to Europe and parts of Asia, widely distributed in temperate parts of the world and found in damp, weedy places, waste grounds and waysides.

Growth A wild plant in Australia and other countries, cultivation is legally restricted.

Parts used Leaves, seeds.

USES Medicinal Hemlock contains the highly toxic alkaloid, coniine, in all parts, but especially in the seeds. At one time it was used as a sedative and powerful pain-reliever – but its toxicity made this a risky business and it is not used medicinally today.

CAUTION All parts of the plant are highly poisonous, and may also cause skin irritations on contact.

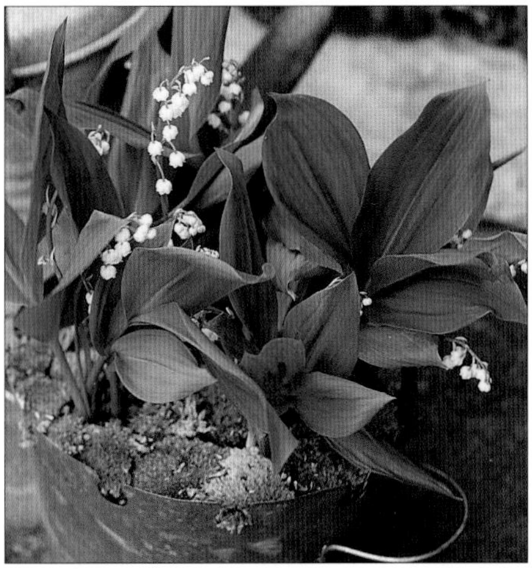

CONVALLARIACEAE

Convallaria majalis

Lily-of-the-valley

History and traditions This pretty cottage garden plant was known to the Anglo-Saxons for its medicinal properties and appeared in early manuscript herbals, including one written in Latin, attributed to Apuleius, AD400. Many of the 16th- and 17th-century herbalists, from Dodoens to Culpeper, took the line that a distillation of the flowers in wine was good for strengthening the memory and comforting the heart. The specific name is a reference to the month of May, when the flowers bloom – or to Maia, Roman goddess of fertility, if you prefer.
Description A hardy perennial with ribbed ovate to lance-shaped leaves and racemes of fragrant white flowers, hanging like little bells, followed by fruits which are round, red berries.
Habitat/distribution Native to Europe, Asia and North America and found in woodlands and alpine meadows.
Growth Prefers humus-rich, moist soil and partial shade. Propagation is easiest by division of the rhizomes in autumn – keep well watered until established and apply a leaf-mould mulch.
Parts used Leaves, flowers.

USES Medicinal It contains glycosides similar to those of foxgloves (*Digitalis* spp.), which affect the action of the heart. It is considered safer than *Digitalis* by some herbal experts and as having less of a cumulative effect.

CAUTION A poisonous plant which should not be eaten. It should be stressed that it is for use by qualified practitioners only.

UMBELLIFERAE/APIACEAE

Coriandrum sativum

Coriander (Cilantro)

History and traditions Seeds of this herb were found in Tutankhamun's tomb of 1325BC. It was known to the Greeks and Romans and features in many medieval herbals – though the authorities were not always in agreement as to its properties. Galen said it was "warm", Dioscorides and Avicenna took it to be "cold". The *Herbarius Latinus,* printed in Mainz in 1484 by Peter Schoeffer, has much to say on the subject. There are recommendations for mixing the juice with houseleek (*Sempervivum tectorum)* and warm vinegar to put on abscesses, for taking it with vinegar soon after dining heavily to "prohibit vapours from rising to the head", and for mixing it with violets for a hangover. If smelled, sniffed or blown up the nostrils, it is claimed, it will restrain a nosebleed, and is effective against St Anthony's fire (erysipelas) and "in tremors of the heart when its powder is given with borage water". William Turner took the strange line that "Coriander taken out of season doth trouble a man's wit with great jeopardy of madness" (*A Newe Herbal,* 1551). From Tudor times until the beginning of this century coriander seeds coated in sugar (comfits) were a popular sweet.
Description An annual 30–60cm/1–2ft tall, with pungent finely divided leaves – the basal ones are pinnatifid (deeply cleft) and wider than the upper ones, which are linear and feathery. Small umbels of white to mauvish flowers are followed by ridged, spherical, pale brown fruits (seeds). There are related species and numerous cultivars, some developed for leaf quality, others for their seeds. A variety with smaller seeds is grown in temperate zones, and one with larger seeds in warmer climates.
Habitat/distribution Originating in northern Africa and the Mediterranean region, it is widely grown in southwest Asia, North and South America and in temperate regions.
Growth A hardy annual, it is propagated from seed sown in spring, preferably *in situ* as it does not transplant well. It succeeds best grown in a well-drained, fertile soil, with ample water in the early stages followed by warmth and sunshine. Young plants quickly run to seed if attempts are made to transplant them in hot, dry spells.
Parts used Leaves, fruits (seeds), essential oil.

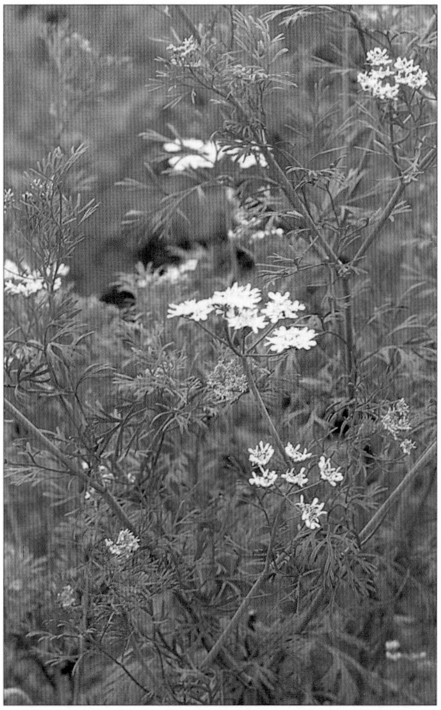

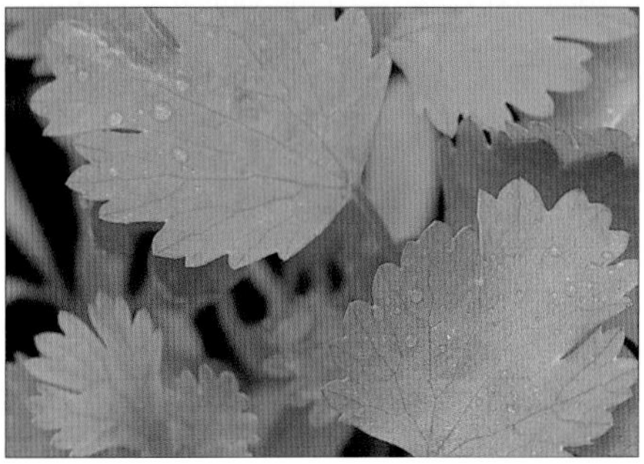

Above *The lower leaves are used in cookery.*

USES Medicinal The leaves and seeds have digestive properties and stimulate appetite. The essential oil has fungicidal, antibacterial properties. Decoctions of the seeds are considered helpful in lowering blood cholesterol levels in Indian herbal medicine. Used as an essential oil in aromatherapy for rheumatism.
Culinary The leaves have a stronger, spicier taste than the seeds, which are milder and sweeter. Both are used in curries, pickles and chutneys and in Middle Eastern, Indian, south-east Asian and South American cuisines. Leaves are added to salads, seeds used in sweet dishes, breads, cakes and to flavour liqueurs.
Aromatic The crushed seeds are added to scented sachets and potpourri. The essential oil has fixative properties.
Commercial The essential oil is used in the pharmaceutical, cosmetic and food industries.
Other name Cilantro.

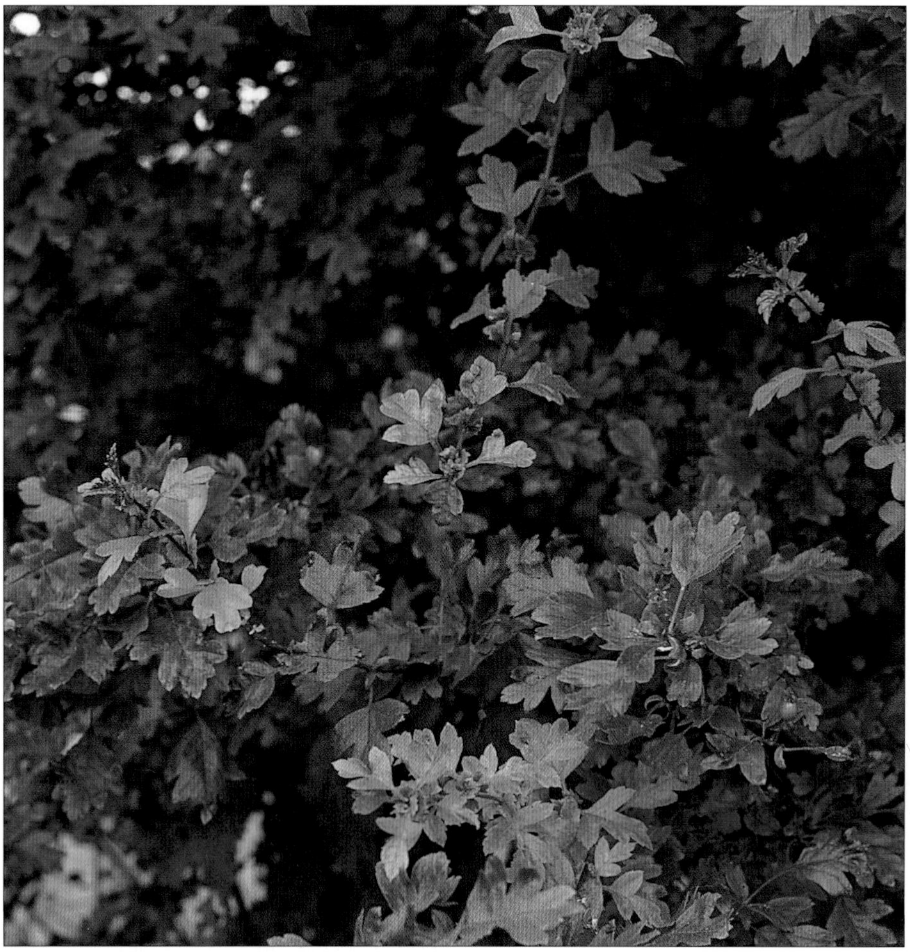

ROSACEAE

Crataegus laevigata

Hawthorn

History and traditions Many superstitions surround this tree, often known as "may", or "mayblossom", for its time of flowering, associations with May Day celebrations and the return of summer. It was considered an omen of both ill and good fortune – unlucky to bring into the house, yet tied outside as a protection from witches, storms and lightning or to stop milk going sour. The strange perfume, with its overtones of decay, contributed to its reputation as an emblem of death and the plague.
Description A deciduous shrub or small tree, growing to 8m/26ft, with thorny branches and small dark green, lobed, ovate leaves. It is densely covered with clusters of white scented flowers with red anthers in spring, followed by red globe-shaped fruit in autumn.
Related species *C. monogyna* is very similar and hybridizes with *C. laevigata.* There are also many ornamental cultivars, some with pink or red flowers, but they lack therapeutic properties.
Habitat/distribution Native to Europe, northern Africa and western Asia, introduced in temperate regions elsewhere. Occurs in hedges and woodland.
Growth A traditional hedging plant, which grows in any soil in sun or partial shade. Propagated from seed, sown in early spring – stratification is necessary for germination.
Parts used Flowers, leaves, fruits.

USES Medicinal An important medicinal herb in Europe, it acts on the circulatory system, strengthens the heart, regulates its rhythm and lowers blood pessure.
Culinary Leaves, sometimes berries, were once eaten in sandwiches, and young shoots cooked in savoury suet puddings.
Other names May, Mayblossom, quickset and quickthorn.

CAUTION Only to be taken on the advice of a qualified herbalist or medical practitioner. Can interact with medication for high blood pressure and heart disorders.

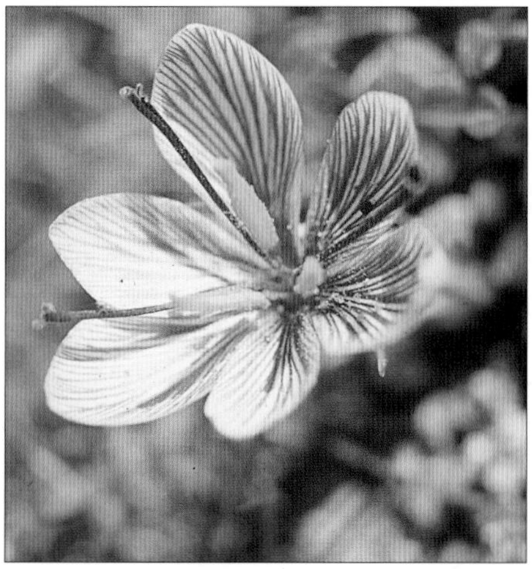

IRIDACEAE

Crocus sativus

Saffron crocus

History and traditions The Greeks called it *krokos,* the Romans *korkum,* and its common name is derived from the Arabic for yellow, *zafran*. In the classical world saffron was appreciated for its scent, flavour, medicinal properties and above all as a luminous yellow dye. In Greece it was a royal colour and in eastern cultures, too, it was reserved for dyeing the clothing of those of high rank or caste. Originating in Persia, it spread to northern India and the Mediterranean by the 10th century. Its popularity in Europe followed the Crusades and it became a valuable trading commodity. So valuable, indeed, that adulteration was always a temptation – but penalties were high. Regular saffron inspections were held in Nuremberg in the 15th century, and records reveal that at least one man was burned in the market place and three others buried alive for tampering with their saffron. Gerard certainly thought highly of its powers: "For those at death's doore," he wrote, "and almost past breathing, saffron bringeth breath again" (*The Herball,* 1597).
Description A perennial, it has linear leaves, growing from the rounded corm. Fragrant, lilac flowers, with deeper purple veins and yellow anthers, appear in autumn. The saffron spice is produced from the three-branched red style.
Habitat/distribution Occurs in southern Europe, northern Africa, the Middle East and India, with major centres of commercial cultivation in Spain and Kashmir, northern India.
Growth Needs well-drained soil, sun and warm summers in order to flower. Plants are sterile and can be propagated only by offsets.

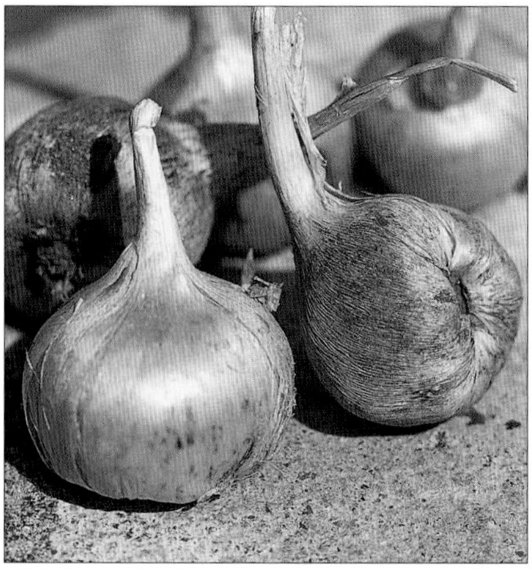

Parts used Flower pistils – dried. It takes over 4,000 flowers to produce 25g/1oz of dried saffron. Cheap or powdered product is often adulterated – the genuine herb is always expensive and should be a dark reddish-yellow in colour.

USES Medicinal Saffron is known to have digestive properties, improve circulation and help to reduce high blood pressure – its high consumption in Spain has been put forward as an explanation for the low incidence of cardio-vascular disease there. It is also the richest known source of Vitamin B^2. Externally it is applied as a paste for inflamed skin and sores.
Culinary It is widely used as a flavouring and colorant in Middle Eastern and northern Indian cookery, in rice dishes, such as the classic Spanish paella, and fish soups including bouilla-baisse from France. It is also used in sweets and cakes – especially in eastern cuisine, and the traditional saffron cakes and loaves of Cornwall in England.

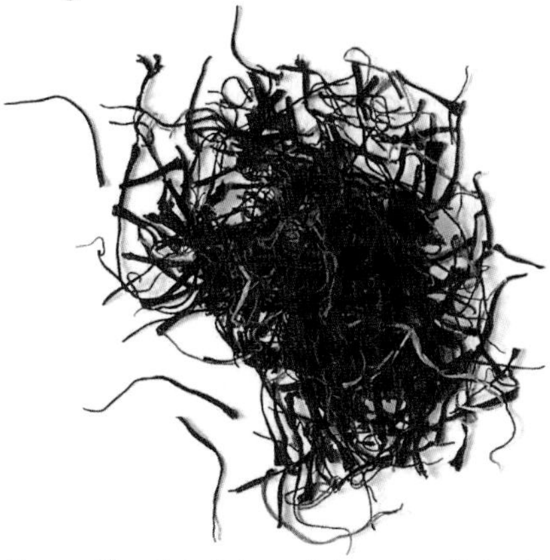

Above *The dried threads have medicinal and culinary uses.*

Top Crocus sativus *corms.*

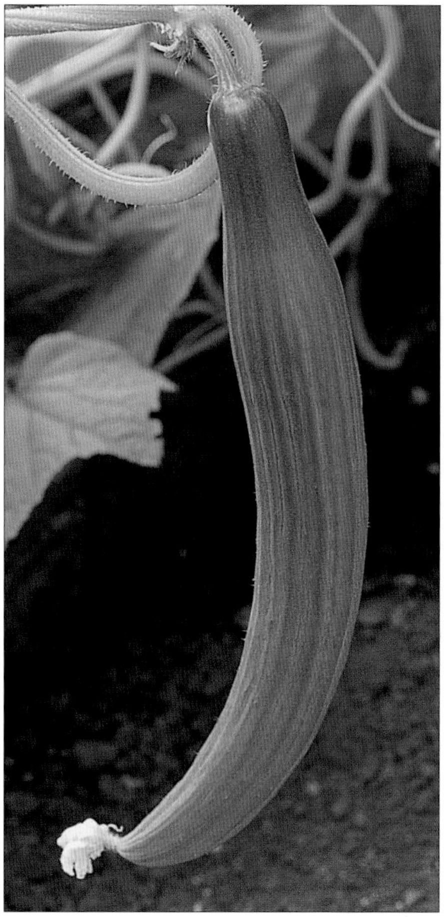

CUCURBITACEAE

Cucumis sativus

Cucumber

History and traditions The cucumber is thought to have originated in northern India, where it has been cultivated for at least 3,000 years. It must have been known in ancient Egypt, as it was one of the luxuries missed by the Israelites after they left Egypt to wander in the desert. It was enjoyed by the Greeks and Romans – the Emperor Tiberius ate it every day, according to Pliny. In Britain it was known from the beginning of the 14th century, but not widely grown there before the 16th century. It features in herbals of the period as being helpful in urinary disorders and was recognized for soothing and cleansing the skin. Gerard believed in its cooling properties and advised eating a cucumber pottage daily for three weeks to "perfectly cure all manner of … copper faces, red and shining fierie noses (as red as Roses) with pimples, pumples, rubies, and such like …" (*The Herball,* 1597).
Description A trailing annual (of the same family as marrows, melons and the creeping wayside plant, bryony, *Bryonia alba*), it has lobed triangular leaves and yellow flowers, followed by the familiar cylindrical fruit with its thick green skin, watery, white flesh and white ovate seeds.
Habitat/distribution Cultivated worldwide.
Growth A tender plant, it must be grown under glass in cool, temperate climates. It is propagated from seed and needs rich, well-drained soil, ample moisture and humidity, with a minimum temperature of 10°C/50°F.
Parts used Fruit, seeds.

USES Medicinal Cucumber is a natural diuretic and laxative and has digestive properties. The seeds are high in potassium and beneficial for diseases associated with excess uric acid, such as arthritis and gout. In traditional Indian medicine, juice from the leaf is combined with coconut milk to restore the electrolyte balance when the body is dehydrated following diarrhoea. When applied externally, the flesh of the cucumber has soothing properties for skin irritations and sunburn.
Culinary The vitamins and minerals (vitamin C, small amounts of vitamin B complex, calcium, phosphorus, iron) which cucumber contains are concentrated in or near the skin, so it should not be peeled. It is also best eaten raw, as cooking destroys the potassium and phosphorus content. A popular salad ingredient, and added to yogurt-based condiments such as the Indian *raita,* Greek *tsatsiki* and Turkish *cacik.*
Cosmetic Soothing and refreshing to the skin, a cucumber face mask helps prevent spots and blackheads. Slices of cucumber, placed over closed eyelids, revive tired eyes.

Cucumber face mask

This recipe doubles up as a lotion to relieve sunburn.

½ cucumber, chopped (but not peeled)
15ml/1 tbsp liquid honey
15ml/1 tbsp rose water
15ml/1 tbsp ground almonds

Liquidize all the ingredients to a pulp in a blender or food processor. Smooth over the face and leave for 15–20 minutes, before wiping off with damp cotton wool (cotton balls).

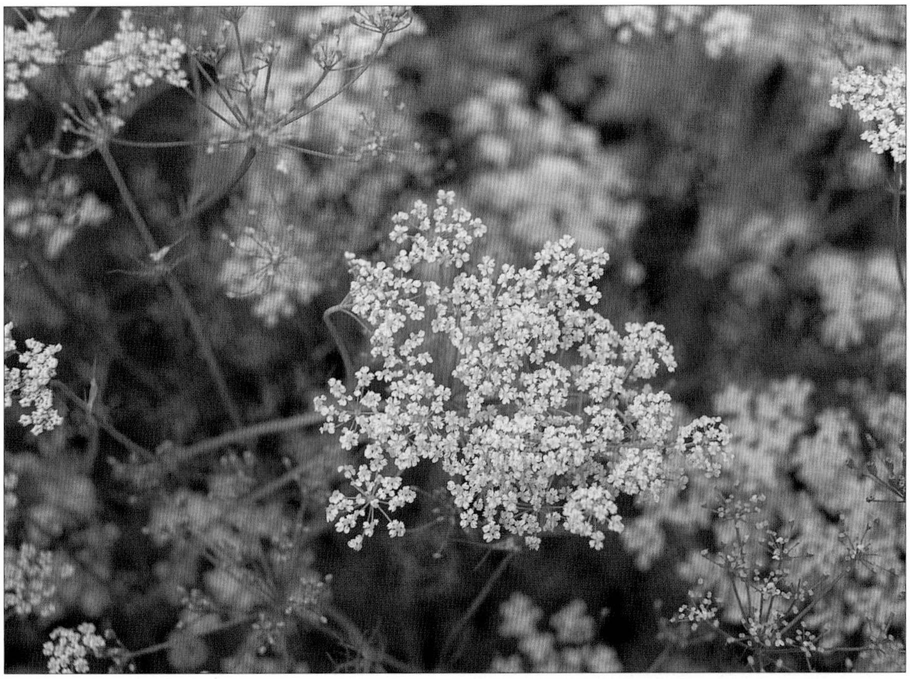

UMBELLIFERAE/APIACEAE

Cuminum cyminum

Cumin

History and traditions Cumin was grown in Arabia, India and China from earliest times. There are descriptions of how it was cultivated in the Bible (Isaiah 28: vv25–27), and the practice of paying it in tithes (a church tax) is referred to in the New Testament. It is mentioned by the Greek physicians, Hippocrates and Dioscorides, and Pliny reports that the ground seed was taken with bread and water or wine as a remedy for "squeamishness". Cumin was a very popular spice in Britain and Europe during the Middle Ages for its strong taste.
Description A half-hardy annual with finely divided, feathery leaves and umbels of very small white flowers. The fruits (seeds) are yellowish brown and ovoid in shape with a distinctive, warm and spicy lingering aroma. The plant is a little like caraway (*Carum carvi*) in appearance, and occasionally confused with it, but quite different in taste.
Habitat/distribution Indigenous to Egypt and the Mediterranean, it is widely grown in tropical and subtropical regions, including northern Africa, India and North and South America.
Growth Grow in a well-drained to sandy soil. Propagated from seed and should be sown under glass in cool temperate regions and transplanted after all frosts. Although it may flower, it is unlikely that fruits will ripen in cool climates.
Parts used Seeds, essential oil.

USES Medicinal Decoctions or infusions of the seeds are taken for digestive disorders, diarrhoea, colds and feverish illnesses. In Ayurvedic medicine it is also used to treat haemorrhoids and for renal colic. The essential oil has antiseptic and antibacterial properties and is applied externally (diluted) for boils and insect bites.
Culinary Widely used in Indian and Middle Eastern cookery to flavour curries, soups, meat and vegetable dishes, bread, biscuits and cheese; and as an ingredient of spice mixtures, pickles and chutneys. There are several species of cumin which produce seeds of varying colour and strength of flavour.

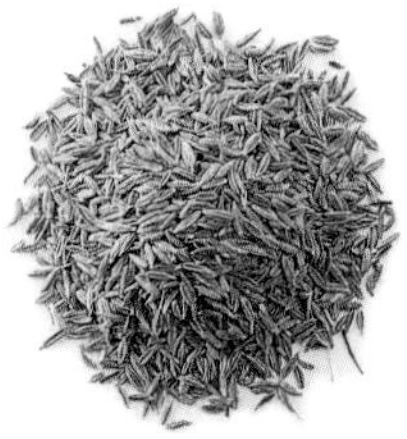

Right *White cumin seeds.*

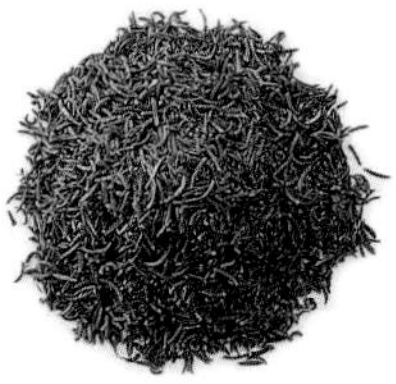

Left *Black cumin seeds.*

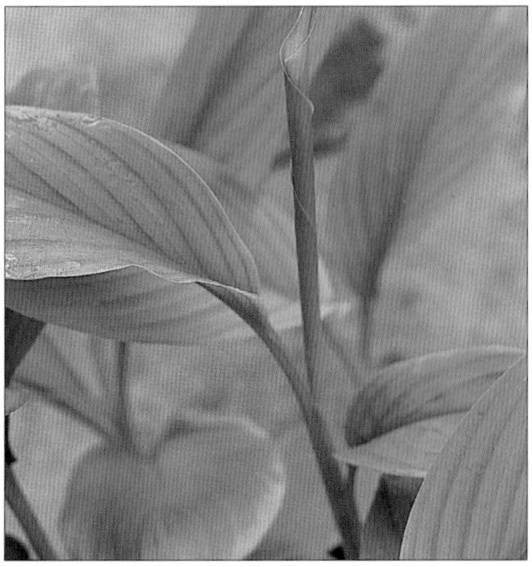

ZINGIBERACEAE

Curcuma longa

Turmeric

History and traditions Turmeric is mentioned in Sanskrit writings and used in Ayurvedic medicine. A native of southeast Asia, it spread across the Pacific, taken by the Polynesians as far as Hawaii and Easter Island. Used as a dye and food flavouring, the generic name is from the word used in ancient Rome for saffron, *korkum*.
Description A perennial, up to 1.2m/4ft tall, it has shiny, lanceolate leaves and dense spikes of pale yellow flowers, enclosed in a sheathing petiole. Grows on a tuberous rhizome.
Growth A tender, tropical plant, it requires well-drained but moist soil, a humid atmosphere and minimum temperatures of 15–18°C/59–64°F. It is propagated by division of the rhizomes.
Parts used Rhizomes – boiled, skinned, dried and ground into bright yellow powder.

USES Medicinal Can treat digestive issues including gallstones, liver conditions and reduce heartburn. The anti-inflammatory actions can support both rheumatoid and osteoarthritis, reducing swelling and joint pain.
Culinary An ingredient of Worcestershire sauce and curry powder, adding colour and a musky flavour to meat, vegetable and savoury dishes.
Cosmetic It makes an excellent skin softener.

CAUTION Only to be taken on medical advice if taking anti-coagulant drugs, such as warfarin, or other medication. Avoid high doses over long periods and excessive sunlight if using topically.

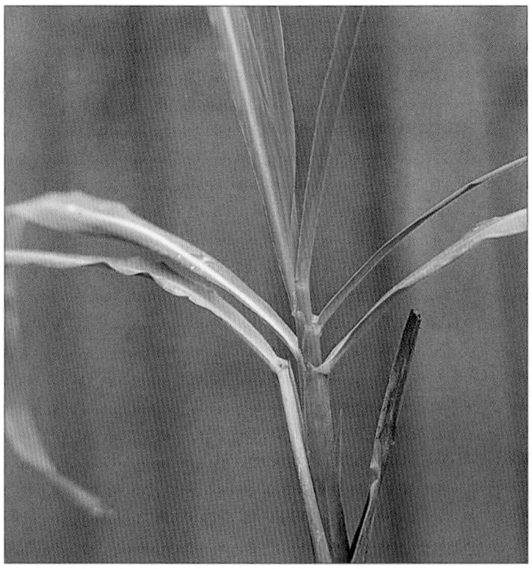

GRAMINEAE/POACEAE

Cymbopogon citratus

Lemon grass

History and traditions Lemon grass did not come to the attention of the west as a medicinal or culinary plant until the modern era. It is now extensively cultivated, in various tropical countries, mainly for distillation of the essential oil, which is used in commercial products. It has also risen in popularity as a culinary herb.
Description A tall, clump-forming perennial, growing to 1.5m/5ft in height, it has linear, grasslike leaves, strongly scented with lemon.
Habitat/distribution Indigenous to southern India and Sri Lanka, found wild and cultivated in tropical and subtropical zones of Asia, Africa, North and South America.
Growth A tender plant, which is grown in fertile, well-drained soil, but needs plenty of moisture and minimum temperatures of 7–10°C/45–50°F. In cool temperate climates it must be grown as a conservatory or warm greenhouse plant, and moved outside in the summer.
Parts used Leaves, young stems, essential oil.

USES Medicinal The essential oil has antiseptic properties and is used externally for rheumatic aches and pains, ringworm and scabies. Internally (in doses of a few drops) it is sometimes taken for indigestion and gastric upsets. The diluted oil is useful to relieve itchy skin.
Culinary The young white stem and leaf base are chopped and used in stir-fry dishes. Leaves may also be infused to make tea.
Aromatic The essential oil is used in home fragrance preparations, in commercial perfumery, soaps and cosmetics and as a flavouring in the food and liquor industries.

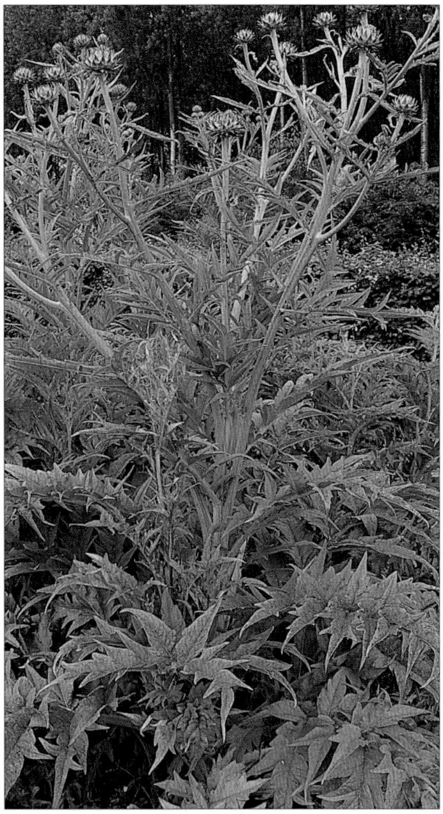

COMPOSITAE/ASTERACEAE

Cynara cardunculus Scolymus Group

Globe artichoke

History and traditions The globe artichoke occurs only in cultivation and was probably developed, by selective breeding in the distant past, from the closely related cardoon (also *Cynara cardunculus).* Both were grown as vegetables by the Greeks and Romans. Medieval Arabian physicians, including Avicenna, knew of its medicinal properties (the common name comes from the Arabic *alkharshuf),* but it does not seem to have been widely grown in Europe before the 16th century, when it was introduced to Britain as a culinary delicacy and ornamental plant. Books of the period abound in recipes for boiling, frying, stewing or potting artichokes and making them into a variety of fancy dishes. Sir Hugh Platt (*Delights for Ladies*, 1594) gives instructions for preserving the stalks in a liquid decoction and for storing the heads (known as apples) throughout the winter.
Description A large perennial, growing to 2m/6ft, with long, greeny-grey, deeply cut leaves, downy on the undersides, ridged stems and large thistle-like flower heads with purple florets and a fleshy receptacle (the heart).

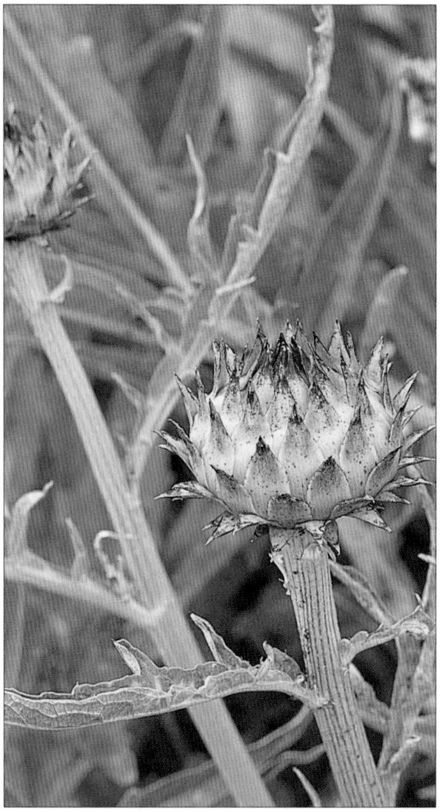

Above *The flower heads are a delicacy.*

Habitat/distribution Native to northern Africa and the Mediterranean, found on light, dry soils. Introduced and widely grown elsewhere.
Growth Tolerates some frost, but does not grow well where temperatures are regularly less than -15°C/5°F, or on heavy, waterlogged soil. Needs humus-rich, well-drained soil and a sunny position. Propagate from seed sown in spring, or by division of sideshoots in spring or autumn.
Parts used Leaves – fresh or dry (medicinal), unopened flowerheads (culinary).

USES Medicinal Artichoke is a bitter tonic, it reduces nausea, and is a diuretic. It is used to influence and protect the liver function, and to treat gout.
Culinary The unopened flower heads are boiled and the tips of the scales eaten, dipped in melted butter or sauce. Hearts are eaten cold with vinaigrette, baked or fried. In Greek, Middle Eastern and Indian cuisines, hearts are eaten raw with lemon juice and pepper.

CAUTION May aggravate conditions such as gallstones. Only to be taken medicinally on professional advice.

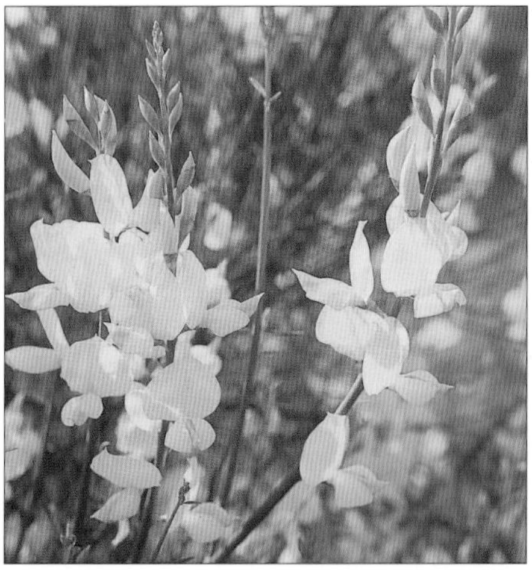

LEGUMINOSAE/PAPILIONACEAE

Cytisus scoparius

Broom

History and traditions Known in medieval times as *planta genista,* common broom gave its name to the Plantagenet royal line. It was the adopted emblem of the father of King Henry II of England, Count Geoffrey of Anjou, who wore a sprig in his helmet when going into battle. Broom is mentioned in Anglo-Saxon writings and the earliest printed herbals make much of its medicinal powers. Pickled broom-buds were a popular ingredient of Tudor salads.

Description An upright, deciduous shrub, growing to 1.5m/5ft, it has arching, twiggy branches, small trifoliate leaves and is covered in a mass of bright yellow pea flowers in spring.

Related species There are many hybrids and cultivars that are not suitable for medicinal use.

Habitat/distribution A native of Europe and western Asia, found in heathlands, woods and scrublands. Introduced elsewhere.

Growth Grows in any well-drained soil in a sunny position. Propagation is by seed or semi-ripe cuttings, but seedlings do not transplant as well as established container-grown plants.

Parts used Leaves, flowers.

USES Medicinal A herb containing alkaloids, similar to those in the poison strychnine, which affect respiration and heart action.

CAUTION The whole plant is toxic and if eaten leads to respiratory failure. Subject to legal restriction in some countries. For use by qualified practitioners only. It is under statutory control as a weed in Australia.

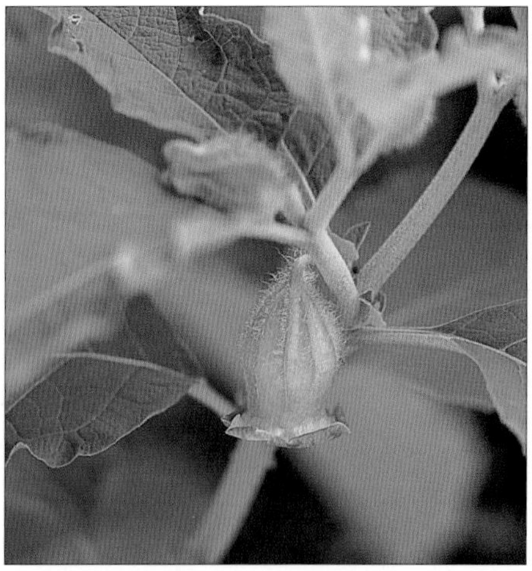

SOLANACEAE

Datura stramonium

Datura

History and traditions A native of North and South America, this plant was brought to Europe by the Spaniards in the 16th century. It was named "devil's apple" after European settlers in America discovered its narcotic effects, and "jimson weed" after Jamestown, Virginia, where they first found it growing. Also indigenous to India, datura appears in ancient Hindu literature of the Vedic period, when its intoxicant and healing powers were well understood and the seeds were smoked as a treatment for asthma.

Description A tall, bushy annual, 2m/6ft tall, it has strong-smelling, triangular, lobed leaves and large white, or violet-tinged, trumpet-shaped flowers.

Habitat/distribution Indigenous to the Americas and temperate, hilly regions of India, now widely grown in other countries.

Growth A half-hardy annual, it does not tolerate frost. Grows in any light soil and is propagated by seed sown in spring.

Parts used Leaves, flowers, seeds.

USES Medicinal Of the same family as *Atropa belladonna,* it contains similar poisonous alkaloids, including atropine. It has been found useful in mitigating the symptoms of Parkinson's disease and for treating asthma.

CAUTION All parts of the plant are highly poisonous. Subject to legal restrictions in some countries. For use by qualified practitioners only.

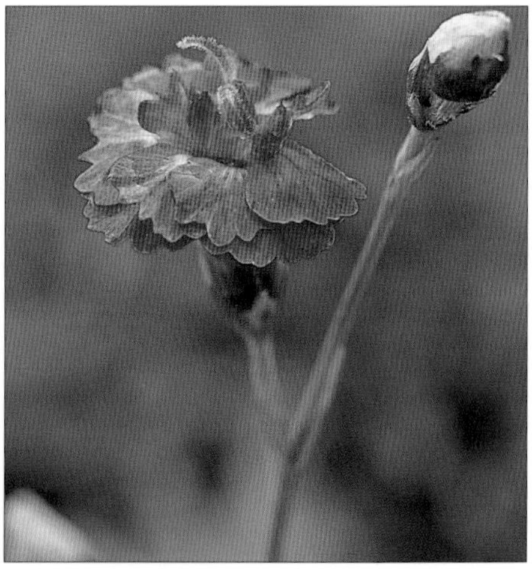

CARYOPHYLLACEAE

Dianthus

History and traditions Pinks are of ancient origin; one species is thought to be represented in the murals at Knossos in Crete and there are records that *D. caryophyllus* was cultivated by the Moors in Valencia in 1460. The Elizabethan name for the pink was gillyflower (or "gillofloure"). This included wild and alpine species and the much-prized clove gillyflower, which seems to have covered any clove-scented pinks. By the 17th century there were many cultivated garden varieties, as featured by Parkinson in his *Paradisi,* 1629, with delightful names like 'Master Tuggie's Princesse', 'Fair Maid of Kent' and 'Lusty Gallant'. Some were known as sops-in-wine after the practice of soaking them in wine to flavour it. Herbals and stillroom books are full of recipes for making

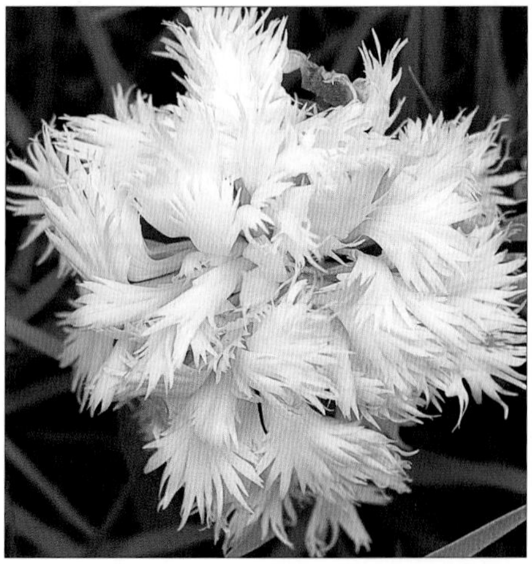

Top Dianthus *'Pink Jewel'.*

Above *An old-fashioned pink* D. *'Mrs Sinkins'.*

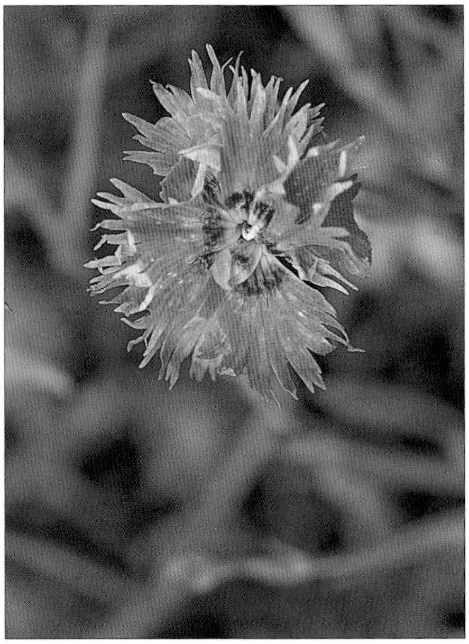

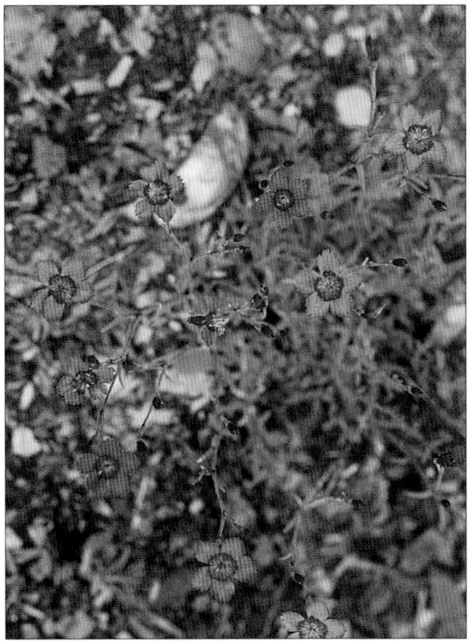

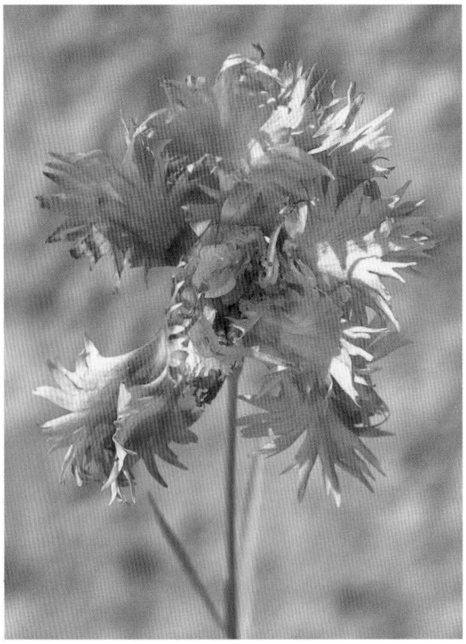

syrups and conserves of gillyflowers, pickled and candied gillyflowers and wine. According to Gerard, a conserve of clove gillyflowers and sugar "is exceedingly cordiall, and wonderfully above measure doth comfort the heart, being eaten now and then" (*The Herball,* 1597).

Description The leaves of all *Dianthus* are linear, lance-shaped and blue grey or grey green in colour, with a waxy texture. The flowers are pink, white or purple (some bi-coloured) with short tubular bases and flat heads with double or single layers of petals, some with toothed or fringed margins. Old-fashioned varieties often have fragrant, clove-scented blooms but only one flowering period in early summer. (Modern varieties repeat-flower.) Garden pinks are 25–45cm/10–18in high, and alpine species a more compact 8–10cm/3–4in high. All are fully hardy.

Habitat/distribution Found in mountains and meadows of Europe, Asia and South Africa.

Species There are about 300 species, with more than 30,000 hybrids and cultivars recorded. Pinks traditionally grown in the herb garden include ***D. deltoides*** (Maiden Pink) with cerise, single flowers with toothed petals (to 20cm/8in high) or the more compact ***D. gratianopolitanus*** **syn.** ***D. caesius,*** which has very fragrant single pink flowers (to 15cm/6in high) or any of the fragrant old-fashioned pinks such as ***D.*** **'Mrs Sinkins'**, with its highly scented double white flowers and fringed petals. There are also numerous modern pinks, with an old-fashioned look, to choose from, such as ***D.*** **'Gran's Favourite'** or the laced ***D.*** **'London Delight'**.

Growth Pinks need a very well-drained neutral to alkaline soil and full sun. In gardens with heavy, clay soils, they can be grown in raised beds to provide sharp drainage. Easily propagated from cuttings of non-flowering shoots in summer or by division in spring or autumn.

Parts used Flowers – fresh or dried.

USES Medicinal At one time thought to have tonic properties, but they are little used today for medicinal purposes.

Culinary Fresh flowers may be added to salads, floated in drinks or crystallized for garnishing cakes and desserts. Before culinary use, remove the bitter petal base.

Aromatic Flowers are dried for inclusion in potpourri and scented sachets. Flowers should be cut when just fully out, the heads twisted off the stems and dried whole.

Other names Pinks, gillyflower, clove gillyflower and sops-in-wine.

Gillyflower vinegar

"Gilliflowers infused in Vinegar and set in the Sun for certaine dayes, as we do for Rose Vinegar do make a very pleasant and comfortable vinegar, good to be used in time of contagious sickness, and very profitable at all times for such as have feeble spirits."

John Evelyn, *Acetaria*, 1719.

Top left D. gratianopolitanus, *known as the Cheddar pink.*

Top centre D. deltoides, *often called the maiden pink.*

Above *A pink-flowering cultivar of* D. *'Mrs Sinkins'.*

Below *Garden pinks, raised from several wild species of dianthus, are a mainstay of the traditional garden. They thrive on an alkaline soil and dislike damp conditions.*

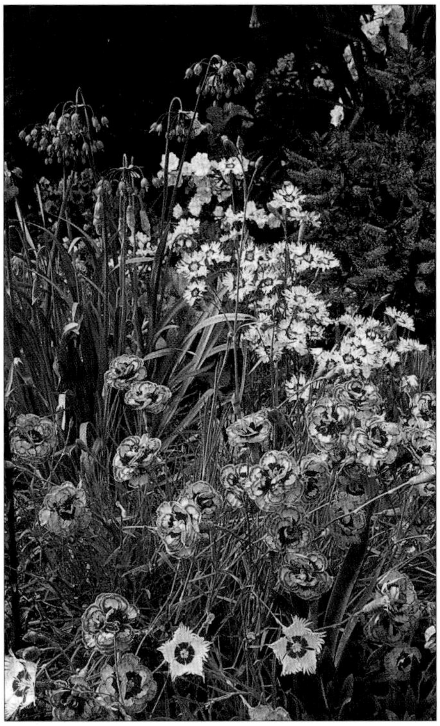

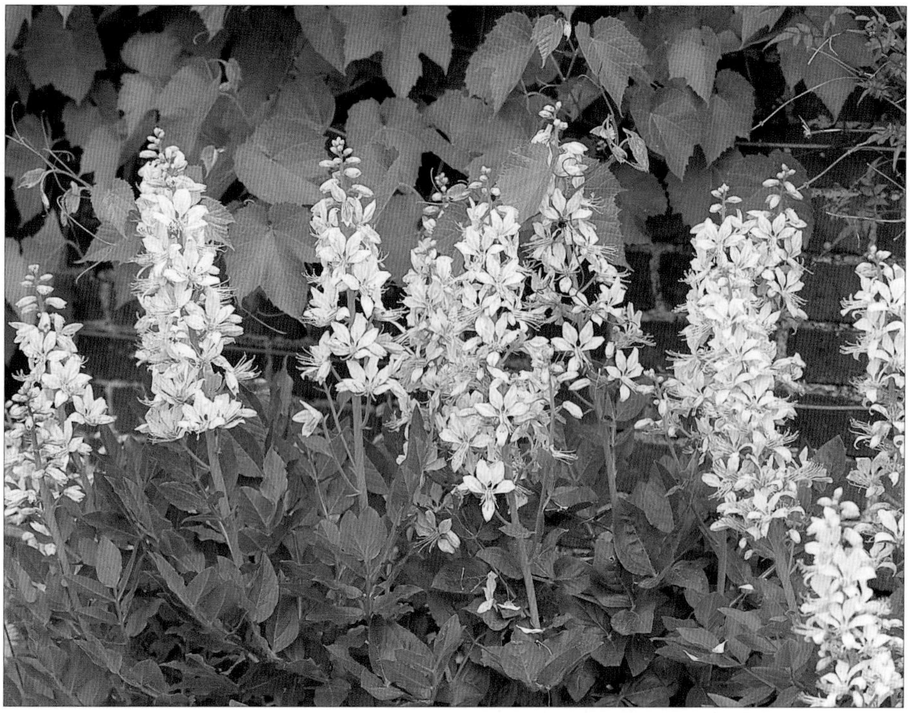

RUTACEAE

Dictamnus albus

Dittany

History and traditions It is called "burning bush" because the whole plant is rich in volatile oil, which can allegedly be set alight as it evaporates, leaving the foliage intact and undamaged. It has a similar lemony, balsamic scent to that of *Origanum dictamnus*, or dittany of Crete, and both plants are probably named after Mount Dicte in Crete. According to Mrs Grieve (*A Modern Herbal,* 1931), *Dictamnus albus* was an ingredient of a number of exotic pharmaceutical preparations available in the early decades of the 20th century, including "Solomon's Opiate", "Guttète Powder", "Balm of Fioraventi" and "Hyacinth Mixture".
Description A clump-forming, aromatic perennial, 40–90cm/16–36in tall, with pinnate leaves, made up of lance-shaped leaflets, and tall racemes of white flowers.
Related species *D. albus* var. *purpureus* has pale pink flowers, striped with darker pink, and is more commonly grown in gardens than the species, but shares its characteristics.
Habitat/distribution Found from central and southern Europe across to China and Korea in dry grasslands and woodlands.
Growth Dittany grows in any well-drained to dry soil in full sun or partial shade. Propagated by seed sown in late summer, in containers and over-wintered in a cold frame. It does not transplant well and is not easy to establish from division.
Parts used Root – dried and powdered.

USES Medicinal It was once prescribed for nervous complaints and feverish illnesses, but is not widely used in Western herbal medicine today. The root bark of a similar species is used in Chinese medicine for its cooling, antibacterial properties.
Horticultural The chief use of this herb today is as an aromatic ornamental in the border or herb garden.
Other name Burning bush.

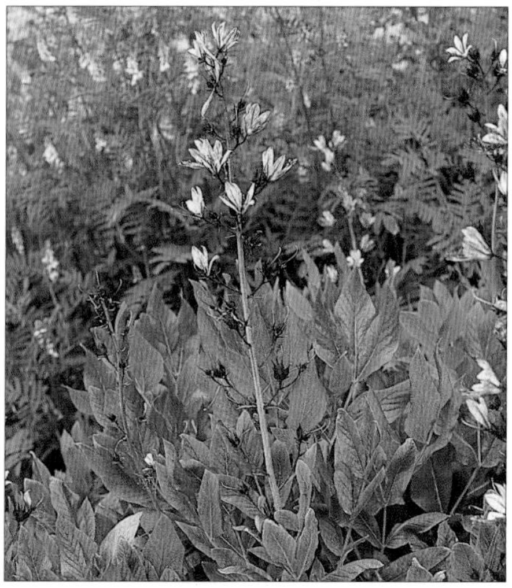

Above Dictamnus albus *var.* purpureus.

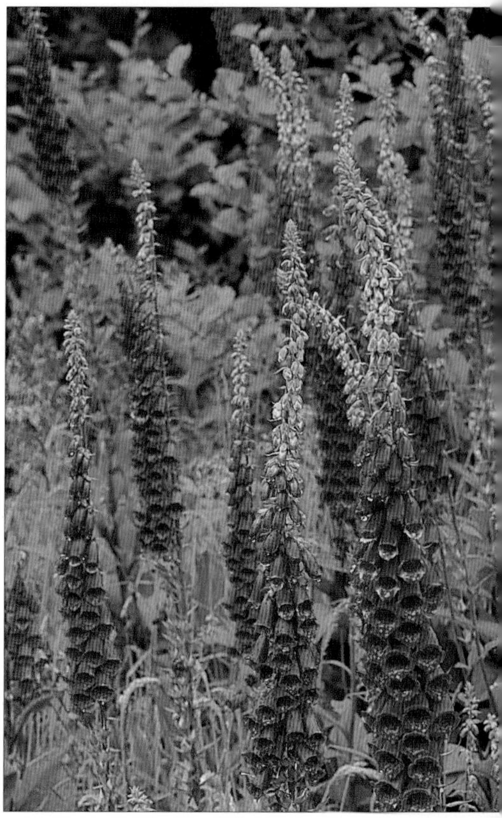

SCROPHULARIACEAE

Digitalis purpurea

Foxglove

History and traditions The foxglove was given its Latin name by the German botanist, Leonard Fuchs, in 1542 (it does not appear in any classical texts). He called it *digitalis,* for its supposed resemblance to fingers (*digit* = finger), and the common name in German, as in several other European languages, is connected with thimbles. Various ingenious explanations have been put forward for what it has to do with foxes: that they wore the flowers on their feet to muffle their tread when on night-time prowls; that it is really from "folksglove" for the "fairy folk"; or from an Anglo-Saxon word "*foxes-glew*" meaning fox-music, for its resemblance to an ancient musical instrument – you can take your pick. Once used in folk medicine for a variety of disorders (despite occasional fatalities), it was its effectiveness as a diuretic against dropsy which led to the discovery of its action on the heart by a Dr Withering, who published his findings in 1785.
Description A biennial or short-lived perennial, reaching 2m/6ft in height. The plant has a rosette of large, downy leaves and spectacular one-sided flower spikes of purple or pink

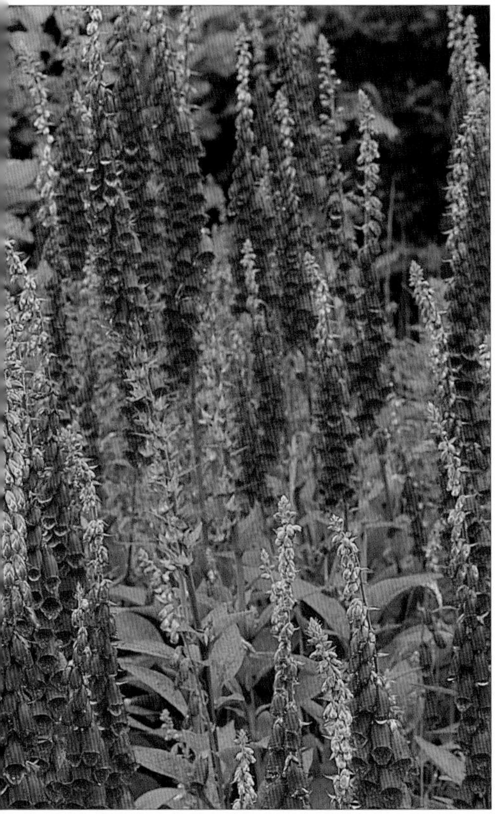

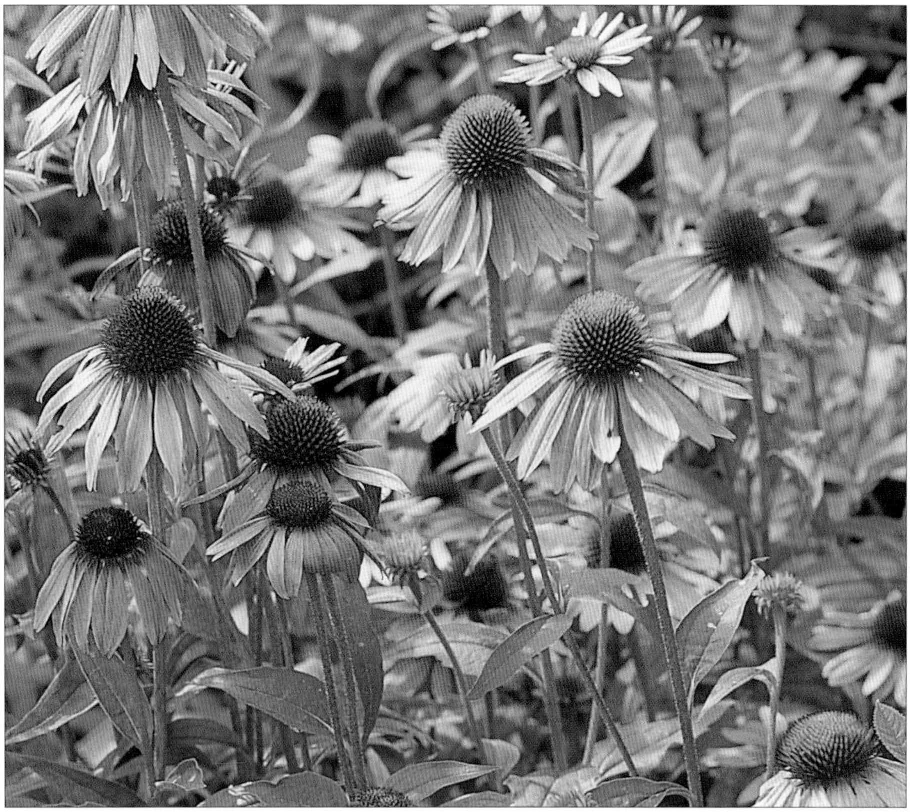

tubular flowers, with crimson on the inside.
Related species *D. purpurea* f. *albiflora* is a white-flowering form and *D. lanata* has fawn-coloured flowers with purplish-brown veins. Both *D. purpurea* and *D. lanata* contain the active principles, though *D. lanata* is most commonly grown in Europe for the pharmaceutical industry.
Habitat/distribution Occurs throughout Europe, northern Africa and western Asia, mostly on acid soil in grassland and woodland.
Growth Although it will grow in most conditions, it prefers moist, well-drained soil in partial shade, with a mulch of leaf mould. Propagate from seed sown in autumn and overwinter in a cold frame. Self-seeds.
Parts used Leaves – from which the active principles digitoxin and digoxin are extracted.

USES Medicinal The foxglove contains glycosides, which affect the heartbeat, and is used in orthodox medicine as a heart stimulant. It should never be used for home treatment.

CAUTION Foxgloves are poisonous and should not be eaten or used in any way for self-medication. A prescription drug only. Legal restrictions apply.

COMPOSITAE/ASTERACEAE

Echinacea purpurea

Purple coneflower

History and traditions Coneflowers were used by Native Americans as wound-herbs, to treat snakebite and as a general cure-all. The early settlers took to them as home remedies for coughs, colds and a variety of infections.
Description A hardy perennial, 1.2m/4ft high, with a rhizomatous rootstock and ovate-lanceolate leaves. The purplish-pink daisy-like flowers have raised conical centres, made up of prickly brown scales. There are also white-flowered cultivars.
Related species *E. angustifolia* and *E. pallida* are species with similar properties, which were also used by the Native Americans.
Habitat/distribution Native to Central and eastern North America, found in dry prairies and open woodlands. Introduced and grown in other temperate regions of the world.
Growth It prefers well-drained, humus-rich soil and a sunny position or partial shade. Cut back the stems as the flowers fade to encourage a second blooming. Propagate by seed sown in spring, under glass at a temperature of 13°C/55°F, or by division of roots in late spring or autumn.
Parts used Roots, rhizomes – dried, powdered or made into capsules.

USES Medicinal Recent research has shown that echinacea has a beneficial effect on the immune system and stimulates the production of white blood cells – and has been used in treating aids. It has antiviral, antifungal and antibacterial properties and is taken internally in the form of capsules or tinctures, for respiratory tract infections, kidney infections, skin diseases, boils, abscesses and slow-healing wounds. A decoction of the roots is applied externally for infected wounds and skin complaints.

CAUTION Only to be taken on the advice of a herbal or medical practitioner if taking other medication. May interact with pharmaceutical drugs. Not for long-term use.

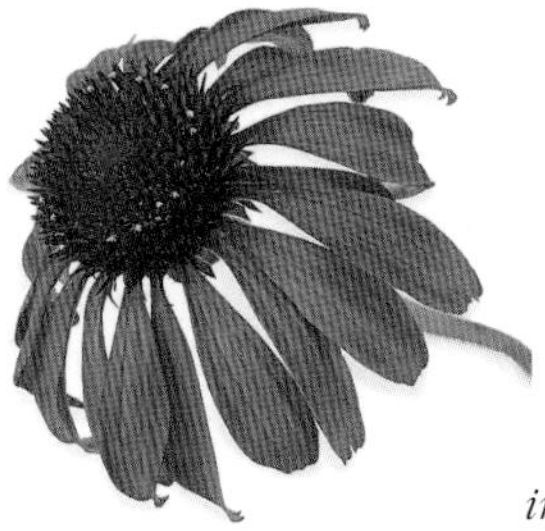

Left Echinacea purpurea *boosts the immune system.*

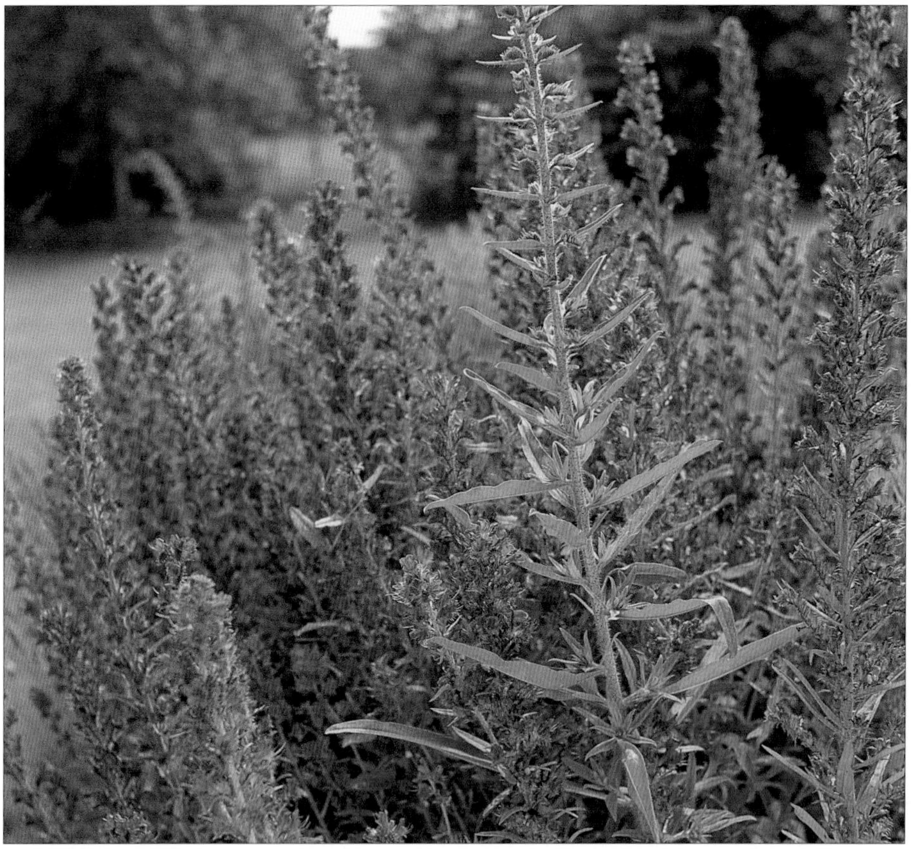

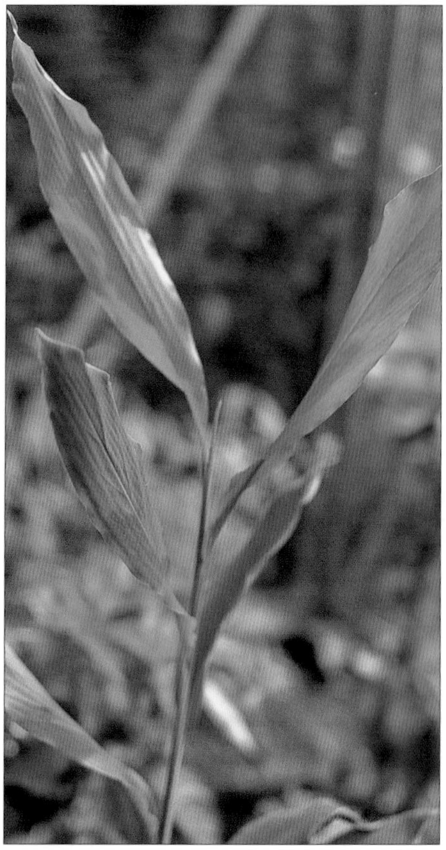

BORAGINACEAE

Echium vulgare

Viper's bugloss

History and traditions Early herbalists thought that the stems, speckled with pustules, looked like snakeskin, the fruits like snakes' heads and the flower stamens like snakes' tongues. So, in line with the medieval Doctrine of Signatures (whereby the appearance of a plant indicates what it can cure) *E. vulgare* was considered an antidote to the bite of an adder, and by extension, to anything else that was poisonous. In the words of William Coles, "a most singular remedy against poyson and the sting of scorpions" (*The Art of Simpling*). It was also widely dispensed against "swooning, sadness and melancholy" (Parkinson). A native of Europe, this attractive but invasive plant spread around the world, and became known as a tiresome weed in many countries, notably Australia and North America – where it is known as "blue devil".

Description A bushy, bristly biennial, 60–90cm/2–3ft tall, with narrow lance-shaped leaves, spotted, hairy stems and dense spires of bell-shaped, violet-blue flowers in summer, opening from pinkish buds.

Habitat/distribution Native to Europe and Asia, it occurs on poor, stony soils and semi-dry grassland. Introduced to, and widespread in, many countries worldwide.

Growth Grows in any well-drained soil, in full sun. Propagated from seed sown in spring or early autumn.

Parts used Leaves, flowers and seeds (formerly).

USES Medicinal Not used currently in herbal medicine.

Horticultural Traditionally grown in herb gardens for its historical associations.

Other names Blue weed and blue devil.

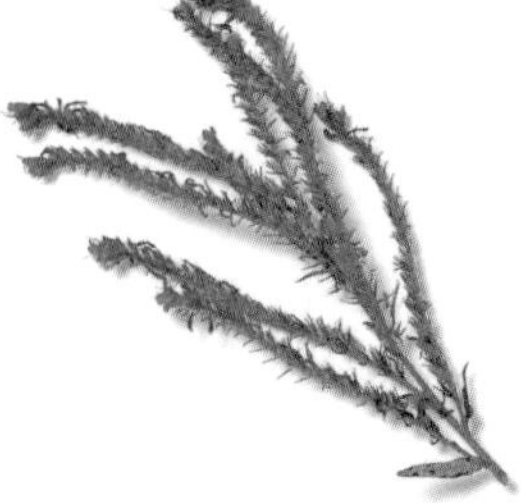

Left *The stems of* Echium vulgare *were thought to resemble snakeskin.*

CAUTION May cause stomach upsets if ingested and irritate skin on contact.

ZINGIBERACEAE

Elettaria cardamomum

Cardamom

History and traditions This pungent spice was known to the Greeks and Romans and mentioned by Theophrastus, Dioscorides and other classical writers. It features in Chinese medical texts, dating from AD270, and has long been used in Ayurvedic medicine as a treatment for impotency. Cardamom is a traditional ingredient of eastern aphrodisiacs and mentioned in this context in the *Arabian Nights* stories. *Elettaria* is taken from an Indian name for this plant, *elaichi*.

Description A large perennial, 2–2.4m/6–8ft tall, with a clump of long lanceolate leaves, growing from a fleshy rhizome. Flowers arise from the base of the plant, followed by pale green capsules, which dry to a pale yellow, containing many small, pungent black seeds.

Related species There are various species, including black cardamom, a taller plant with large, dark-brown seed capsules, containing small black seeds with a strong eucalyptus aroma.

Habitat/distribution Native to southern India and Sri Lanka, it is also grown in Thailand, Central and tropical South America.

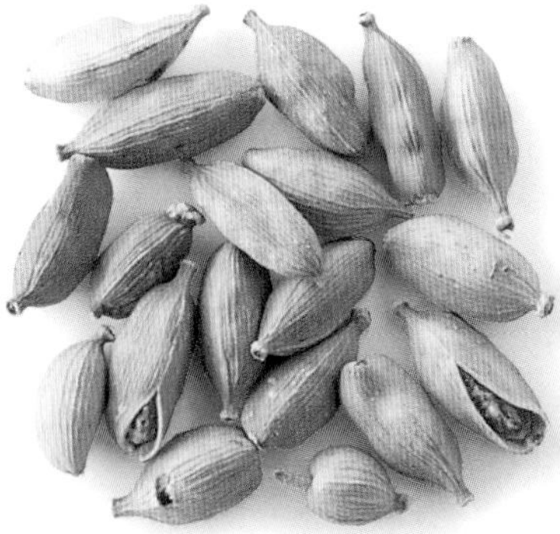

Above *Green cardamom seed pods.*

Growth It needs a minimum temperature of 18°C/64°F, well-drained, rich soil, partial shade, plenty of rain and high humidity. Propagated by seed or division of the rhizomes.
Parts used Seeds, essential oil.

USES Medicinal A warm, stimulating herb, it acts as a tonic and has antidepressant properties. It is also used as a digestive. Seeds are chewed to freshen the breath. Oil of cardamom is antiseptic.
Culinary A major curry spice, the seeds are also used to flavour hot wine punches, sweet, milky rice puddings and egg custard.
Aromatic The pleasant-smelling essential oil is used in perfumery and pharmaceutical products.

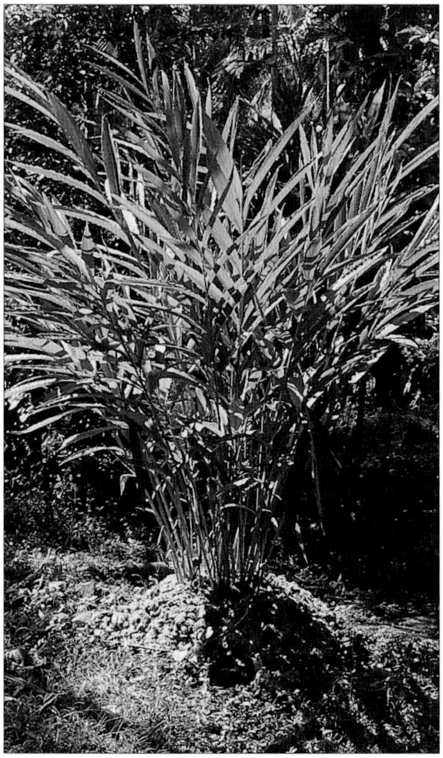

Above *Black cardamom.*

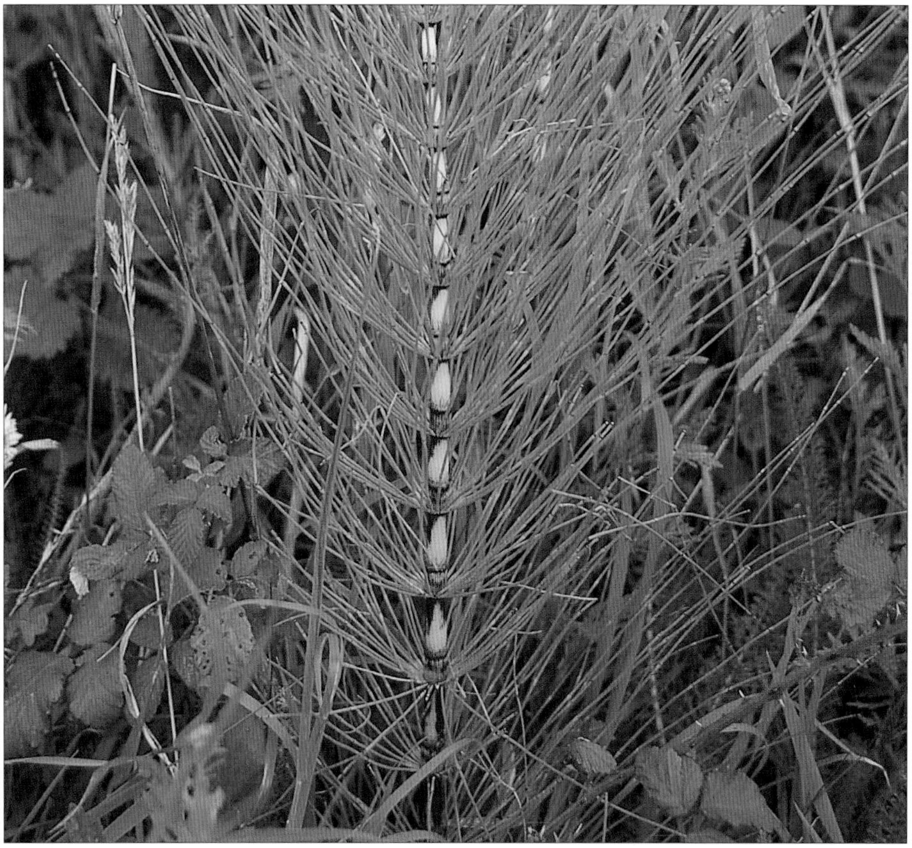

EQUISETACEAE

Equisetum arvense

Horsetail

History and traditions The Latin generic name comes from *equus*, a horse, and *seta*, a bristle. In former times this strange-looking, bottle-brush plant was used to clean pewter vessels and scour wooden kitchen utensils – the stems contain silica, which has a polishing action, as well as being a healing agent. In northern counties of England until the 19th century horsetail was commonly employed by milkmaids for cleaning out their pails. The Swedish botanist, Carl Linnaeus, claims that in his country it was eaten by both cattle and reindeer, though inclined to provoke diarrhoea. There are no records as to whether poor Romans, who were reputed to have eaten it (as an ubiquitous asparagus substitute), were similarly affected. Rich Romans, presumably, did not have to put it to the test. Culpeper lists many medicinal uses for horsetail, and declares that "it solders together the tops of green wounds and cures all ruptures in children".
Description A relic from prehistory, closely related to the vegetation which decayed to form modern coal seams, it is a perennial, which grows on a creeping rhizome to about 50cm/20in in height. Brown stems, topped by cones, release spores and then wither, the method of reproduction of this plant being very similar to that of ferns. The mass of branched green stems, with black-toothed sheaths, are sterile.
Habitat/distribution Occurs throughout Europe from the arctic region to the south, also in Asia and China, and is found in moist waste ground. In some countries, where it has been introduced, it is regarded as a pernicious weed.
Growth A hardy plant, it grows in most conditions, although it prefers moist soil and sun or partial shade. It is propagated by division, but is invasive – and it would be wise to take this into account before introducing it into the garden.
Parts used Stems – fresh or dried.

USES Medicinal It has astringent, diuretic properties and is said to be helpful for prostate problems, cystitis and urinary infections, but it can be an irritant, and self-medication is not advised. It is also said to be beneficial, when applied externally, for haemorrhages and ruptured ligaments.
Other names Bottle-brush and paddock pipes.

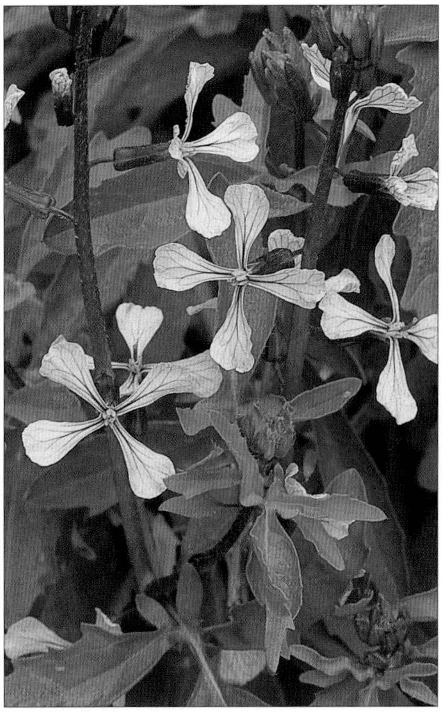

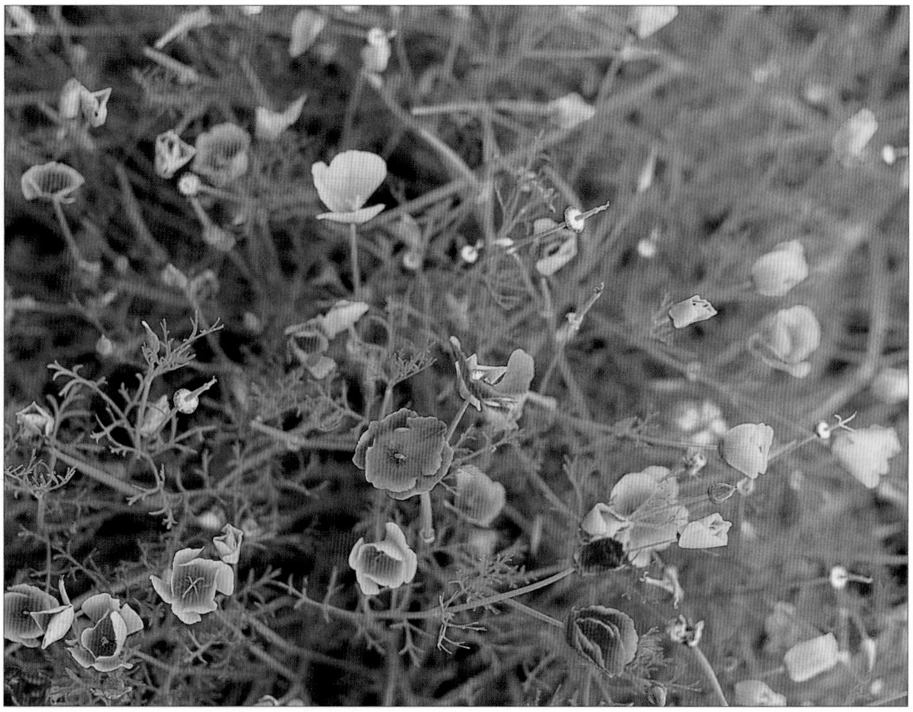

CRUCIFERAE/BRASSICACEAE

Eruca vesicaria subsp. *sativa*

Rocket (Arugula)

History and traditions Rocket (arugula) has been a salad herb since Roman times. Its strong, mustard-like taste is indicated by the generic Latin name, which comes from *urere,* to burn. Various claims were made for it in the past as a painkiller. William Turner said the seed was effective "against the bitings of the shrew-mouse and other venemous beasts". Gerard made the claim that "whosoever taketh the seed of Rocket before he be whipt, shall be so hardened that he shall easily endure the paines" (*The Herball*, 1597). Culpeper declared it to be "celebrated against diseases of the lungs" and that "the juice is excellent in asthmas ... as also against inveterate coughs". But none of this has stood the test of time and salad rocket (arugula) is no longer used medicinally.
Description A frost-hardy annual, 60–100cm/2–3ft tall, with dentate, deeply divided leaves. Small, four-petalled, white flowers, streaked at the centre of each petal with violet, appear in late winter to early summer. Originally a wild plant, rocket (arugula) has been cultivated for so long that it is now classified as a subspecies.
Habitat/distribution Native to the Mediterranean and Asia, introduced and widely grown elsewhere.
Growth Propagate from seed, sown successionally, *in situ*, from late winter to early summer. When grown on poor, dry soil, with plenty of sun, it has a more pungent taste than if grown on moist soil in cooler conditions.
Parts used Leaves.

USES Culinary A pungent herb that lends interest to lettuce and other bland-tasting leaves as a salad ingredient.
Other name Salad rocket (arugula).

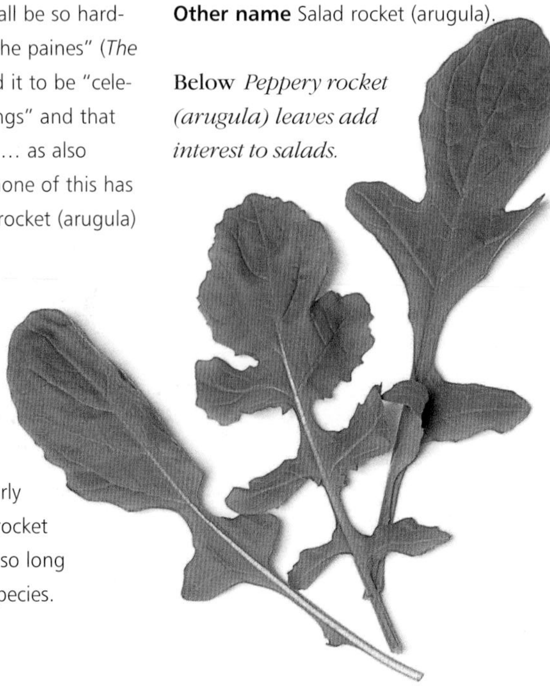

Below *Peppery rocket (arugula) leaves add interest to salads.*

PAPAVERACEAE

Eschscholzia californica

Californian poppy

History and traditions This bright yellow poppy is the state flower of California. It was used by Native Americans as a gentle narcotic and pain reliever, especially against toothache.
Description A hardy annual up to 60cm/2ft tall, with finely divided, feathery leaves. A mass of shallow-cupped flowers in orange, yellow, red and occasionally white appear in early summer, followed by long curved seedpods.
Habitat/distribution Native to western North America and widely grown in many countries.
Growth Grow this plant in well-drained to poor soil and full sun. Propagated by seed sown *in situ* in spring or autumn.
Parts used Whole plant – dried as an ingredient for infusions and tinctures.

USES Medicinal The Californian poppy is a sedative herb that relieves pain and it is taken internally as an infusion, for anxiety, nervous tension and insomnia. It also has diuretic properties and promotes perspiration. It is safe for children and is used traditionally for bedwetting.

CAUTION Only to be taken on professional advice.

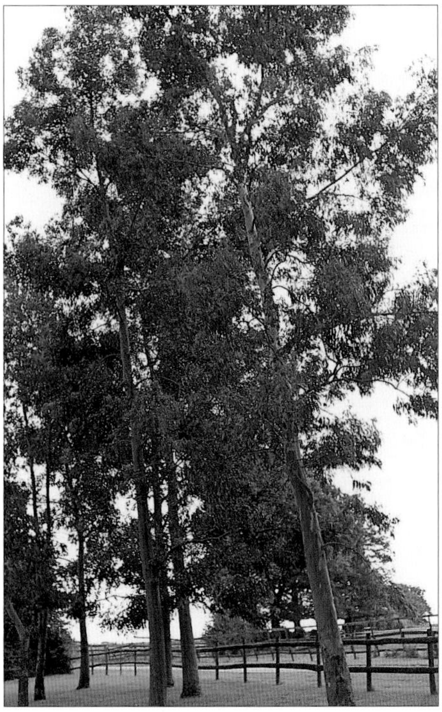

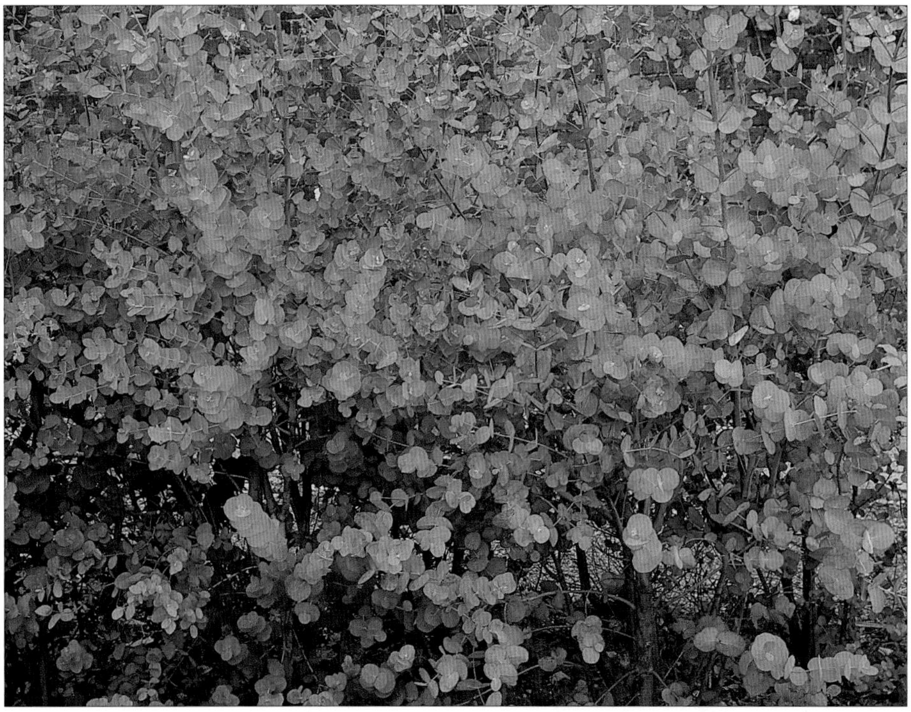

MYRTACEAE

Eucalyptus spp.

Gum tree

History and traditions Eucalyptus trees are native to Australia and were used by the Aborigines in their traditional medicine. They have been widely adopted by other countries, including Africa, the Americas, India and southern Europe, as timber and shade trees, for planting in marshy ground to dry out malaria-inducing swamps, and for their volatile (essential) oil content. Commercial production of eucalyptus essential oils began in Australia in the second half of the 19th century, coinciding with their introduction to the West.

Description Large, fast-growing evergreen trees which grow to considerable heights in warm climates, averaging 70m/230ft, with varying estimates for the record, dating from 1872 between 97m/318ft and 132.5m/434ft. Many have distinctive, rounded juvenile foliage, adult leaves of *E. globulus* and *E. gunnii* are lanceolate, blue grey and studded with oil-bearing glands. Clusters of fluffy cream-coloured flowers appear in summer, followed by globe-shaped fruits.

Species There are over 500 species and all contain antiseptic essential oils, though constituents and properties vary. ***E. globulus*** (blue gum) has been most widely cultivated around the world and has attractive, juvenile leaves much sought after in floristry. *E. gunnii* is one of the hardiest and most suited to growing in cool temperate regions.

Habitat/distribution: Native to Australia, *E. globulus* is found in moist valleys of New South Wales and Tasmania, *E. gunnii* in Tasmania. All are native to Australia.

Growth *Eucalyptus* spp. vary from tender to fully hardy – but none will stand prolonged low temperatures, especially when immature. *E. globulus* is half-hardy, -5°C/23°F, and *E. gunnii* is frost-hardy, -15°C/5°F. Grow in well-drained soil and full sun. Propagate from seed, sow under cover in spring or autumn.

Parts used Leaves, essential oil.

USES Medicinal Eucalyptus has decongestant, expectorant properties and helps to lower fever. The essential oil is highly antiseptic. Leaf or oil is used in steam inhalations and vapour rubs to ease the symptoms of colds, catarrh, sinusitis and respiratory-tract infections. Essential oil is used in massage oils and compresses for inflammations, rheumatism and painful joints. Used as a tea or tincture to relieve upper respiratory infection.

Above left *Eucalyptus trees are rich in volatile oils.*

Above *Immature foliage of* Eucalyptus gunnii.

Lavender and eucalyptus vapour rub

50g/2oz petroleum jelly
15ml/1 tbsp dried lavender
6 drops eucalyptus essential oil

Melt the petroleum jelly in a bowl over a pan of simmering water. Stir in the lavender and heat for 30 minutes.

Strain the liquid jelly through muslin, leave to cool slightly, then add the eucalyptus oil. Pour into a clean jar and leave to set.

Use as a soothing decongestant rub for throat, chest and back.

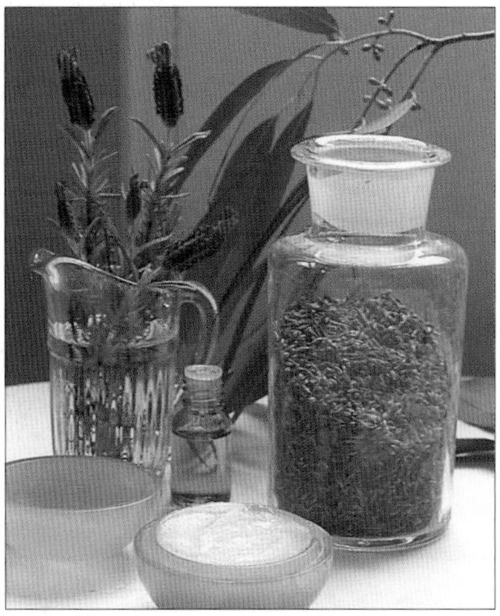

COMPOSITAE/ASTERACEAE

Eupatorium

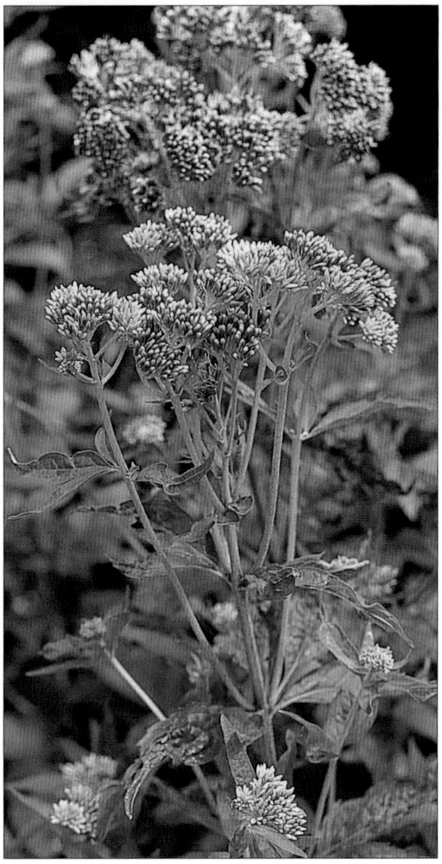

Eupatorium cannabinum Hemp agrimony

History and traditions The Latin specific name and common name are taken from the words *cannabis* and *hemp*, because of a similarity in the shape of the leaves. Hemp being used for rope fibre, by extension *E. cannabinum* gained the name "holy rope" – a plant with beneficent characteristics was often arbitrarily associated with holiness. But it was never in fact a source of rope and shares none of the properties of *Cannabis sativa*. It has a history of medicinal use as a diuretic, purgative, cure for dropsy, general spring tonic and antiscorbutic (counteracting scurvy). Herbalists in the 17th century also recommended it for healing "fomenting ulcers" and "putrid sores".
Description A woody-based, hardy perennial, up to 1.2m/4ft tall, leaves are opposite and mostly subdivided into 3–5 leaflets. A froth of pinky-white flowers, borne in corymbs (flat-topped flower clusters), appear in midsummer – giving rise to another of the herb's country names, "raspberries and cream".
Habitat/distribution Indigenous to Europe, found in damp, rich soils, marshy places and fens.
Growth Grow in moist soil, in full sun or partial shade. Propagate by division in spring or sow seed in containers in spring.
Parts used The whole plant – the flowering tops are dried for use in infusions, extracts and other preparations.

USES Medicinal It has long been known for its diuretic properties, as a tonic for debility and a treatment for influenza-like illnesses, but the wider medicinal action of this herb is complex, even contradictory. Recent research suggests that it contains compounds that are capable of stimulating the immune system and combating tumours, but it also contains alkaloids that are potentially dangerous to the liver and in large enough doses could cause liver damage. Externally, it is applied, as in previous times, to ulcers and sores.
Other names Holy rope, St John's herb and ague weed.

Eupatorium perfoliatum Boneset

History and traditions Boneset was an important herb in the traditional medicine of native Americans, used for fevers, digestive disorders, rheumatism and as a powerful emetic and laxative. It also had magical protective properties assigned to it – infusions were sprinkled to keep evil spirits away. The name has nothing to do with its ability to mend bone fractures, but refers to its efficacy in treating "break bone fever", a virulent flu-like illness, from which the early settlers suffered. It was listed in Dr Griffith's *Universal Formulary* (1859) to be administered in combination with sage and cascarilla bark "for a hectic fever".
Description A tall, hardy perennial, growing to 1.5m/5ft, with lanceolate, rough-textured leaves surrounding the stems (perfoliate), and large clusters of white flowers in late summer.
Habitat/distribution A native of North America in open, marshy regions – introduced in other countries.
Growth Grow in moist soil in full sun or partial shade. Propagate by seed sown in containers in spring or by division in spring or autumn.

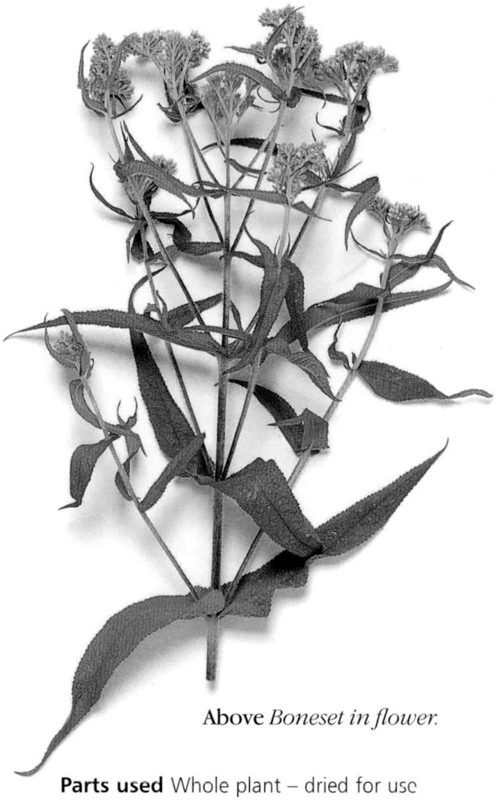

Above *Boneset in flower.*

Parts used Whole plant – dried for use in infusions, extracts and tinctures.
USES Medicinal A popular herb used to manage fevers and infections, taken internally for colds, influenza and bronchitis. It is also thought to stimulate the immune system, as is *E. cannabinum*.
Other names Feverwort, ague weed, thoroughwort, Indian sage, sweating plant.

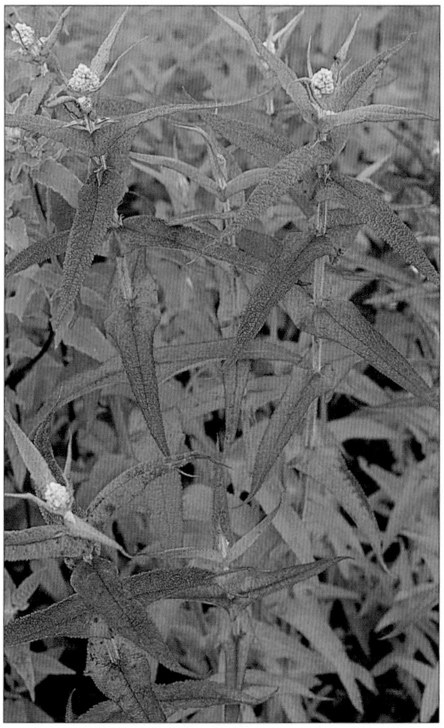

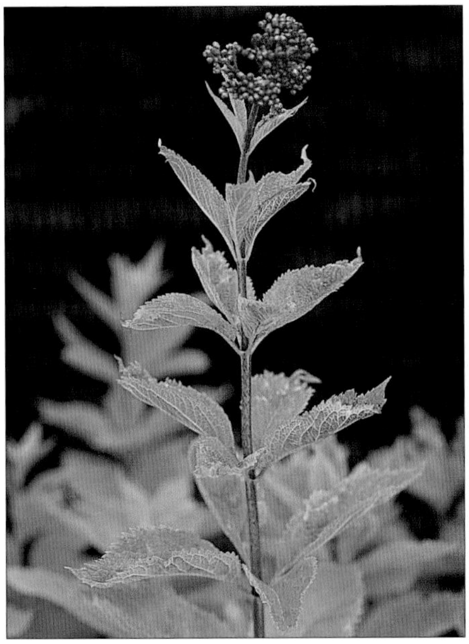

Eupatorium purpureum
Joe Pye weed

History and traditions Joe Pye is said to have been a traditional healer from New England, with a reputation for successful cures, who swore by *E. purpureum,* using it in his remedies. The name 'gravel root' pertains to the herb's ability to clear urinary stones, for which it is still used today, and the name 'queen of the meadows' is because the massed plants, when in flower, are a truly splendid sight.
Description A handsome hardy perennial which grows to at least 2.1m/7ft tall, with purplish stems, whorls of slender, finely toothed, ovate leaves and dense, domed corymbs of purple-pink flowers in late summer to autumn. It makes a magnificent plant for the border and is often sold as an ornamental.
Habitat/distribution A North American native, found in woodland and grassland on moist or dry soils.
Growth Grows best in moist, well-drained soil in partial shade or sun. Propagated by seed sown in containers in spring, or by division when dormant.
Parts used Rhizomes, roots – dried for use in decoctions and tinctures.

USES Medicinal It has a restorative, cleansing action, mainly used in modern herbal medicine for kidney and urinary disorders, including stone, cystitis and prostate problems. Also used for painful menstruation, rheumatism and gout.
Other names Gravel root, queen of the meadows.

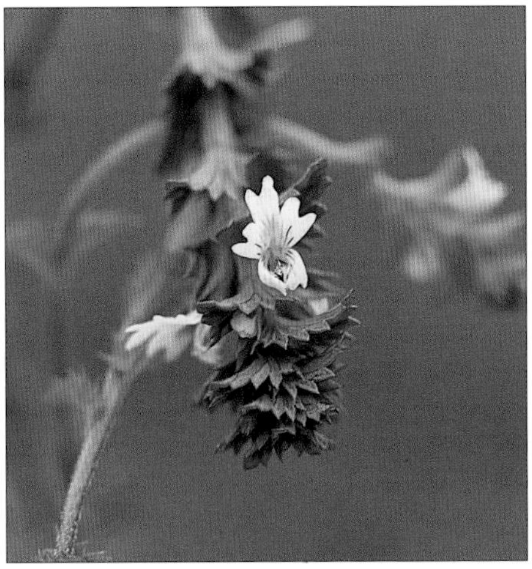

SCROPHULARIACEAE
Euphrasia officinalis
Eyebright

History and traditions The botanical name of this plant comes from the Greek for gladness. It was first introduced as an "eye" herb by Hildegard of Bingen, in 1150. In the 16th century, Fuchs and Dodoens promoted it for eye complaints. The Doctrine of Signatures had a considerable bearing on the matter, as the markings on the little white flower were supposed to resemble a bloodshot eye.
Description An annual semi-parasitic herb, 5–30cm/2–12in in height, it attaches itself to the roots and stems of grasses, absorbing mineral substances from them. Leaves are rounded, toothed and small – 1cm/½in long – and the tiny white flowers are double-lipped with yellow throats and dark-purple veins.
Habitat/distribution Native to northern Europe, found also in Siberia and the Himalayas in meadowland and pastures on poor soil.
Growth A wild plant that is difficult to cultivate because of its semi-parasitic habit. If propagation is to be attempted, seeds should be sown near to potential host grasses.
Parts used Whole plant – dried for use in infusions and herbal preparations.

USES Medicinal A herb which reduces inflammation and is said to be helpful, taken as an infusion, for hayfever, allergic rhinitis, catarrh and sinusitis. For external use it is made into washes for sore, itchy eyes and conjunctivitis, or for skin irritations and eczema.

CAUTION May cause eye irritation.

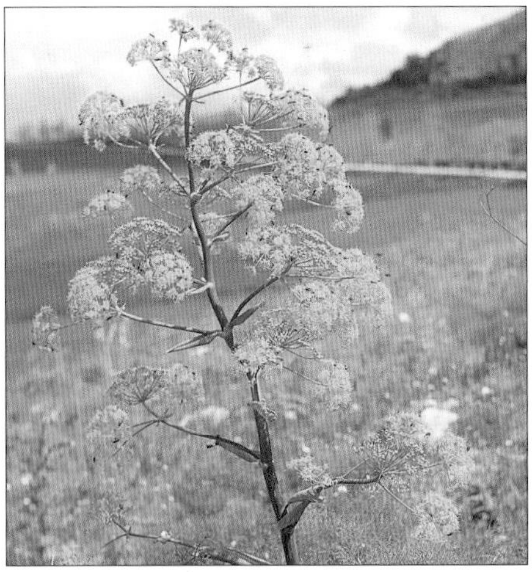

UMBELLIFERAE/APIACEAE
Ferula assa-foetida
Asafoetida

History and traditions The specific name refers to the strong, fetid smell of the gum resin obtained from the roots of this plant. It was valued throughout the Middle Ages as a prophylactic against plague and disease, and a piece was sometimes hung around the neck for this purpose. Asafoetida is still popular in India today as a flavouring and condiment and for its medicinal properties.
Description A herbaceous perennial, growing to 2.3m/7ft, it has a thick, fleshy taproot, finely divided, feathery leaves and yellow flower umbels in summer – and looks like giant fennel.
Habitat/distribution Occurs in western Asia from Iran to Afghanistan and Kashmir, on rocky hillsides and open ground.
Growth It is frost hardy, withstanding temperatures to -5°C/23°F and should be grown in well-drained, reasonably rich soil. Propagated by seed sown in autumn as soon as it is ripe.
Parts used Gum resin – produced from the base of the stems and root crown when the plant is cut down, drying as reddish tears. Sold whole, in powdered form, or as a tincture.

USES Medicinal It has a long tradition of use in Ayurvedic medicine for many complaints, including digestive disorders, respiratory diseases, impotence, painful menstruation, and problems following childbirth, and is said to counteract the effects of opium.
Culinary Despite its strong, sulphurous aroma, when added in small quantities, this herb enhances the flavour of curries and spicy food. The green parts are used as a vegetable.

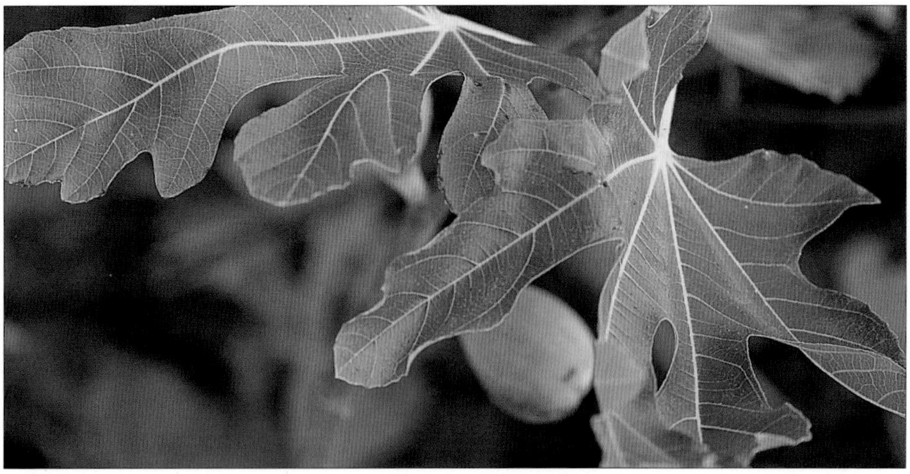

MORACEAE
Ficus carica
Fig

History and traditions Figs originally came from Caria, a region of modern Turkey, which is the source of the species name. They were widely cultivated in ancient Greece and Rome and there are many references to them in classical writings from Homer to Theophrastus, Dioscorides and Pliny. Greek athletes ate figs to improve their strength and performance and the Romans fed them to their slaves (presumably for similar reasons). In Roman mythology the fig was dedicated to Bacchus and renowned as the tree which gave shelter to the wolf that suckled Romulus and Remus. Figs have been grown in the rest of Europe since they were popularized by the Emperor Charlemagne in the 9th century.
Description A deciduous tree, growing to 10m/33ft with deeply lobed, palmate leaves. The flowers are completely concealed within fleshy receptacles and are followed by small green, pear-shaped fruits, ripening to dark purple, when the flesh surrounding the seeds becomes sweet and juicy.
Habitat/distribution Native to Turkey and southwest Asia, naturalized throughout the Mediterranean region and grown in many warm temperate zones worldwide.
Growth Although fig trees will withstand temperatures to -5°C/23°F, they need some protection from prolonged frost and cold. Warm, sunny summers are necessary to produce good fruit. Grow in well-drained, rich soil in a sunny position, and provide a sheltered place in cool areas. Propagated from semi-ripe cuttings in summer.
Parts used Fruits – fresh or dried.

USES Medicinal Well known for their laxative properties – syrup of figs is a traditional remedy for constipation – they are also highly nutritious, containing vitamins A, C and minerals, including calcium, phosphorus and iron, and are considered restorative and strengthening to the system. The milky juice, or sap, from green figs helps to soften corns and calluses on the skin.
Culinary The fruits are delicious raw, or as a cooked ingredient of sweet pies, pastries, desserts and conserves. Dried figs are stewed, or eaten as they are.

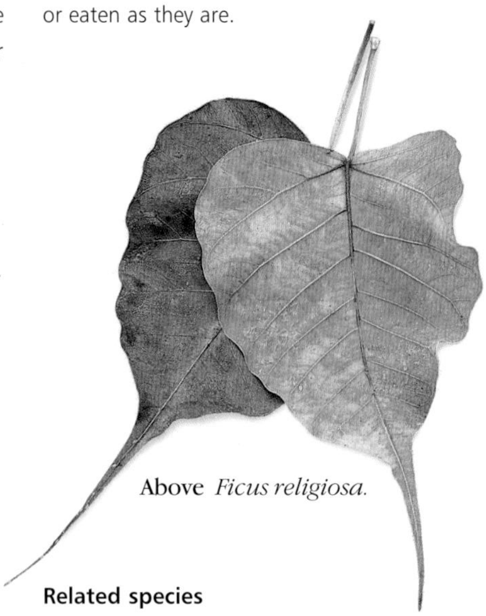

Above *Ficus religiosa.*

Related species

MORACEAE
Ficus religiosa
Peepal

Ficus religiosa is a large, spreading tree with distinctive, broad oval leaves, each tapering to a point. It was while meditating beneath a peepal tree that the Buddha attained enlightenment, and it is revered by both Hindus and Buddhists. In Ayurvedic medicine it is used to treat various diseases, including dysentery and skin disorders.

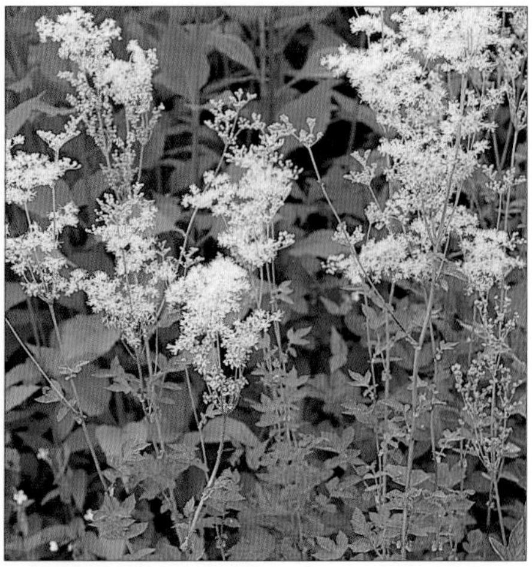

ROSACEAE
Filipendula ulmaria
Meadowsweet

History and traditions The Dutch named this herb *"reinette"* (little queen) and it is known in several European languages as queen of the meadows. It features in the poetry of Ben Jonson as "meadow's queen" and John Clare celebrates its beauty in his poem "To Summer".
Description A herbaceous perennial, on a stout rootstock, 1–1.2m/3–4ft tall, with irregularly pinnate, inversely lance-shaped leaves and dense corymbs of fluffy, creamy flowers in summer. Leaves have a more pleasant, aromatic scent than the sickly, hawthorn-like smell of the flowers.
Habitat/distribution Native to Europe and Asia, introduced and naturalized in North America. Widely grown in temperate regions, in marshlands and meadows, by ponds and streams.
Growth Grow in moist to boggy soil, in sun or partial shade – dislikes acid soil. Propagated by seed sown in spring or in autumn and overwintered in a cold frame, or by division in autumn or spring.
Parts used Leaves, flowers – fresh or dried.

USES Medicinal Taken as an infusion for heartburn, excess acidity and gastric ulcers. Also said to be helpful for rheumatism, arthritis and urinary infections. It is rich in salicylic acid, which has pain-relieving properties. Salicylic acid is then synthesised into acetylasalicylic acid, the active ingredient in apsirin.

CAUTION Not to be used if allergic to aspirin. May cause gastric upsets.

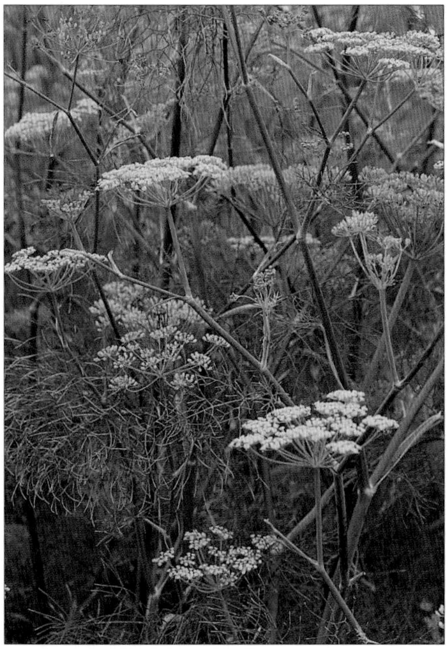

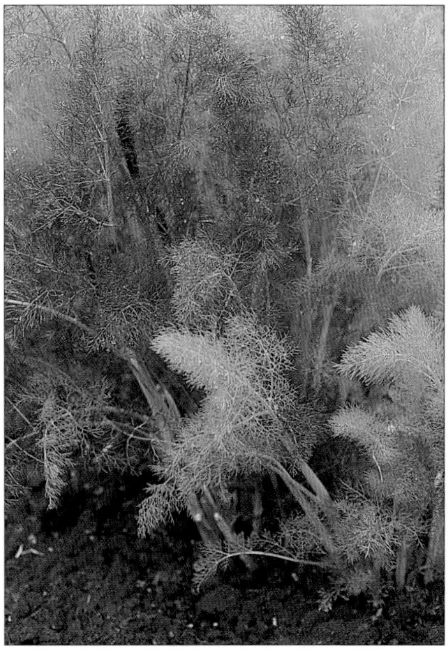

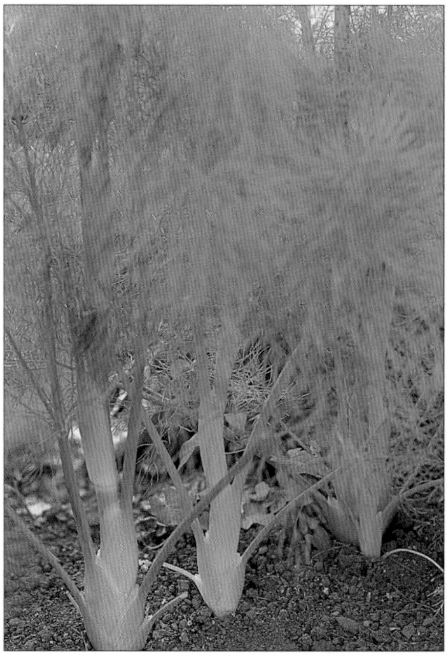

UMBELLIFERAE/APIACEAE

Foeniculum vulgare

Fennel

History and traditions The Romans enjoyed fennel both as a culinary plant, eating the stems as a vegetable, and for its medicinal properties – Pliny listed it as a remedy for no fewer than 22 complaints. It appears in early Anglo-Saxon texts and European records of the 10th century and was associated with magic and spells, being hung up at doors on Midsummer's Eve to deter witches. It was also used as a slimming aid and to deaden the pangs of hunger. William Coles wrote that it was "much used in drinks and broths for those that are grown fat, to abate their unwieldiness and cause them to grow more gaunt and lank" (*Nature's Paradise* (1650). A use which is still valid today, it may be relevant that the chemical structure of fennel bears certain similarities to that of amphetamines.

Description A graceful aromatic perennial, up to 2m/6ft tall, with erect, hollow stems and mid green, feathery foliage – the leaves are pinnate, with threadlike leaflets. Umbels of yellow flowers are borne in summer, followed by ovoid, ridged, yellow-green seeds. The whole plant is strongly scented with aniseed.

Related species *F. v.* 'Purpureum' has bronze foliage and makes an attractive ornamental. *F. v.* var. *dulce* (Florence fennel, sweet fennel, finocchio) is cultivated for its bulbous, white stem bases.

Habitat/distribution Native to Asia and the Mediterranean, and occurs in much of Europe on wasteland, on dry sunny sites and in coastal areas. Widely naturalized in other countries.

Growth Grow *F. vulgare* and *F. v.* 'Purpureum' in well-drained to sandy soil in a sunny position. Does not always survive severely cold or wet winters, especially if grown on heavy soil. *F. v.* var. *dulce* needs a richer but well-drained soil, and plenty of water to produce the requisite swollen stems, which are blanched by earthing up around them. Propagation is from seed sown in spring.

Parts used Leaves, stems, roots, seeds, essential oil.

USES Medicinal An infusion of the seeds soothes the digestive system, and is said to increase the production of breast milk in nursing mothers as well as being settling for the baby. Also used as a mouthwash for gum disorders and a gargle for sore throats.

Culinary Leaves and seeds go well with fish, especially oily fish, such as mackerel. Seeds lend savour to stir-fry and rice dishes. The bulbous stems of Florence fennel are eaten raw in salads or cooked as a vegetable.

Aromatic The essential oil is used in perfumery, to scent soaps and household products, and as a flavouring in the food industry.

CAUTION Not suitable for pregnant women as in large doses fennel is a uterine stimulant.

Above centre *Fennel foliage.*

Above F. v. *var.* dulce, *florence fennel.*

Fennel tea

Drinking fennel tea can have a good effect when on a slimming regime. Try taking a cup before meals to reduce appetite, or at any time instead of tea or coffee laced with milk and sugar.

250ml/½ pint/1 cup of boiling water
5ml/1 tsp of fennel seeds
½ thin slice of fresh orange

Put the fennel seeds in a cup, crush them lightly and pour over the boiling water. Cover and leave to infuse for 5 minutes. Strain before pouring and add the orange for extra flavour.

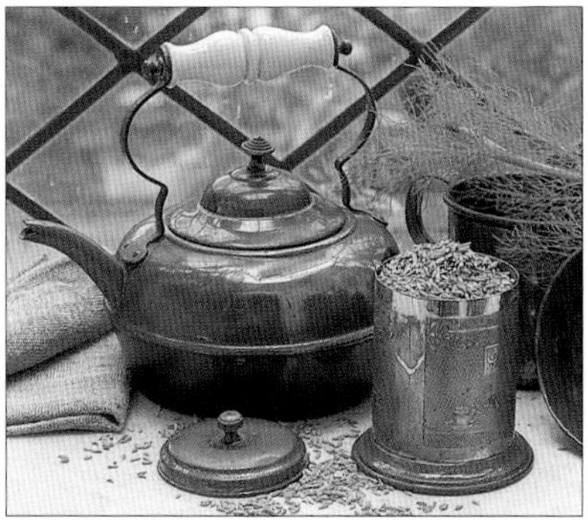

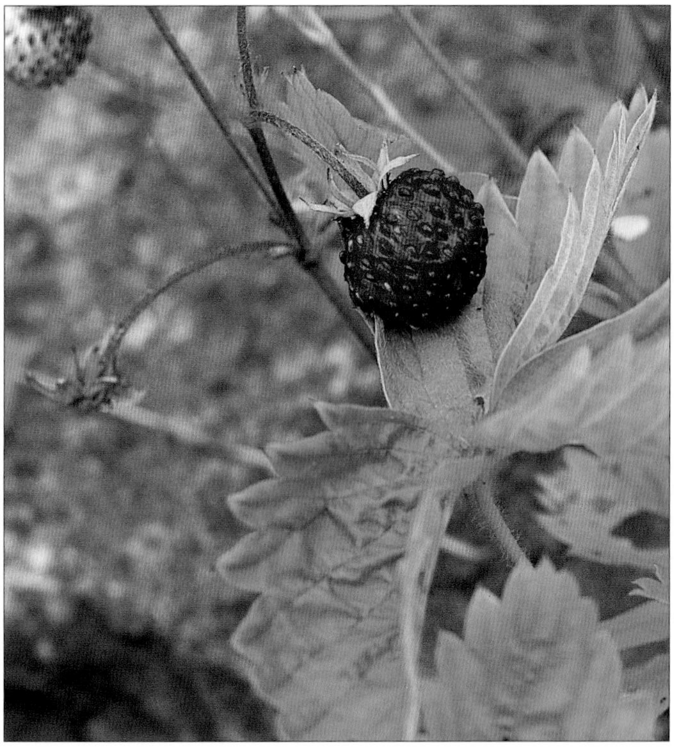

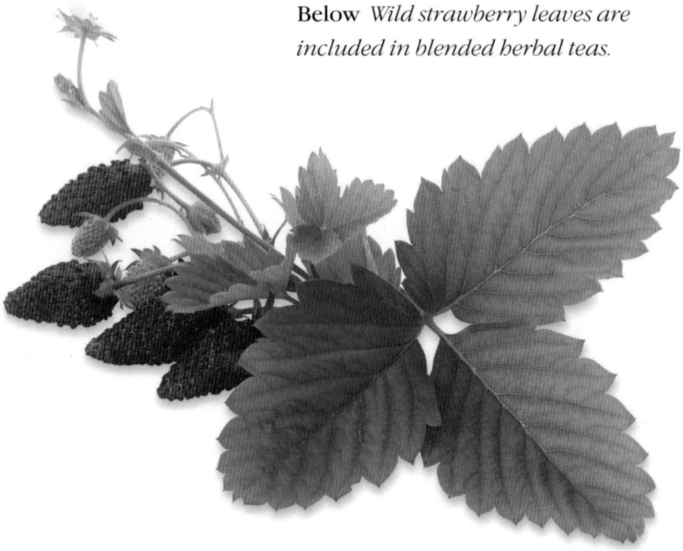

Below *Wild strawberry leaves are included in blended herbal teas.*

ROSACEAE

Fragaria vesca

Wild strawberry

History and traditions The large garden strawberry was not developed until the end of the 18th century by cross-breeding with American species. Until then, wild strawberries were the only kind known, although they were cultivated – when "by diligence of the gardener" the fruits were "as big as the berries of the Bramble in the hedge", as Thomas Hill puts it in *The Gardener's Labyrinth*,1590. Hill recommended eating them with cream and sugar, or, preferably in his view, with sugar and wine. Old stillroom books give recipes for strawberry teas and cordials, and for beauty aids, such as a face wash of strawberries, tansy and new milk. Culpeper had great faith in the powers of this plant to counteract all manner of disorders, from cooling the liver, blood and spleen, refreshing and comforting fainting spirits and quenching thirst, to washing foul ulcers, fastening loose teeth and healing spongy gums.

Description A low-growing perennial, 25cm/10in tall, which spreads by sending out rooting runners. It has shiny, trifoliate leaves, made up of ovate, toothed leaflets, and small white, yellow-centred flowers, followed by red ovoid fruits with tiny yellow seeds embedded in the surface.

Related species Alpine strawberries are cultivars of the species, *F. vesca,* and have smaller, but more distinctively aromatic fruits.

Habitat/distribution Found in Europe, Asia and North America, in grassland and woodland. Widely grown in temperate and subtropical regions.

Growth Grow in fertile, well-drained soil (on the alkaline side), in sun or partial shade. Propagate by separating and replanting runners – or by seed sown in containers at a temperature of 13–18°C/55–64°F.

Parts used Leaves, roots, fruits.

USES Medicinal Infusions or decoctions of the leaves and root are traditionally recommended for gout, are also taken for digestive disorders and used as a mouthwash to freshen breath. (Leaves of large, garden varieties do not have medicinal properties.) Leaves are diuretic and the fruits are mildly laxative. Preparations made with the fruits can be applied externally for skin inflammations, irritations and sunburn.

Culinary Rich in vitamin C, fruits are eaten fresh or made into desserts, conserves and juices. Dried leaves are included in blended herbal teas to improve taste and aroma.

Cosmetic The wild strawberry fruits have a cleansing, astringent action on the skin and are often added to face masks, skin toners and cleansing lotions.

Strawberry cleansing milk

A soothing lotion suitable for any skins.

225g/8oz fresh, ripe strawberries
150ml/¼ pint/⅔ cup milk

Mash the strawberries to a pulp and mix with the milk. Pour into a clean bottle and keep in the refrigerator. Apply to the face on pads of cotton wool (cotton balls). Lotion does not keep and should be used within two days.

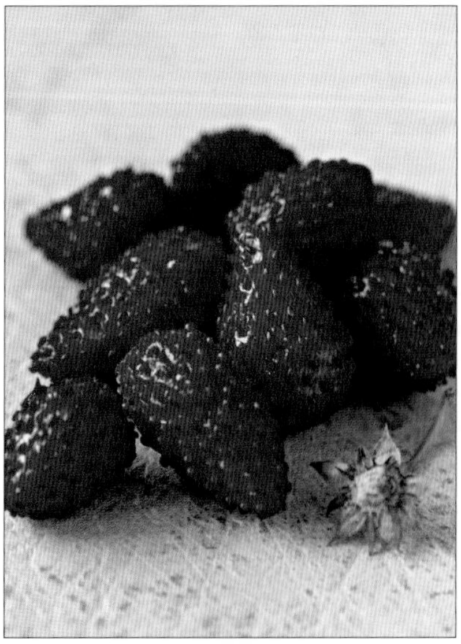

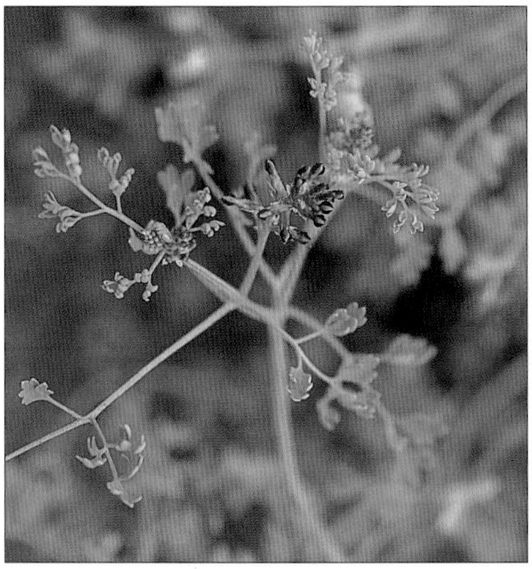

PAPAVERACEAE

Fumaria officinalis

Fumitory

History and traditions Shakespeare had no high opinion of this plant, referring to it twice as "rank fumitory" – it was one of the "idle weeds" with which King Lear crowned himself when mad, and a plant which grew in "fallow leas", left uncultivated because of war (*Henry V*). *Fumaria* is from the Latin for smoke, *fumus*. Various explanations have been put forward for its application to this plant – from the leaves having a "smoky appearance" to smoke from the plant, when burnt, dispatching evil spirits; or the view, attributed to Pliny, that putting the juice in the eyes makes the tears run to such an extent that it is like being blinded by smoke.
Description An annual herb, 15–30cm/6–12in tall, with trailing stems, small, finely divided grey-green leaves and racemes of tubular, pink flowers from midsummer to autumn.
Habitat/distribution A European native, also found in western Asia and naturalized in North America, occurs on weedy ground, in fields and gardens (once a common cornfield weed).
Growth A wild plant, it will grow in any light soil, in sun or shade. Propagated from seed sown in spring, it also self-seeds readily.
Parts used Whole plant; cut in flower and dried.

USES Medicinal Contains small amounts of similar alkaloids to those found in poppies. Formerly used internally for digestive complaints and externally for eczema, skin disorders and conjunctivitis, but is little used today.

CAUTION Mildly toxic – not for self-medication.

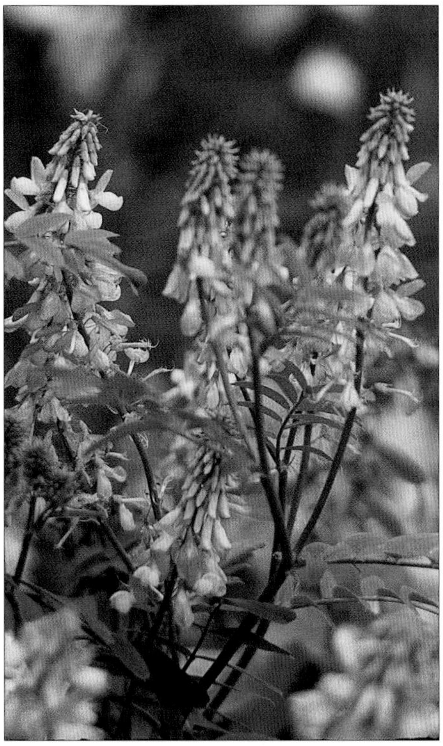

LEGUMINOSAE/PAPILIONACEAE

Galega officinalis

Goat's rue

History and traditions The generic Latin name is said to come from the Greek for milk, *ghala*. The reputation of this herb for increasing the milk supply of cattle and other animals who eat it was established at the end of the 19th century by studies carried out in France. It was, at one time, thought to be helpful in cases of plague and was a favourite choice for fevers. Culpeper advised that "a bath made of it is very refreshing to the feet of persons tired of over-walking". The common name "goat's rue" is possibly because the crushed leaves have a rank smell.
Description A bushy, hardy perennial, up to 1.5m/5ft tall, with lax stems, pinnately divided leaves and racemes of mauve, white or bi-coloured flowers borne throughout the summer – it makes an attractive plant for the border or herb garden.
Related species *G. offinalis* 'Alba' is a white-flowering cultivar.
Habitat/distribution Native to Europe and western Asia, introduced in other countries, found in moist meadows and pasturelands.
Growth Goat's rue will grow in most soils, but prefers moist conditions, thrives and spreads rapidly in rich, fertile soil. Plant in full sun or partial shade. Propagated from seed sown in spring (soaking seeds overnight, or scarifying them, encourages germination).
Parts used Flowering tops – dried.

USES Medicinal An infusion of the herb is supposed to improve lactation for humans, just as eating the plant does for animals. It also has digestive properties and is said to lower blood-sugar levels, making it helpful for late-onset diabetes.
General High in nitrogen, it makes a useful "green manure" when ploughed into the soil.
Other name French lilac.

Below Galega officinalis *'Alba'*.

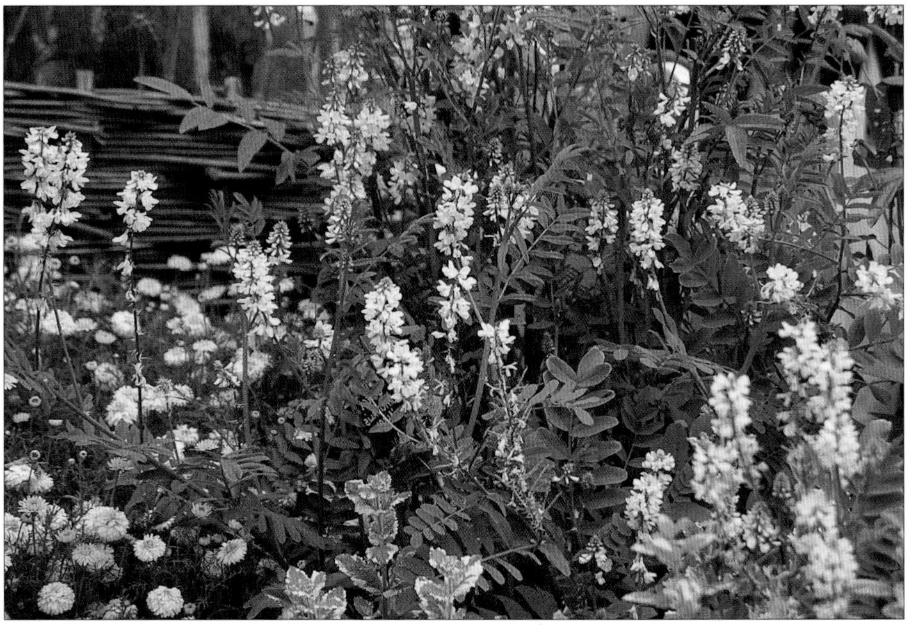

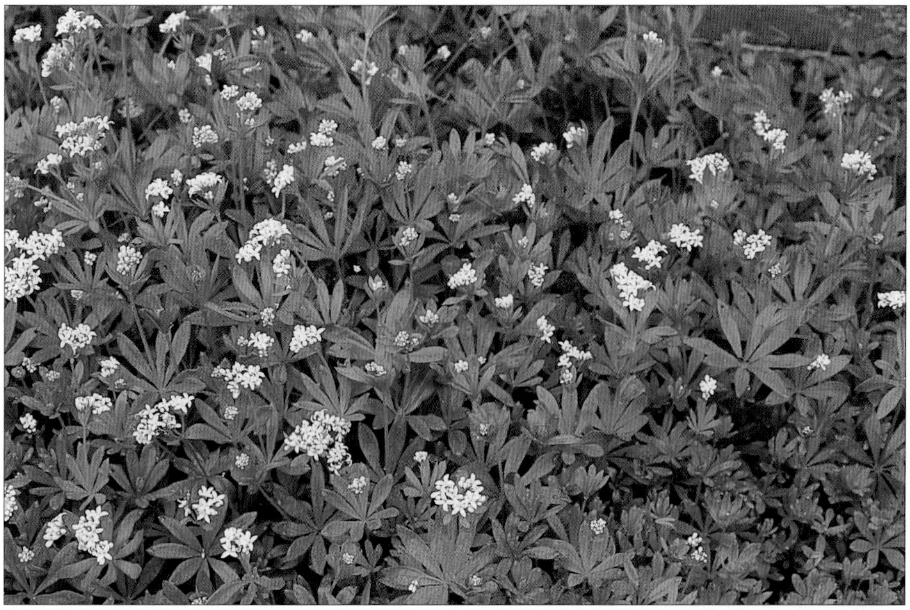

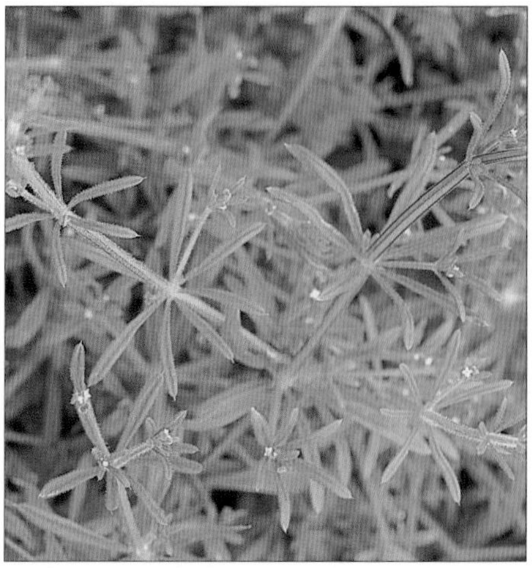

RUBIACEAE

Galium

Galium odoratum syn. *Asperula odorata*
Sweet woodruff

History and traditions A strewing herb since medieval times, it is one of many species containing compounds which release coumarin, with its characteristic scent of new-mown hay, as the plant dries. Thomas Tusser called it "sweet grass" and recommended it for making a water to improve the complexion as well as for strewing. Gerard recommended it as a kind of air conditioning: "The flowers are of a very sweet smell as is the rest of the herb, which, being made up into garlands or bundles, and hanged up in houses in the heat of summer, doth very well attemper the air, cool and make fresh the place" *(The Herball,* 1597). The dried leaves were put into sachet mixtures to deter moths, used to stuff pillows and mattresses and placed between the pages of books.
Description A spreading perennial, growing on a creeping rhizome, about 40cm/16in tall, it has four-angled stems, whorls of rough-textured, lanceolate leaves and a mass of tubular, star-shaped, scented, white flowers in summer.
Habitat/distribution Native to Europe and Asia, also found in northern Africa and naturalized in North America. Found on loamy, nutrient-rich soils in mixed woodland.
Growth Grow in humus-rich soil in partial shade. Propagation is easiest by division of runners in spring or autumn. Can also be grown from seed, sown as soon as ripe in late summer.
Parts used Whole plant – cut when in flower and dried.

USES Medicinal Coumarin gives it sedative properties and infusions are taken for nervous irritability and insomnia. Modern research has found that two of its coumarin molecules join to produce dicoumarol, which prevents blood-clotting and strengthens capillaries, and it is taken internally for varicose veins and thrombo-phlebitis. It is a diuretic and said to improve liver function and have a tonic effect on the system.
Aromatic The coumarin smell intensifies and improves with keeping, so the dried herb is added to potpourri or sachets for the linen cupboard – it helps repel insects.

Galium verum
Ladies' bedstraw

This member of the *Galium* genus has the characteristic four-angled stems and whorls of clinging, bristled leaves, but the flowers are bright yellow and smell of honey. It too emits the sweet, coumarin scent when dry and was much used in the past as a mattress stuffing – hence its popular name. Dioscorides wrote about it as a "milk" plant and it was used in his time and for centuries afterwards as an agent for curdling cheese and colouring it yellow – it does in fact contain a rennin enzyme.

Galium aparine
Goosegrass

This familiar, creeping, clinging plant may look like a tiresome weed (and all too often behave like one) but is not without its uses. It is a traditional springtime tonic in central Europe, taken as an infusion of the fresh green parts, or as a pulped juice, and is said to help eliminate toxins from the system.
Other name Cleavers.

USES Medicinal Some herbalists recommend it for debilitating conditions such as myalgic encephalomyelitis (ME) and glandular fever. It is a lymphatic tonic, helping to clear lymphatic swelling and enlarged lymph nodes, especially in the pelvis. Galium is also demulcent for the urinary tract. It can be used topically for inflammation of the skin, minor injuries and conditions such as eczema and psoriasis.

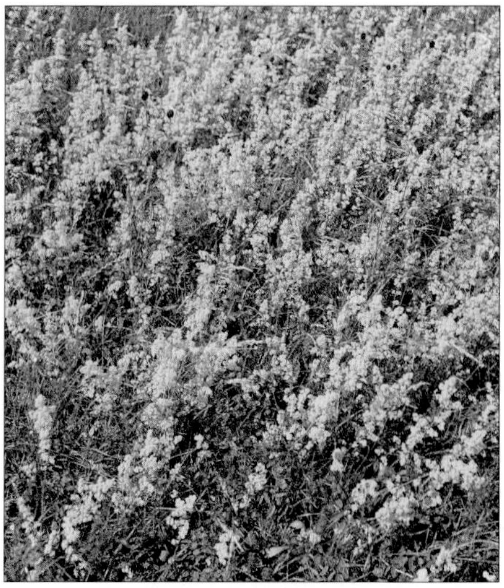

Above *Ladies' bedstraw.*

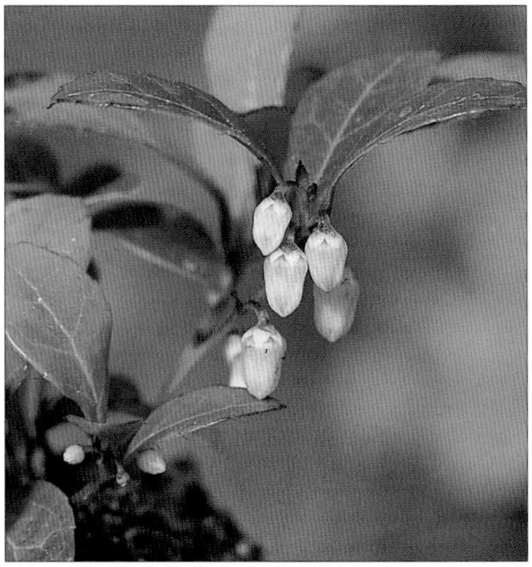

ERICACEAE

Gaultheria procumbens

Wintergreen

History and traditions This shrub is the source of the original wintergreen, later extracted from a species of birch, *Betula lenta,* and nowadays mostly produced synthetically. It was used as a tea and medicinally by Canadian Indians for aching muscles and joints. Its Latin name comes from Dr Jean-Francois Gaulthier, who worked in Quebec in the mid-1700s. The leaves were officially in the United States *Pharmacopoeia* until towards the end of the 19th century and wintergreen oil is still listed.
Description A prostrate shrub, 15cm/6in high, it has dark green, glossy, oval leaves and clusters of small, white, drooping, bell-shaped flowers in summer, followed by scarlet berries.
Habitat/distribution A North American native, found in woodlands and mountainous areas.
Growth Grow in a moist soil, on the acid side of neutral, in partial shade. Dividing the rooted suckers is the easiest way to propagate this plant. Semi-ripe cuttings can be taken in summer, or seeds can be sown in containers and overwintered in a cold frame.
Parts used Leaves, essential oil – obtained by distillation of the leaves.

USES Medicinal The leaves contain methyl salicylate, an anti-inflammatory with similar properties to aspirin. The essential oil has antiseptic properties and is used for massaging aches and pains, for rheumatism and arthritis. Infusions of the leaves are used as gargles.

CAUTION The oil is toxic in excess.

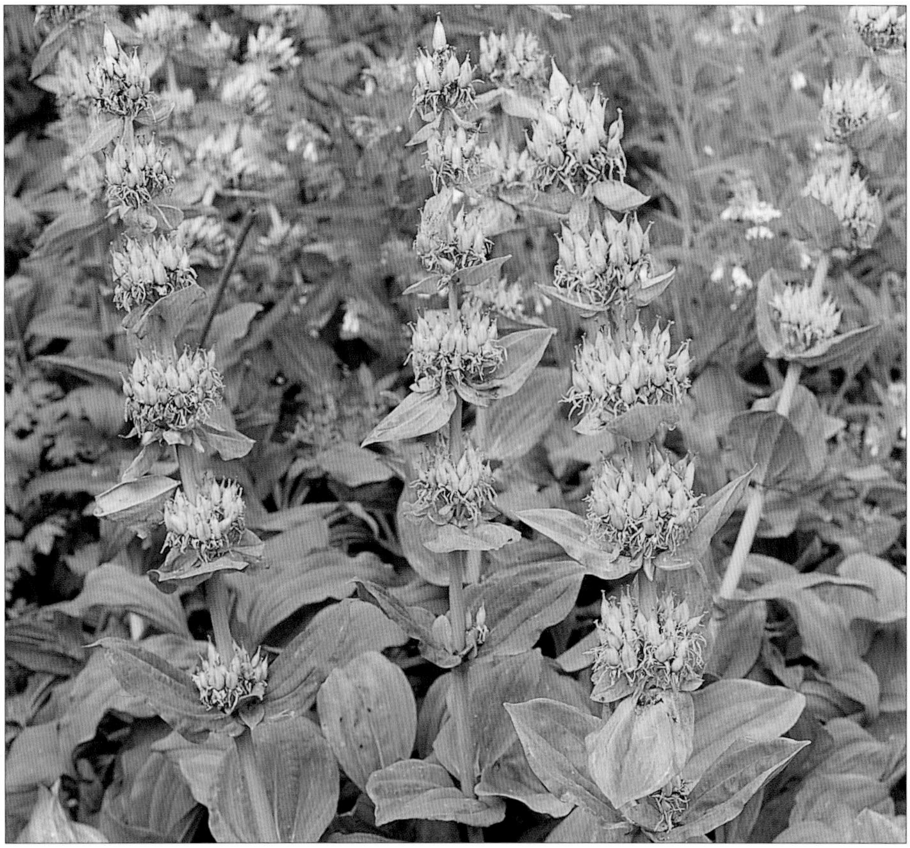

GENTIANACEAE

Gentiana lutea

Yellow gentian

History and traditions Gentians are said to be named after a King Gentius of Illyria (an ancient country of the East Adriatic), who was credited by Pliny and Dioscorides as having been the first to recognize its medicinal properties. In the Middle Ages it was popular as a counter-poison and the German physician and botanist Hieronymus Bock in his *Neue Kraüter Buch*, 1539, refers to the use of the roots in dilating wounds. Nicholas Culpeper, inventive as ever, recommends it as a healing decoction for cows unlucky enough to be bitten on the udder by venomous beasts. It is not certain which species were used in former times, but *G. lutea* has proved to be the most important from a medicinal point of view. In former times gentian wine was taken as an aperitif.
Description A hardy herbaceous perennial, it grows on a thick taproot, to a height of 1–2m/3–6ft. Erect stems have fleshy, ribbed leaves in pairs, joined at the base, and bright yellow flowers, with short, tubular petals, borne in clusters in the leaf axils. It usually flowers about three years after planting.
Habitat/distribution Native to Europe and western Asia. Found in mountainous pastures and woodlands.
Growth Grow in well-drained, humus-rich soil, in sun or partial shade, and keep fairly moist – heavy, waterlogged soil is likely to induce root rot. Propagated by division or offshoots in spring, or by seed sown in autumn.
Parts used Roots, rhizomes – dried for use in decoctions, tinctures and other preparations.

USES Medicinal The most bitter of herbs, yellow gentian has been used in tonic medicines for centuries. It is said to be anti-inflammatory and to reduce fevers and is taken internally for digestive complaints and loss of appetite.
General An ingredient of commercially produced tonics and bitter aperitifs.

CAUTION It should not be used without advice from a qualified practitioner, as it could have adverse effects on some gastric disorders. Not to be taken by anyone with high blood pressure, or by pregnant women. Avoid long-term use internally and externally due to high tannin content.

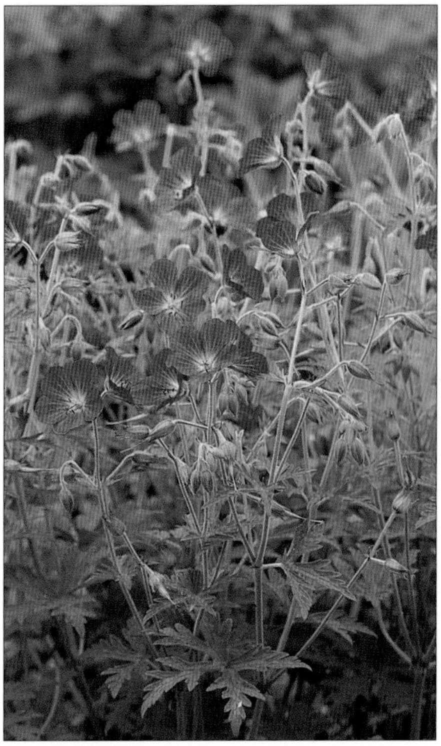

GERANIACEAE

Geranium maculatum

Cranesbill

History and traditions The common name refers to the beak-like shape of the fruit, and the generic name is from the Greek word for a crane, a stork-like bird with a long bill. The leaves become distinctively speckled as they age, and the specific name *maculatum* means spotted. Traditionally used in the folk medicine of Native Americans, it was at one time listed in the United States *Pharmacopoeia*.

Description A hardy, clump-forming perennial, it grows to 75cm/30in and has deeply divided palmate leaves. Large, round, purple-pink flowers appear in the axils in late spring to early summer, followed by the beak-shaped fruits.

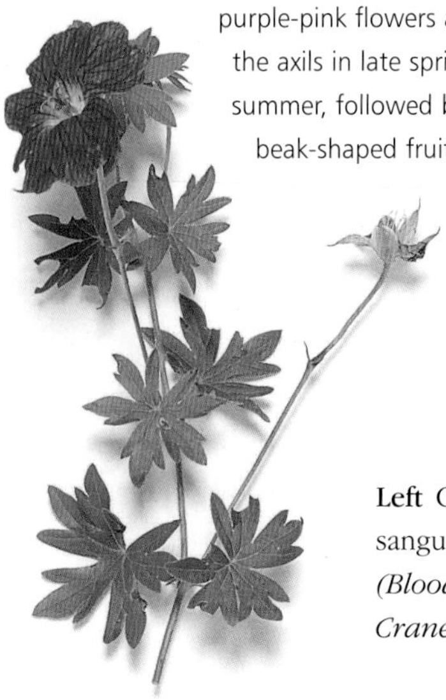

Left Geranium sanguineum, *(Bloody Cranesbill)*

Related species *G. robertianum* (herb Robert) is a common wild plant, growing to 50cm/20in, with a creeping decumbent habit and soft, downy, reddish stems. Leaves have three pinnately-lobed leaflets and small five-petalled, rose-pink flowers, striped in white. It gives off an unpleasant smell when crushed.

Habitat/distribution *G. maculatum,* native to North America, and found in a variety of habitats. Widely grown in temperate regions elsewhere. *G. robertianum* is native to Europe, North America, Asia and northern Africa in poor, dry soils.

Growth *G. maculatum* prefers moist soil and a sunny position or partial shade. Most easily propagated by division in early spring or late winter, seeds may be sown in spring or autumn. *G. robertianum* is a wild plant and grows best in poor, dry soil.

Parts used *G. maculatum* – whole plant, roots – dried for use in infusions, powders, tinctures and other preparations.

USES Medicinal *G. maculatum* is an astringent herb, which is said to control bleeding and discharges. It was formerly used in the treatment of diarrhoea, dysentery and cholera. Externally it is applied to wounds and used as a gargle for sore throats and mouth ulcers.

Other names American cranesbill and spotted cranesbill.

CAUTION Avoid long-term use.

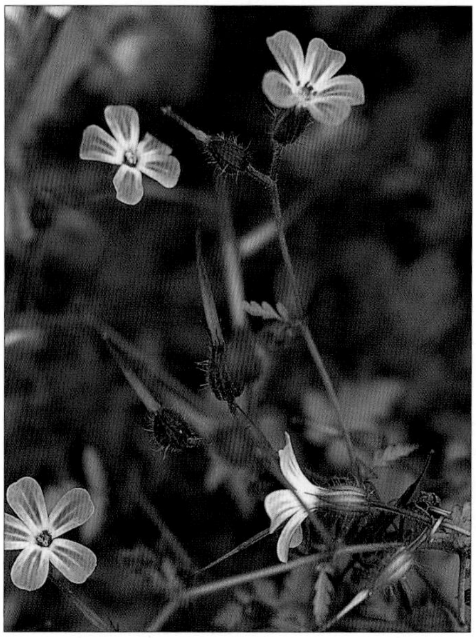

Above Geranium robertianum.

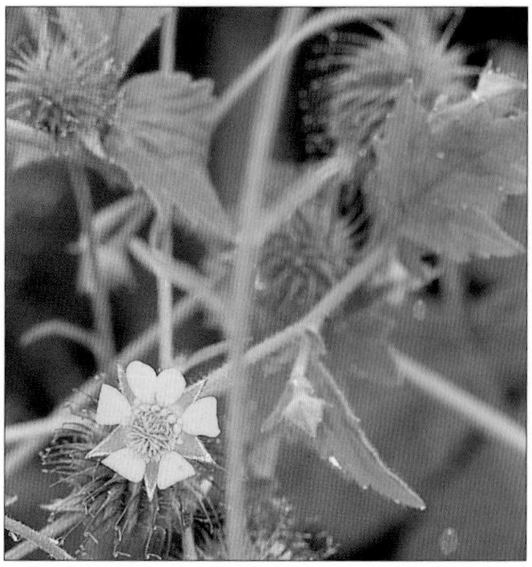

ROSACEAE

Geum urbanum

Wood avens

History and traditions The medieval name was *herba benedicta*, or the blessed herb, for its supposed ability to repel evil spirits – and the second part of one of its common names, herb bennet, is a contraction of *benedicta*. The three-part leaf and the five petals of the flower supposedly represented the Holy Trinity and five wounds of Christ, and it appears as a carved decoration in 13th-century churches. As a medicinal herb, there were rules laid down as to the time and season for digging up the root for maximum efficacy, and it was included in cordials to be taken as a plague preventive.

Description A rather undistinguished, hardy perennial plant, growing from 20–60cm/8–24in, with downy stems, three-lobed leaves and tiny, yellow, five-petalled flowers in summer, followed by fruits with brown, hooked bristles.

Habitat/distribution Native to Europe and found in wasteland, hedgerows and woodlands on moist, high-nitrogen soils.

Growth A wild plant, it grows best on rich, moist soils and self-seeds freely.

Parts used Whole plant, roots – the flowering tops are dried for use in infusions, roots used fresh or dried in decoctions.

USES Medicinal Another herb with astringent properties resulting from the high levels of tannins in the plant. *Geum* is indicated for the treatment of diarrhoea.

Culinary The roots were formerly used for their supposed clove-flavouring in soups and ale.

Other name Herb bennet.

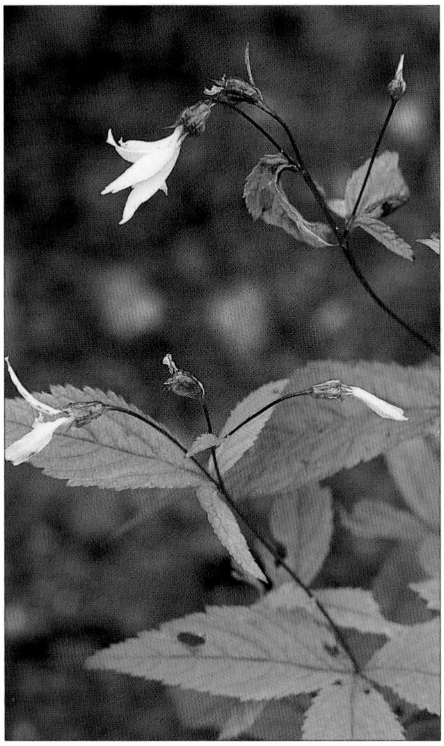

ROSACEAE

Gillenia trifoliata

Indian physic

History and traditions A medicinal plant of Native Americans with emetic, purgative properties. Also known as "bowman's root", for its wound-healing effects, and "American ipecacuanha". The early colonists adopted it and it was formerly listed in the United States *Pharmacopoeia*.

Description A graceful hardy perennial, growing to 1m/3ft, with red-tinged, wiry stems, bronze-green, three-palmate leaves and irregularly star-shaped flowers, with narrow white petals and red-tinted calyces.

Habitat/distribution Native to eastern North America, found in moist woodlands, introduced and widely grown as a garden plant in Europe and temperate regions.

Growth Grow in humus-rich, moist soil in partial shade. Propagated by division in spring or autumn, or by seed sown in autumn in containers and overwintered in a cold frame.

Parts used Root bark – dried for use in decoctions and powders.

USES Medicinal It is used as a purgative and expectorant.

Right Gillenia trifoliata.

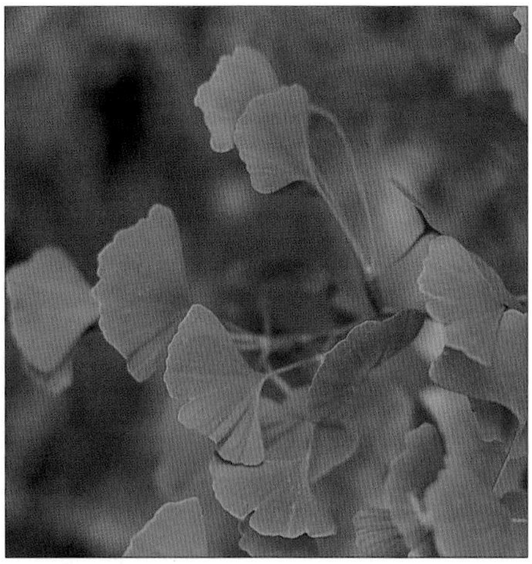

GINKGOACEAE

Ginkgo biloba

Ginkgo

History and traditions Identical in appearance to tree fossils 200 million years old, ginkgo has always been a sacred tree in China – it was grown for centuries in temples, some specimens reaching a great age, with circumferences up to 9m/29ft. It has been cultivated in Europe since the early 18th century with seeds brought from China or Japan. The seeds have long been used in traditional Chinese medicine, and modern research has discovered constituents in the leaves of potential therapeutic importance, unknown in any other plant species.

Description There is only one species in the genus. A deciduous tree growing to 40m/130ft, it has lobed, fan-shaped leaves (similar in appearance to maidenhair fern foliage, but larger), which turn yellow in autumn. Flowering takes place after 20 years, with male and female flowers and fruits borne on separate trees. Male trees have an earlier leaf-fall and less spreading form; female fruits have a rancid smell when fallen. Ginkgo is a very robust tree and suffers from few pests, tolerates pollution or a salty atmosphere well.

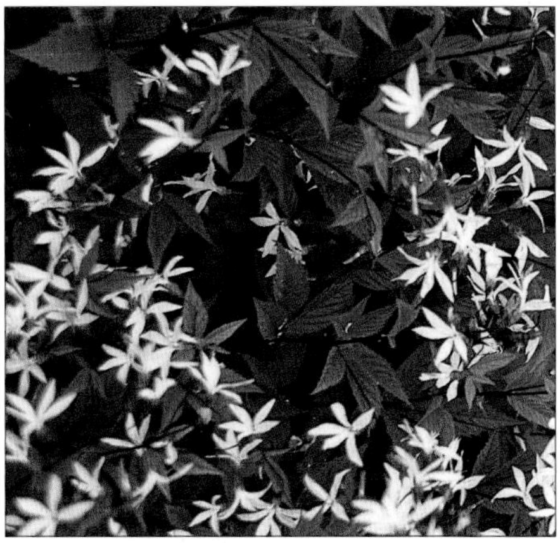

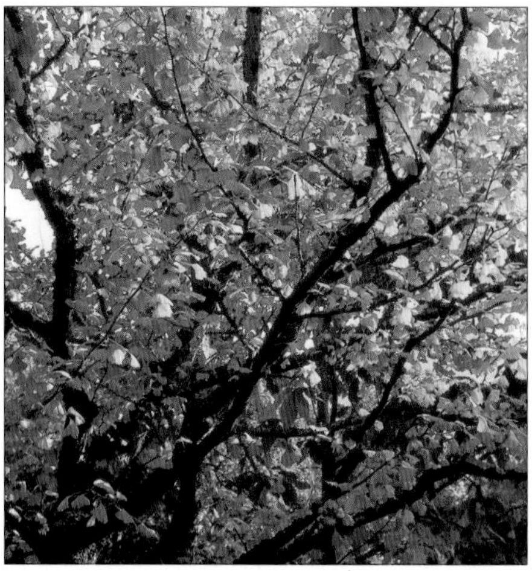

Habitat/distribution Originating in China and Japan, it is no longer found in the wild, but is cultivated as specimen and shade trees, and now widely grown in other countries.

Growth Fully hardy, it does best in well-drained but fertile soil and a sunny position. Propagated from seed sown in containers in autumn or from cuttings taken in summer. It should not be pruned as this leads to die-back.

Parts used Leaves – picked in autumn and dried. Seeds – used in decoctions.

USES Medicinal The leaves have recently been discovered to contain compounds called ginkgolides. Gingko leaf promotes blood flow and inhibits allergic reactions. The seeds have anti-fungal and antibacterial properties, and are used in Chinese medicine for asthma and coughs. Recent studies shows the neuroprotective properties of Gingko can be used to aid memory loss and can be used in dementia treatment, under the supervision of a medical herbalist.

Culinary Ginkgo nuts (the female fruits with the outer unpleasant layer removed) are roasted and sometimes served in Chinese cuisine.

General Seeds produce oil, which may cause dermatitis in sensitive people, and leaves contain insecticidal compounds.

CAUTION Only to be taken on the advice of a qualified herbalist or medical practitioner. Can interact with pharmaceutical drugs, including anti-coagulants, such as warfarin. May cause headaches and gastric upsets. Not for long-term use.

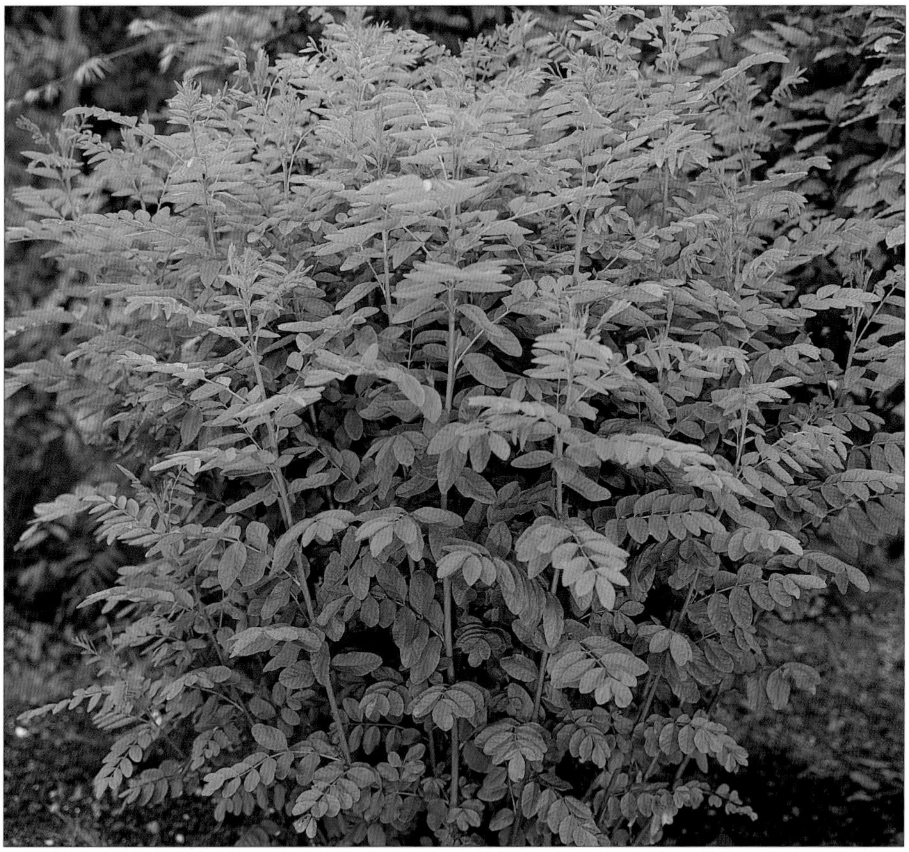

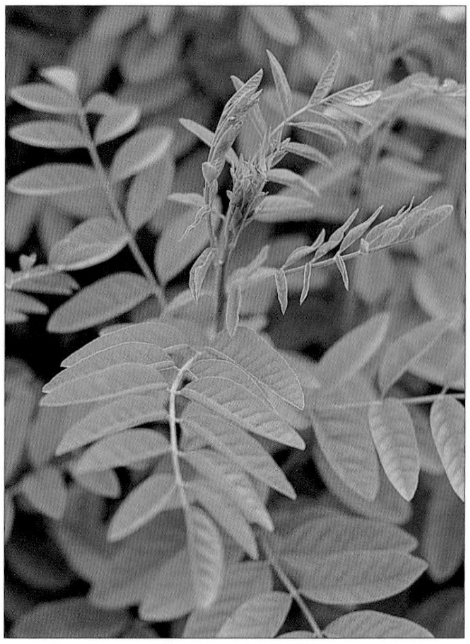

LEGUMINOSAE/PAPILIONACEAE

Glycyrrhiza glabra

Liquorice

History and traditions Liquorice has been valued for thousands of years for the sweetness of its root (it contains glycosides, including glycyrrhizin, that are 50 times sweeter than sugar) and for its medicinal powers. The generic name is from the Greek *glykys* (sweet) and *rhiza* (a root). This became corrupted to "*gliquiricia*" and thence to "liquorice". The Egyptians put it into funeral jars and some was found in the burial chamber of Tutankhamun. The Chinese believed it was rejuvenating and gave them long life and strength. Roman legionnaires chewed it on the battlefield – a habit taken up by Napoleon. It did not reach Europe until the 15th century, when it soon became established as a remedy for many ailments, including coughs, chest infections and digestive disorders. In 1760 a Pontefract apothecary, George Dunhill, thought of adding sugar and flour to the liquorice essence to produce the well-known confectionery. Liquorice confectionery is still made from the plant and it is an ingredient of many pharmaceutical products.

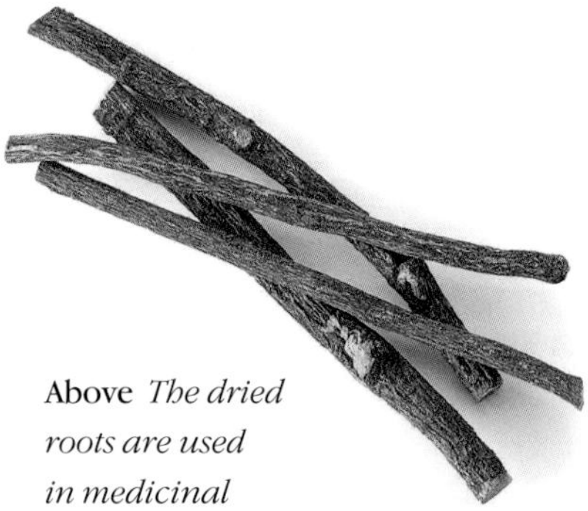

Above *The dried roots are used in medicinal preparations and to make confectionery.*

Description A hardy perennial, growing up to 1.2m/4ft, the leaves are pinnate, divided into 9–17 oval leaflets; the violet, pea-like flowers are borne in short racemes, followed by long seed pods.

Related species *G. lepidota* is a North American wild species of liquorice, used by Indian tribes to ease childbirth.

Habitat/distribution Originally from the Middle East, Asia and China, it is now cultivated in temperate regions worldwide, including parts of Australia, North and South America.

Growth It requires a deep, rich, moisture-retentive soil and a sunny position. Propagated by division of roots in autumn or spring. Germination from seed is slow. To encourage strong root growth, remove flower heads.

Parts used Roots – lifted in autumn, when plant is 3–4 years old, and dried for use in decoctions, liquid extracts and powders. Roots are boiled to extract the essence used in confectionery.

USES Medicinal An important herb in Ayurvedic medicine for stomach disorders, sore throats, respiratory infections and as first aid for snake or scorpion bites. In Chinese herbal medicine, it is used for sore throats and food poisoning. It has soothing anti-inflammatory properties and is added to proprietary cough mixtures, lozenges and laxatives. Liquorice will soothe gastrointestinal inflammation and irritations such as acid reflux, gastritis, irritable bowel disorder and ulcers. It is also used to treat rheumatism, muscle spasm and cramps and joint inflammation. Naturally sweet, it is helpful in Type 2 Diabetes helping to balance blood sugar levels. Liquorice root should not be used for self-medication.

General As well as being used in confectionery production, liquorice is used to flavour beers and tobacco.

CAUTION Avoid high dosages for prolonged periods without professional advice. Do not use with digoxin, diuretics, laxatives and other drugs that may reduce potassium. Seek help if taking prescribed medication.

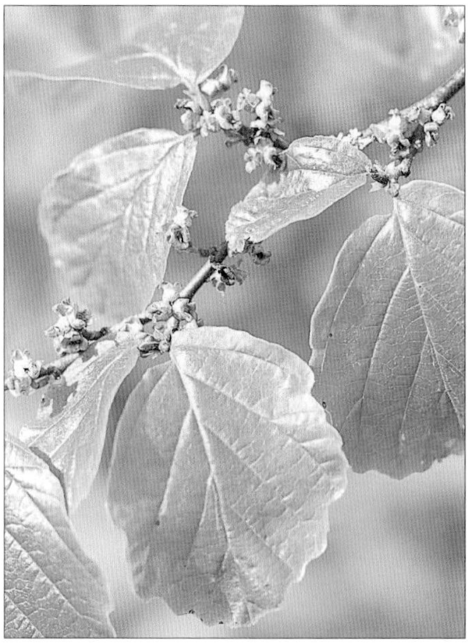

HAMAMELIDACEAE

Hamamelis virginiana

Witch hazel

History and traditions Native American tribes used decoctions of the bark to reduce swellings and bruises. Colonists took note and it was listed in the United States *Pharmacopoeia* from 1860 onwards. It was also thought to have supernatural properties and the forked branches were used as divining rods in the search for water and gold.

Description A deciduous tree or shrub, up to 5m/16ft in height, it has smooth brown bark and obovate leaves. Clusters of fragrant, yellow flowers appear in late autumn to early winter.

Habitat/distribution Native to North America, now widely cultivated in other countries as a garden ornamental.

Growth A hardy shrub, it requires moderately fertile, moist but well-drained soil and a sunny or partially shady position. Propagation is from seed sown in containers in autumn.

Parts used Twigs – cut after flowering, to make the distilled extract. Bark – used in tinctures and extracts. Leaves – dried for use in powders, liquid extracts, ointments.

USES Medicinal Distilled witch hazel is available for external use on bruises and sprains. The tincture is much stronger and should be used only under the guidance of a qualified practitioner. Witch hazel extract is a constituent of proprietary haemorrhoid ointments and other pharmaceutical preparations.

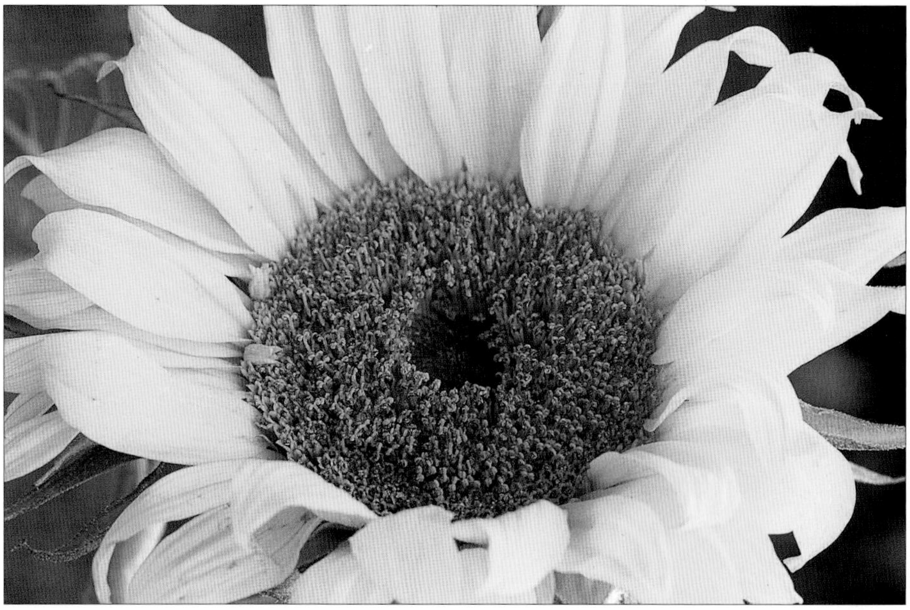

COMPOSITAE/ASTERACEAE

Helianthus annuus

Sunflower

History and traditions The sunflower originated in the Americas, probably Mexico. There is evidence that before 1000BC it was grown there for its seeds. It was among the many plants introduced to Europe from the New World in the 16th century, but did not become a major food plant and source of oil until large-scale cultivation began in Russia two centuries later (by the 1970s it was second only to soya bean as an oil crop). At some point it gained a reputation for being antimalarial and was used in Russian folk medicine for reducing fevers. The common name is a translation of the generic term, which is taken from the Greek for sun, *helios,* and flower, *anthos* – both for its sunlike appearance and because it turns its head to follow the sun's direct rays.

Description A tall, impressive annual, up to 3m/10ft in height, with erect stems and oval, hairy leaves. The showy daisy-shaped flower heads, up to 30cm/1ft across, have bright yellow ray florets, and brown disc florets at the centre, followed by the striped black-and-white seeds, about 1,000 per head.

Habitat/distribution Native to Central, North and South America, introduced and widely grown in Europe and other countries in open sunny sites.

Growth A hardy annual which tolerates most soils, as long as reasonably well-drained. Propagate by seed sown in spring.

Parts used Whole plant – cut when flowering begins for use in extracts and tinctures. Seeds are collected when ripe in autumn, and used fresh or pressed to produce a fatty oil.

USES Medicinal Sunflower seeds and oil are a good source of vitamin E, which has anti-oxidant properties. They are high in polyunsaturates, especially linoleic acid, needed for the maintenance of cell membranes – they also help lower blood cholesterol levels. Formerly, preparations made from the seeds were used for treating coughs and bronchial infections, applied externally to bruises and for easing rheumatic pains.

Culinary Seeds are eaten fresh or roasted in salads, bread and bakery products. Oil is used for cooking and in salad dressings. Also a constituent of margarine.

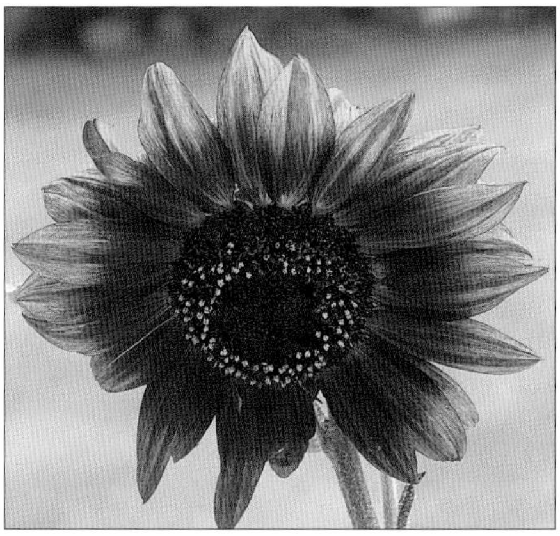

Above Helianthus annuus *'Velvet Queen' is an attractive cultivar.*

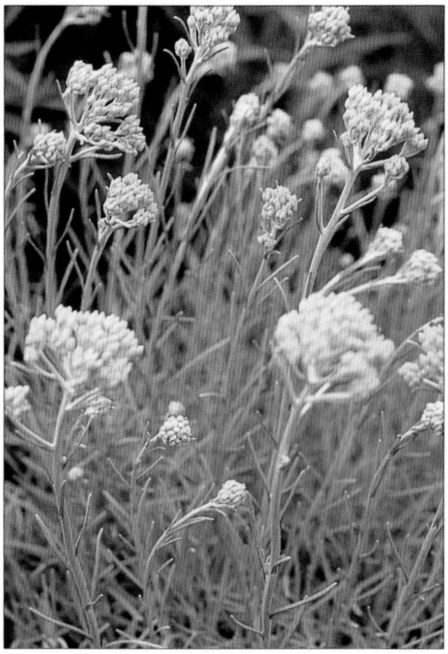

COMPOSITAE/ASTERACEAE

Helichrysum italicum syn.
H. angustifolium

Curry plant

History and traditions A native of southern Europe, it seems to have crept into modern herb gardens, where it is now firmly established, because of the popular name, curry plant, relating to its strong smell. But it is not a culinary plant and has nothing to do with curry – or curry leaves (see *Murraya koenigii*). It is one of the "everlasting" flowers (most of which have a papery texture and retain form and colour when dried). It justifies its position as a herb because it is included in potpourri and has insect-repellent properties.

Description An evergreen subshrub, 60cm/2ft in height, it has linear, silver-grey leaves and clusters of yellow button-shaped flowers in summer.

Habitat/distribution Native to the Mediterranean and grown throughout Europe, other species occur in Africa and Asia.

Growth Although frost hardy, it does not tolerate prolonged cold, wet winters. Grow in light, well-drained soil in full sun. Propagated by semi-ripe or heel cuttings in summer.

Parts used Leaves, flowers.

USES Aromatic Dried flowers and foliage may be added to potpourri and insect-repellent sachet mixtures. The essential oil is said to be antiviral, but it is not confirmed.

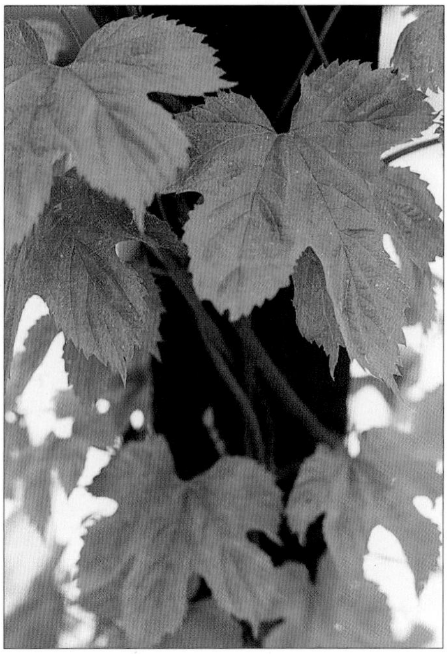

CANNABACEAE

Humulus lupulus

Hops

History and traditions The hop plant was described by Pliny, who named it "*lupus salictarius*", or "willow wolf", for its habit of twining round willow stems and strangling them "as a wolf does a lamb". The Romans ate the young shoots as vegetables. Its major significance was that it changed the character of beer, acting as a preservative and giving it a bitter flavour. It was first used for this in Flanders in the 14th century, but there was great opposition to it in Britain, where it was thought to "spoil" the traditional ales, so it was not in general use there before the 17th century. Even then John Evelyn wrote, "Hops transmuted our wholesome ale into beer. This one ingredient … preserves the drink indeed, but repays the pleasure in tormenting diseases and a shorter life" (*Pomona,* 1670). But it did become established as a medicinal plant and Culpeper's view was that a "decoction of the tops cleanses the blood, cures the venereal disease, and all kinds of scabs, itch, and other breakings out of the body; as also tetters, ringworms, spreading sores, the morphew, and all discolourings of the skin".

Description A hardy, twining, herbaceous climber, it has clinging hairy stems and 3–7 lobed palmate leaves. Male and female flowers are borne on different plants – the male ones are in small inconspicuous clusters, the female in conelike, pale green inflorescences, which are the hops used in beer making.

Related species *H. lupulus* 'Aureus' has golden-green foliage and it makes an attractive and vigorous ornamental climber for the herb garden.

Habitat/distribution Its country of origin is not certain, but it is found in Europe, western Asia and North America and widely distributed in northern temperate zones. Naturalized in woodland and hedgerows.

Growth Prefers moist, fertile, well-drained soil and a sunny position or partial shade, but is a vigorous plant that grows under most conditions. Propagated by softwood cuttings in spring.

Parts used Female flowers (cone-like) – dried; oil distilled from flowers; fresh young shoots.

USES Medicinal Has sedative, digestive and antibacterial properties. Taken internally in infusions or tinctures for insomnia, nervous tension and anxiety and to support peri and menopausal symptoms, such as hot flushes and night sweats; used externally for skin complaints.

Culinary Young shoots can be cooked and eaten like asparagus.

Aromatic Dried flowers are added to sleep pillows, distilled oil used in perfumes. Thought to help prevent ageing of skin and brittleness of hair. Flowers or essential oil are included in rejuvenating baths and hair treatments.

General Flowers (hops) used to flavour beers and ales, distilled oil and extracts used in the food industry.

CAUTION Avoid in pregnancy or if depressed.

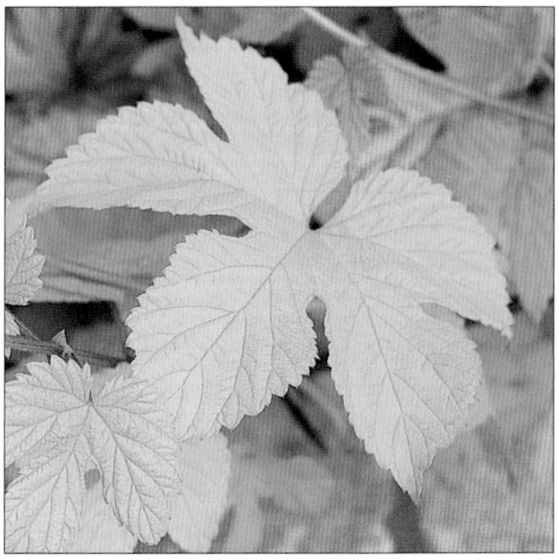

Above Humulus lupulus *'Aureus', golden hops.*

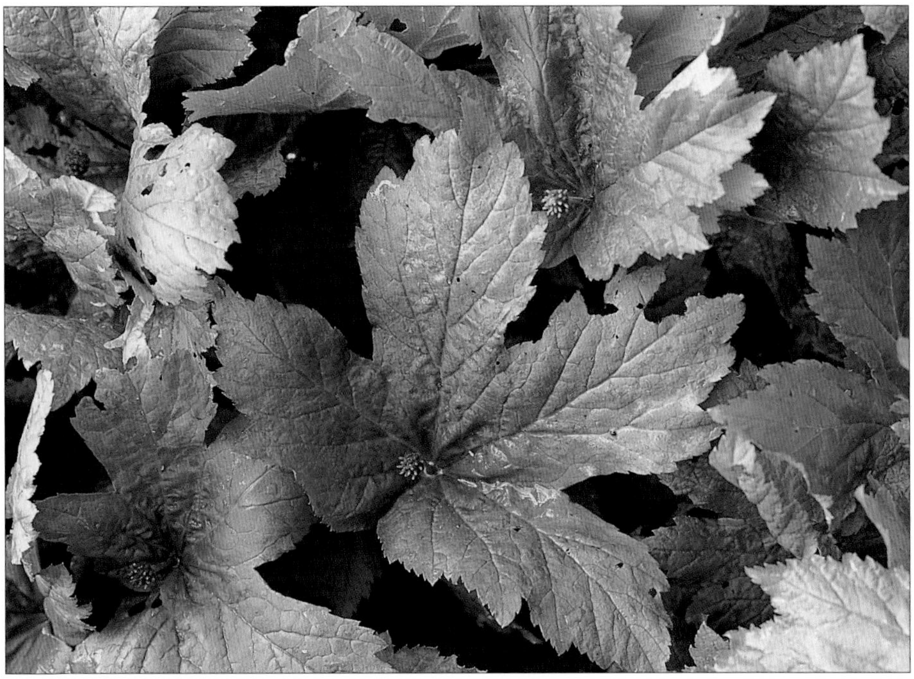

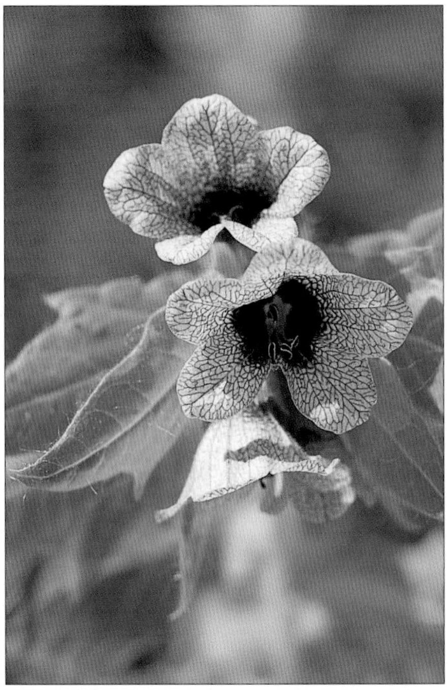

RANUNCULACEAE

Hydrastis canadensis

Golden seal

History and traditions This was once a very common herb in North America, its orange root being variously used to make a yellow dye, in medicinal remedies for digestive problems, bruises and swellings and also as an insect repellent. Early settlers were impressed by its properties and it was listed in the United States *Pharmacopoeia* from 1831 to 1936. Its continued popularity has led to overexploitation: it is now rare in the wild, from which all trade supplies come (cultivation is difficult).

Description A hardy perennial, 20–30cm/8–12in in height, it has a thick, knotted, yellow rhizome, palmate, deeply lobed leaves, and single greenish-white flowers, with no petals, in late spring to early summer. Fruits are red and raspberry-like, but inedible.

Habitat/distribution Native to north-eastern North America, found in damp forests.

Growth It requires moist, humus-rich soil and a shady position. Propagation is by seed sown in autumn, though germination is slow and erratic, or by division in early spring or late autumn. Plants do not establish easily.

Parts used Rhizome – dried for use in tinctures, decoctions and pharmaceutical preparations.

USES Medicinal It has anti-inflammatory properties, helps to check bleeding, is also antibacterial, decongestant and mildly laxative. Popular in North America for boosting the immune system, taken as a tea in combination with other herbs, such as *Echinacea purpurea*.

CAUTION This plant is poisonous in large doses. It should not to be taken if pregnant, breast-feeding, or by anyone with high blood pressure.

SOLANACEAE

Hyoscyamus niger

Henbane

History and traditions This is a poisonous herb with a long history. It appears in the works of Dioscorides, Pliny and other classical writers as a sleep-inducing and pain-relieving drug and is mentioned in Anglo-Saxon herbals under the name of "Henbell". In Greek mythology the dead, consigned to the underworld kingdom of Hades, were crowned with wreaths of henbane. Its narcotic properties, inducing giddiness and stupor, made it a sought-after herb for witches' brews and sorcerers' spells. It is thought to have provided the "leprous distillment" poured into the ear of Hamlet's father as he lay sleeping. Seventeenth-century herbals recognized its deadly nature, recommending it for external use only, and dental practitioners of the time burned seeds of henbane in chafing dishes to produce analgesic fumes as they treated their patients.

Description An annual or biennial, growing to 60–90/cm/2–3ft, it has a rank, unpleasant smell and coarsely toothed, grey-green, sticky leaves. Bell-shaped, creamy-yellow flowers, veined with purple, grow from the leaf axils and appear throughout the summer, followed by fruit capsules containing many seeds.

Habitat/distribution Probably originated in the Mediterranean region, now widely distributed in Europe and Asia, found in sandy waste ground and coastal sites.

Growth Grow in poor, stony or sandy soils. Propagated from seed sown *in situ* in spring, often self-seeds.

Parts used Leaves, flowering tops – dried for use by the pharmaceutical industry.

USES Medicinal It contains toxic alkaloids hyoscyamine, hyoscine and atropine (as in *Atropa bella-donna*) which affect the central nervous system. These constituents are included in some pharmaceutical drugs for asthma and nervous disorders. Also for muscle spasms and tremors as suffered in senility and diseases associated with old age.

Other name Hogbean.

CAUTION All parts are highly poisonous. Henbane is for use by qualified practitioners only and should never be used for self-medication. Legally restricted in some countries.

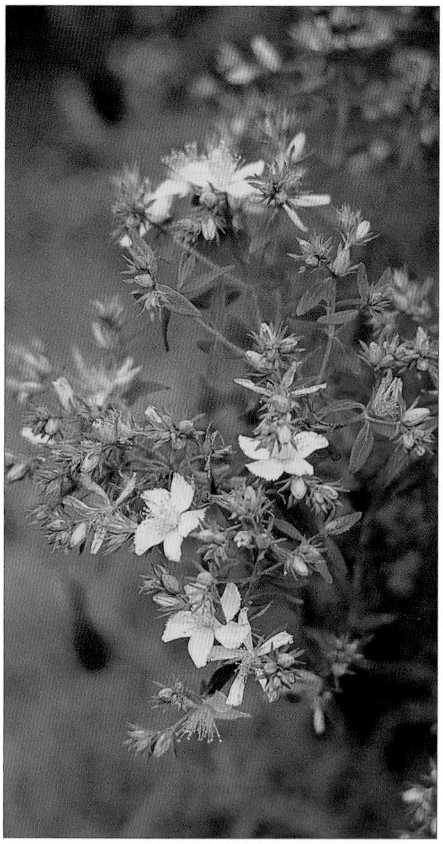

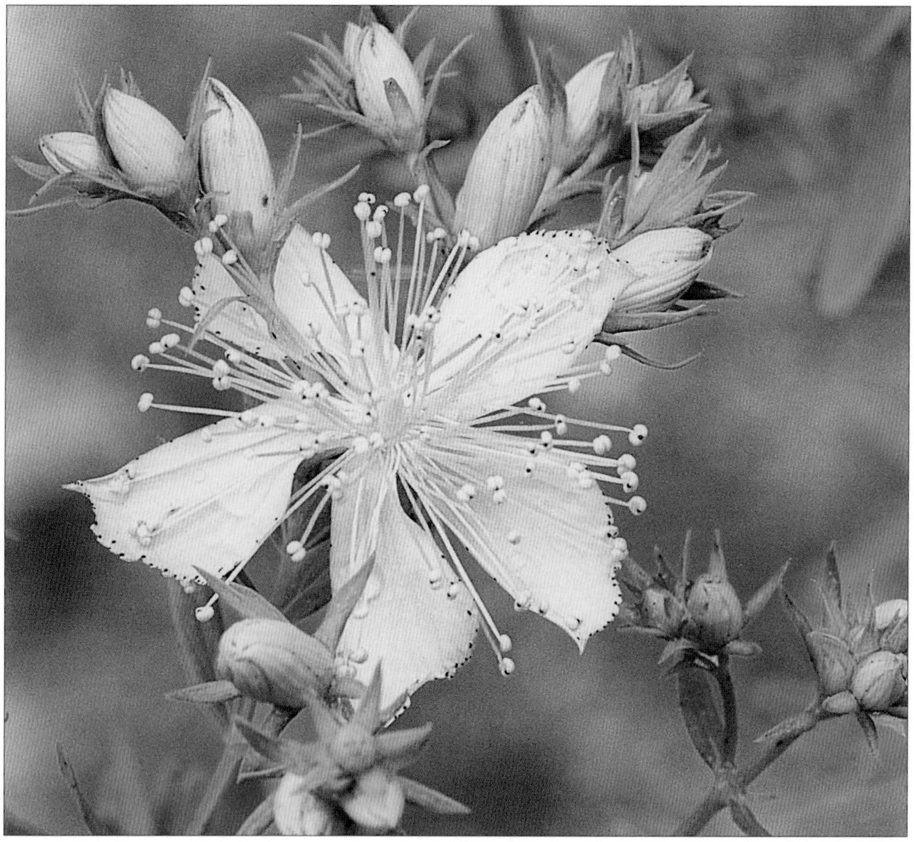

GUTTIFERAE/CLUSIACEAE

Hypericum perforatum

St John's wort

History and traditions This is a herb that has attracted a wealth of folklore over the centuries and been ascribed many magical and mystical properties. It is named after St John the Baptist, the red pigment, hypericin, which exudes from the crushed flowers signifying his blood. It is in full flower on St John's Day, 24 June, which also coincides with northern hemisphere midsummer rituals, and it was ascribed the power to drive away ghosts and witches and protect from thunderbolts and lightning. Many superstitions surrounded it, including gathering it on St John's Eve with the dew still on it in order to find a husband, or as a childless wife, gathering it naked to ensure a speedy conception. It has, in fact, been discovered recently to be an effective antidepressant, being effective for mild to moderate depression, without the side effects of conventional drugs. In Germany it has a medical licence and has been widely prescribed for depressive states, outselling Prozac eight times over. But as with many beneficial plants, there are contra-indications which should be taken into account (see CAUTION).

Description It is a hardy perennial, about 30–60cm/1–2ft in height; the stems are erect, woody at the base, with small linear-oval leaves, dotted with glands, which can be seen as little pinpricks when held up to the light. The flowers have five petals, edged with glands.

Habitat/distribution A native of Europe and temperate Asia, found in woodlands, and in hedgerows on semi-dry soils. Naturalized in America and Australia.

Growth Grow in well-drained, dryish soil in full sun or partial shade. Propagation by division is the easiest method; it can also be grown from seed sown in spring or autumn, and spreads rapidly once established.

Parts used Flowering tops – fresh or dried for use in infusions, creams, oils, and as liquid extracts for use in pharmaceutical preparations.

USES Medicinal It is said to have calming properties. Infusions are taken for anxiety and nervous tension. It also has antiseptic and anti-inflammatory properties and promotes healing; creams and infused oils are applied to burns, muscular pain, neuralgia and sciatica.

Above *The flowers of* Hypericum perforatum *contain the active principle hypericin.*

St John's wort oil

To make an infused massage oil to help ease inflammation and joint pain:

25g/1oz flowering tops of St John's wort
600ml/1 pint/2½ cups sunflower oil

Put the flowering tops into a bowl and crush them lightly. Pour in the oil. Stand the bowl over a pan of barely simmering water and heat gently for 1 hour. Strain off the herb by pouring it through muslin fixed over a jug, then transfer to a clean, airtight bottle.

CAUTION May interact with pharmaceutical drugs. Only to be taken on medical advice if on other medication and under the care of a medical herbalist. Can cause sensitivity to sunlight. Harmful if eaten, poisonous to livestock, statutorily controlled in some countries.

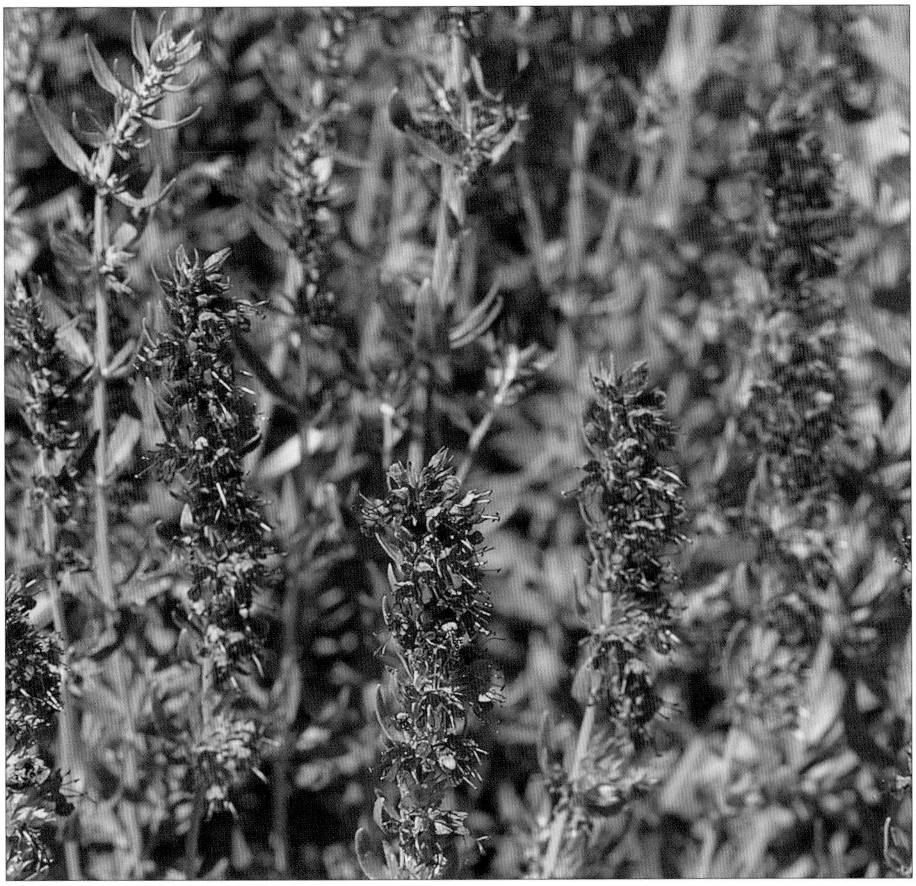

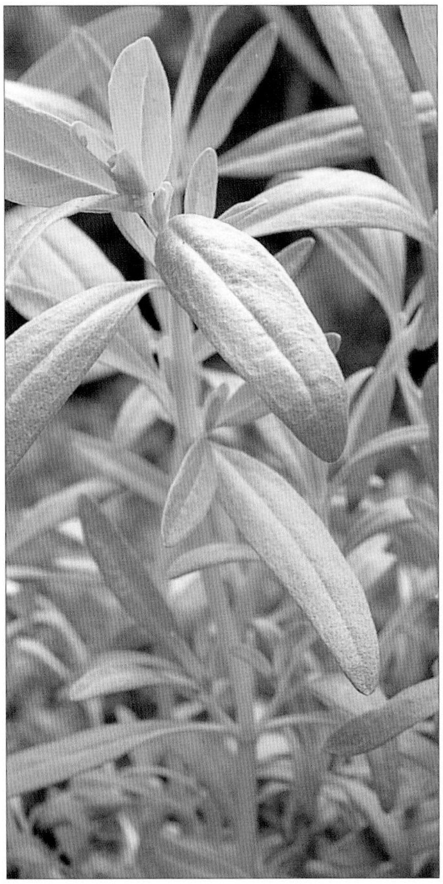

Above left *Hyssop flowers add colour to the garden in mid to late summer.*

Above *The leaves have a pungent flavour, popular in Elizabethan culinary dishes.*

LABIATAE/LAMIACEAE

Hyssopus officinalis

Hyssop

History and traditions The name is an ancient one – it is virtually the same in all European languages and comes from the Greek, *hyssopos.* In Hebrew it is *ezob,* meaning a "holy herb", though it is not certain whether the hyssop we know is the plant referred to in the Bible. Hippocrates and Dioscorides rated it highly as a medicinal herb, recommending it for respiratory disorders – as it is still used in herbal medicine today. Its strong, aromatic smell meant it was suitable for strewing in rooms in the house – and is included for this purpose in Thomas Tusser's list (*Five Hundred Points of Good Husbandry,* 1580). It frequently featured in designs for knot gardens of the 17th century, was a popular culinary herb used in "pottages" (soups) and salads, and was taken as a tea, or made into syrups and cordials for coughs and colds. It was one of the original ingredients of the liqueur, Chartreuse.

Description Classed as a semi-evergreen, because it loses some foliage in winter, mainly if weather is severe. It is a bushy perennial, about 60–90cm/2–3ft high. The stems are woody at the base with small, dark green, linear leaves and dense spikes of deep blue flowers in late summer, which are very attractive to bees. There are also forms with pink and white flowers.

Habitat/distribution Native to the Mediterranean region and western Asia, found on dry, rocky soils. Introduced and widely grown throughout Europe and North America.

Growth Grow in well-drained to dry soil in a sunny position. Propagated by seed sown in spring, or by cuttings taken in summer. Prune back hard in spring to prevent it becoming straggly (it will regenerate from the old wood).

Parts used Leaves, flowers – fresh or dried.

USES Medicinal Hyssop has expectorant properties, promotes sweating and is anti-catarrhal and antibacterial. Infusions are taken for coughs, colds and chest infections.

Culinary The leaves have a strong, slightly bitter flavour and may be added to soups and cooked meat and vegetable dishes with discretion. The attractive blue flowers make a pretty garnish for salads.

Old recipes for hyssop

• A Water to Cause an Excellent Colour and Complexion: Drink six spoonfuls of the juice of Hyssop in warm Ale in a Morning and fasting. From *The Receipt Book of John Nott*, cook to the Duke of Bolton, 1723.

• To Make Syrup of Hysop for Colds: Take an handful of Hysop, of Figs, Raysins, Dates, of each an ounce, French Barley one ounce, boyl therein three pintes of fair water to a quart, strain it and clarifie it with two Whites of Eggs, then put in two pound of fine Sugar and boyl it to a Syrup.

The Queen's Closet Opened, W. M., cook to Queen Henrietta Maria, 1655.

COMPOSITAE/ASTERACEAE

Inula helenium

Elecampane

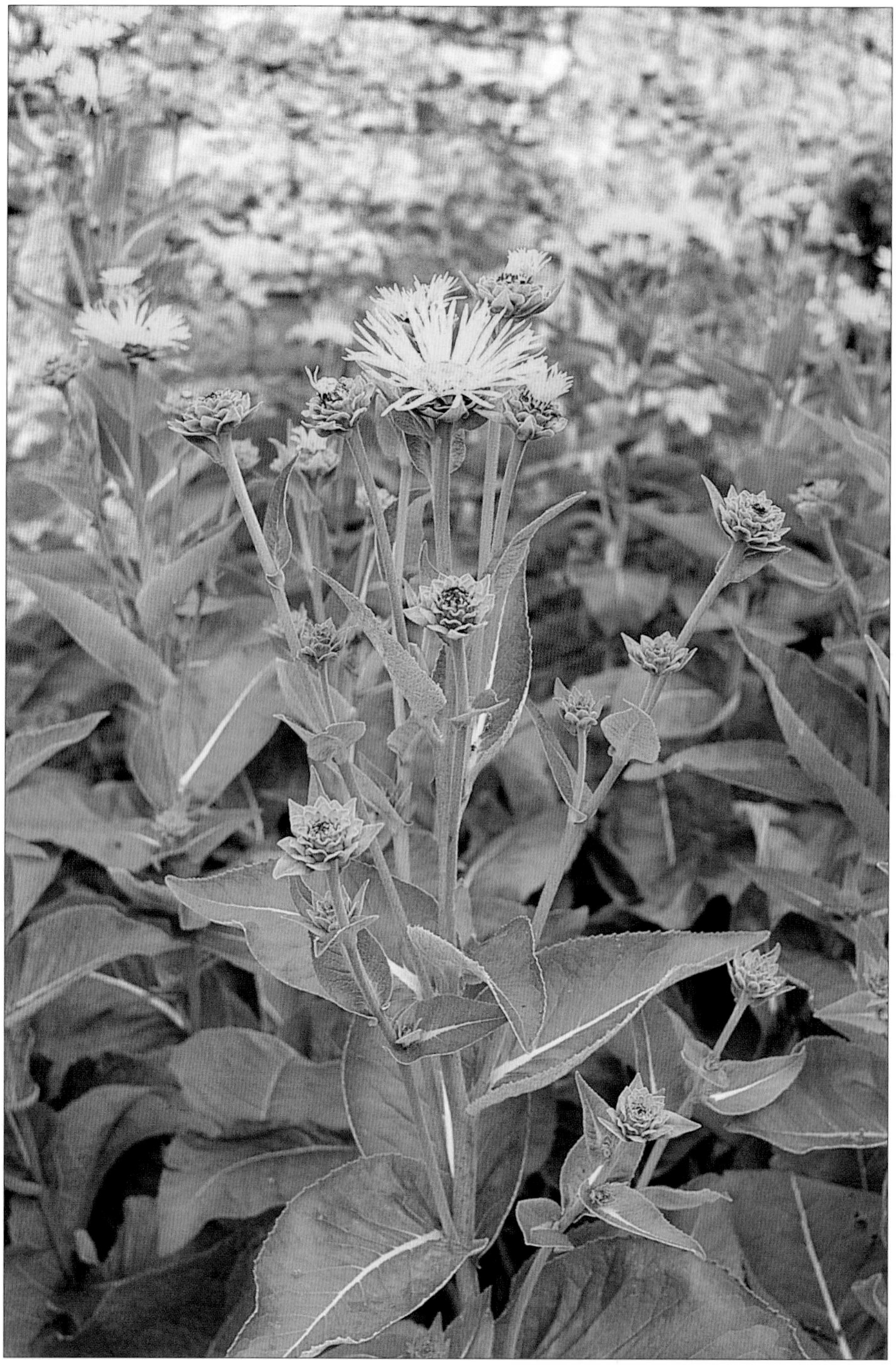

History and traditions It is said to be named after Helen of Troy, who was gathering this herb when abducted by Paris, or, according to another version, it grew from her tears on the same occasion. In any case it is an ancient herb, well known to the Greeks and Romans, who ate it as a bitter vegetable and digestive after a heavy meal. They also appreciated its medicinal properties – Galen recommended it for sciatica and Pliny thought that the root "being chewed fasting, doth fasten teeth". It appears frequently in Anglo-Saxon medical texts and in the writings of Welsh physicians of Myddfai in the 13th century. It remained popular in folk medicine as a cough and asthma remedy over the centuries, and was grown in cottage gardens. The roots were often candied and old herbals contain many recipes for conserves, cough remedies and tonics made of this plant. John Lindley in his *Flora Medica*, 1838, remarks, "The plant is generally kept in rustic gardens, on account of many traditional virtues."

Description A hardy perennial, with tall, erect, softly hairy stems, to 2/m/6ft in height, it has ovate, pointed leaves, toothed at the edges, and terminal yellow flower heads, shaped like shaggy daisies, in late summer.

Habitat/distribution Native to southern Europe and western Asia, naturalized in North America, introduced elsewhere in warm and temperate zones. Found on damp soils, near ruins, in woodland and field edges.

Conserve of elecampane root

Cleanse and scrape the root. Cut them into thin round slices, letting them soke in water over the hot embers ... boil them till all the liquor be wasted. Beat them in a stone mortar, very fine. Boyle the whole with a like weighte of honey or sugar two or three times over. All other roots may in like manner be candied ... but far pleasanter in the eating if to the confection a quantity of cinnamon be added. Candy the roots in October.
From *The Gardener's Labyrinth*, by Thomas Hill, 1577.

Growth Grow in rich, moist soil in a sunny position. Propagated by division of roots in spring or autumn, or by seed, which may be slow to germinate.

Parts used Roots, flowers – fresh or dried.

USES Medicinal The constituents of this herb include up to 40 per cent insulin. But its chief use in herbal medicine is for coughs, hay fever, asthma, catarrh and respiratory infections, taken as infusions or decoctions (these must be filtered to exclude irritant fibres). Elecampane is also said to have a beneficial effect on the digestion when taken internally. Applied externally it is said to relieve many skin inflammations and irritations and has sometimes been recommended as an embrocation, or rub, for the relief of sciatica and neuralgia.

CAUTION Not to be taken in pregnancy or while breastfeeding. May cause allergic reaction or gastric upsets.

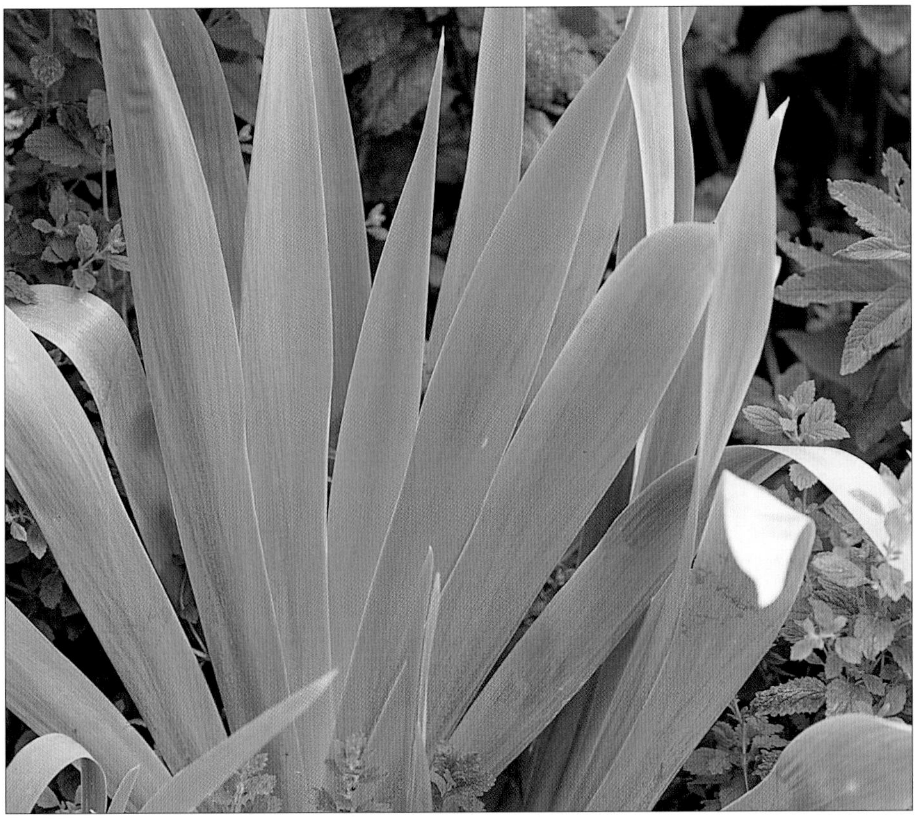

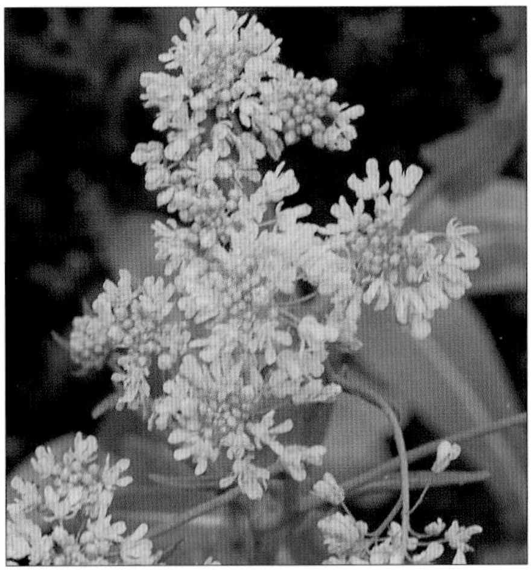

IRIDACEAE

Iris germanica var. *florentina*

Orris

History and traditions Orris, taken directly from the Greek *iris*, is the name for the powdered rhizome of the Florentine iris, which has been valued since ancient Egyptian times for its faint violet scent and fixative properties in perfumery and potpourri. During the 18th century it was incorporated in many cosmetic powders for wigs, hair and teeth. This variety of iris has been associated with Florence, in Italy, since the 13th century, when it was first cultivated there on a large scale, and can still be seen on the city's coat of arms.
Description A hardy perennial, growing on a stout rhizome, 60–90cm/2–3ft tall, with narrow, sword-shaped leaves. Flowers are white, with outer petals mauve-tinged and yellow-bearded, or occasionally pure white.
Habitat/distribution Native to southern Europe, naturalized in central Europe, the Middle East and northern India, introduced elsewhere. Found in sunny, stony, hilly locations.
Growth Grow in well-drained soil in full sun. Propagated by division of rhizomes and offsets in late summer to early autumn.
Parts used Rhizomes – dried and powdered.

USES Aromatic An indispensable ingredient for making potpourri and scented sachet mixtures. It enhances the scent of the other ingredients and gives the whole preparation a more lasting quality. Also used in commercial potpourri products and perfumery.
Cosmetic Occasionally seen as an ingredient of home-made toothpowders. A constituent of commercial dental preparations and scented dusting powders.
Other name Florentine iris.

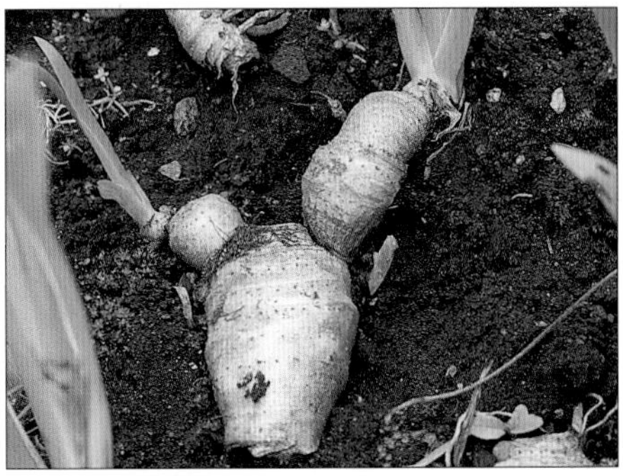

Above *The rhizome of the Florentine iris is dried to make orris root powder.*

CAUTION All parts of the plant are harmful if eaten – the powdered root causes vomiting. May cause skin irritations.

CRUCIFERAE/BRASSICACEAE

Isatis tinctoria

Woad

History and traditions Woad was the source of the blue body paint of the ancient Britons, described by Pliny and other Roman writers. Although largely replaced by indigo, from the subtropical *indigofera* species, in the 1630s and then by synthetics at the end of the 19th century, a factory producing dye from woad existed in England until the 1930s.
Description A hardy biennial (or short-lived perennial if flower heads are cut before seeding), it grows on a taproot, from 0.5–1.2m/20in–4ft tall. In the first year it produces a rosette of ovate leaves, from which branching stems with lanceolate leaves topped by racemes of yellow flowers grow in summer, followed by pendulous black seeds.
Habitat/distribution Indigenous to Europe and western Asia, introduced elsewhere. Found on chalky (alkaline) soils in sunny, open sites.
Growth Grow in humus-rich, moist but well-drained soil, in full sun. Propagated by seed sown in containers in spring, maintaining a temperature of 13–18°C/55–64°F or in autumn for overwintering in a cold frame. Does not flourish in the same ground for more than a few years.
Parts used Leaves – dried, fermented and also powdered for use as a dye. Leaves and roots – dried for Chinese herbal preparations.

USES Medicinal Traditionally a wound-healing herb, as well as a dye, it has long been used in Chinese herbal medicine and recently discovered to have antiviral properties.
General The leaves yield a very fast blue dye.

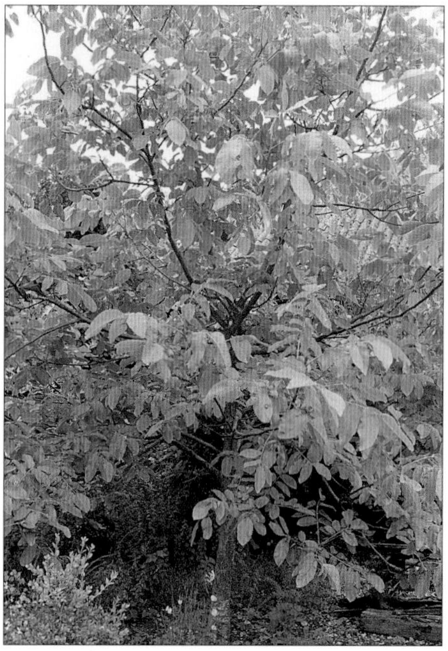

JUGLANDACEAE

Juglans regia

Walnut

History and traditions The walnut tree has been valued since ancient Greek times for its medicinal properties and many uses. It was known to the Romans as a fertility symbol and Pliny was the first to give directions for making it into a dye for restoring grey hair to brown – a use which lasted into the 20th century.

Description A variable deciduous tree, growing to about 30m/99ft, it has pinnate leaves, with 7–9 ovate leaflets. Male catkins and female flowers are followed by dark green fruits, each containing a wrinkled brown nut.

Habitat/distribution Native to south eastern Europe, Asia, China and the Himalayas, widely introduced elsewhere.

Growth Walnut trees require deep, rich soil and a sunny position.

Parts used Leaves, bark, fruit, oil.

USES Medicinal Infusions of the leaves are taken internally as a digestive tonic and applied externally for cuts, grazes and skin disorders, such as eczema. Decoctions of the inner bark are used for constipation and of the outer nut rind for diarrhoea.

Culinary The nuts are included in many dishes. Oil from the seeds is popular for salads, especially in France.

Cosmetic An infusion of the nut rind is said to make a hair restorer.

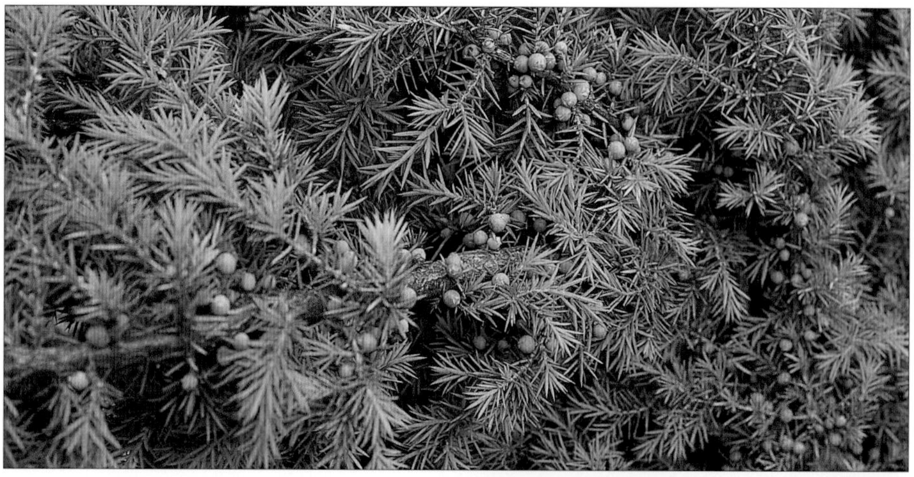

CUPRESSACEAE

Juniperus communis

Juniper

History and traditions From biblical times juniper has symbolized protection, and there are many references to people using it for shelter. "Elijah went a day's journey into the wilderness and came and sat down under a juniper tree" (I Kings 19:4). In medieval Europe a fire of juniper wood was burned to discourage evil spirits and protect from plague – and it was thought that felling a tree would bring a death in the family within a year. Its medicinal properties were recorded by the ancient Greek and Roman physicians. Culpeper recommended it, among many other uses, as "a counter-poison, resister of the pestilence and excellent against the biting of venomous beasts". It is famous as a flavouring ingredient of gin – the English word being an abbreviation of "Holland's Geneva" as gin was first known, from the Dutch word for juniper, *jenever.*

Description A hardy, coniferous, evergreen shrub or small tree, 2–4m/6–13ft tall, of upright or prostrate form with needle-like leaves. The small, spherical fruits, borne on the female plants, are green at first, and take two years to ripen to blue black.

Related species Various junipers were used medicinally by Native Americans, including *J. virginiana*, which produces the extremely toxic red cedar oil. *J. sabina* has poisonous berries and should not be confused with those of *J. communis.*

Habitat/distribution Widely distributed in the northern hemisphere of Europe, Asia and North America on heaths, moors and mountain slopes. Those grown in warmer regions, with longer, sunnier summers, such as the Mediterranean, have sweeter, more aromatic berries.

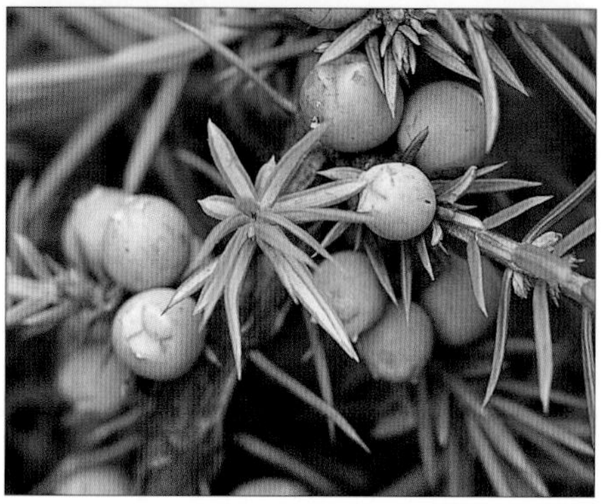

Above *Unripened juniper berries.*

Growth Tolerant of most soils. For berry production grow female plants in a sunny position. Propagated by heel cuttings in late summer, or by seed sown in containers under cover in spring or autumn.

Parts used Fruits – collected from wild plants for use fresh, dried or for distillation of the volatile oil.

USES Medicinal The berries have antiseptic, anti-inflammatory and digestive properties and are thought to be helpful for rheumatism, gout, arthritis and colic. This is a strong herb and should only be used for short periods of time.

Culinary Juniper is added to pickles, chutneys, sauces, marinades, meat and game dishes, pâtés and sauerkraut.

General Used to flavour gin. Oil is used in cosmetics and perfumery.

CAUTION The berries are not given to patients with kidney disease, or to pregnant women, as they are a uterine stimulant.

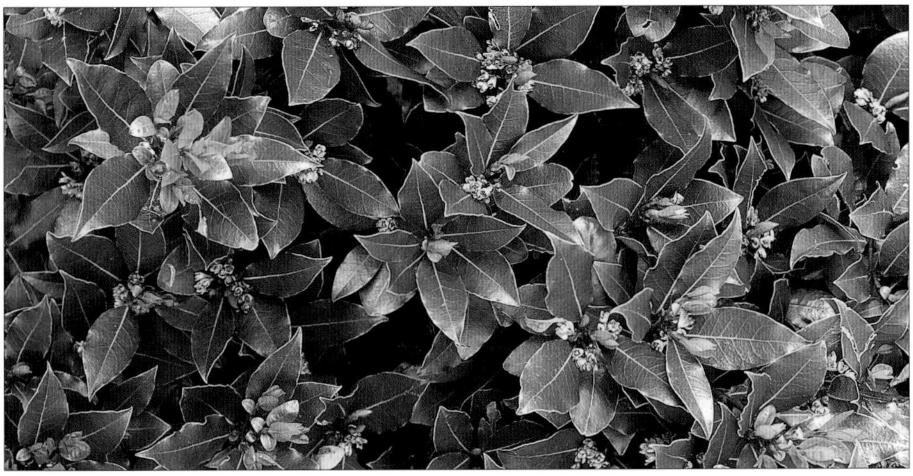

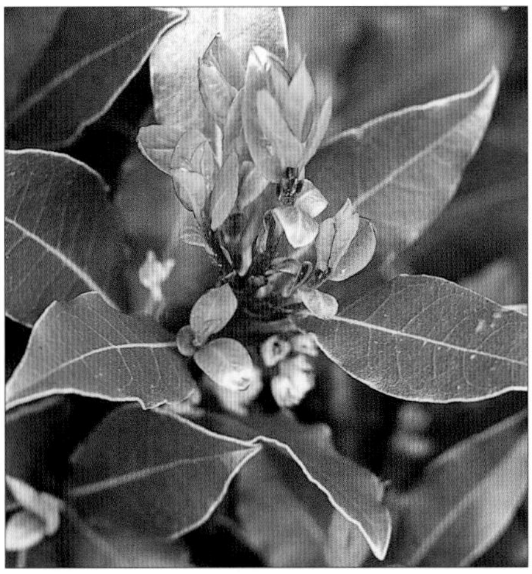

LAURACEAE

Laurus nobilis

Bay

History and traditions This is the plant from which the victor's crown of laurels was made – the Latin name is from *laurus* (praise) and *nobilis* (renowned or noble). It was dedicated to Apollo, Greek god of music, healing, light and truth, and many superstitions arose as to its powers. In the writings of Theophrastus there is a reference to the custom of keeping a bay leaf in the mouth to prevent misfortune and by Roman times it had gained a reputation for preventing lightning strikes – the emperor Tiberius always wore a laurel wreath on his head during thunderstorms as a precaution. Bay trees were also thought to purify the air where they grew. During a plague epidemic, the Roman emperor Claudius moved his court to Laurentium, named after the bay trees that grew there, because of the protection they would provide. Introduced to Britain from the Mediterranean, the sweet bay tree brought its reputation with it. Writing in the 17th century, Culpeper said of it, "Neither witch nor devil, thunder nor lightning will hurt a man where a bay tree is." A wreath of bay leaves was the traditional garnish for the boar's head, centrepiece of the Yuletide feast.

Description An evergreen shrub, or small tree, 3–15m/10–50ft tall, it has aromatic dark green, glossy ovate leaves. Clusters of small creamy-yellow flowers, opening from tight round buds, appear in spring, followed by purple-black berries.

Related species *L. n.* 'Aurea' is an attractive cultivar with golden-yellow foliage.

Habitat/distribution Native to southern Europe, the Mediterranean and North Africa, introduced and widely grown in other warm temperate regions.

Growth Grow in fertile, reasonably moist but well-drained soil in a sheltered, sunny position. Although frost hardy, it needs winter protection when immature; and foliage is sometimes damaged by severe frosts and cold winds. Propagated by semi-ripe cuttings in summer.

Parts used Leaves – fresh or dried. Essential oil.

USES Medicinal Bay is not widely used in modern herbal medicine. But studies carried out in the late 1980s on the ability of herbs to inhibit bacterial growth showed bay to be one of the most effective.

Culinary A first-rate culinary herb, a bay leaf is always included in a *bouquet garni,* and adds flavour to marinades, casseroles, stews, soups and dishes requiring a long cooking time. Also used to flavour sweet sauces and as a garnish for citrus sorbets.

Above *Bay leaves for culinary use have a more agreeable, less bitter flavour when dried.*

Below *A standard bay tree in a pot.*

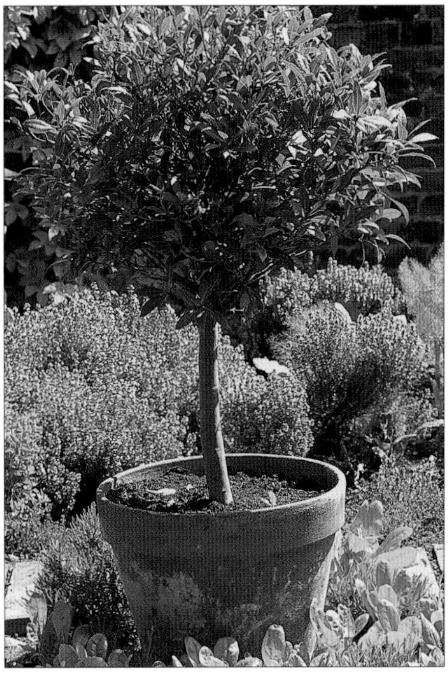

Decorative bay

The Romans embellished their houses with branches of bay for the festival of Saturnalia, celebrated between 17th and 23rd December, to coincide with the winter solstice. With Christianity, bay became a symbol of eternal life, as did other evergreens, and was once widely used as a decoration for homes and churches during the Christmas season. The aromatic, dark green leaves make it ideal for festive decorations today.

- Bay leaves make an impressive and welcoming wreath for the front door. Push them into a base of floral foam, in a circular holder, and decorate with fir cones, shiny red apples and ribbon.
- A glass bowl filled with floating candles surrounded by bay leaves makes a spectacular, fragrant table-centre.
- A mophead bay (tree-form standard), studded with baubles, makes an attractive alternative to a fir Christmas tree.

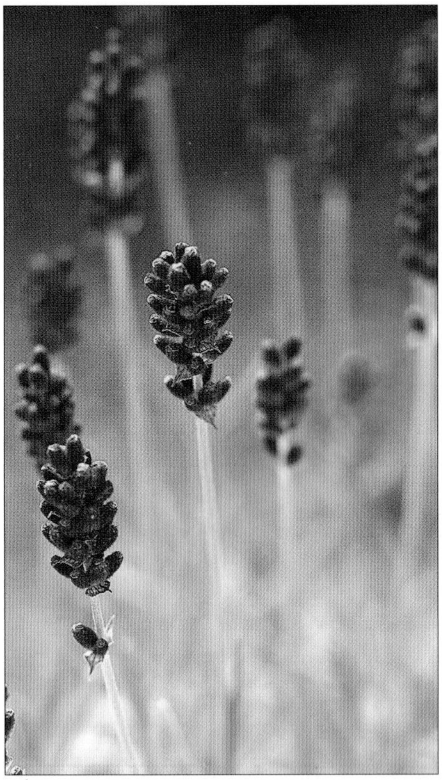

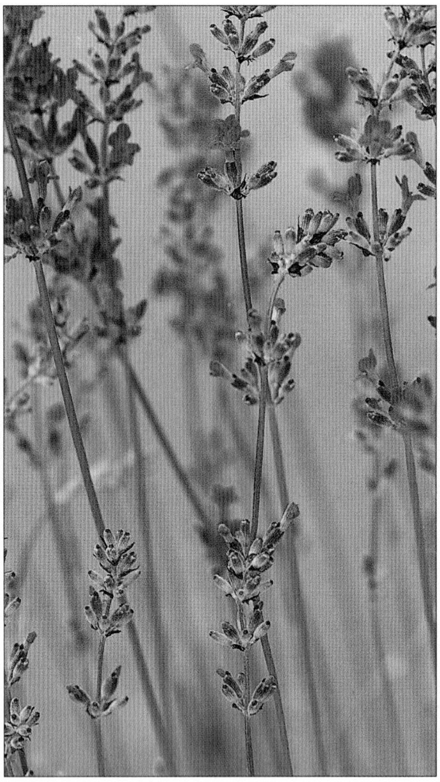

LABIATAE/LAMIACEAE

Lavandula

History and traditions The Romans are said to have scented their bathwater with lavender (the Latin name is from *lavare,* to wash) and its inimitable fragrance has ensured its lasting popularity. Its medicinal and insecticidal properties were also recognized early and have been largely vindicated since. In 1387 at the court of Charles VI of France all the cushions were stuffed with lavender both for its pleasant scent and to deter insects. It was an essential ingredient of "Four Thieves' Vinegar", which is supposed to have given immunity to those who robbed the bodies of plague victims, and William Turner had the idea "that the flowers of Lavender quilted in a cap and dayly worne are good for all diseases of the head that come of a cold cause and that they comfort the braine very well" (*A New Herball,* 1551). In the early years of this century, René Gattefosse, one of the founders of aromatherapy, discovered the powers of lavender when his badly burned hand was healed after it had been immersed in undiluted essential oil of lavender. And since then, modern scientific research has established the antiseptic, antibacterial properties of this herb.

Description and species Lavender has been cultivated for so long that accurate identification is not always easy, and most of those grown in gardens are hybrids or cultivars. There are three important groups of lavenders (but this by no means provides a definitive list or complete explanation of lavender nomenclature):

1. ***L. angustifolia*** **(common lavender, English lavender)** – Has small purple flowers, grows to 60–90cm/2–3ft, and is said to be effective for medicinal purposes. It has many attractive cultivars, which may not have the same degree of medicinal qualities, but are probably more suitable for fragrant, culinary and decorative purposes. These include ***L. a.*** **'Hidcote'** – with a neat, erect habit and strongly scented, deep violet flowers, 30–60cm/1–2ft. *L. a.* 'Munstead' is more compact, 30–45cm/12–18in, with paler, purple flowers. ***L. a.*** **'Nana Alba'** is a dwarf, white-flowered cultivar, 15–30cm/6–12in. There are also some pink-flowered cultivars, such as ***L. a.*** **'Rosea'**.
2. *L.* x ***intermedia*** **'Grey Hedge'** are hybrids of ***L. angustifolia*** and ***L. latifolia*** and include ***L.*** **x *intermedia*** **'Grappenhall'**, which has long spikes of lavender-blue flowers, and ***L.*** x ***intermedia*** **'Twickel Purple'**, with shorter, bushier flowers.
3. *L.* ***stoechas*** **(French or Spanish Lavender)** – This is a species that is also considered to have medicinal value – and was probably the type of lavender known to the Greeks and Romans. It has short, fat spikes of dark purple flowers, topped by butterfly wing bracts, and grows from 30–90cm/1–3ft.

Habitat/distribution Lavender is native to the Mediterranean and Middle East, introduced and widely grown elsewhere.

Growth Requires a very well-drained soil and plenty of sun. Lavenders hybridize easily; most do not come true from seed and they are best propagated from heel cuttings taken in mid- to late summer. *L. angustifolia* and cultivars are hardy, so are *L.* x *intermedia* and cultivars. *L. stoechas* is frost-hardy. (Some other species of lavender are tender or half-hardy).

Parts used Flowers – fresh or dried, and the essential oil.

USES Medicinal Infusions of the flowers may be applied as a compress to ease headaches, and are sometimes taken internally (made weak) for anxiety and nervous exhaustion. As an embrocation an external stimulant and antiseptic.

Above left Lavandula angustifolia *'Hidcote'.*

Above right Lavandula angustifolia *'Munstead'.*

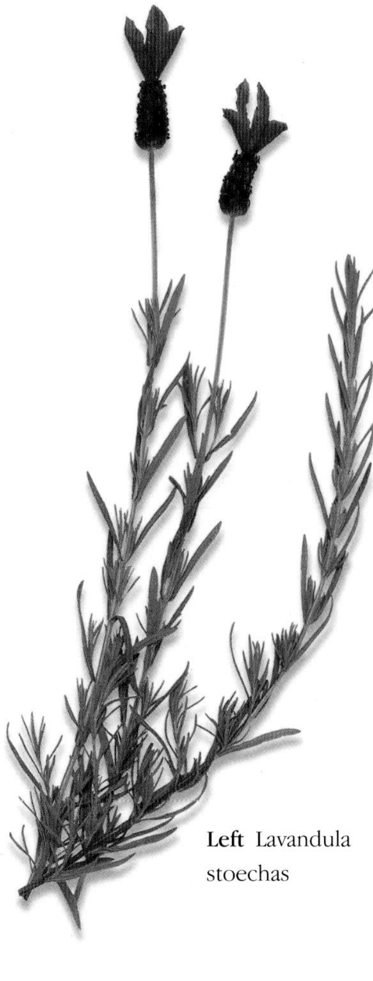

Left Lavandula stoechas

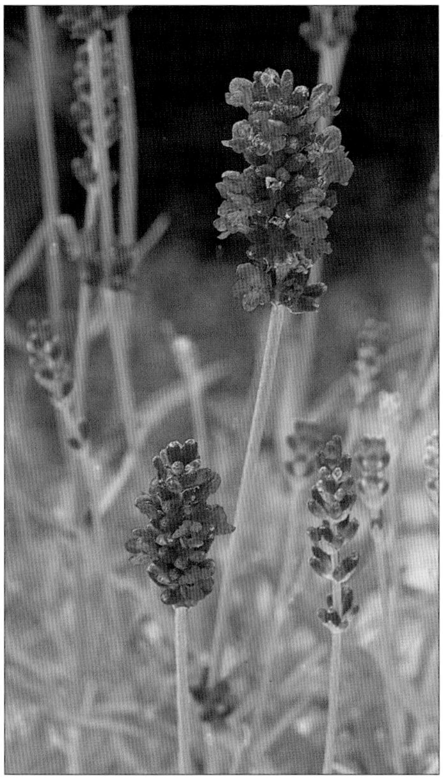

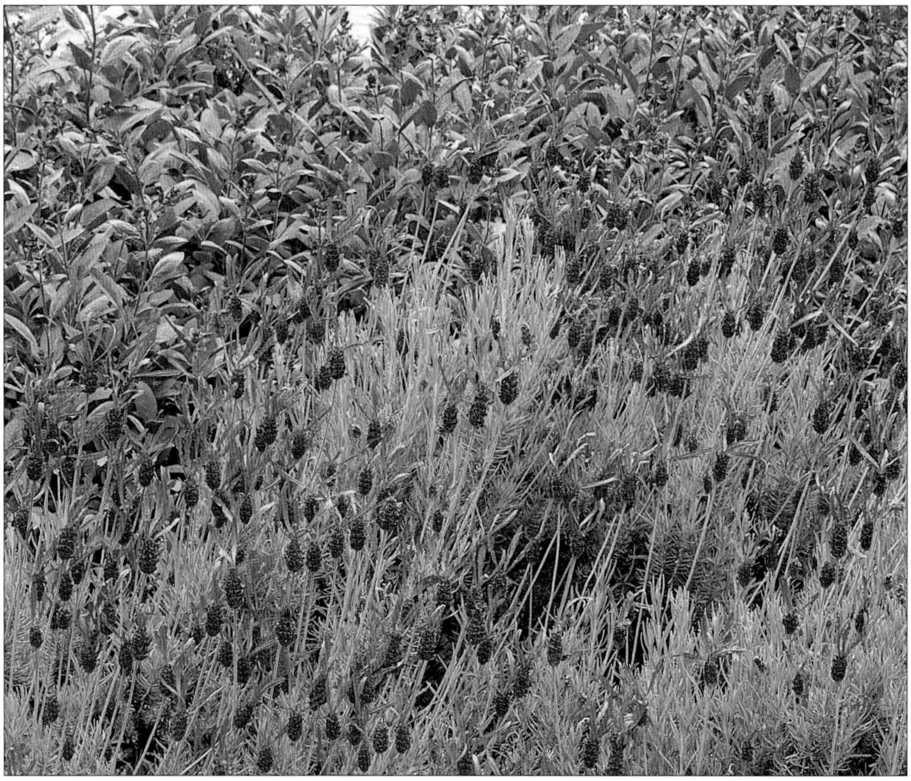

Essential oil (diluted in a carrier oil) is applied to sunburn, burns and scalds, or used as a massage oil for tension headaches, migraine and muscular aches and pains. Inhaling the fragrance of flowers or oil can be very calming, anti-depressive and may help relieve insomnia. The oil is applied to prevent and relieve insect bites and discourages head lice when applied to the comb.

Culinary Flowers are used to flavour sugar for making cakes, biscuits, meringues, ice creams and desserts. They can be added to vinegar, marmalade or jam, or cooked (tied in a muslin bag) with blackcurrants or soft fruit mixtures.

Cosmetic Infusions of fresh flowers make a fragrant hair rinse, or they can be tied in bags to scent bathwater. Drops of essential oil are also added to baths or included in home-made beauty preparations. Lavender oil is widely used in commercial perfumery.

Aromatic Flowers are dried for potpourri and scented sachets.

Top left Lavandula x intermedia *'Twickle Purple'*.

Top right Lavandula pedunculata *subsp.* pedunculata *with purple sage.*

Centre right Lavandula angustifolia *'Rosea'*.

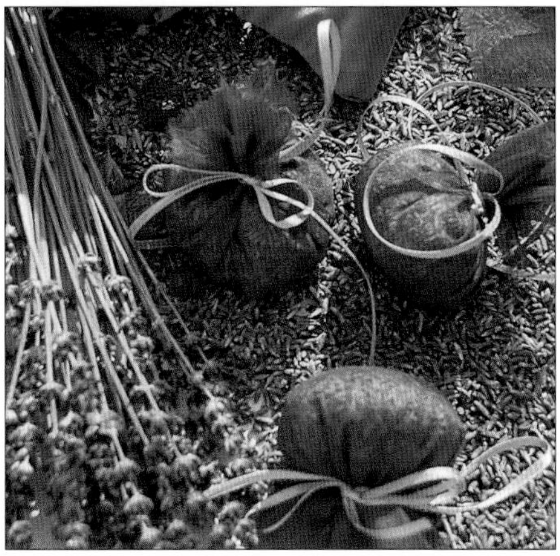

Above *Dried lavender is a traditional filling for scented sachets.*

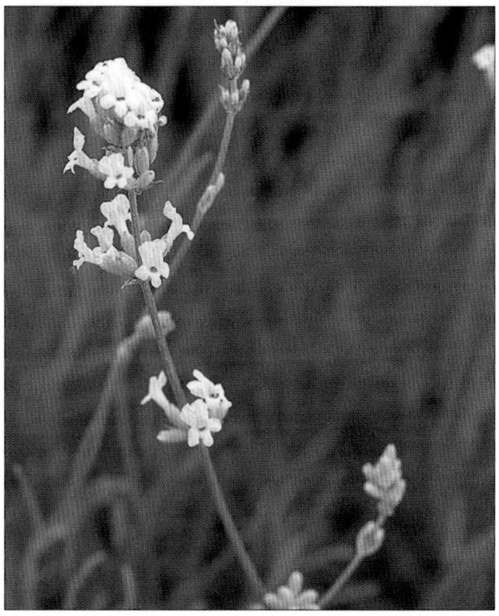

Lavender sachets

The flowers of lavender have been used for centuries to scent clothes and deter moths and insects.

• **To dry your own lavender:** Cut the flowers with long stalks, as soon as they are fully open, on a dry day, but before the essential oils evaporate in the sun. Tie with raffia or string, in small bunches and hang up in a warm, dry place, with the heads suspended in paper bags – to keep off dust and catch petals as they fall. When fully dry, this will take about a week, depending on humidity and air temperature, rub the petals off the heads.

• **To make the sachets:** Cut circles of muslin, or any fine see-through fabric, put a small handful of dried lavender in the centre, gather up to form a bundle and fasten at the neck with an elastic band. Finish with a ribbon.

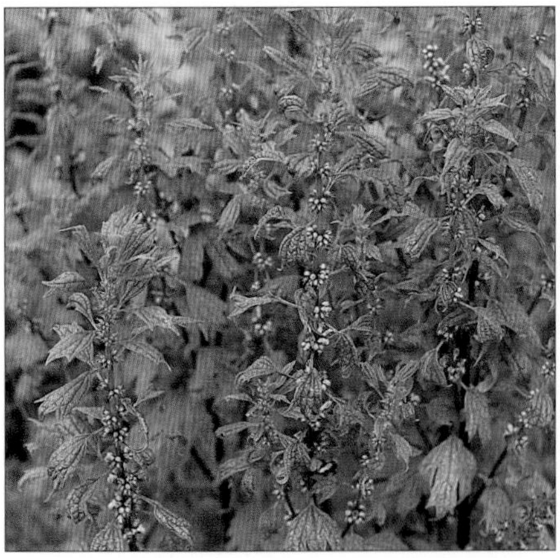

LABIATAE/LAMIACEAE

Leonurus cardiaca

Motherwort

History and traditions In ancient Greece, this herb was given to pregnant women to calm their anxieties. The generic name, *Leonurus,* refers to the plant's supposed resemblance to a lion's tail, but the specific name, *cardiaca,* comes directly from the Greek word for heart because of its widespread use in former times for treating heart palpitations and afflictions. *Macer's Herbal*, 1530 attributes to it supernatural powers against wicked spirits.

Description A tall, hardy, strong-smelling perennial, growing to 1.2m/4ft, it has square, hollow stems, with deeply lobed, prominently veined leaves, set opposite each other. The mauve-pink, double-lipped flowers appear in the upper leaf axils throughout summer. Widely grown in herb gardens for its attractive foliage.

Habitat/distribution Indigenous to Europe and western Asia. Introduced elsewhere. Found on roadsides and waste grounds on light, calcareous soils.

Growth Grow in moist but well-drained soil in a sunny position. Propagated by seed sown in spring, or by division in spring or autumn.

Parts used Flowering tops – dried for use in infusions, liquid extracts and tinctures.

USES Medicinal Research has shown that this herb has a beneficial and calming effect on the heart, and is mildly sedative. It is used to influence the menstrual cycle.

CAUTION Only to be taken on the advice of qualified herbalist or medical practitioner. Not to be taken in pregnancy.

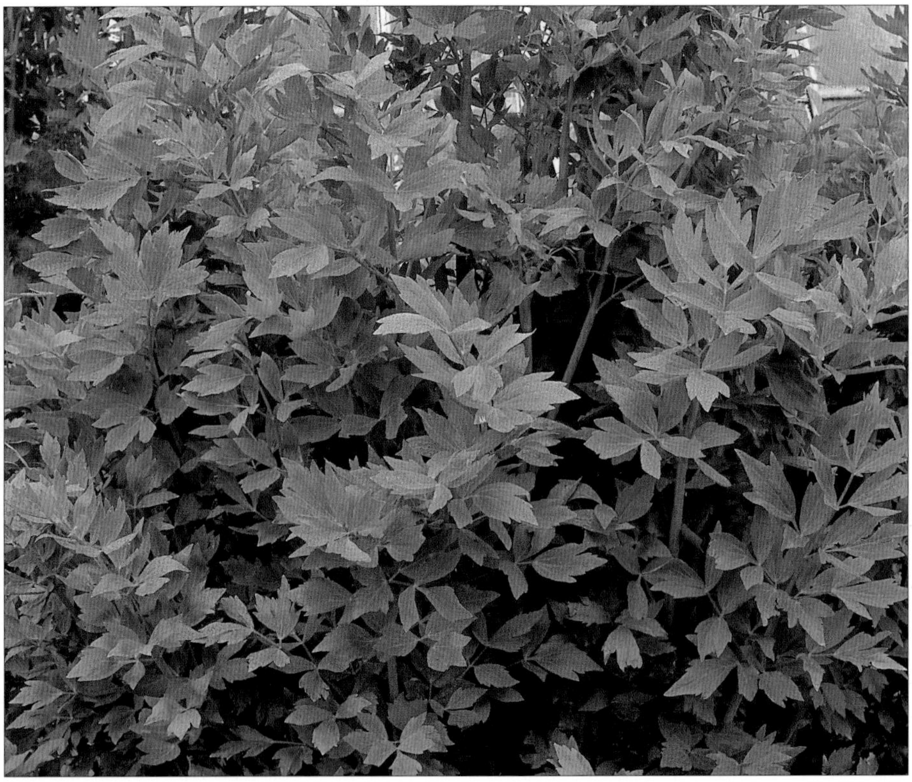

UMBELLIFERAE/APIACEAE

Levisticum officinale

Lovage

History and traditions Lovage has been cultivated since the time of Pliny as a seasoning and digestive herb. The Greeks and Romans chewed the seed to aid digestion, a practice followed by Benedictine monks of the Middle Ages, and Parkinson refers to its "hot, sharpe, biting taste" and culinary usage: "The Germans and other Nations in times past used both the roote and seede instead of Pepper to season their meates and brothes and found them as comfortable and warming" (*Paradisi,* 1629). An earlier writer mentions lovage as a bath herb for its aromatic scent: "This herbe for hys sweete savoure is used in bathe" (*The Gardener's Labyrinth,* 1577). Its former medicinal uses, referred to by many herbalists, included "expelling stone of the kidneys and bladder". All of which remains broadly valid today, though the leaves are used in preference to seeds and roots for culinary purposes.

Description A hardy herbaceous perennial, growing on deep fleshy roots to 2m/6ft in height, it has glossy, deeply divided leaves with a spicy, celery-like scent, and umbels of undistinguished, dull yellow flowers in summer, followed by small seeds.

Habitat/distribution Lovage probably originated in Europe, but has long been widely cultivated throughout the world. Rarely found in the wild, except as a garden escape.

Growth A vigorous, spreading plant, it will grow in most soils (except heavy clay), but thrives best in well-manured, moist but well-drained soil, in sun or partial shade. Propagated from seed sown in spring or by division of the roots in spring or autumn.

Parts used Leaves – fresh or dried for culinary use and infusions; stems – fresh; roots, seeds – dried for use in decoctions and other medicinal preparations; essential oil – distilled from leaves and roots.

USES Medicinal It is taken internally for digestive disorders, colic and flatulence, also for cystitis and kidney stones. Lovage tea was formerly taken for rheumatism. Do not use medicinally during pregnancy.

Culinary Leaves are used to flavour soups, stews, meat, fish or vegetable dishes; young shoots and stems are eaten as a vegetable (like braised celery) and may be candied like angelica; seeds are added to biscuits and bread. Lovage cordial used to be a popular drink.

Aromatic Essential oil is used in perfumery, and as a flavouring in the food and drink industry.

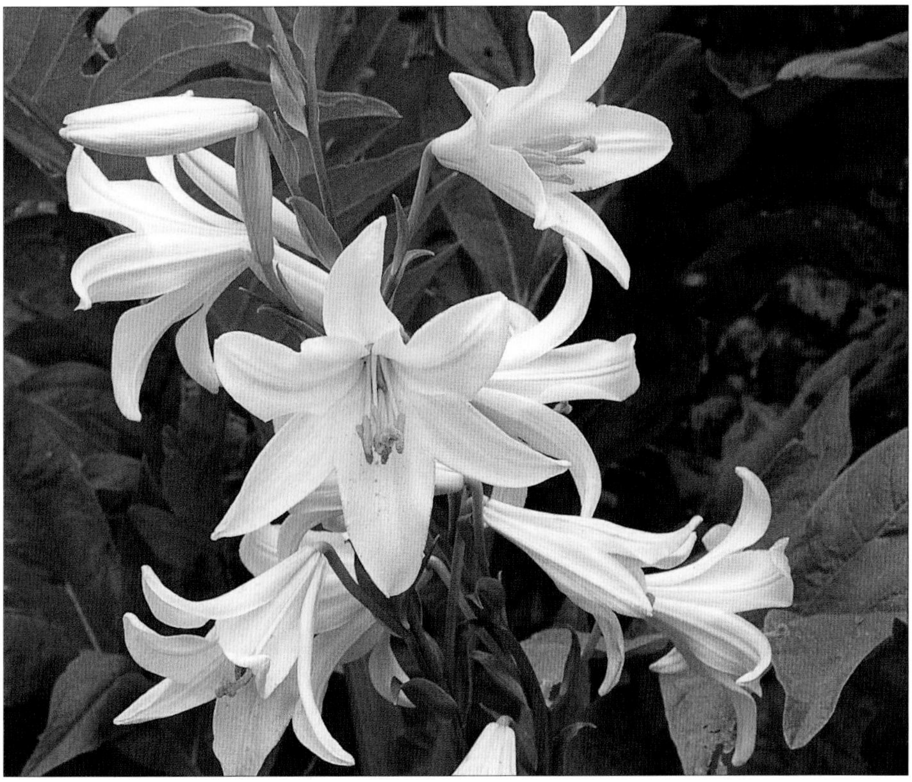

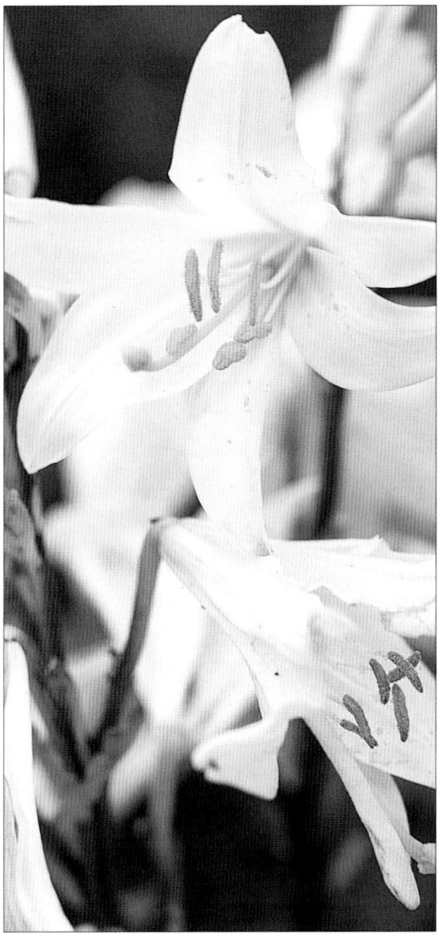

Above *The flawless white blooms of* Lilium candidum *were considered a symbol of purity from earliest times and were closely associated with the Madonna.*

LILIACEAE

Lilium candidum

Madonna lily

History and traditions *L. candidum* appears in Cretan frescoes dating to 3000BC and has been cultivated since at least 1500BC for its scent and its medicinal properties. The flawless white flowers ensured its place as a symbol of purity and its association with the Virgin Mary and it is frequently featured in religious paintings. Shakespeare makes endless references to the whiteness of the "unsullied lily", the "sweetest and the fairest", and Gerard records that the white lily was known as "Juno's Rose" because it grew from her milk, which had fallen to the ground (*The Herball,* 1597). He also writes of using the bulbs of the white lily, mixed with honey, to heal wounds, but makes it clear that a variety of lilies were used for medicinal purposes. He ascribes many virtues to the "red lily", including its ability to remove facial wrinkles, and reveals that Pliny recommended it as a corn remover. *L. candidum* is little used in modern herbalism, but the flowers are cultivated commercially in some countries for their perfumed essence, and it remains a traditional herb garden ornamental.

Description A perennial, growing from a scaly bulb to 1–1.5m/3–5ft in height, it has stiff, erect stems with small, lance-shaped leaves and racemes of 5–20 fragrant, trumpet-shaped, white flowers, tinged inside with yellow, and with bright yellow anthers. It is the only lily to have overwintering basal leaves.

Habitat/distribution A Mediterranean native, widely cultivated in other countries.

Growth Can be difficult to grow and requires conditions that suit it exactly before it will flourish. All lilies dislike heavy, clay soils.

Parts used Roots, flowers – juice is used fresh in ointments and herbal preparations.

USES Medicinal It has soothing, healing properties and is used externally (but only rarely) for burns, skin inflammations and disorders.

Growing Madonna lilies

Lilium candidum is one of the oldest flowering plants in cultivation and the flowers are strongly fragrant. These beautiful white lilies can be unpredictable to grow, but the following guidelines will help to ensure success:

- Plant bulbs immediately they arrive. If there is a delay, keep it as short as possible, and meanwhile store bulbs in peat in a dark place – if exposed to light, they soften and deteriorate quickly.
- Good drainage is essential. Prepare soil thoroughly. Dig out to two spades' depth, put in a layer of coarse gravel, then replace the top soil, mixing it with sand and leaf mould. Alternatively, plant in containers, putting in a layer of coarse gravel, topped by a gritty, open compost (soil mix).
- Plant in early autumn (preferably at the beginning of September, no later than October, in the northern hemisphere).
- Bulbs should be only just covered – unlike other lilies, which require deeper planting.
- Once planted and established, do not disturb – Madonna lilies resent being moved.

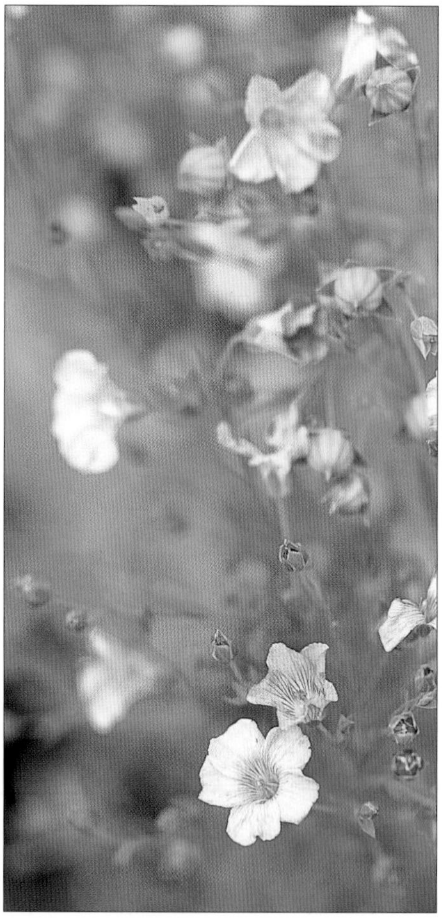

LINACEAE

Linum usitatissimum

Flax

History and traditions Flax has been an important economic crop since 5000BC, valued for its fibre in making linen and for its oil-producing seeds. The Bible has many references to linen woven from flax, and both seeds and cloth have been found in Egyptian tombs. In medieval Europe it was promoted by the Emperor Charlemagne for the health-giving properties of the seeds, and there are detailed descriptions in old herbals of the process of turning flax stems into fibre for making clothing, sheets, sails, fishing nets, thread, rope, sacks, bags and purses. Many superstitions have arisen, especially concerning its cultivation: sitting on the seed bag three times and facing east before planting, ringing church bells on Ascension Day and jumping over midsummer fires were all thought to ensure a good crop – and of course the seeds provided protection from witchcraft. It has also been a valued medicinal herb since Hippocrates recommended it for colds and is still used in herbal medicine.

Description A hardy, slender annual, about 90cm–1.2m/3–4ft in height. It has narrow, lanceolate, greeny-grey leaves and simple, five-petalled, pale blue flowers borne in summer, followed by spherical seed capsules, rich in oil.

Related species *L. usitatissimum* is thought to be a cultivar of *L. bienne* in the distant past. Tall cultivars have been developed for textiles, and shorter ones for the production of seeds for linseed oil. *L. perenne,* grown in Europe and North America, is a perennial species. *L. catharticum* (purging flax) is a white-flowered annual with oval leaves; used homeopathically to treat bronchitis and haemorrhoids.

Habitat/distribution Probably of Middle Eastern origin, it is widely distributed in temperate and subtropical regions of the world and found as a cultivated escape on sunny waste ground and waysides.

Growth Grow in dry, sandy soil in full sun. Propagated from seed sown *in situ*. Sow in late spring or early summer.

Parts used Whole plant – used fresh in infusions, cut after flowering for fibre; seeds – collected when ripe – dried for use whole, in infusions and other preparations, or extracted for linseed oil.

USES Medicinal Seeds are used as laxatives, in infusions and macerations for coughs, sore throats and gastric disorders, in poultices for boils and abscesses. Linseed oil contains linolenic essential fatty acids, necessary for many bodily functions, as well as vitamins A, B, D, E, minerals and amino acids. It is said to be helpful for many disorders, including rheumatoid arthritis, menstrual problems, menopausal symptoms and skin complaints. The unripe seeds are toxic.

General Stem varieties are soaked ('retted') in water to release fibres for making linen cloth. Linseed oil from seed varieties is one of the most important commercial drying oils, used in paints, varnishes and putty.

Other name Linseed.

> CAUTION Contains traces of prussic acid, but this plant is not thought to be harmful unless taken in very large doses. Some *Linum* species have been suspected of poisoning stock in Australia. Artists' linseed oil should not be taken medicinally.

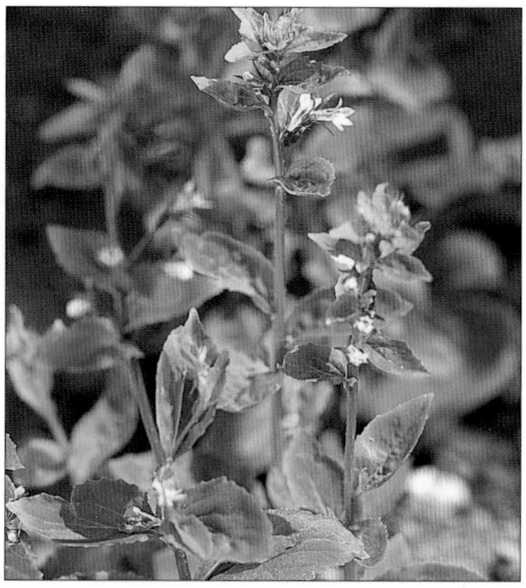

CAMPANULACEAE

Lobelia inflata

Indian tobacco

History and traditions This North American plant gained its common name from the local tradition of smoking it to relieve chest infections and asthma. It was enthusiastically adopted by early settlers as a cure-all for a wide variety of complaints and promoted in the early 19th century by the herbalist Samuel Thomson, who was charged with murder after one of his patients died from its effects. The generic name *Lobelia* (there are over 350 species) is named after the Flemish botanist Matthias de L'Obel (1538–1616). The specific name is a reference to the inflation of the seed capsule as it ripens.

Description A hardy annual, 20–60cm/8–24in, it has hairy stems and ovate leaves, toothed at the edges. Inconspicuous flowers borne in terminal racemes are pale violet, tinged with pink, followed by two-celled, oval capsules.

Habitat/distribution Native to North America.

Growth Grow in rich, moist soil in full sun or partial shade. Propagated by seed.

Parts used Whole plant – cut when flowering.

USES Medicinal It contains alkaloids that increase the rate of respiration and induce vomiting. It is also an expectorant and emetic. In small doses it dilates the bronchioles and is used for conditions such as bronchitis, asthma and pleurisy, but is for use by qualified practitioners only. Used in proprietary cough medicines. It can also help with smoking cessation.

> CAUTION Poisonous and can cause fatalities.

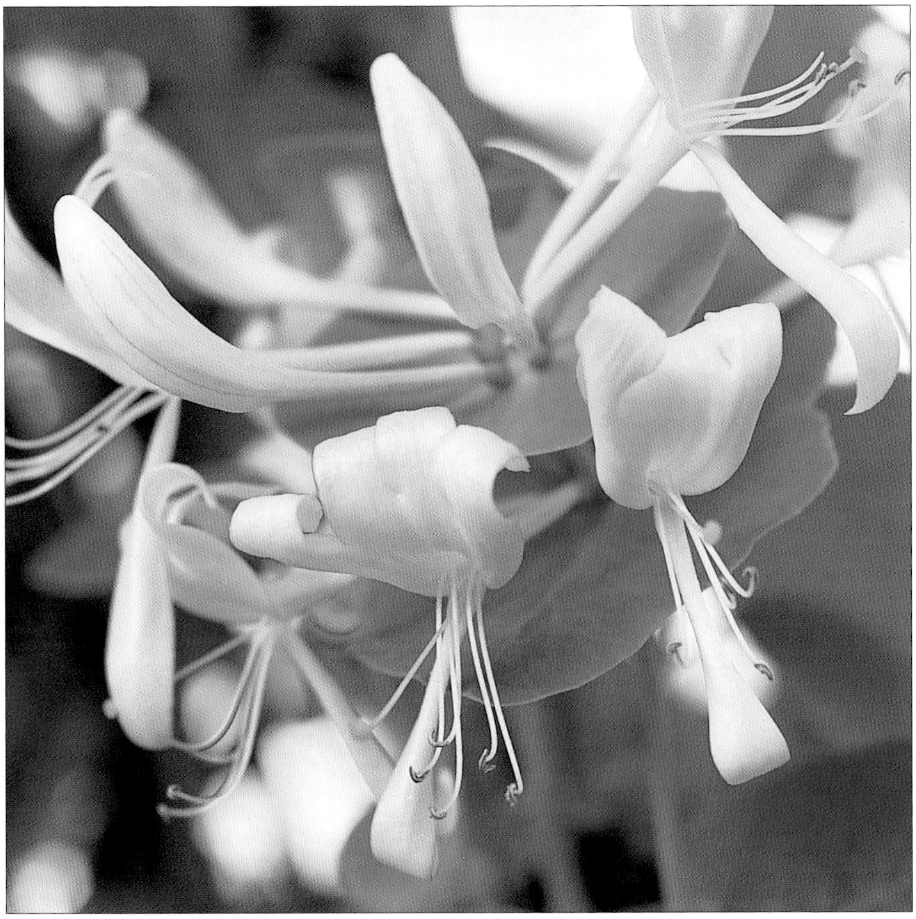

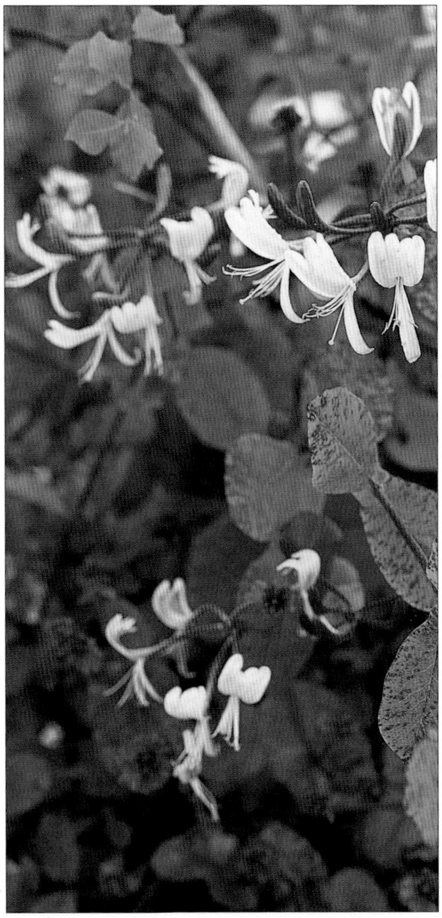

CAPRIFOLIACEAE

Lonicera spp

Honeysuckle

History and traditions Various species of honeysuckle have been used since ancient Greek times for their medicinal properties. Dioscorides is quoted by Gerard as recommending the seeds for "removing weariness" and "helping the shortness and difficulty of breathing" and a syrup of the flowers for diseases of lung and spleen. Little used medicinally today, honeysuckle keeps its place in the herb garden as a fragrant climber, memorably described by Shakespeare as the "lush woodbine" and "sweet honeysuckle" which "over-canopied" Titania's bower (*A Midsummer Night's Dream*). The name honeysuckle comes from the old practice of sucking the sweet nectar from the flowers.

Description and species Two species were most often recommended for medicinal purposes: ***L. periclymenum*** **(woodbine, wild or common honeysuckle)** has whorls of very fragrant, creamy-white to yellow, tubular two-lipped flowers, followed by red berries; and ***L. caprifolium*** **(Italian, Dutch** or **perfoliate honeysuckle)** has upper leaves surrounding the stem and creamy-white to pink flowers. Both are fully hardy, ***L. periclymenum*** grows to 7m/23ft, ***L. caprifolium*** to 6m/19ft. ***L. japonica*** **(Japanese honeysuckle)** often has violet-tinged white flowers, followed by black berries.

Habitat/distribution Widely distributed in the northern hemisphere, in woodlands, hedgerows and rocky hillsides.

Growth Grow in fertile, well-drained soil in full sun or partial shade. Propagated by seed sown in late summer to autumn in containers and overwintered in a cold frame, or by semi-ripe cuttings taken in summer. Prune out straggly or overgrown branches.

Parts used Flowering stems.

USES Medicinal *L. caprifolium* and *L. periclymenum* were formerly used for their expectorant, laxative properties. *L. japonica* (*jin yin hua*) is used in traditional Chinese medicine for clearing toxins from the system.

CAUTION Honeysuckle berries are poisonous.

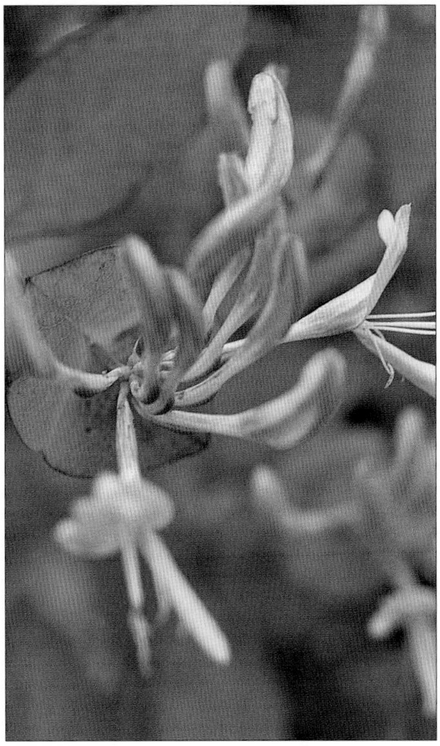

Above *The flowers contain sweet nectar.*

Top right *A cultivar of* Lonicera periclymenum.

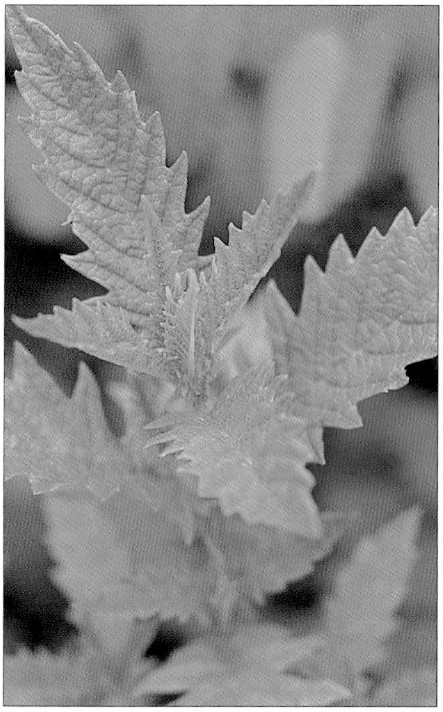

LABIATAE/LAMIACEAE

Lycopus europaeus

Gipsyweed

History and traditions This herb is said to have gained its name because gipsies used it to stain their skins darker. It was also effective in dyeing fabrics and at one time was a valuable medicinal plant.
Description A perennial, mint-like herb, but with no aroma, it grows on a creeping rootstock to about 60cm/2ft in height. It has single stems with opposite, deeply toothed, pointed leaves and whorls of small, pale mauve flowers in the leaf axils in late summer.
Related species *L. virginicus* (Virginia bugle weed), also known sometimes as gipsyweed, is native to North America. It is a very similar plant to *L. europaeus* and shares the same properties.
Habitat/distribution *L. europaeus* is a native of Europe and western Asia.
Parts used Whole flowering plant – it can be used fresh or dried.

USES Medicinal Gipsyweed is reputed to have sedative properties. Traditionally it is used to treat hyperthyroidism. Avoid if trying to conceive. Do not take alongside preparation containing thyroid hormone.
General It produces a black or dark grey dye on woollen and linen fabrics.

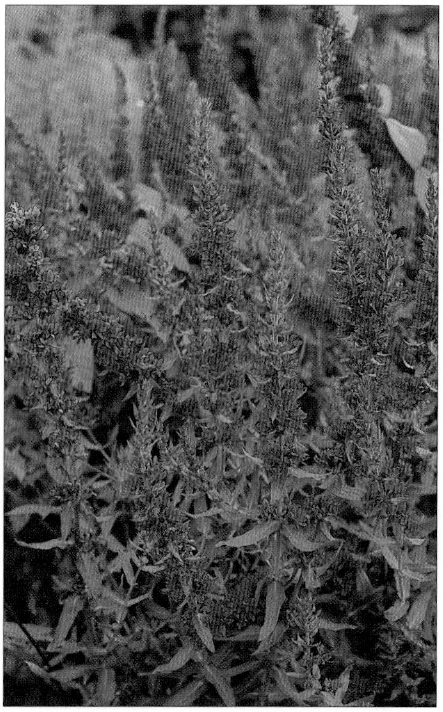

LYTHRACEAE

Lythrum salicaria

Purple loosestrife

History and traditions The name loosestrife is connected to this herb's old reputation for soothing ill-behaved animals. Gerard, in his *Herball* of 1597, writes of it "appeasing the strife and unruliness which falleth out among oxen at the plough, if it is put about their yokes". As it was also supposed to drive away flies and gnats, perhaps this was the reason for its calming influence. The generic name is from the Greek, *luthron*, meaning blood, a reference to the colour of the flowers, and it was considered by herbalists of old to be effective against internal haemorrhages, excessive menstruation and nosebleeds. John Lindley, in *Flora Medica*, 1838, refers to it as "an astringent, which has been recommended in inveterate cases of diarrhoea," and it was often used in his day to treat outbreaks of cholera.
Description Purple loosestrife is a perennial which grows on a creeping rhizome with erect stems reaching 0.6–1.5m/2–5ft in height. It has long, lanceolate leaves and crimson-purple flowers borne on whorled spikes in mid to late summer.
Habitat/distribution A European native, it occurs widely in Asia, northern Africa, Australia and North America. It is usually found in wet and marshy places.
Growth It grows best in moist to wet soil in sun or partial shade and is propagated by seed or division in autumn or spring. It often self-seeds and spreads rapidly. It is classed as a noxious weed in some countries and imports of the plants and seeds are forbidden.
Parts used The whole flowering plant – it is used fresh or dried in infusions, decoctions and ointments.

USES Medicinal It has been found in modern research to have antibacterial properties and is still recommended by modern herbalists for diarrhoea and dysentery as well as for haemorrhages and excessive menstrual flow. It is said to be soothing, when applied externally, to sores, ulcers, skin irritations and eczema.

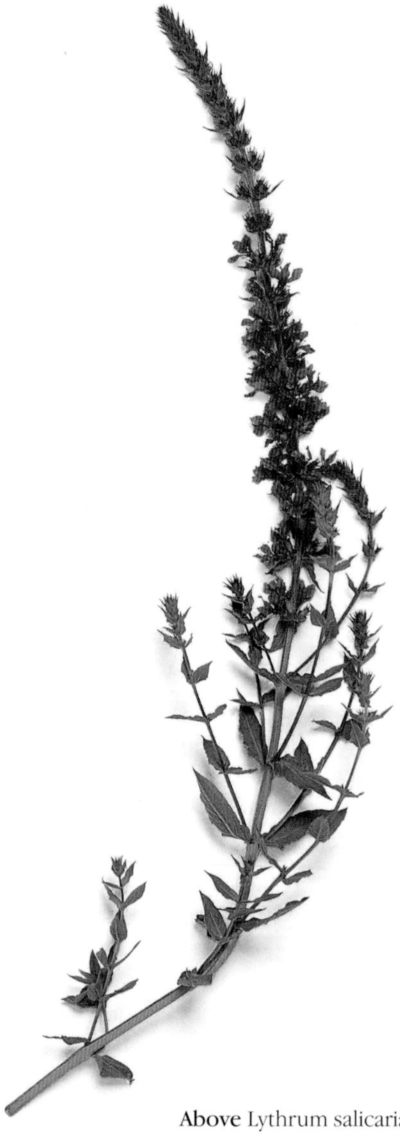

Above Lythrum salicaria

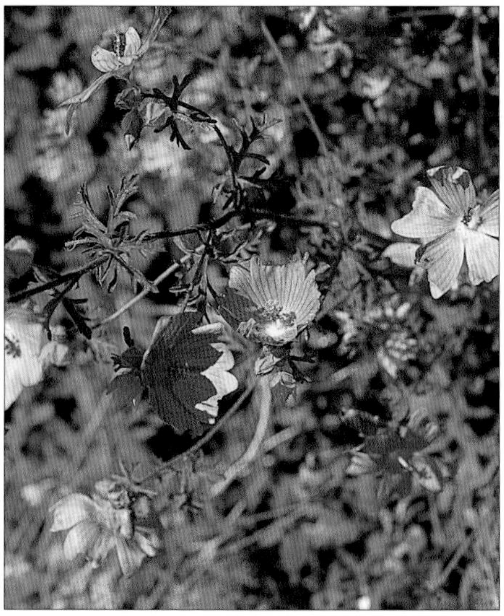

MALVACEAE

Malva sylvestris

Mallow

History and traditions The common mallow was cultivated by the Romans as a medicinal and culinary herb, the leaves being cooked as a vegetable and seeds added to salads and sauces. By the 16th century it had gained a reputation as a cure-all, commended for its gentle purgative action, a process that was thought to rid the body of disease. But its culinary uses remained paramount, and herbals and household books of the period are full of recipes for cooking the leaves with butter and vinegar, making "suckets" (candy) of the stalks, and, even more imaginatively, cutting and rolling them into balls and passing them off as green peas (*Receipt Book of John Nott,* 1723). The generic name, *Malva,* meaning soft, refers to the downy leaves and soothing properties of the plant.

Description A perennial, growing from 45–90cm/18in–3ft, it has much-branched erect or trailing stems, with 5- to 7-lobed leaves, and pink, five-petalled flowers, streaked with darker veins, borne throughout summer.

Related species *M. moschata* (musk mallow) grows to 90cm/3ft and has purple-spotted stems, heart-shaped basal leaves and narrowly divided upper leaves, both scented faintly with musk. Solitary pale pink flowers are borne in the leaf axils. It is weaker in effect than *M. sylvestris,* but with the same uses. The closely related plant *Althaea officinalis* (marshmallow) is considered more medicinally effective than either of the *Malva.*

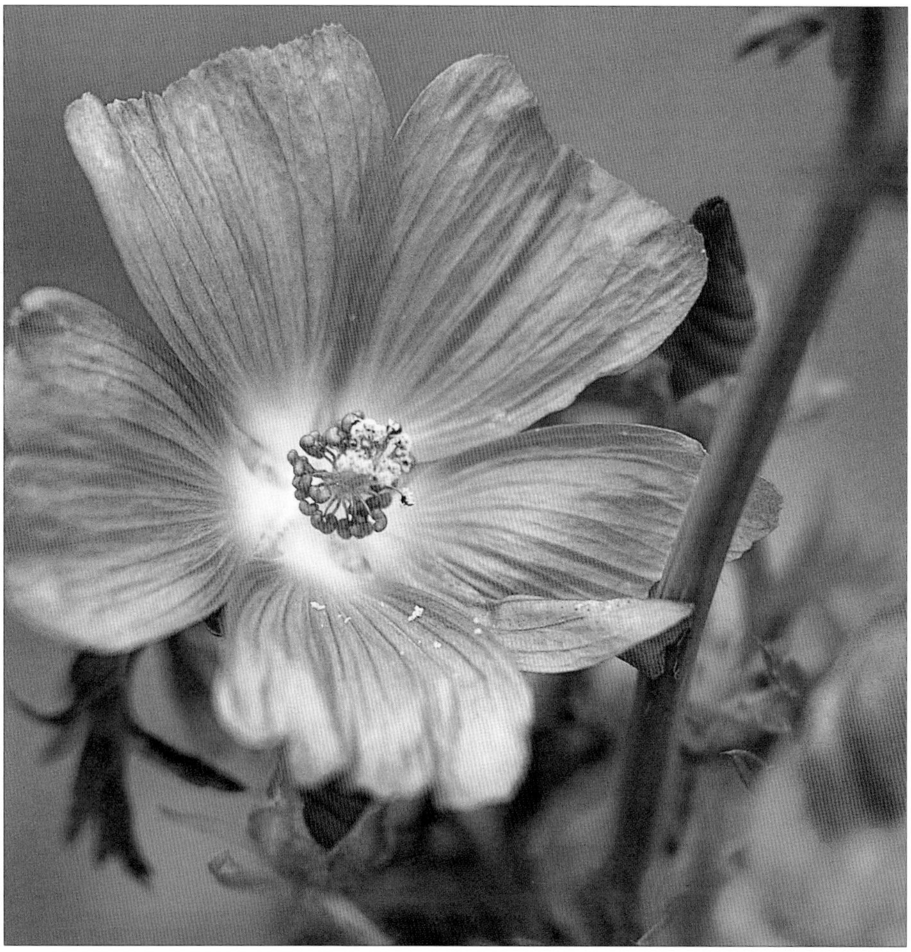

Above *A flower of the musk mallow,* Malva moschata.

Habitat/distribution Native to Europe, western Asia and North America. Found at field edges, embankments and on waste ground, in porous soils and sunny situations.

Growth Grow in well-drained to dry soil, in a sunny position. Propagated by seed sown in the spring or by division of the roots in late autumn or early spring.

Parts used Leaves, flowers – used fresh or dried. Fruits (seed capsules) – picked unripe and used fresh.

USES Medicinal Mallow contains a high proportion of an emollient mucilage, reduces inflammation and calms irritated tissues. Infusions are taken internally for coughs, sore throats and bronchitis. The leaves are applied externally as a poultice for skin complaints, eczema and insect bites. It is also an expectorant herb and large doses can have a laxative effect.

Culinary Young leaves and shoots contain vitamins A, B^1, B^2 and C and can be eaten raw in salads or cooked as vegetables. Unripe fruits are sometimes added to salads.

Other name Common mallow.

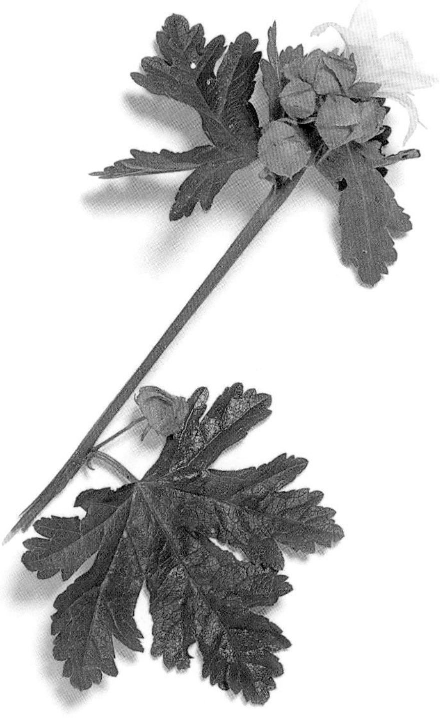

Above Malva moschata *f.* alba

SOLANACEAE

Mandragora officinarum

Mandrake

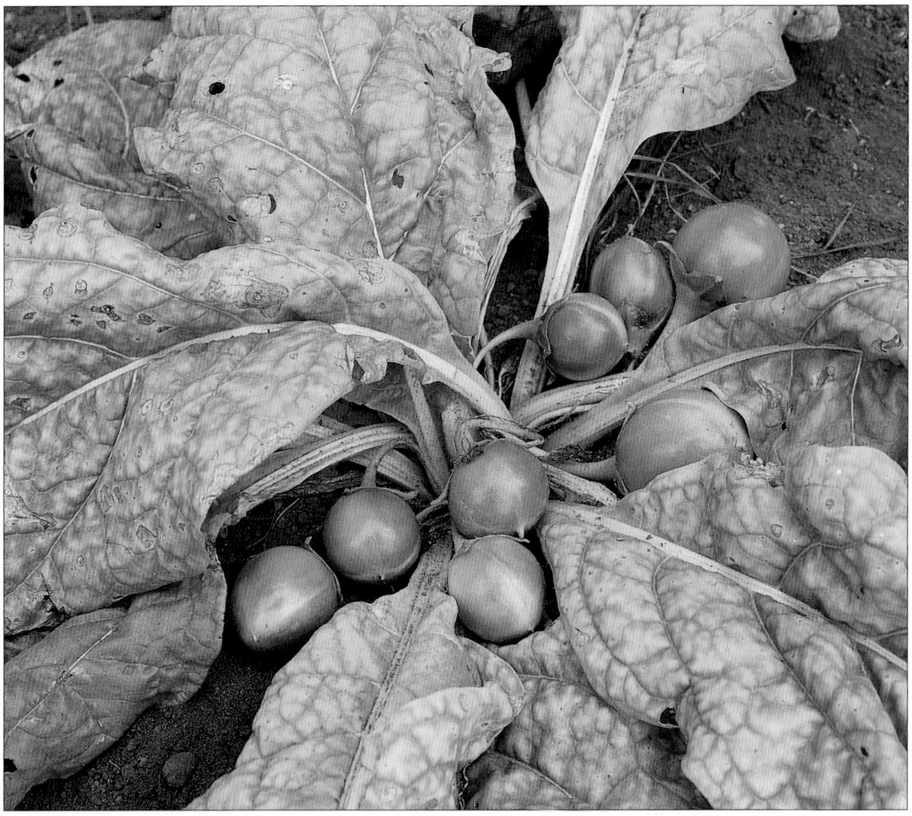

History and traditions Mandrake has attracted more stories and superstitions than almost any other herb – perhaps because of its hallucinogenic properties, coupled with its strange appearance and forked roots, fancifully thought to resemble the human form. Closely related to *Atropa belladonna* and *Hyoscyamus niger* (henbane), it contains the toxic alkaloids atropine and hyoscyamine and has been used since the ancient Greek and Roman period as a powerful sedative, when it was first found to deaden the pain of surgery. An early introduction to Britain, it features in many Anglo-Saxon medicinal texts and was mentioned by Turner in 1551 for its anaesthetic properties. Just holding the fruit (mandrake apple) in the hand was said to be a cure for insomnia. At the end of the 19th century it became an official homeopathic preparation but is rarely used today and retains its place as a "herb" because of its historical interest.

Description A low growing perennial, 15cm/6in in height, it has a basal rosette of broad, oval, veined and rough-textured leaves, with wavy margins, which start erect and spread flat as they grow. Clusters of bell-shaped, greenish-white flowers, flushed with purple, arise from the base and are followed by large, spherical green fruits ripening to yellow.

Habitat/distribution Originated in the Himalayas and southeast Mediterranean, introduced into western Europe, Britain and other countries. Found on sunny sites, in poor, sandy soil.

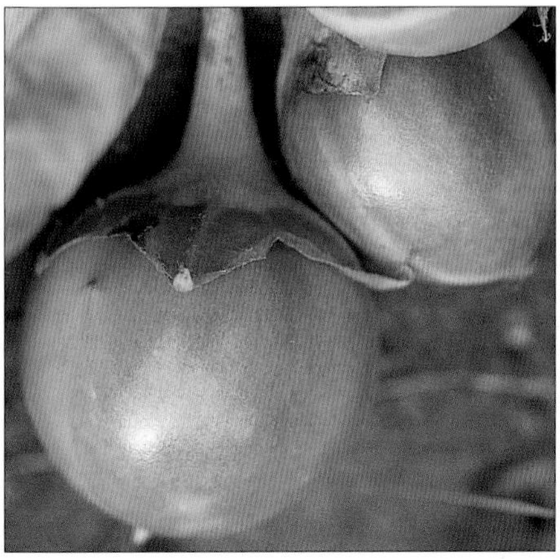

Above *Mandrake fruits, sometimes known as the devil's apples.*

Growth Although hardy to -10°C/14°F, mandrake needs protection from prolonged cold and wet weather in winter. Grow it in a sheltered, sunny spot such as at the base of a wall, or in a rockery, in well-drained, reasonably fertile soil. It resents disturbance once properly established and is propagated by seed in autumn, root cuttings in winter.

Parts used Roots.

USES Medicinal Formerly used as a sedative and painkiller.

Other name Devil's apples.

CAUTION A dangerously poisonous plant, which should not be used internally or externally. Can be fatal. Subject to legal restrictions in some countries.

Mandrake myths

One of the most popular superstitions about mandrake was that its unearthly shrieks, when pulled up, sent people mad if it did not kill them. As Shakespeare records: "And shrieks like mandrakes torn out of the earth/That living mortals hearing them run mad" (*Romeo and Juliet*) or "Would curses kill as doth the mandrakes groan" (*Henry VI*, Part 2).

An ingenious way to avoid death on digging up the plant was to tie it to a hungry dog, with a dish of meat just out of reach, so that he would die instead as he pulled the root from the ground. Once dug up it could be handled with impunity.

The fancied resemblance of the roots to people meant they were sought after as amulets to protect from witchcraft and bring prosperity. This led to a lucrative scam (scathingly described by Turner in his *New Herbal*, 1551) of false mandrake manikins being sculpted out of bryony roots and sold to the gullible at high prices. The sensible Gerard, too, dismissed the mandrake myths with these words: "There have been many ridiculous tales brought up of this plant, whether of old wives or runnegate surgeons, or phisick mongers, I know not, all which dreames and old wives tales you shall from henceforth cast out your bookes of memorie." (*The Herball*, 1597).

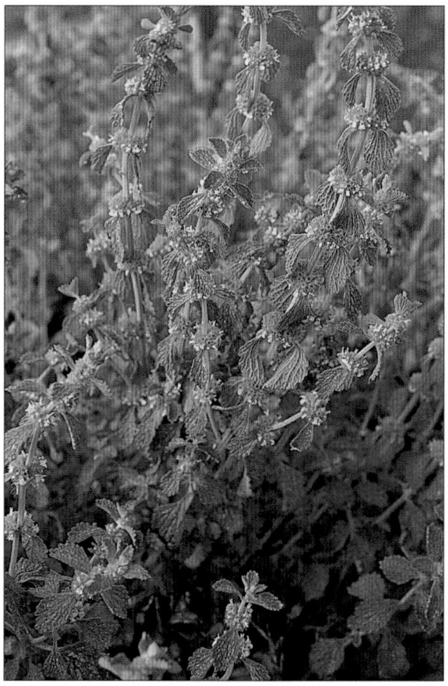

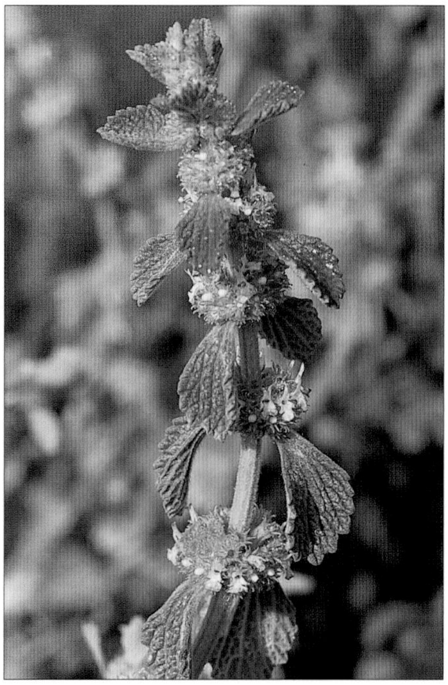

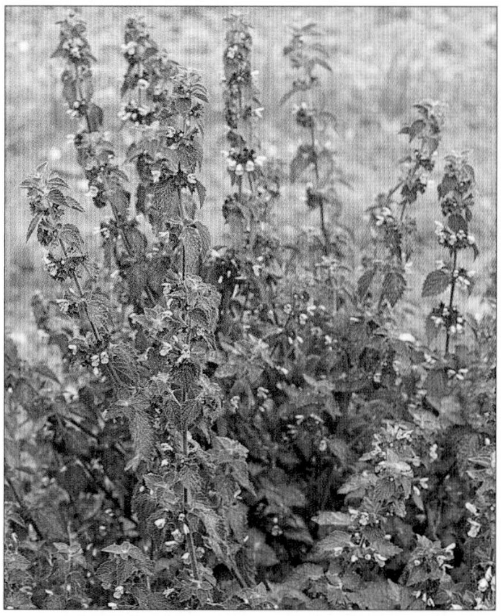

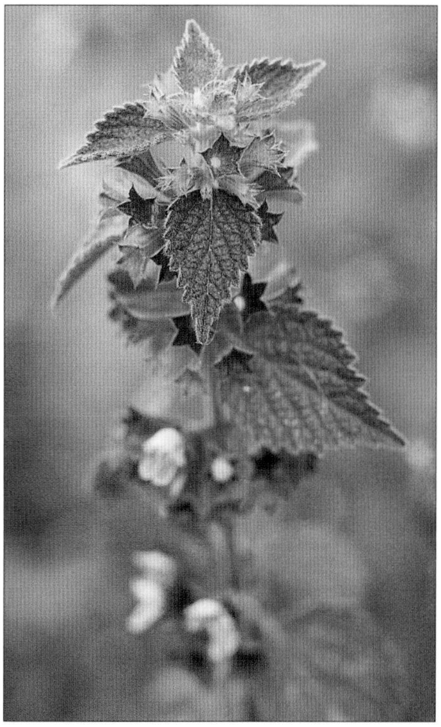

LABIATAE/LAMIACEAE

Marrubium vulgare

Horehound

History and traditions This herb has been known since Egyptian times, and is thought to be one of the bitter herbs which the Jews consumed at the Feast of the Passover.

The generic name *Marrubium* comes from the Hebrew word *marrob* – a bitter juice. Its reputation as a remedy for coughs and colds goes back to at least Pliny's time. Several 16th-century herbalists, including Gerard, use almost the same words to recommend a syrup of the fresh leaves in sugar as a "most singular remedie against the cough and wheezing of the lungs." Horehound candy was still being made to the old recipes well into the 20th century.

Description A hardy perennial growing to 60cm/2ft, with erect, branched stems and greeny-grey, soft, downy, ovate leaves, bluntly toothed, arranged opposite. Whorls of small, white, tubular flowers appear in the leaf axils in summer.

Related species *Ballota nigra,* although from a different genus, is known as black horehound, and was once used for similar purposes. However, it has an unpleasant smell and is considered less effective and has been superseded by *M. vulgare.*

Habitat/distribution Native to Europe, northern Africa and Asia, introduced elsewhere. Found on dry grassland, pastures and field edges.

Growth Grows in any soil and prefers a sunny situation. Propagated from seed sown in spring, but can be slow to germinate, or by division of roots in spring. (It is under statutory control as a weed in Australia and New Zealand.)

Parts used Flowering stems – fresh or dried.

USES Medicinal Taken as an infusion for coughs, colds and chest infections. Combined with hyssop, sage or thyme to make a gargle for sore throats. Made into cough candy.

Above Marrubium vulgare*, or white horehound.*

Top right and right Ballota nigra *is considered inferior as a medicinal plant.*

Horehound recipes

• **Horehound and ginger tea – for a cold**

15g/½ oz fresh horehound leaves
5ml/1 tsp powdered ginger
600ml/1 pint/2½ cups boiling water
honey to taste

Put the roughly chopped leaves into a pot or jug with the ginger, pour in the boiling water, cover and leave to infuse for 5–7 minutes. Strain off the leaves and sweeten with honey to taste before drinking.

• **A Recipe for horehound candy from *The Family Herbal* (1810)**

Boil some horehound till the juice is extracted. Boil up some sugar to a feather height, add your juice to the sugar, and let it boil till it is again the same height. Stir it till it begins to grow thick, then pour it on to a dish and dust it with sugar and when fairly cool cut into squares. Excellent sweetmeat for colds and coughs.

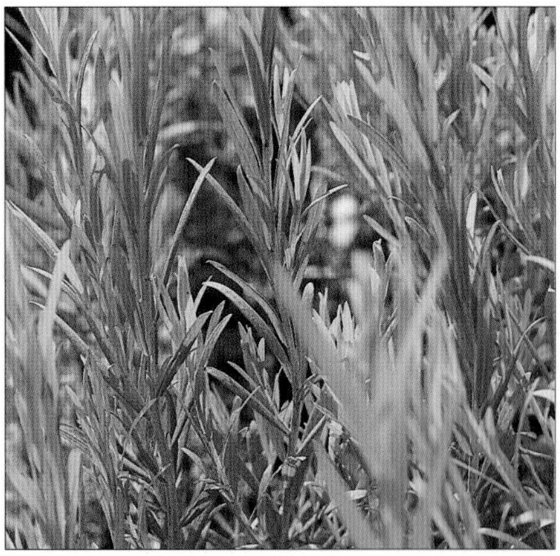

MYRTACEAE

Melaleuca alternifolia

Tea-tree

History and traditions Tea-tree was named by Captain Cook's crew when, following local custom, they drank it as a tea substitute. The Australian Aborigines used it medicinally, and in World War II tea tree oil, distilled from *M. alternifolia,* was used in Australia as a powerful germicide. It has since gained ground in herbal medicine for its remarkable healing properties.
Description Melaleucas are half-hardy to tender evergreen trees, 15–40m/50–130ft, with thin, peeling, corky bark, narrow, pointed, leathery leaves and bottle-brush-shaped flowers.
Related species Several species of melaleuca are used medicinally. *M. leucadendron* produces distilled cajuput oil, which has similar uses to eucalyptus oil. *M. viridiflora* is the source of niaouli oil used in perfumery.
Habitat/distribution Native to Australia and Malaysia, introduced in other tropical regions. Often found in swampy areas.
Growth *M. alternifolia* is half-hardy, *M. leucadendron* is tender. Grow in moisture-retentive to wet soil, in full sun. They must be grown as conservatory plants in cool, temperate regions. Propagated by seed or by semi-ripe cuttings.
Parts used Essential oil.

USES Medicinal Strongly antiseptic, antibacterial and antifungal, tea-tree oil is used diluted in a carrier oil and applied externally for healing cuts, burns, stings, insect bites, acne, and athlete's foot. It is also said to be effective against warts, verrucas and head lice eggs when used undiluted.
General A constituent of many pharmaceutical and cosmetic industry products.

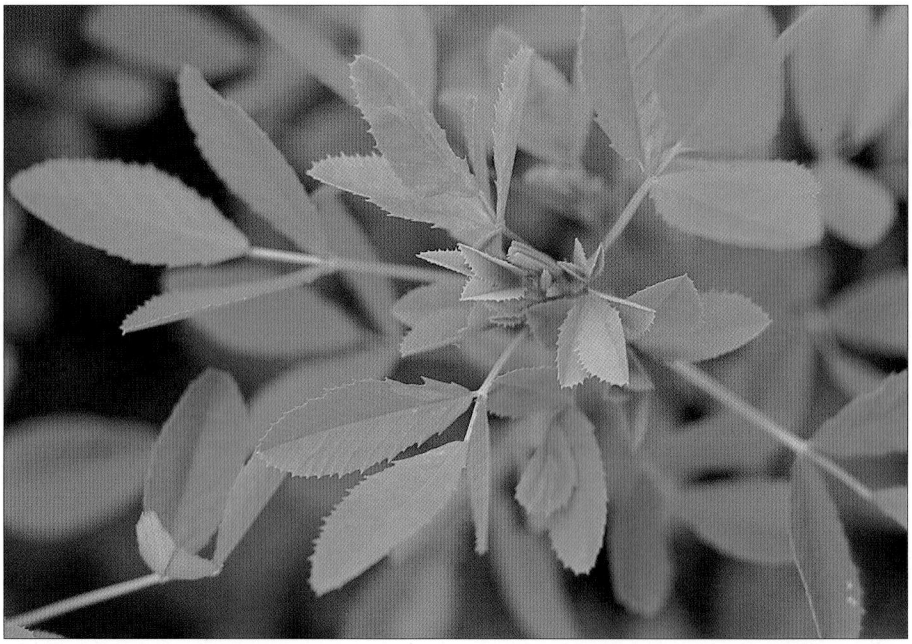

LEGUMINOSAE/PAPILIONACEAE

Melilotus officinalis

Melilot

History and traditions Once popular as a strewing herb for the haylike scent it develops when drying, due to the coumarin content, the name of the genus means "honey-lotus" for the sweet smell of its nectar and it is very attractive to bees. It was used in the Greek physician Galen's time, AD130–201, as an ingredient of ointments for reducing swellings, tumours and inflammations, and appears in later European herbals for similar purposes. Culpeper adds that "the head often washed with the distilled water of the herb and flowers is good for those who swoon, also to strengthen the memory".
Description An erect, straggly biennial, 0.6m–1.2m/2–4ft high, it has ridged, branched stems with trifoliate leaves and narrow ovate leaflets. The yellow, honey-scented flowers are borne in slender axillary racemes, from midsummer to autumn.
Habitat/distribution Native to Europe and Asia, naturalized in North America. Found in dry, chalky embankments, wastelands and roadsides.
Growth Grow in well-drained to dry soil, in a sunny situation. Propagated by seed sown in spring or autumn.
Parts used: Flowering stems – dried for use in herbal preparations.

USES An aromatic herb with sedative, anti-inflammatory properties, it was formerly taken as an infusion or tincture for insomnia, tension headaches and painful menstruation, and applied externally to wounds and skin inflammations. It also has a reputation for helping to prevent thrombosis and has been used for bronchial complaints and catarrh.
Aromatic It has insect-repellent properties and the dried herb is sometimes included in scented sachets for the wardrobe.
Other names Yellow melilot and yellow sweet clover.

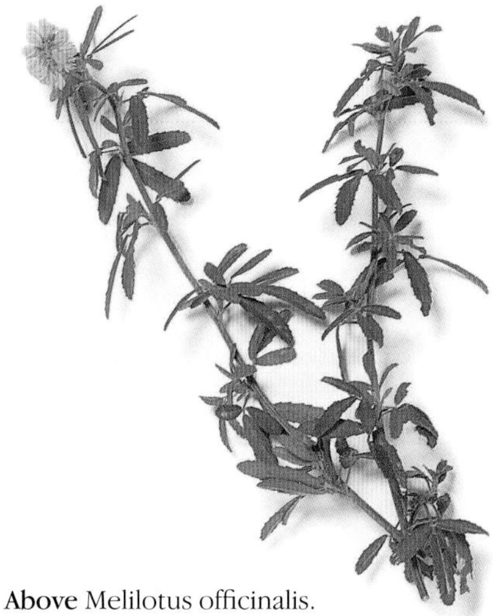

Above Melilotus officinalis.

CAUTION Dicoumarol, a powerful anticlotting factor, is sometimes produced during the drying process. It is emetic in large doses. Do not use concurrently with warfarin or other anti-coagulants. Harmful to livestock.

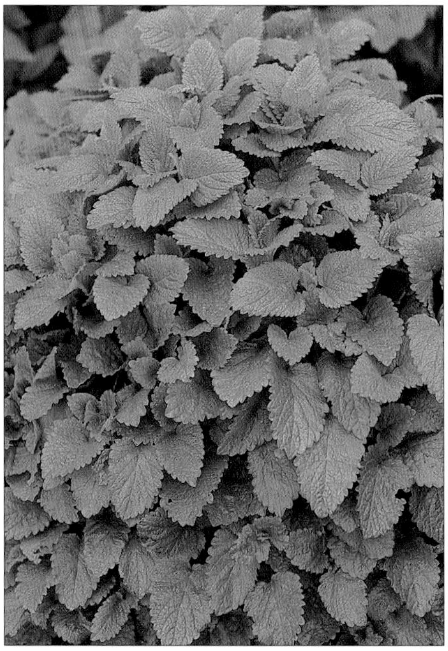

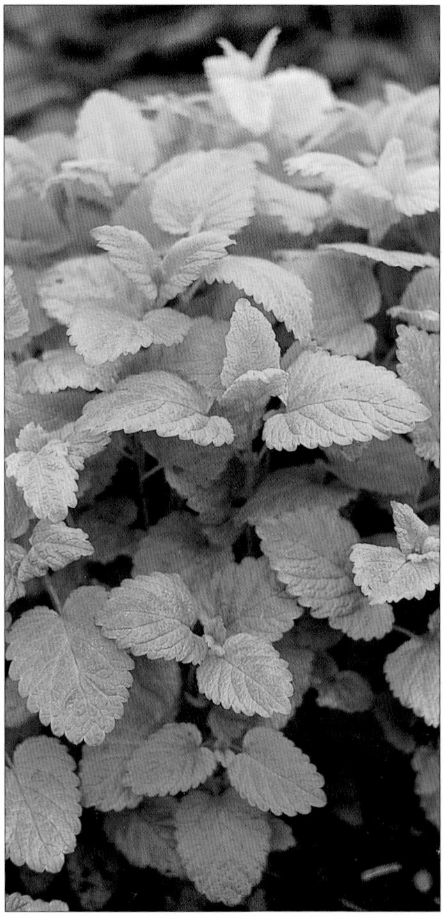

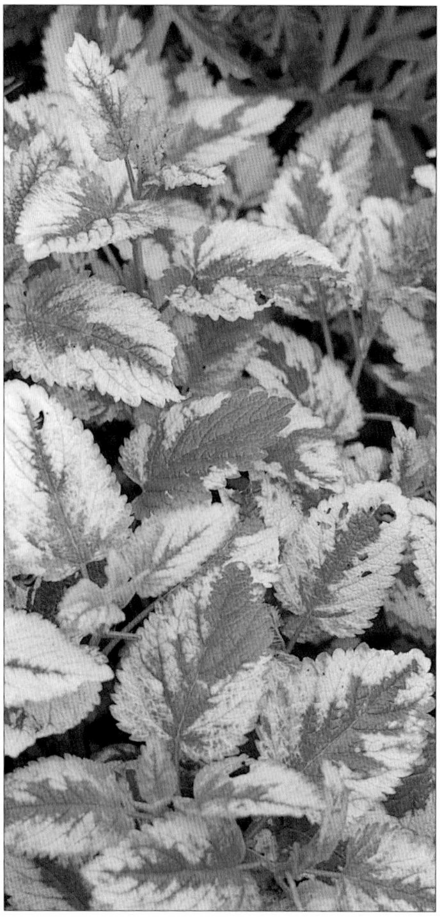

LABIATAE/LAMIACEAE

Melissa officinalis

Lemon balm

History and traditions Lemon balm has been cultivated as a bee plant for over 2000 years, bunches being put into empty hives to attract swarms. It is thought that the leaves contain the same terpenoids as found in glands of honey bees. The Arab physicians of the 1st and 2nd centuries are credited with introducing it as an antidepressant medicinal herb. John Parkinson wrote that "the herb without question is an excellent help to comfort the heart" (*Paradisi*, 1629) and many of the old herbalists refer to it as driving away "all melancholy and sadnesse". It has been taken as a calming tea for its gently sedative effects ever since. Unsubstantiated stories of regular drinkers of balm tea living into their hundreds have been perpetuated by modern herbal writers.

Description A vigorous, bushy perennial, 30–80cm/12–32in in height, it has strongly lemon-scented, rough-textured, ovate, toothed leaves. Inconspicuous clusters of pale yellow flowers appear in the leaf axils in late summer.

Related species *M. officinalis* 'Aurea' is a cultivar with bright gold and green variegated leaves. It is inclined to revert as the plant matures, so cut back after flowering to encourage new variegated growth. *M. officinalis* 'All Gold' has bright yellow foliage, but should be planted in partial shade, as it is inclined to scorch in a position where it receives full sun.

Habitat/distribution Native to southern and central Europe, introduced and widely distributed in northern temperate zones. Often found as a garden escape.

Growth Grows in any soil in sun or partial shade. Spreads and self-seeds freely. The easiest method of propagation is by division in spring. The species can be grown from seed, but cultivars must be vegetatively propagated.

Parts used Leaves – best used fresh, as scent and therapeutic properties are lost when dried and stored; essential oil – distilled from leaves.

USES Medicinal Lemon balm has sedative, relaxing, digestive properties and infusions are taken internally for nervous anxiety, depression, tension headaches and indigestion. It also has insect-repellent properties, is antiviral and antibacterial, and is applied externally, in infusions, poultices or ointments, for sores, skin irritations, insect bites and stings. It can be particularly helpful for reducing cold sores (*herpes simplex* virus). The essential oil is used in aromatherapy for anxiety states.

Culinary Fresh leaves add lemon flavour to sweet and savoury dishes as well as drinks.

Above centre Melissa officinalis *'All Gold'*.

Above Melissa officinalis *'Aurea'*.

Recipes for lemon balm

- **Chicken lemon balm**

Use handfuls of the fresh leaves to stuff the body cavity of a chicken, and sit it on a further bed of leaves before roasting it, to keep flesh moist and impart a subtle lemon flavour.

- **Orange and lemon balm salad**

Snip fresh lemon balm over peeled, thinly sliced oranges, sprinkled with a mixture of fresh orange and lemon juice, sweetened with honey.

CAUTION Mixed opinions whether lemon balm is safe to use in pregnancy. If using, do so in low dosages. Safe in lactation. Use caution if taking central nervous system depressants or thyroid medications.

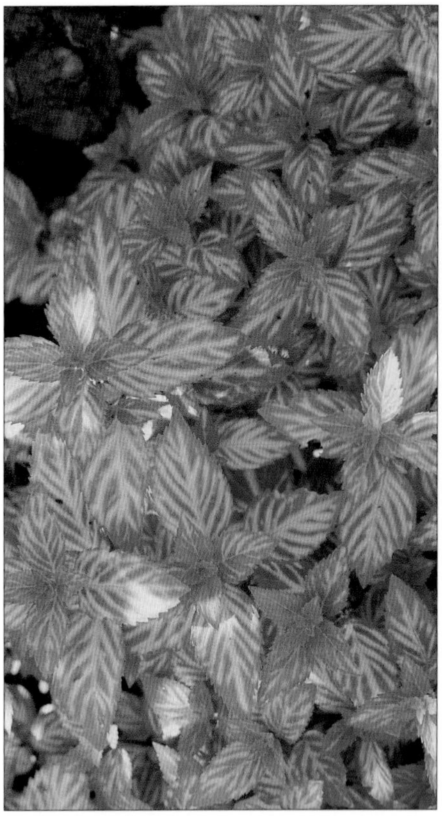

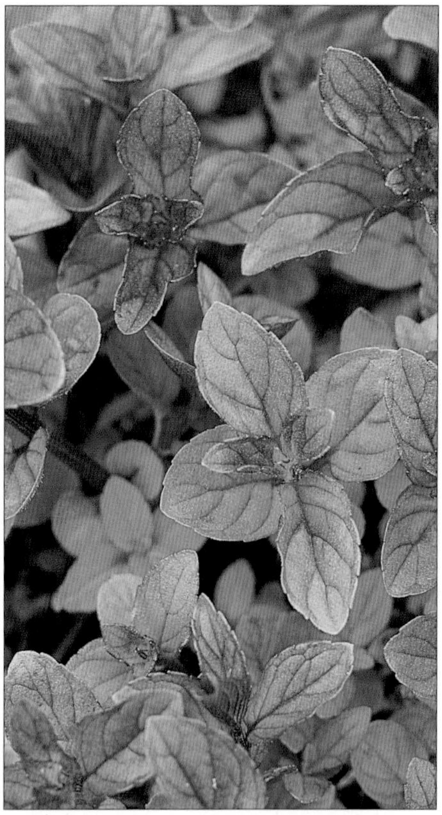

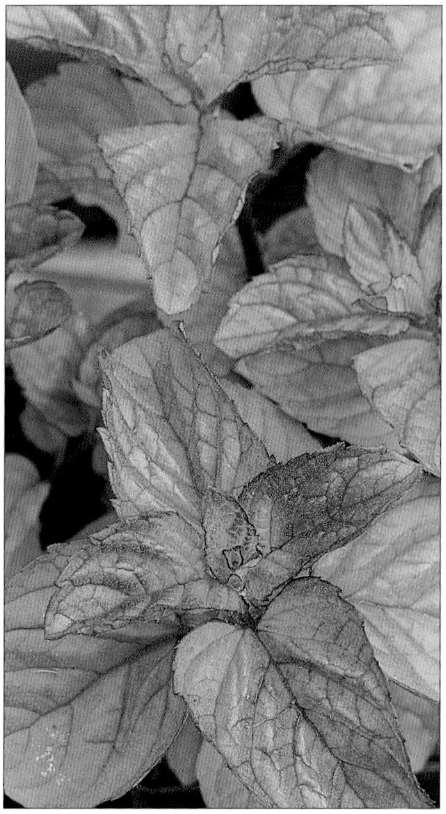

LABIATAE/LAMIACEAE

Mentha

History and traditions The Romans made great use of mint for its clean, fresh scent, putting it in their bathwater and making it into perfumes. The poet Ovid describes scouring the boards with "green mint" before setting out food for the gods, and Pliny has been attributed with the view that the smell of mint stirs up the taste buds "to a greedy desire of meat". This conflicts with a modern study, carried out in the United States in 1994, which found that the smell of mint helped alleviate hunger pangs. The Romans introduced spearmint to Britain, where it soon became established. In the late 16th century, Gerard talks of its popularity as a strewing herb "in chambers and places of recreation". It is now one of the most popular herbs.

Habitat/distribution Mints are widely distributed in Europe, Asia and Africa, introduced and naturalized elsewhere, often found in damp or wet soils. Cultivated as a crop in many countries including Europe, North America, the Middle East and Asia.

Species There are 25 species of mint in all, but they are often variable and individual plants can be difficult to identify because mints hybridize readily. The following hardy perennials are top favourites for the herb garden. Most are vigorous, the variegated ones less so, and spread rapidly on creeping rootstocks.

M. **x** ***gracilis*** **'Variegata' (gingermint)** – Has gold and green variegated, smooth, ovate leaves, scented with a hint of ginger, and grows 30cm–1m/1–3ft tall. Tiny, pale lilac flowers are borne in whorls in the leaf axils.

M. **x** ***piperita*** **(peppermint)** – Has dark green (often tinged with purple) lanceolate to ovate, toothed leaves and whorls of pale pink flowers in summer. It grows to 30–90cm/1–3ft tall. Peppermint is a variable hybrid of *M. spicata* and *M. aquatica*, sometimes assigned two different forms as black peppermint, *M.* x *piperita* f. *rubescens,* and white peppermint, *M.* x *piperita* f. *pallescens.* It is rich in menthol, which gives it the characteristic cooling, slightly numbing, peppermint taste, but is too dominant for general cookery and is used to flavour sweet foods.

M. **x** ***piperita*** **f.** ***citrata*** **(eau-de-Cologne mint)** (bergamot, lemon or orange mint) – A cultivar with large, toothed, ovate leaves, 30–90cm/1–3ft tall. The scent is reminiscent of lavender water with citrus overtones.

M. pulegium **(pennyroyal)** – There are creeping (to 10cm/4in) and upright (to 40cm/16in) varieties. Both have small, elliptic to ovate, usually smooth-edged leaves, and prolific, distinctive whorls of mauve flowers in the leaf axils. The high concentration of pulegone gives it a pleasantly antiseptic smell, but it is toxic in very large doses and abortifacient.

Mentha requienii (**Corsican mint)** – A creeping, mat-forming mint, 2.5–10cm/1–4in, with very small, smooth and shiny, rounded leaves and tiny, mauve flowers in summer. It makes a good ground cover herb for a damp, shady situation.

M. spicata **(spearmint)** – This has bright green, wrinkled, finely toothed leaves, with a fresh, uncomplicated, not too overpowering mint scent. White or pale mauve flowers are borne in terminal spikes in mid- to late summer. A popular culinary mint, used since the time of the Romans; 30–90cm/1–3ft tall.

M. suaveolens **'Variegata' (variegated applemint** also known as **pineapple mint)** – This has soft, downy, cream and white variegated leaves and a sweet, apple scent. 30–90cm/1–3ft tall. Pineapple mint makes a very attractive ornamental and container plant.

M **x** ***villosa*** **var.** ***alopecuroides*** **(Bowles' Mint)** – Formerly known as *M. rotundifolia* var. 'Bowles', it is in fact a variety of a sterile hybrid between *M. spicata* and *M. suaveolens.*

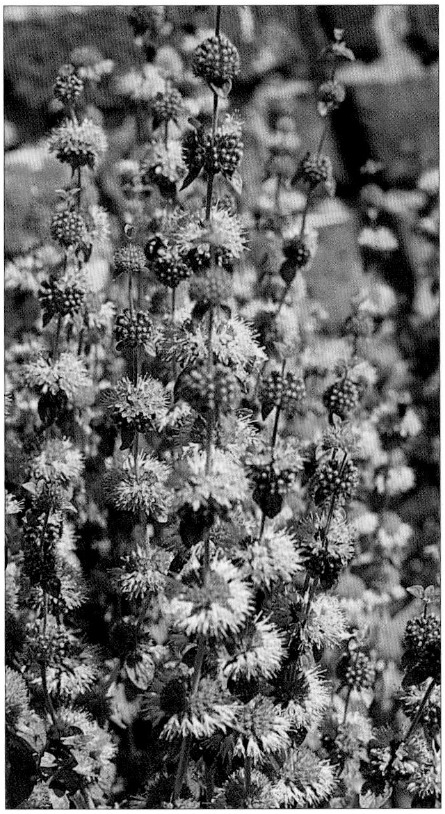

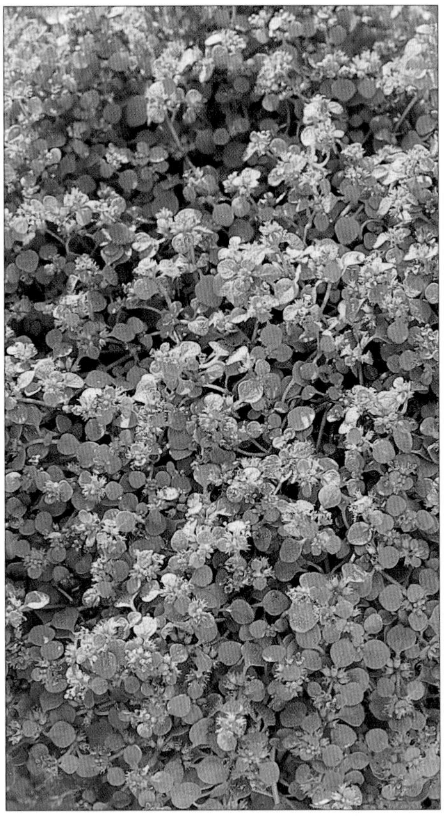

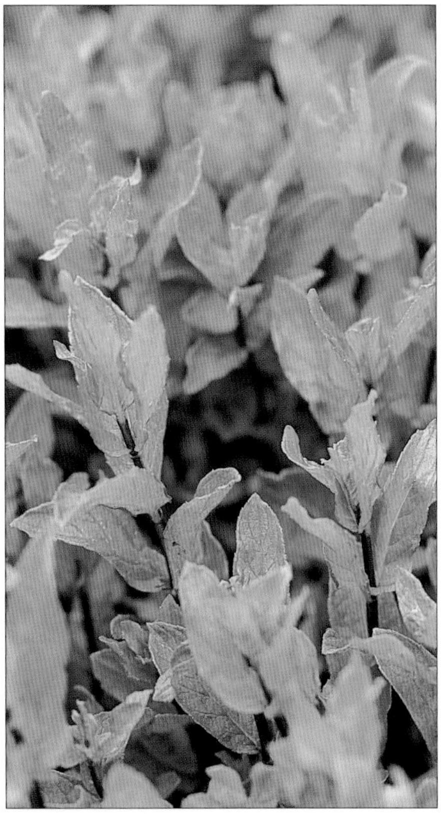

The rounded, ovate, toothed leaves are greyish green; soft and downy, lilac-pink flowers are borne in terminal, branched spikes. It is popular for culinary use; the clean mint flavour has overtones of apple.

Growth Mints grow best in rich, damp soil and partial shade. Most do not come true from seed or are sterile hybrids. They are easily propagated by division or by taking root cuttings from early spring throughout the growing season.

Parts used Peppermint, spearmint – leaves, essential oil; pennyroyal, gingermint, Bowles' mint, eau-de-Cologne mint – leaves.

USES Medicinal Peppermint can be taken as a tea for colds and to aid digestion. The essential oil has decongestant, antiseptic, mildly anaesthetic effects and is used externally, often as an inhalant to relieve colds, chest infections, catarrh and asthma. It also has insect-repellent properties. Excess use may cause allergic reactions. Pennyroyal is taken internally as an infusion for indigestion and colic. Stimulates the uterus and should not be given to pregnant or breastfeeding women. Toxic in large doses. An insect-repellent plant, used to deter ants when planted in the garden. Spearmint can be taken as a tea for digestive disorders; it is less pungent than peppermint and a non-irritant.

Culinary Spearmint and Bowles' mint are used in sauces, mint jelly, to flavour yoghurt as a savoury dip or side dish, in salads, rice dishes, meat, fish or vegetable dishes, as a garnish, to flavour herb teas and drinks. Peppermint is used to flavour sweets and chocolates, icings, cakes, desserts, ice creams, cordials and as a tea. Gingermint leaves may be floated in summer drinks. Pennyroyal is traditionally used to flavour black pudding (an old name is pudding grass).

Aromatic Fresh leaves or essential oils are added to baths, cosmetics and fragrant household preparations.

General Essential oils are used in food, pharmaceutical and cosmetic industries.

CAUTION Do not use during pregnancy or when breast-feeding.

Top, from left to right Mentha x gracilis *(ginger mint);* M. x piperita *f.* rubescens *(black peppermint)*; M. x piperita *f.* citrata *(eau-de-Cologne mint);* M. pulegium *(pennyroyal);* M. requienii *(Corsican mint);* M. spicata *(spearmint).*

Above right M. suaveolens *'Variegata' (variegated applemint).*

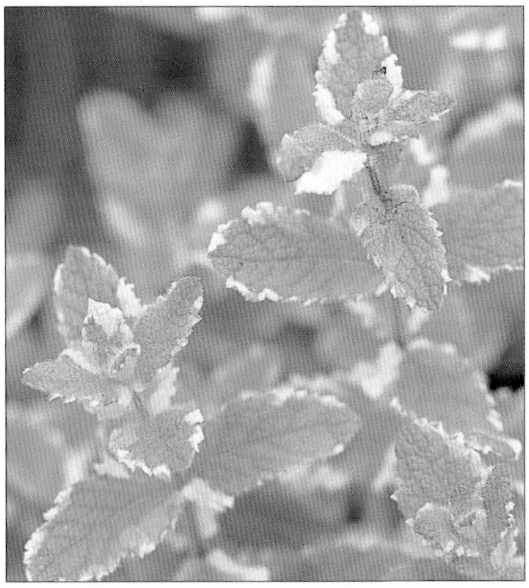

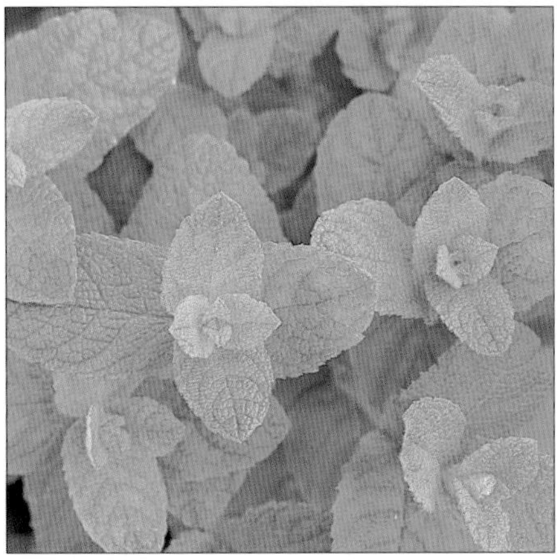

Above Mentha suaveolens, *or applemint.*

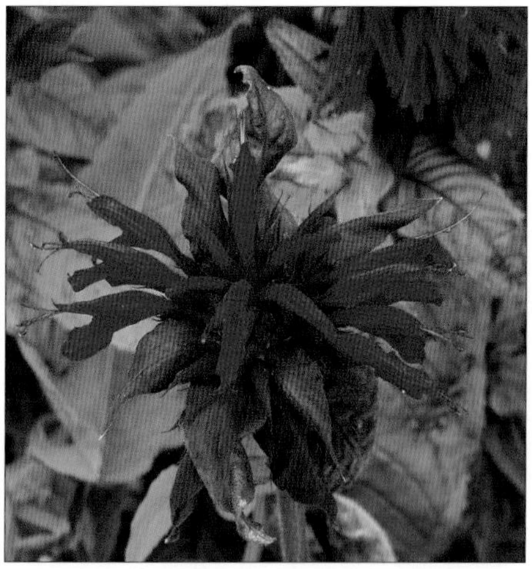

LABIATAE/LAMIACEAE

Monarda didyma

Bergamot

History and traditions Native Americans used several monarda species medicinally. *M. didyma* became known as "Oswego tea" after the Oswego river, near Lake Ontario, where it was found growing by European settlers. Its refreshing taste made a good tea substitute. The scent of flowers and leaves is similar to the Bergamot orange, which is how it gained its common name.
Description An aromatic, hardy perennial, 40–90cm/16in–3ft in height, it has soft, downy, greyish-green, ovate leaves, with serrated edges, and red or mauve flowers in solitary terminal whorls in late summer.
Related species: *M. fistulosa* (wild bergamot) is closely related and has purple flowers – also called "Oswego tea". There are many attractive hybrids including 'Cambridge Scarlet' (above) and 'Croftway Pink'.
Habitat/distribution Native of eastern North America, found in damp woodlands, introduced and widely grown elsewhere.
Growth Grow in humus-rich, damp soil. Prefers partial shade, but tolerates full sun if kept moist. Prone to mildew in dry conditions. Propagated by division or by seed sown in spring.
Parts used Leaves, flowers – fresh or dried.

USES Medicinal Taken as a digestive tea. It has expectorant and antiseptic qualities and helps to relieve wind. It is useful as a diluted essential oil for the treatment of shingles.
Culinary Fresh leaves are added to wine cups, fruit drinks and to China tea to give it an "Earl Grey" flavour.
Aromatic Flowers are dried for potpourri.

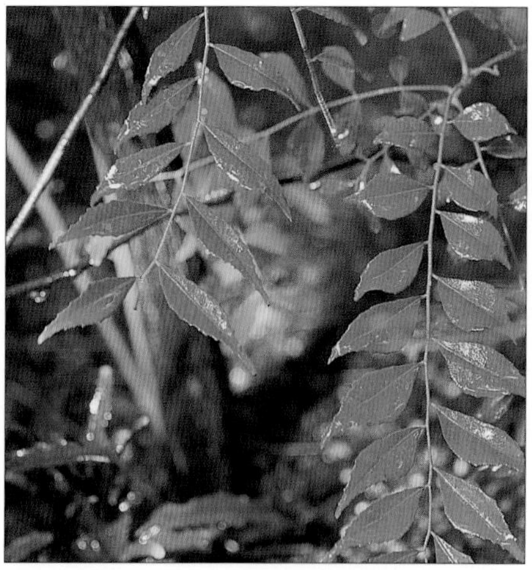

RUTACEAE

Murraya koenigii

Curry leaves

History and traditions The Indian name for the leaves of this shrub is "curry patta" and they have long been used in southern India and Sri Lanka in local dishes as well as for their medicinal properties. Curry leaves are not widely used in the West because much of the flavour is lost on drying – but they are imported fresh by wholesalers for use in the food industry.
Description An aromatic, more or less deciduous shrub, growing to 6m/20ft in height, it has bright green pinnate leaves, with smooth, ovate leaflets. Clusters of small white flowers are followed by edible berries, which turn from green to purple as they ripen.
Habitat/distribution Native to southern India and Sri Lanka, introduced and grown in all tropical zones, found in rich soils.
Growth A tender, tropical shrub, it is grown in humus-rich, moist but well-drained soil in sun or partial shade. Propagated by seed or cuttings.
Parts used Leaves – picked and used fresh; seeds; essential oil – distilled from leaves.

USES Medicinal Contains alkaloids with anti-fungal activity. The juice of the leaves contains vitamin C and minerals, including calcium, phosphorus and iron and is used as a herbal tonic for digestive disorders. Eating the fresh leaves is reputed by some to help prevent the onset of diabetes and to encourage weight loss. Juice of the crushed berries, mixed with lime juice, is applied to insect bites and stings.
Culinary Used in Indian cookery to flavour a variety of dishes, including curries and chutneys.
General Essential oil used in the soap industry.

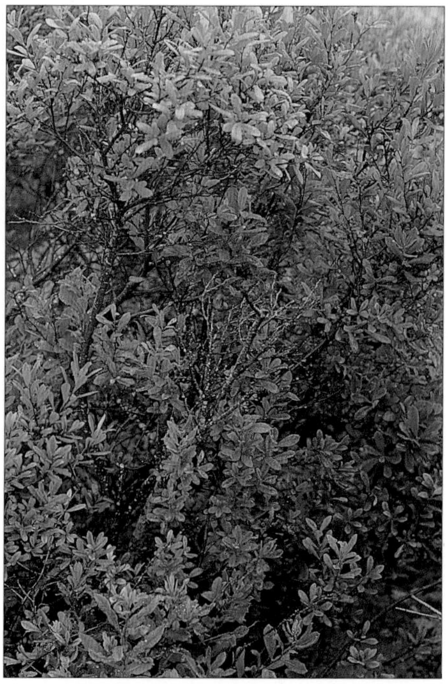

MYRICACEAE

Myrica gale

Bog myrtle

History and traditions This was once an indispensable plant in much of northern Europe for its many household uses. It was used as a hops substitute to flavour beer and improve its foaming; the fruits were boiled to produce wax for making candles; it made a yellow dye; and its insect-repellent properties meant it was often put into mattress stuffings, which gave it the former name "flea wood".
Description Hardy, deciduous shrub, growing to 1.5m/5ft, it has narrow, bright green, oval to lanceolate leaves and yellowish-green flowers, borne in dense catkins in late spring to early summer, followed by flattened yellow brown fruits.
Habitat/distribution Native to North America, northwest Europe and northeast Siberia, found in wet heathlands.
Growth Prefers a damp, acid soil (tolerates boggy conditions) and partial shade, but can be grown in full sun. Propagated by separating suckers, by cuttings, or by seed sown in spring or autumn.
Parts used Leaves – dried.

USES Aromatic Strongly insecticidal. Dried leaves can be added to insect-repellent mixtures and sachets.
Other name Sweet gale.

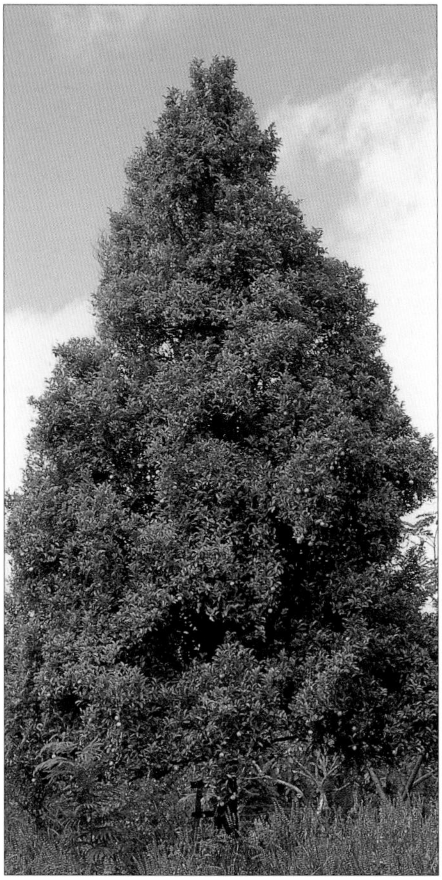

MYRISTICACEAE

Myristica fragrans

Nutmeg / Mace

History and traditions Nutmeg and mace are different parts of the same fruit of the nutmeg tree. The scent of the nutmeg has variously been compared with myrrh and musk. The common name comes from "nut" and the Latin, *muscus,* or old French, *mugue,* meaning musk. Nutmegs were probably introduced to Europe in about the 6th century by Arab or Indian traders, who brought them to the Mediterranean from the Far East. The Portuguese set up a trade monopoly in this valuable spice at the beginning of the 16th century after taking possession of the Moluccan islands where the trees grew. This was taken over by the Dutch, who limited cultivation of nutmeg to the Moluccas and continued the monopoly into the 19th century. Today nutmeg is widely grown in tropical regions, with Indonesia and the West Indies as leading world producers. It has been used over the centuries as a medicinal tonic and culinary spice, its hallucinogenic properties have long been recognized and it acquired a reputation as an effective aphrodisiac.

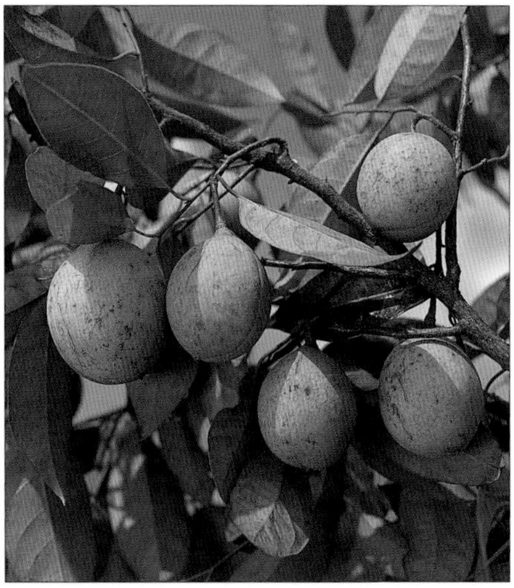

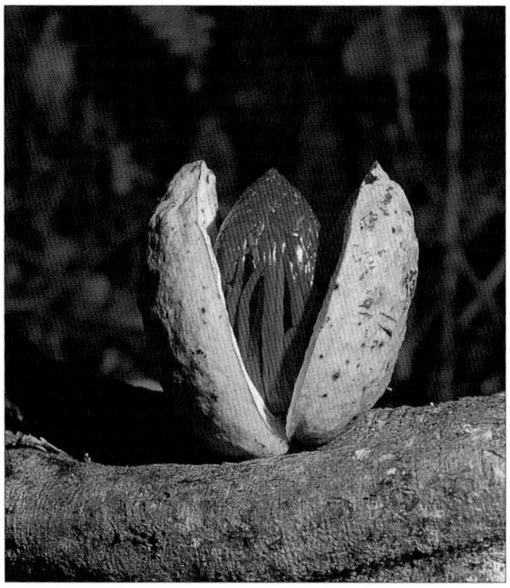

Above left *Whole nutmeg fruits on the tree.*

Above *The outer shell splits to reveal the nutmeg seed, enclosed in a red aril.*

Description An evergreen dioecious tree, usually 9–12m/29–39ft but occasionally up to 15–20m/49–65ft tall, with glossy, pointed oval leaves and inconspicuous pale yellow flowers, male in clusters with numerous fused stamens, the female solitary or in groups. Brownish-yellow globular fruits each containing an ovoid brown seed (nutmeg), surrounded by a shredded crimson aril (mace), do not appear before the tree is 9–10 years old.

Habitat Indigenous to Molucca (Maluku) and Banda islands, now widely grown in Indonesia, Sri Lanka, India, the West Indies, Brazil and elsewhere in tropical zones, frequently on volcanic soils in areas of high humidity.

Growth A tender, tropical tree, grown in sandy, humus-rich soil. Prefers shade or partial shade. Propagated by seed or cuttings. May be grown as a conservatory or hothouse plant in temperate regions, with a minimum temperature of 18°C/64°F and a humid atmosphere.

Parts used Seed (nutmeg), aril (mace) – dried and used whole or powdered; volatile oil distilled from fruits; fatty oil compressed from mace (nutmeg butter, mace oil).

USES Medicinal Nutmeg is taken internally, in small doses, for digestive disorders, nausea and insomnia. Applied externally for toothache and rheumatic aches and pains.

CAUTION Nutmeg should always be used sparingly. It contains a toxic compound, myristicin, whose chemical structure has similarities with mescaline, and can cause hallucinations and convulsions even in moderate doses.

Culinary Both nutmeg and mace are ground or grated and used in a wide range of sweet and savoury dishes, but mace is less pungent. Added to soups, sauces, milk and cheese dishes, meat and vegetable dishes, biscuits, fruit cakes, puddings and drinks.

General Volatile oil and fatty oil (nutmeg butter) are used in the pharmaceutical and perfumery industries.

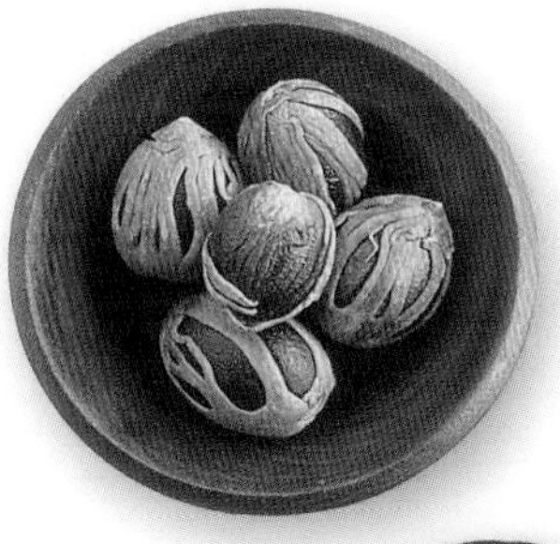

Top *Nutmegs with outer covering of mace (dried aril).*

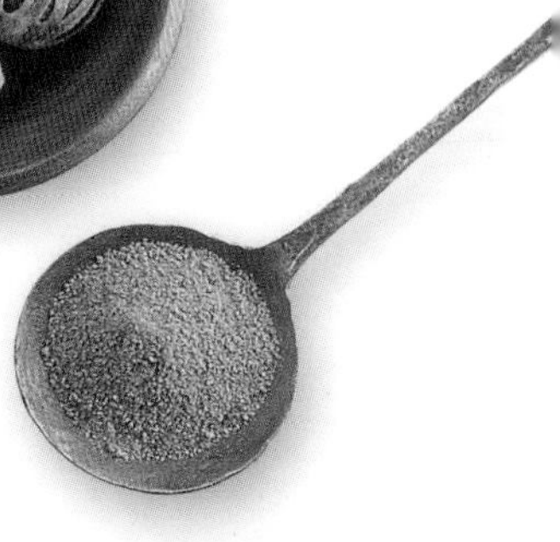

Centre *Ground nutmeg.*

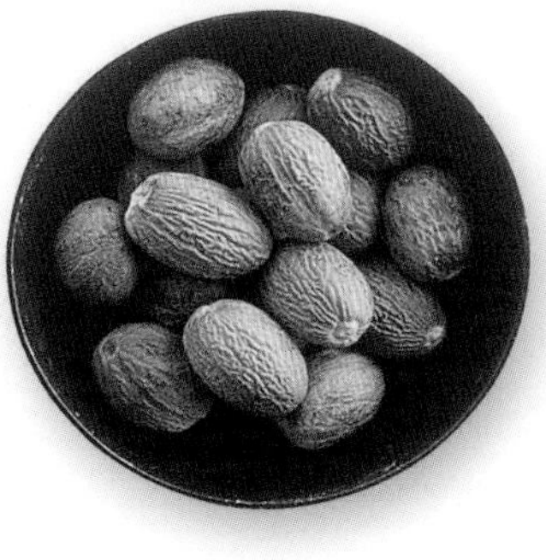

Right *Dried nutmeg seeds.*

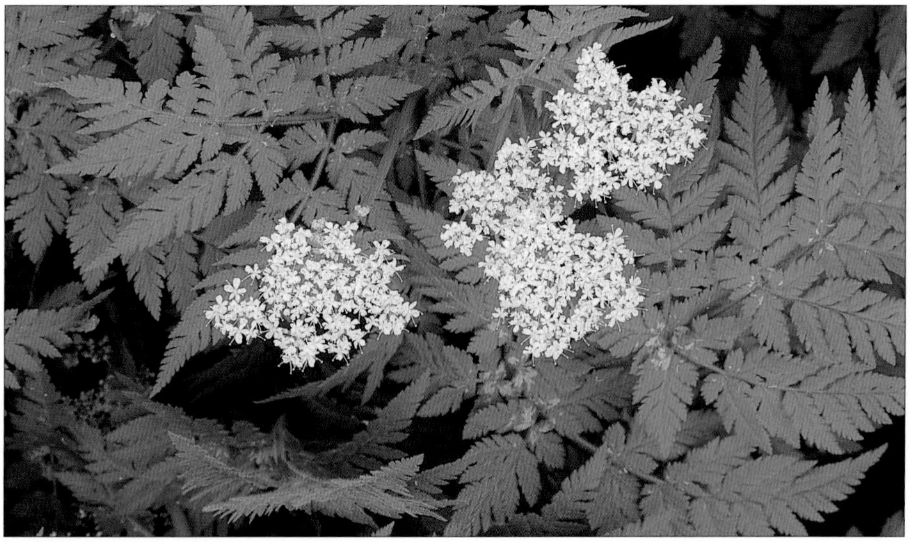

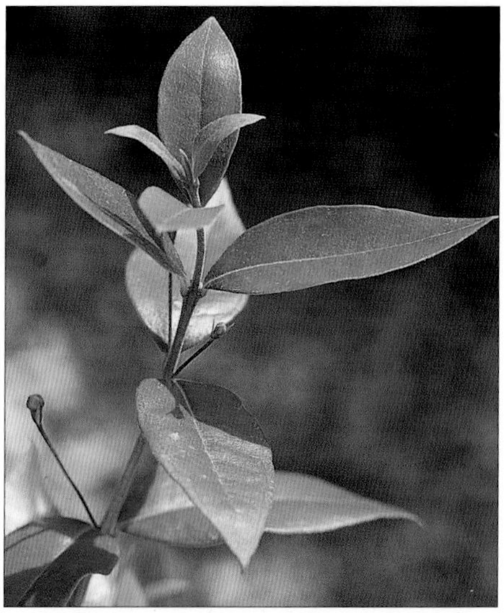

UMBELLIFERAE/APIACEAE

Myrrhis odorata

Sweet cicely

History and traditions The Latin name refers to the sweet aniseed smell of this herb, said to resemble myrrh – *Myrrhis* comes from the Greek word for fragrance. It is probable that the "wild chervil", or "sweet chervil", referred to in old herbals is the same plant. *The Leech Book of Bald, c.* AD950, gives a salve of wild chervil for the treatment of tumours. It was used as a medieval strewing herb, and the roots and leaves were cooked as a pot-herb. Recent scientific research has found that compounds isolated from *M. odorata* are related in chemical structure to podophyllotoxin, the highly poisonous active ingredient of *Podophyllum peltatum* (American may-apple). However, this does not mean that *M. odorata* as a whole plant, or the isolated compounds, have the same high level of toxicity as *Podophyllum peltatum*, and it is not thought to be harmful as a culinary herb.

Description A vigorous, hardy, herbaceous perennial, with a strong taproot, grows 0.9–1.2m/3–4ft tall, with hollow stems and soft, downy fernlike leaves. Compound umbels of white flowers appear in late spring, followed by large, distinctively beaked and ridged brown fruit. The whole plant is pleasantly scented.

Habitat/distribution Native to Europe, introduced and naturalized in other temperate regions, found in hedgerows and field edges often in shady positions.

Growth Grows under any conditions, in sun or shade, but said to prefer moist, humus-rich soil.

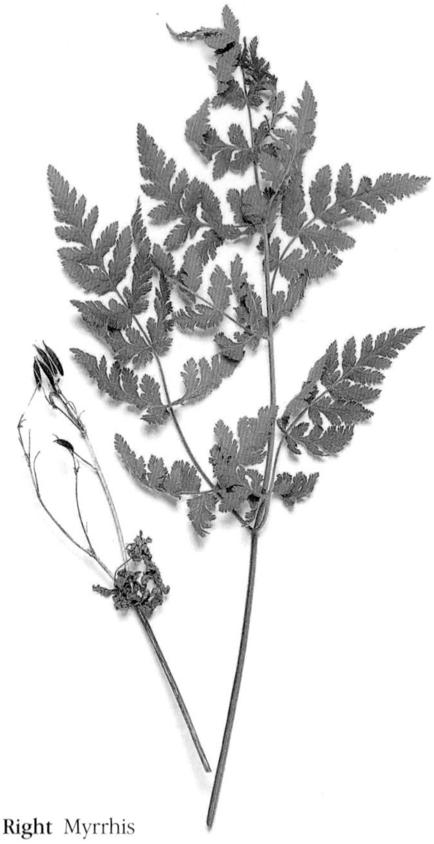

Right Myrrhis odorata

An invasive plant which self-seeds and spreads rapidly and is virtually impossible to eradicate once established. Propagated by seed, after vernalization, or by division of roots in spring.

Parts used Leaves – fresh.

USES Culinary Traditionally used as a sweetening agent and flavouring for stewed soft fruits and rhubarb. Leaves also make a pretty garnish for sweet and savoury dishes.

MYRTACEAE

Myrtus communis

Myrtle

History and traditions This sweet-smelling shrub from the Mediterranean was dedicated to Venus, goddess of love. Myrtle has long been associated with weddings and included in bridal bouquets. After the ceremony, sprigs were often planted as cuttings in the garden of the marital home or beside the front door, to ensure peace and love within, which happy states would be lost if the plants died or were dug up.

Description An evergreen shrub, to 3m/10ft tall, with glossy ovate to lanceolate leaves, dotted with oil glands. Fragrant white five-petalled flowers, which appear in early summer, are followed by blue-black berries.

Related species *M. communis* subsp. *tarentina* is a compact variant, 0.9–1.5m/3–5ft tall.

Habitat/description Native to the Mediterranean region and western Asia, introduced and widely grown elsewhere.

Growth Frost-hardy, but does not tolerate prolonged cold spells and waterlogged soils. Propagated by semi-ripe cuttings in late summer.

Parts used Leaves – fresh for culinary use, dried for infusions; fruits – fresh or dried; volatile oil.

USES Medicinal Myrtle has antiseptic, decongestant properties and it is taken internally, in infusions, for colds, chest infections, sinusitis and for urinary infections.

Culinary The leaves and fruits are used in Middle Eastern cookery with lamb and game.

General The essential oil is used in perfumery, cosmetic and soap industries.

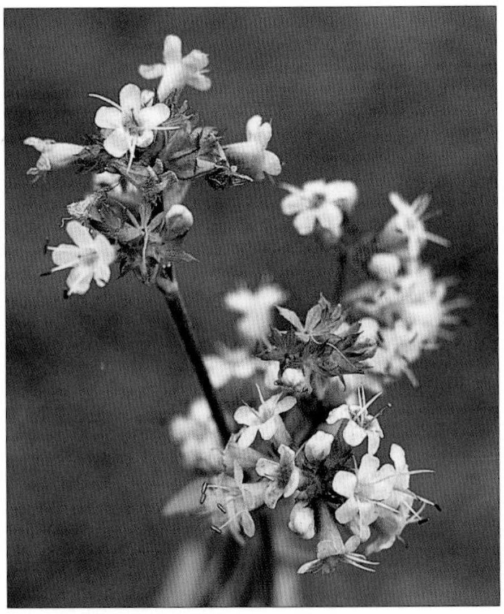

VALERIANACEAE

Nardostachys grandiflora

Spikenard

History and traditions This plant was an ingredient of the expensive perfumed unguents of the Romans and ancient Eastern nations, prized for the durability of its scent. It was the "very costly" ointment of spikenard with which Mary wiped the feet of Jesus (John 12:3–5). The Indian name *jatamansi* refers to the bearded appearance of the fibrous rhizomes, or "spikes", which were supposed to resemble ears of corn.
Description An erect perennial, 25–30cm/10–12in in height, with a fibrous rootstock, crowned by nearly basal lanceolate leaves and from which stems bearing pale pink flowers in terminal clusters arise.
Habitat/distribution Native to the Himalayas from Kumaon to Sikkim and Bhutan, at altitudes of 3,000–5,000m/9,800–16,400ft, where the atmosphere is cool and moist, on poor, stony soil and rocky ledges.
Growth Fully hardy; grow in gritty, well-drained, poorish soil, in a rockery or similar situation, but provide midday or partial shade and plenty of moisture to keep roots cool.
Parts used Roots – dried for use in decoctions; volatile oil distilled from roots.

USES Medicinal: An important herb in Ayurvedic medicine for over 3,000 years, the root has antiseptic, bitter tonic properties and is soothing to the nervous system. It is used for insomnia and as a gentle tranquillizer, for menopausal problems, respiratory disorders and in the treatment of intestinal worms.

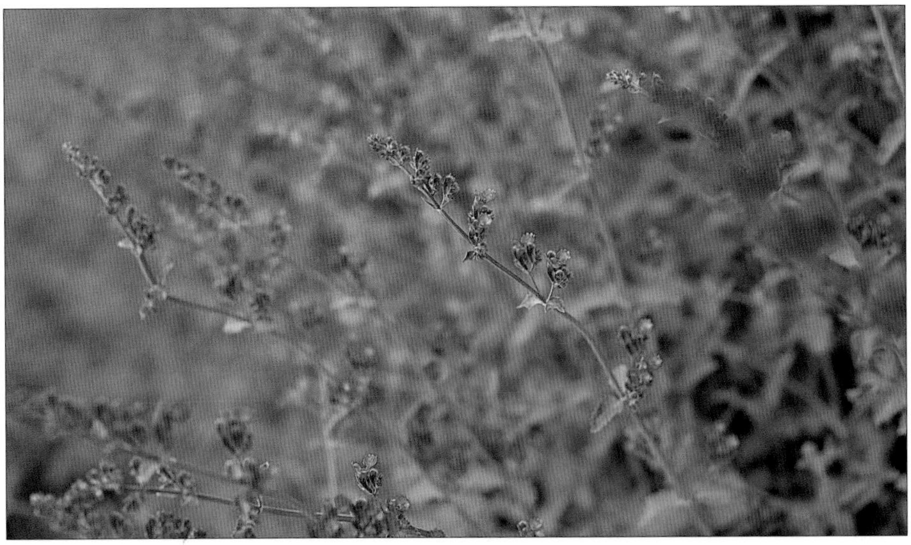

Above Nepeta x faassenii.

LABIATAE/LAMIACEAE

Nepeta cataria

Catmint

History and traditions This herb often proves irresistible to cats. It is mildly hallucinogenic, which could be the attraction, but another theory is that the plant has overtones of tomcats' urine and is associated with courtship behaviour. It is also said to be hated by rats. Chewing the root is reputed to make humans aggressive, and one old British story recalls that a reluctant hangman used it to give him courage to carry out his duties. There are references to its medicinal properties in old herbals, it was occasionally used for flavouring, and found its way into herbal tobaccos, but it does not seem to be widely used today, except perhaps to make toys for cats.
Description A hardy perennial, 30–90cm/1–3ft tall, it has coarse-textured, ovate, grey-green leaves, with serrated edges. Pale mauve flowers in terminal or axillary whorls are borne from midsummer to autumn. The whole plant has a strong, antiseptic, mintlike odour, similar to pennyroyal.
Related species The hybrid *N.* x *faassenii*, commonly known as *N. mussinii*, is a more attractive plant, frequently grown in herb gardens for its prolific, soft-blue flowers, which bloom over a long period. It has no medicinal virtues – but cats have been observed rolling in it.
Habitat/distribution Occurs in Europe, Asia and Africa, introduced and naturalized in North America and temperate zones. Found in moist, calcareous soils, on roadsides, in hedgerows and field edges.

Growth Catmint prefers moist soil and a sunny position. Propagated by root division in spring or autumn or by cuttings in summer.
Parts used Leaves and flowering stems – dried or fresh.

USES Medicinal Catmint lowers fever, increases perspiration and is mildly sedative. It is sometimes taken as an infusion for feverish colds, influenza, nervous tension, anxiety and gastric upsets, or applied externally to cuts and bruises.
Culinary It makes a stimulating, minty tea.
Household The dried herb is used to stuff toys for cats.
Other names Catnip and catnep.

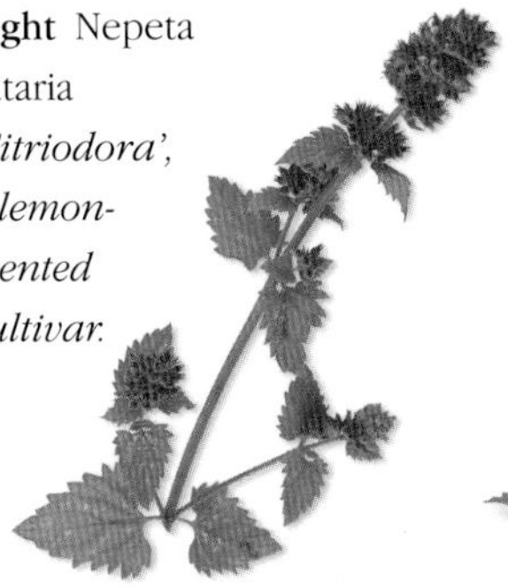

Right Nepeta cataria *'Citriodora', a lemon-scented cultivar.*

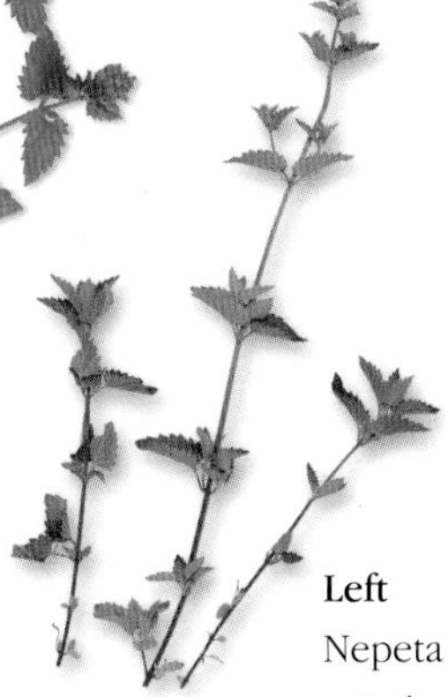

Left Nepeta cataria

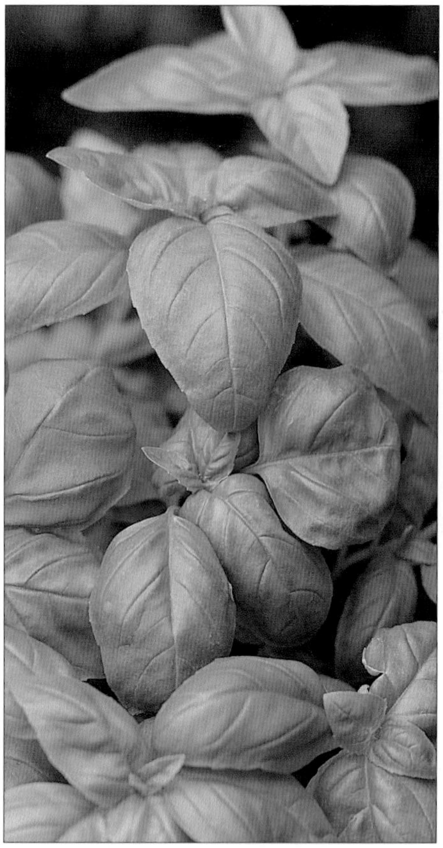

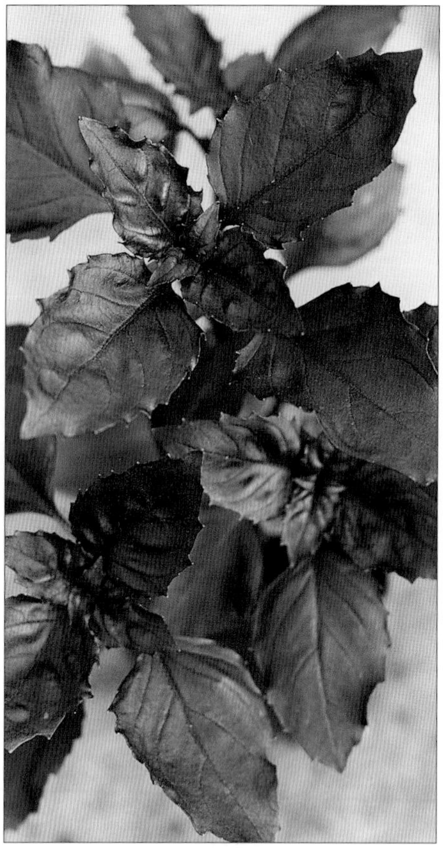

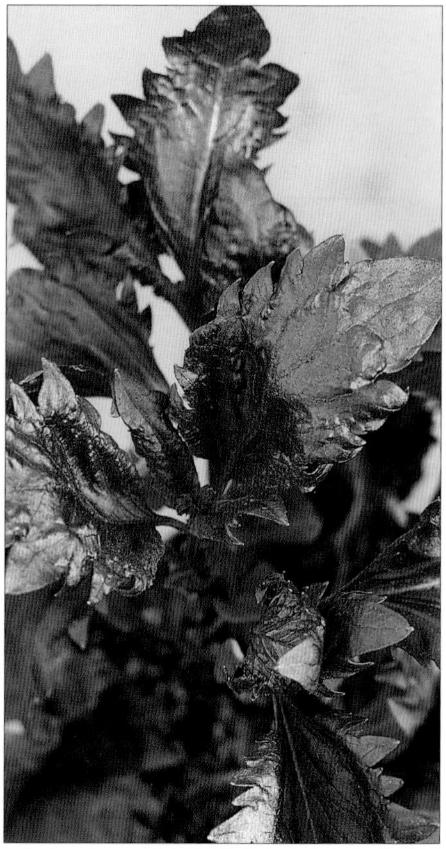

LABIATAE/LAMIACEAE

Ocimum basilicum

Basil

History and traditions A native of India, basil first came to Europe in the 16th century. In India, where it is known as *tulsi,* it is sacred to the god Vishnu. It is thought to protect from misfortune and is planted in temple gardens and offered at Hindu shrines. Traditionally, a basil leaf was placed on the chest of a corpse, after the head had been washed in basil water. In other Eastern cultures it became a funeral herb, planted or scattered on graves. Basil has a mass of conflicting associations. As Culpeper remarked, "This is the herb which all authors are together by the ears about and rail at one another (like lawyers)" (*The English Physician*, 1653). The Greeks and Romans thought it represented hate and misfortune, and that shouting abuse at it encouraged it to grow. In some later European cultures it represented sympathy and the acceptance of love. In Crete, it stood for love washed with tears, taking a middle line. There was no agreement on its properties either, in former times. Some said it was poisonous, others that it was health-inducing. In 16th-century Britain it was appreciated for its scent. Thomas Tusser listed it as a strewing herb and John Parkinson wrote, "The ordinary Basil is in a manner wholly spent to make sweete or washing waters among other sweete herbs, yet sometimes it is put into nosegays" (*Paradisi,* 1629). Today it is among the most popular and widely grown of culinary herbs.

Description A much-branched half-hardy annual, to 20–60cm/8–24in tall, with soft, ovate, bright green leaves and whorls of small white flowers, borne in terminal racemes in mid to late summer.

Related species Basils are extremely variable. Even within the same species, the pungency and flavour vary considerably, according to the composition of their volatile oils, which depends on soil, climate and growing conditions. They also hybridize easily under cultivation and many that are sold commercially are not recognized as distinct varieties or cultivars by botanists. ***O. glabrescens*** **'Dark Opal'** is a reliable cultivar with purple leaves and bright cerise-pink flowers. ***O. g.*** **'Purple Ruffles'** has large crinkled, purplish leaves with curly edges and makes a vigorous bush. ***O. basilicum.*** **var. *crispum*** **(curly basil)** has coarse, curled, dark green leaves, and is sometimes known as "Neapolitana". ***O. b.*** **'Genovese'** has soft but broader leaves than the species, is strongly aromatic, and frequently offered as a culinary variety – popular in pesto sauce. ***O. b.*** **var. *minimum*** **(bush basil, Greek basil)** is very compact and bushy, growing 15–30cm/6–12in tall, and has small, but pungent leaves and tiny white flowers. ***O. sanctum*** **(holy basil, tulsi)** is a shrubby perennial, 45–60cm/18–24in, with green, slightly hairy, ovate leaves and thin white to pale mauve flower spikes. Other cultivars with interesting flavours include ***O. b.*** **'Horapha'**, often used in oriental cuisines; and ***O. b.*** **'Cinnamon'**, which is from Mexico, about 30–60cm/12–24in high, with pink flowers and a distinctive cinnamon scent.

Habitat/distribution Native to India and the Middle East, naturalized in parts of Africa and other tropical and subtropical regions, introduced and widely grown elsewhere.

Growth Basil requires well-drained, moist, medium-rich soil and full sun. It is propagated from seed, which must be sown after any danger of frost in cool regions. In cold, wet, northern summers it may need to be grown on under glass, but flourishes as a container plant and should be kept outside in hot, dry spells to develop the best flavour.

Parts used Leaves – fresh, essential oil.

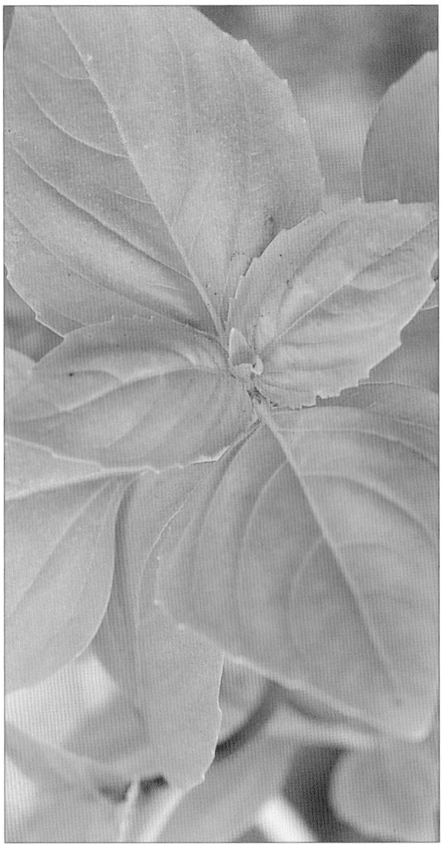

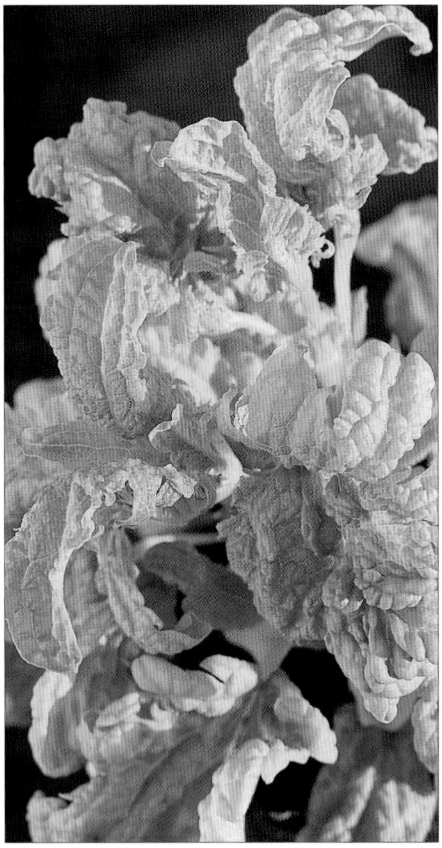

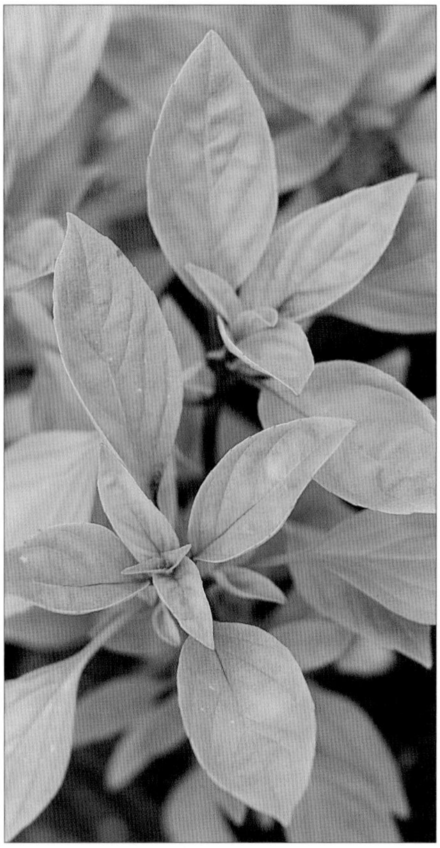

Top, from left to right Ocimum basilicum; O. glabrescens *'Dark Opal'*; O. g. *'Purple Ruffles'*; O. b. *'Cinnamon'*; O. b. *'Green Ruffles'*; O. b. *'Thai'*.

Right Ocimum basilicum *var.* minimum.

Below right Ocimum sanctum.

USES Medicinal Has antidepressant, antiseptic, soothing properties. The fresh leaves are rubbed on insect bites and stings to relieve itching, made into cough syrups, and taken as an infusion for colds. The leaves or essential oil are used in steam inhalations as a decongestant for colds; diluted essential oil makes an insect repellent or massage oil for depression and anxiety. **Culinary** The leaves do not retain their flavour well when dried and are better used fresh. They have an affinity with tomatoes and aubergines (eggplants), and add a distinctive fragrance to tomato-based dishes. Fresh basil should be added towards the end of the cooking process so that its fragrance is not lost. Basil is a good choice for planting in a kitchen herb garden. **Aromatic** The essential oil is used in aromatherapy and as a perfumery ingredient. **Other name** Sweet basil.

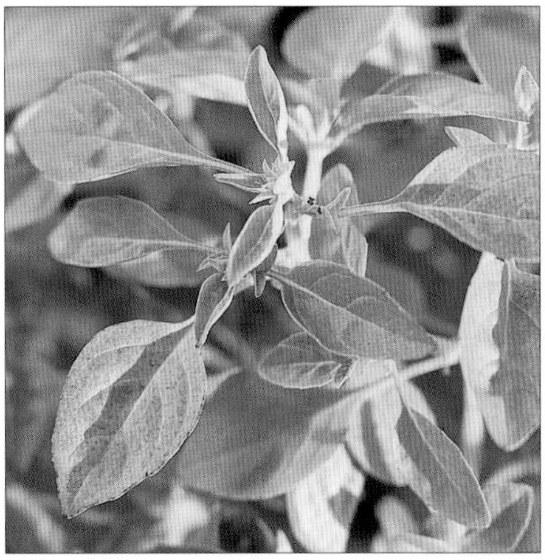

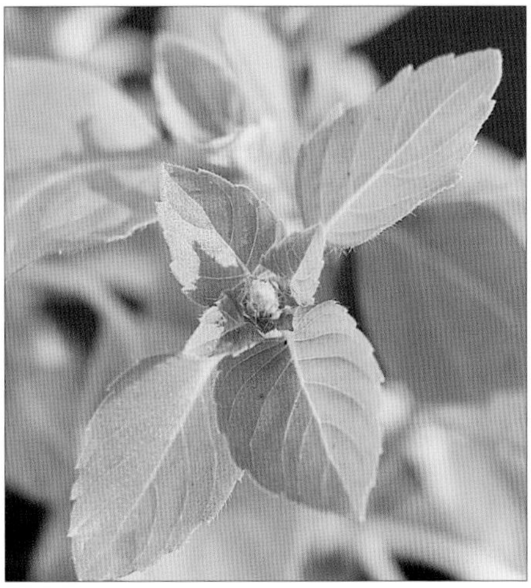

Pesto sauce

The traditional way of making this sauce was to pound the ingredients with a pestle and mortar.

Serves 4
50g/2oz fresh basil leaves
25g/1oz fresh parsley
2–3 cloves of garlic
8 tbsp extra virgin olive oil
25g/1oz grated Parmesan cheese
salt and ground black pepper

Put the basil, parsley, garlic and olive, into a food processor or blender and blend until smooth. Scrape down the mixture from time to time. Decant into a bowl. Stir in the grated Parmesan and season to taste. Keep refrigerated for up to two weeks.

CAUTION Essential oil should not be used during pregnancy. *Ocimum sanctum*, Holy Basil, should only be taken on professional advice and is not to be taken by diabetics.

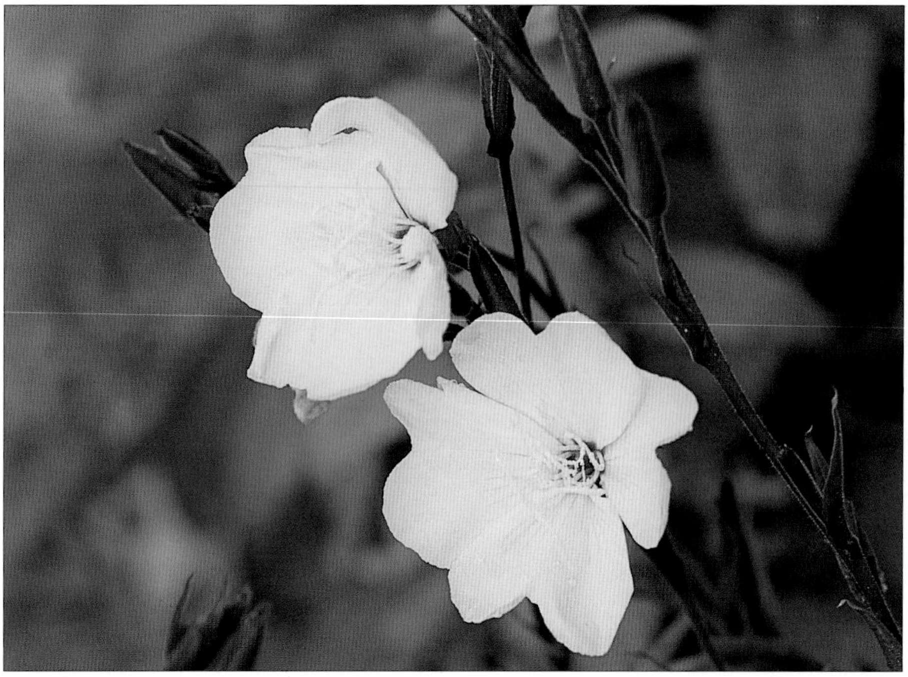

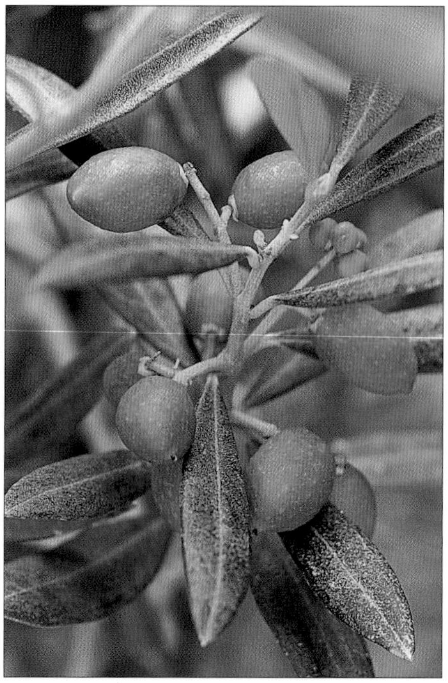

ONAGRACEAE

Oenothera biennis

Evening primrose

History and traditions An American native, the evening primrose was introduced to Europe in 1619, when seeds were brought to the Padua Botanic Garden in Italy. Although it had some place in the folk medicine of Native Americans, in Europe it was used more as a culinary than a medicinal herb – leaves were put into salads and roots cooked as vegetables. It came to prominence after modern research in the 1980s established that oil from the seeds contains GLA, or gamma-linolenic acid, an unsaturated fatty acid which assists the production of prostaglandins, hormone-like substances, which act as chemical messengers and regulate hormonal systems. It is not related to the primrose (*Primula vulgaris*).

Description An erect biennial, up to 1.5m/5ft tall, with a thick, yellowish taproot and a rosette of basal leaves from which the flowering stems arise. These have alternate, lanceolate to ovate leaves, and are topped by bright yellow flowers, which open at night to release their fragrance and are pollinated by moths. Downy pods follow, containing tiny seeds.

Habitat/distribution Originated in North America, introduced and naturalized throughout Europe and in temperate zones. Found on poor, sandy soils, waste ground and embankments, as a garden escapee.

Growth Grow in open, sandy soil in a warm sunny position. This plant self-seeds freely once established. Propagated from seed sown in autumn or spring.

Parts used Seeds – pressed to produce oil.

USES Medicinal The oil is thought to benefit the immune system and regulate hormones. It is taken internally for premenstrual tension, menopausal problems, allergies, skin complaints, such as eczema and acne, and to counteract the effects of excess alcohol. It may also be helpful for high blood pressure, arthritis and multiple sclerosis.

Cosmetic The fresh flowers are often made into face masks to improve skin tone. The oil is an ingredient in commercial cosmetics and pharmaceutical products.

CAUTION Only to be taken on medical advice if other prescribed medication is being taken. Can interact with epilepsy drugs. Not to be taken in pregnancy.

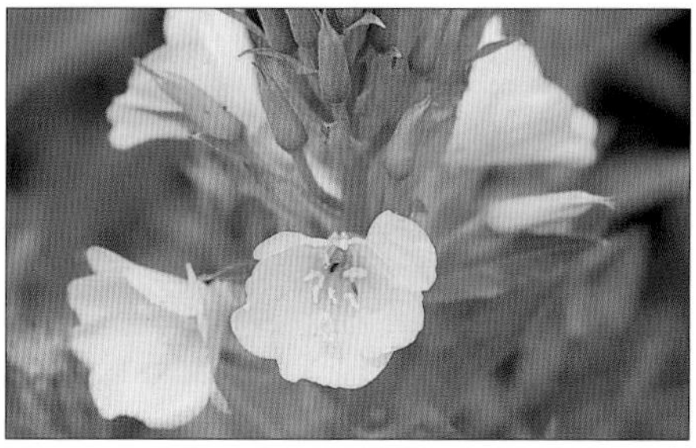

OLEACEAE

Olea europaea

Olive

History and traditions There is evidence that the olive tree has been cultivated north of the Dead Sea since 3700–3600BC. Known to the Egyptians, it was always prized for the quality of the oil from the fruits. The Romans called the tree *"olea"*, from *oleum,* meaning oil, the Greek word being *elaio.* The olive branch has been a symbol of peace and reconciliation since the biblical story of the dove returning to Noah's Ark with a sprig of olive in its beak after the flood had subsided.

Description An evergreen tree, 9–12m/29–40ft tall, it has pale grey bark and pendulous branches, with smooth, leathery, grey-green, lanceolate to oblong leaves. Creamy-white flowers are borne in short panicles in summer, followed by green, ripening to dark purple fruits, known as drupes.

Habitat/distribution Native to the Mediterranean region, introduced in warm temperate regions of Africa and Asia.

Growth Requires well-drained to dry soil and full sun. Although frost hardy, it can be grown outside successfully only in Mediterranean climates. Propagated by seed sown in autumn or by semi-ripe cuttings in summer.

Parts used Leaves – dried for use in infusions and other herbal preparations; fruits – harvested in autumn and winter, by beating them from

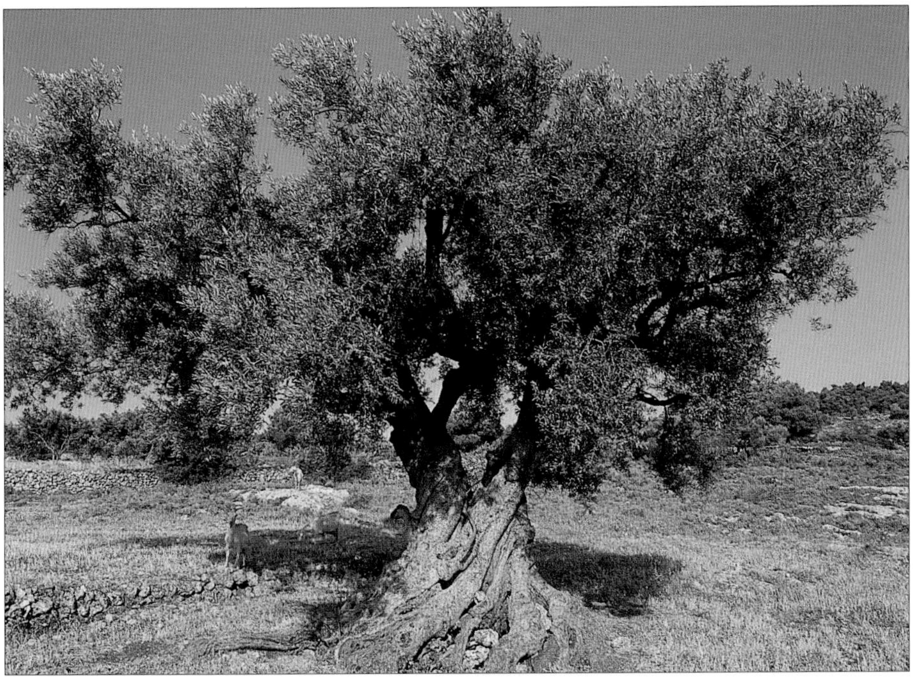

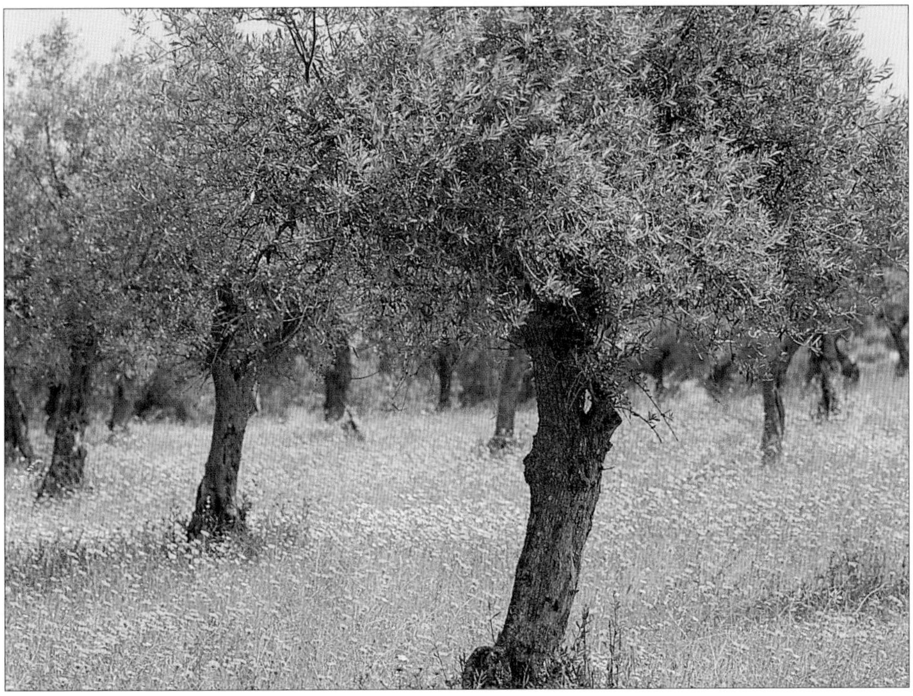

the trees on to groundsheets; oil – pressed from the fruit. Extra virgin, cold-pressed oil, extracted without heat or chemical solvents, has the best flavour and properties.

USES Medicinal The oil is monounsaturated and its consumption is thought to help lower cholesterol levels and blood pressure, reducing risk of circulatory diseases. Leaves are antiseptic and astringent, taken internally in infusions for nervous tension and high blood pressure and applied externally to cuts and abrasions. The oil is thought to be helpful when taken internally for constipation and peptic ulcers.
Culinary The fruits of the olive tree are eaten as appetizers, made into *tapenade* spread, added to salads, sauces, bread, pizzas, pasta and many other dishes. The oil is used in salad dressings, sauces, mayonnaise and as a general cooking oil.

Top *The olive tree is slow growing and often attains a great age.*

Above *An olive grove in Extremadura, Spain.*

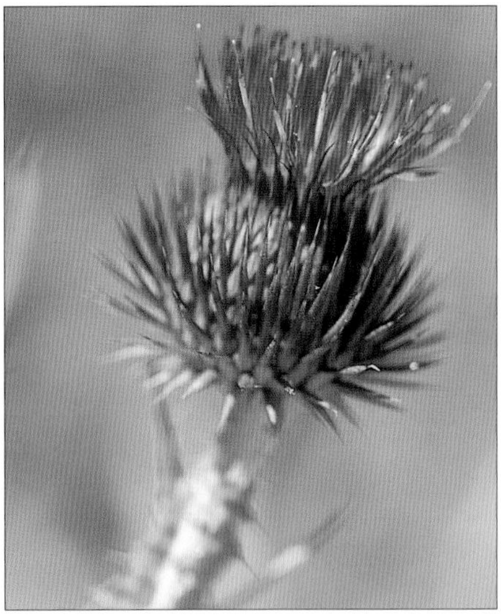

ASTERACEAE/COMPOSITAE

Onopordum acanthium

Scotch thistle

History and traditions This is thought to be the thistle that is the national emblem of Scotland, dating from the time of James III of Scotland (d. 1488). It is also the emblem of the ancient, knightly Order of the Thistle, inaugurated by James V of Scotland, 1513–1542. Some bizarre claims were made for the properties of this plant. Pliny recommended it for baldness and Dioscorides as "a remedy for those that have their bodies drawne backwards".
Description A hardy biennial, growing on a strong taproot, the spiny, toothed, dark green leaves have a striking cobweb-effect pattern of white veins, with purple thistle-head flowers rising on long stems to 1.5m/5ft.
Habitat/distribution Occurs in the Mediterranean, Europe and Asia, introduced and naturalized in other countries.
Growth Grows in most conditions, but flourishes in reasonably fertile, well-drained soil and a sunny position. Propagated by seed sown in autumn or spring.
Parts used Leaves, stems, flowers.

USES Medicinal Scotch thistle is rarely used medicinally currently.
Culinary The whole plant is edible if not very palatable. Young stems can be boiled as a vegetable; flower receptacles are said to be substitutes for artichoke hearts.
Horticultural It is widely grown as a herb garden ornamental.
Other names Cotton thistle and woolly thistle.

LABIATAE/LAMIACEAE

Origanum

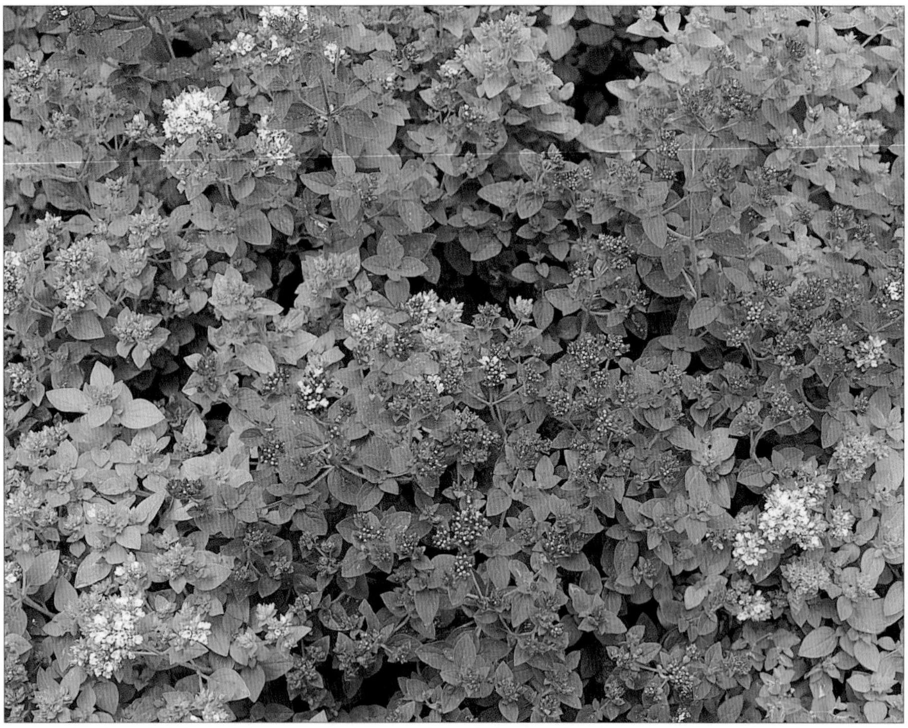

Above Origanum onites, *or pot marjoram, surrounded by Golden marjoram.*

History and traditions *Origanum* means "joy of the mountains" from the Greek *oros,* a mountain, and *ganos,* brightness or joy. According to legend, Aphrodite, Greek goddess of love, found this herb in the depths of the ocean and took it to the top of a mountain where it would be close to the sun's rays. Ever since, it has been associated with the return of sunshine and warmth, with love and the banishing of sorrow. It found a place at both weddings and funerals, being used to crown newly married couples and to provide comfort to mourners. The tradition arose that planting *Origanum* on a grave ensured a happy afterlife for the deceased and Gerard recommends it for those "given to over much sighing" (*The Herball,* 1597). It is one of the most versatile herbs, variable in form, and valued through the centuries for its fragrant, medicinal and culinary properties alike.

Species and nomenclature There is often confusion about the difference between oregano and marjoram. Marjoram is the common English name for the *Origanum* species, but *O. vulgare*, or 'wild marjoram', is widely known as 'oregano' and *O. onites* is sometimes called 'Greek oregano'. To complicate matters further, there are many hybrids among cultivated marjorams, which are difficult to identify and variously named.

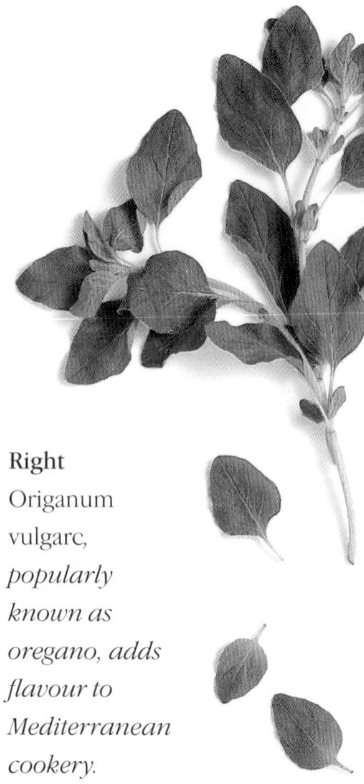

Right Origanum vulgare, *popularly known as oregano, adds flavour to Mediterranean cookery.*

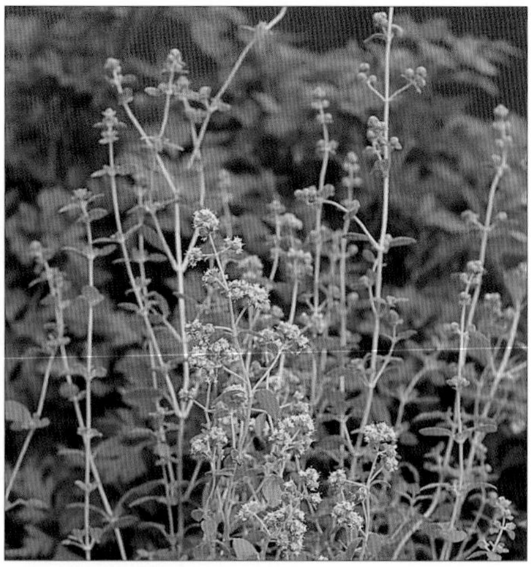

Origanum majorana
Sweet marjoram

Description A half-hardy perennial, often grown as an annual, 60cm/2ft tall, with elliptic pale greyish-green leaves, arranged opposite. The small, white, sometimes pinkish, flowers grow in distinctive knotlike clusters, surrounding the stems, giving it the once popular name "knotted marjoram".

Habitat/distribution *O. majorana* originated in the Mediterranean and Turkey and is widely naturalized in northern Africa, western Asia, parts of India and introduced to many places elsewhere. Found on dryish but often nutrient-rich soils in sunny positions.

Growth Requires well-drained, but not too dry, fertile soil and full sun. Propagated by seed sown in spring, after danger of frost in cool temperate regions.

Parts used Leaves, flowering stems – fresh or dry; essential oil distilled from leaves.

USES Medicinal A warming, relaxing herb with antiseptic properties, taken internally as an infusion for nervous anxiety, insomnia, tension headaches, colds and bronchial complaints, digestive complaints and painful menstruation. Dilute oil is applied externally for muscular aches and pains, sprains and stiff joints.

Culinary It is said to have the most delicate flavour of the marjorams and is widely used in Italian, Greek and Mediterranean cookery, especially in pasta sauces, pizza toppings, tomato sauces, vegetable dishes, and to flavour bread, oil and vinegar.

Aromatic Dried flowering stems add fragrance to potpourri. Essential oil is used in food and cosmetic industries.

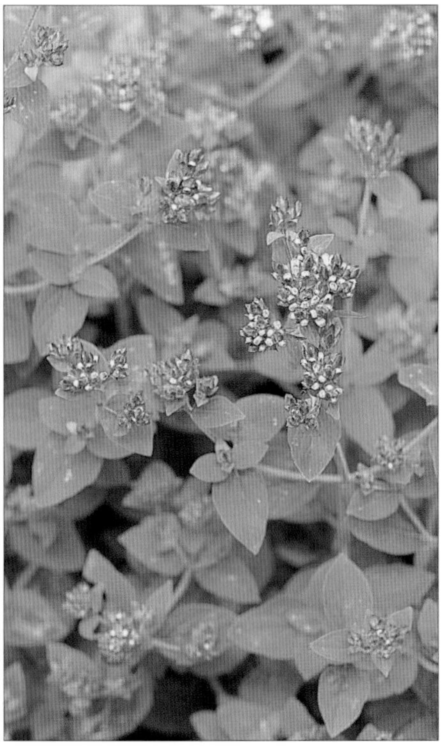

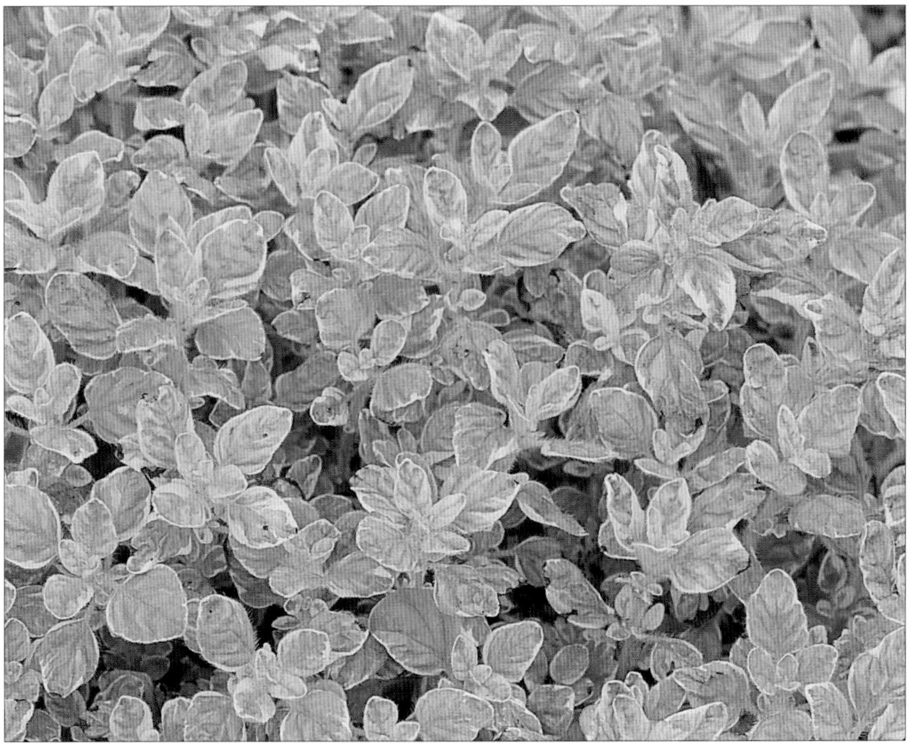

Origanum onites
Pot marjoram

Description A hardy to frost-hardy perennial, 60cm/2ft tall, with hairy stems, and ovate-elliptic, bright green, downy leaves. White or purple flowers are borne in dense clusters in mid to late summer.
Habitat/distribution Native to the Mediterranean and the Middle East, introduced and widely grown in other countries. Grows on light, well-drained soils and open hillsides.
Growth Grow in well-drained soil in a sunny position. Propagated by division or by cuttings taken in summer.
Parts used Leaves, flowers – fresh or dried.

USES Culinary The flavour is less delicate than *O. majorana,* and not as pungent and aromatic as most *O. vulgare*, but it makes an acceptable alternative for similar culinary uses.
Aromatic Dried leaves and flowers are added to potpourri.

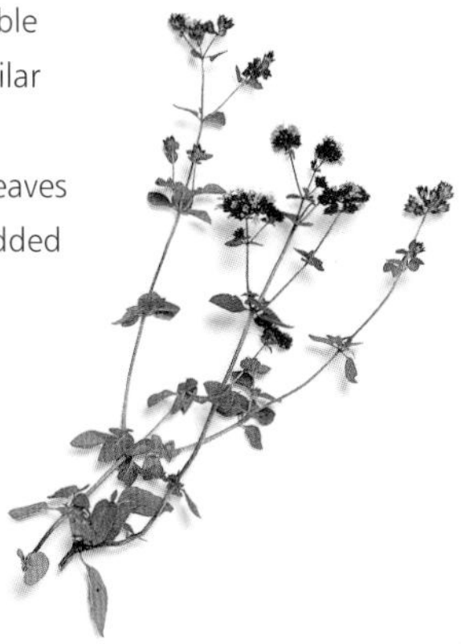

Right Origanum onites

Origanum vulgare
Oregano

Description A variable, bushy, hardy perennial, to 60cm/2ft, with aromatic, ovate, dark green leaves and panicles of pink to purple tubular flowers in summer. It usually has a higher proportion of thymol than *O. majorana,* giving it a more thyme-like scent. The composition of the essential oils and flavour of the plant varies according to soil, sun and general growing conditions. Oregano grown in cooler, wetter regions does not have the same intensity of flavour as that grown in a Mediterranean climate.
Related species There are many attractive, ornamental cultivars of *O. vulgare,* which are not suitable for culinary and medicinal use but are frequently grown in herb gardens, including *O. v.* 'Aureum', a golden marjoram, and *O. v.* 'Polyphant', a variegated marjoram.
Habitat/distribution Native to the Mediterranean, found in dry soils on sunny, open hillsides. Introduced and widely grown in other countries.
Growth Requires well-drained soil and a sunny position. *O. vulgare* is best propagated by division or by cuttings taken in summer – the cultivars must be vegetatively propagated.
Parts used Leaves, flowers – fresh or dried; essential oil distilled from the leaves.

Top Origanum vulgare *'Polyphant'.*

Below Origanum vulgare *'Aureum', an attractive ornamental.*

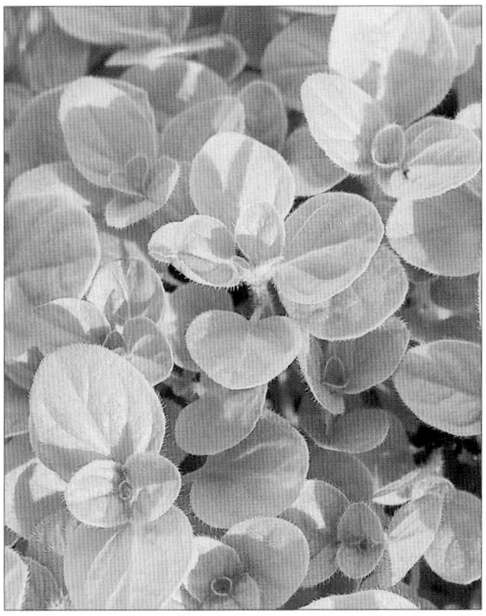

USES Medicinal Similar uses to *O. majorana.*
Culinary Similar uses to *O. majorana.*
Other name Wild marjoram.

CAUTION Marjorams are only to be taken on medical advice if other prescribed medication is being taken. Can interact with other drugs. Not to be taken in pregnancy.

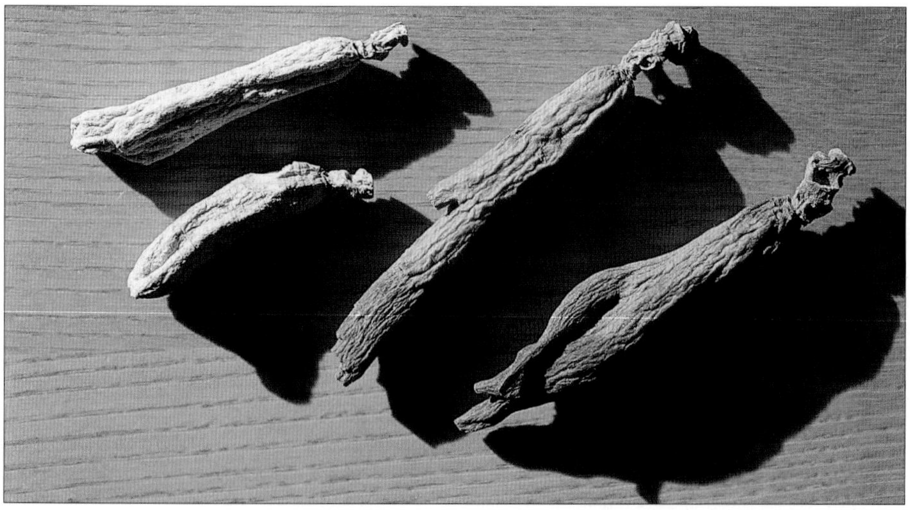

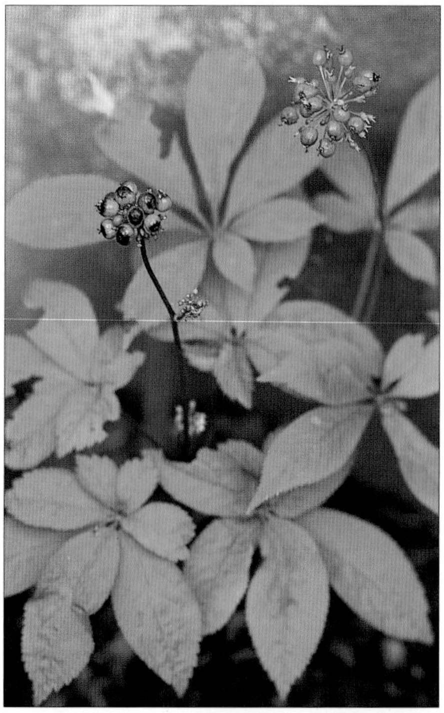

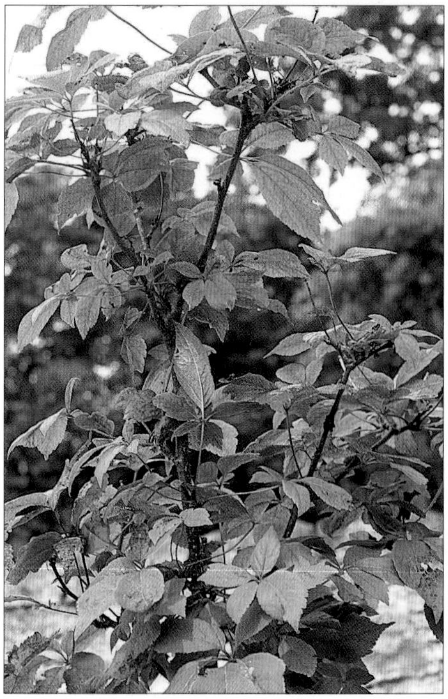

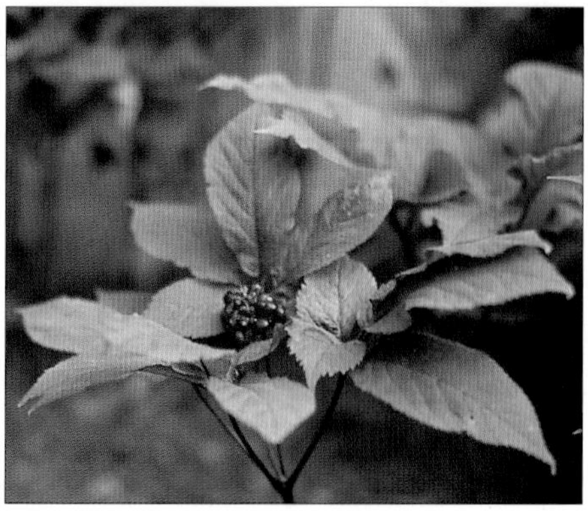

ARALIACEA

Panax ginseng

Ginseng

History and traditions Used as a tonic and "vital essence" in Chinese medicine for thousands of years. It was so highly prized for its medicinal properties that emperors set up monopolies and wars were fought over the rights to harvest ginseng. First introduced to Europe as early as the 9th century, it did not catch on until the 1950s when scientific studies discovered that its active principles have a "normalizing" effect on various bodily functions. The name *panax* comes from *pan,* all, and *akos*, a remedy. The Chinese name, from which the word ginseng is adapted, means man root, or like a man. Various *Panax* species are cultivated in Asia, China, Russia, Japan, the United States and Britain.

Description A hardy perennial, 70–80cm/28–31in tall, it usually has a forked root, erect stems, with fleshy scales at the base and whorls of palmate leaves, with finely serrated leaflets. Insignificant greenish-yellow flowers are followed by bright red berries.

Related species There are several species of ginseng with similar medicinal properties, and as the plants look very alike they are often confused. These include *P. japonicus*, which grows wild in wooded areas of central Japan; *P. quinquefolius* (American ginseng); *Eleutherococcus senticosus* (Siberian ginseng), which has almost identical properties to the Panax species, but is stronger and considered very beneficial. *P. pseudoginseng* refers to several sub-species found in Asia, from the Himalayas to China.

Habitat/distribution The *Panax* species are native to China, Korea and Japan. Found in damp, cool, woodlands. *Eleutherococcus senticosus* is from Siberia.

Growth For successful cultivation, well-drained, sandy loam, with added leaf mould, is essential. Propagation is from seed, but germination is often erratic.

Parts used Roots – processed from 6–7-year-old plants for use in tablets, extracts, tea and medicinal preparations.

USES Medicinal Ginseng is said to stimulate the nervous and immune systems, improve and regulate hormonal secretion, increase general stamina and strength, lower blood sugar and blood cholesterol levels. It is a true adaptogen herb, improving the body's adaptability to stress. Adaptogens have an overall tonifying effect on the body, and it has been found that the combined action of ginseng's many constituents has a general tonic effect on the whole body.

Top left Panax ginseng *roots.*

Top right Panax japonicus.

Centre right Eleutherococcus senticosus.

Right Panax quinquefolius.

CAUTION Should only be taken under medical supervision for short periods. Excess or regular intake may cause headaches, giddiness, nausea, double vision and raised blood pressure. Do not use if you have high blood pressure or in pregnancy.

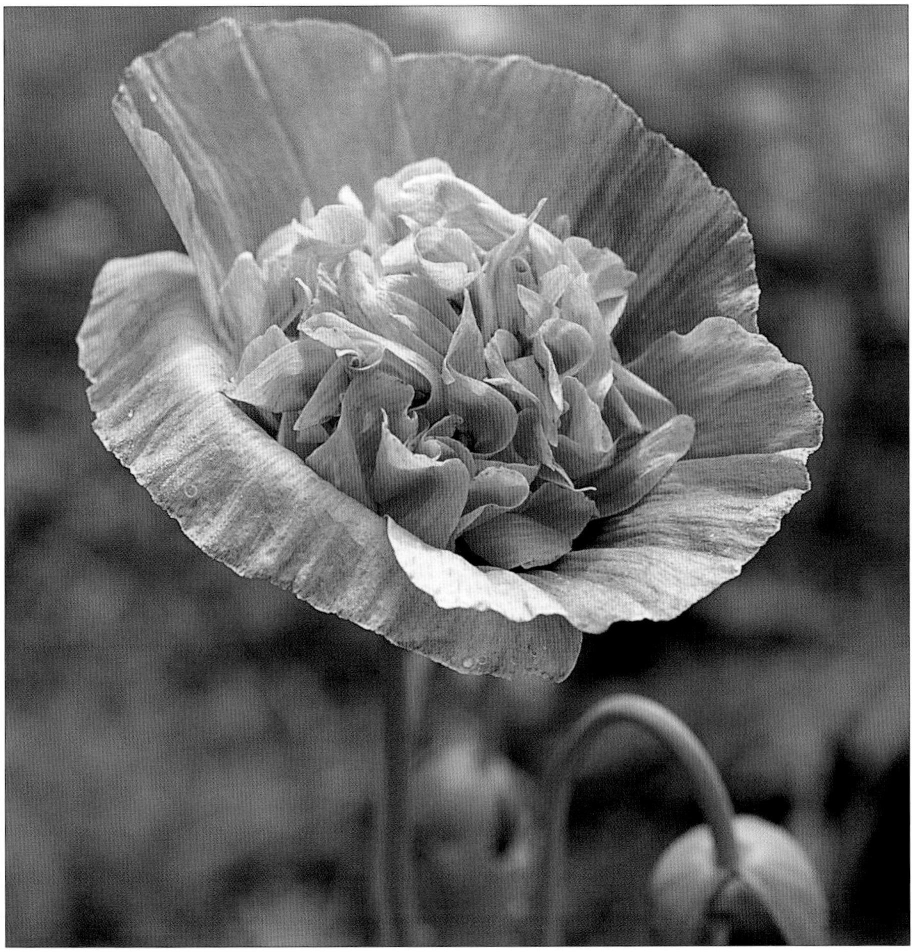

PAPAVERACEAE

Papaver somniferum

Opium poppy

History and traditions Opium, made by lancing the green seed capsule to extract the milky latex, has been used for medicinal purposes since earliest times, and the Greek authorities Theophrastus and Dioscorides wrote of it in this context. It was probably introduced to Europe by early Arabian physicians, and a cough syrup made from the opium poppy, widely recommended by the Arabian, Mesue, in the 11th century, was adopted as a standard for many centuries following. But as a highly addictive, powerful narcotic, opium caused as many problems as it solved. Opium poppies are now cultivated on a large scale as the source of powerful pain-killing drugs, including morphine and codeine (two of the most important of its 25 alkaloids), as well as to produce the drug heroin (diamorphine). The flowers are frequently grown in herb gardens as ornamentals.
Description A hardy annual, up to 1.5m/5ft tall, it has oblong, deeply lobed, blue-green leaves. Large, lilac, pink or white flowers, with papery petals, borne in early summer, are followed by blue-green seed pods.
Habitat/distribution Native to southeast Europe, the Middle East and Asia. Introduced elsewhere. Grows on shallow, chalky (alkaline) soils in sunny positions.
Growth Prefers well-drained soil and full sun. Propagated by seed sown in spring, often self-seeds once established.
Parts used Fruits, seeds.

USES Medicinal Proprietary drugs and pharmaceutical products are made from the fruits. Not for home remedies or self-treatment.
Culinary The seeds do not contain any of the alkaloids found in the capsules. They are dried for use whole or ground in breads, biscuits, bakery products and as a garnish. Commercially produced seed is from a subspecies of *P. somniferum*, developed for its seed production.

CAUTION Legal restrictions apply to this plant and its products in most countries.

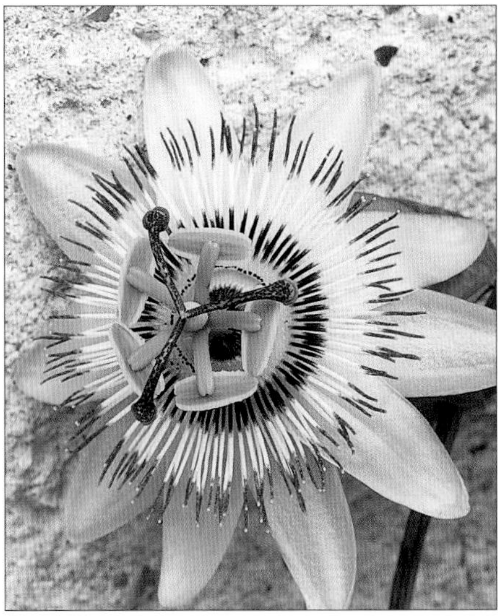

PASSIFLORACEAE

Passiflora incarnata

Passion flower

History and traditions A plant of tropical and subtropical regions of the Americas, it was imaginatively dubbed "Calvary Lesson" by Roman Catholic missionaries in South America, taking the intricate form of its flower to represent Christ's crucifixion. The three styles are for the nails used on the cross; the five anthers for the five wounds; the corona is the crown of thorns; and the ten sepals are for ten of the twelve apostles – leaving out Peter and Judas Iscariot, who betrayed him. It has a long history of being a folk remedy to treat anxiety.
Description A hardy perennial, climbing plant on a woody stem, to 8m/26ft, it clings to its support with axillary tendrils and has deeply lobed leaves and attractive creamy-white to lavender flowers, with purple calyces.
Habitat/distribution Native to tropical regions of North and South America, occurs in Asia and Australia, introduced and grown elsewhere.
Growth Requires well-drained, sandy soil and a sunny position. Propagation is easiest from semi-ripe cuttings taken in summer. Seed requires heat to germinate and can be slow and erratic to grow.
Parts used The whole plant – cut when fruiting and dried for use in infusions and medicinal preparations.

USES Medicinal Has sedative and nervine properties, useful for nervous conditions such as anxiety, heart palpitations, sleep disturbances, including insomnia.

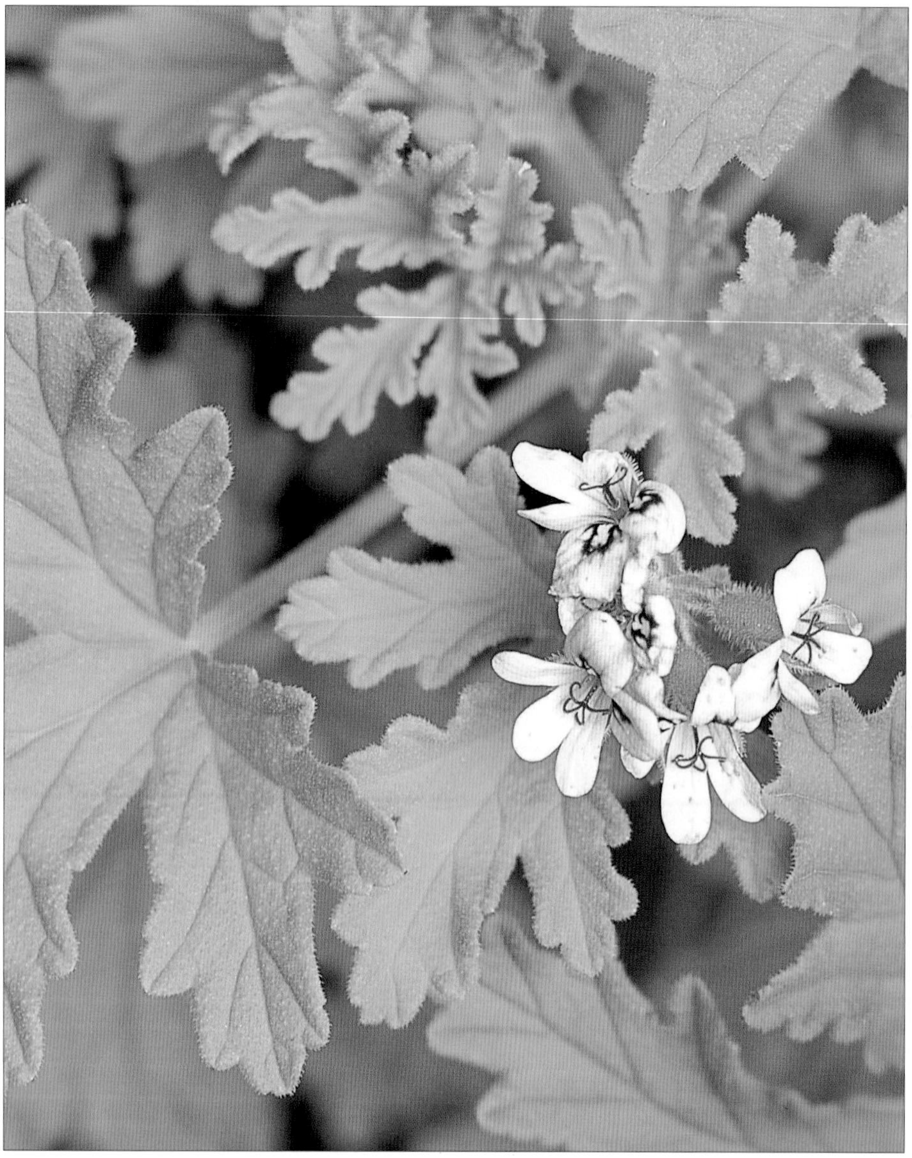

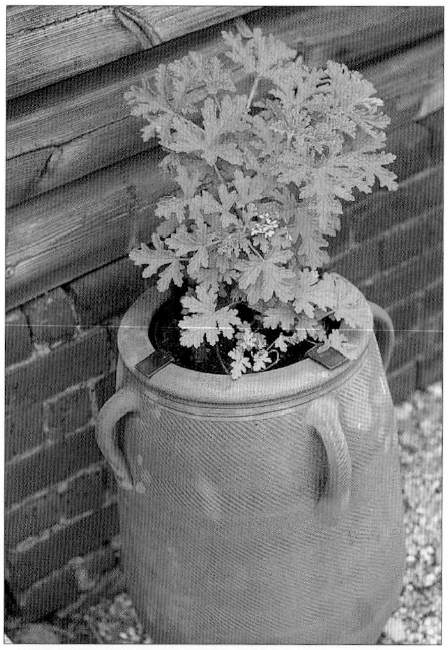

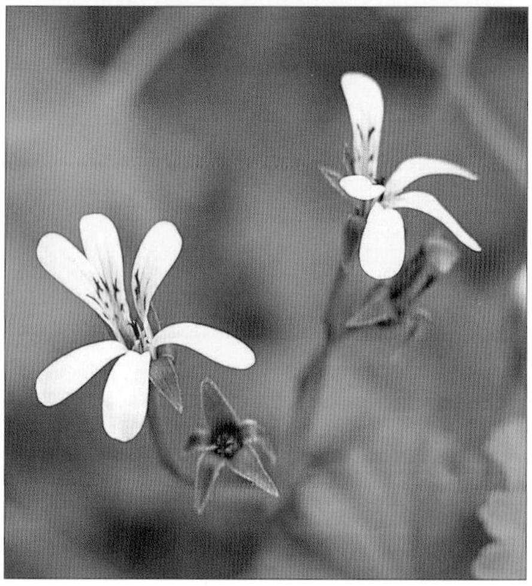

GERANIACEAE

Pelargonium

History and traditions Most scented pelargoniums, often familiarly known as "geraniums", come from South Africa and were introduced to Europe some time in the 17th century. The scented-leafed varieties were very popular in Britain with the Victorians, who grew them as house plants, and in France distilled oil from the "rose-scented" group became an important perfume ingredient in the mid-19th century.

Description and species There are numerous hybrids and cultivars with differing foliage, habits of growth and types of fragrance. It is the leaves that are scented. The flowers, appearing in summer, are virtually unperfumed, smaller and more insignificant than those of regal and zonal pelargoniums, grown as colourful bedding plants. These are some of the most popular scented-leafed pelargoniums:

P. graveolens – An upright shrubby plant, it grows 60–90cm/2–3ft tall, and has deeply cut, triangular, rough-textured, bright green leaves and small pink flowers. It grows vigorously and is slightly hardier than most of the others. This is the original "rose geranium", though the scent is much harsher and more spicy than a true rose fragrance, with strong overtones of lemon.

P. odoratissimum – A low-growing, species – 30cm/1ft – with a trailing habit and little white flowers borne on long stems. The soft, rounded, bright green leaves are wavy at the edges and apple-scented.

P. crispum – Has a neat, upright habit, and grows 60–70cm/24–28in tall. It has pink flowers and clear green, three-lobed, crinkly leaves, which are coarse to the touch and pungently lemon-scented.

***P. crispum* 'Variegatum'** – Is an attractive variegated cultivar, with crisply curled leaves, edged with creamy yellow and the same, strong lemon scent as the species.

P. tomentosum – Is a lovely trailing, or prostrate species, 0.9–1.2m/3–4ft, which makes a good container plant, if grown on a stand and allowed to drape downward. It has small white flowers and soft, downy, grey-green leaves with a strong peppermint fragrance.

***P.* 'Fragrans'** – A small, upright subshrub, 45cm/18in tall, it has clusters of small, greyish-green, rounded leaves, with finely cut, crinkled edges and a smooth, silky texture.

The flowers are white and the foliage pleasantly pine-scented with overtones of nutmeg.

P. 'Lady Plymouth' – An attractive hybrid, 0.6–1.5m/2–5ft tall, it has triangular, deeply lobed, crisp-textured leaves, with a cream and green variegation, little pink flowers and a citrus fragrance with a hint of rose.

Habitat/distribution Most pelargoniums are natives of South Africa; a few come from tropical Africa, the eastern Mediterranean, the Middle East, India, western Asia and Australia. Cultivated in France, northern Africa and Réunion for essential-oil production.

Growth All are tender and must be grown as conservatory plants in cool, temperate regions, though they are best kept outside in the summer months. A few (including *P. graveolens* and *P.* 'Fragrans') may survive a mild winter in a cold greenhouse. They make good container plants and should be given a gritty, loam-based compost. Cut back in autumn and prune lightly in spring to maintain a neat, bushy habit. Pelargoniums grown outside need free-draining soil and a sunny position. They are easily propagated by softwood cuttings taken in summer.

Parts used Leaves, essential oil – distilled from the leaves.

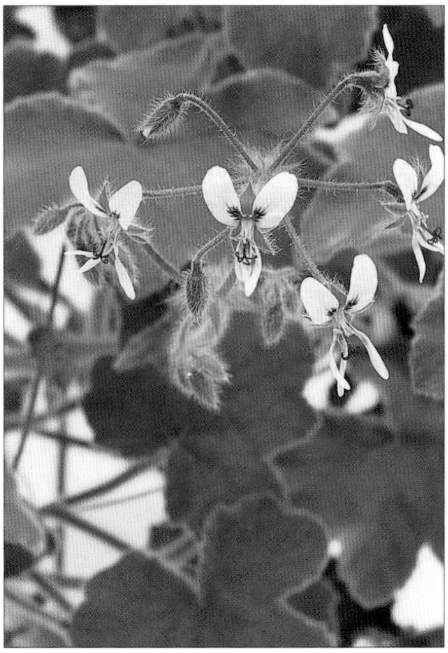

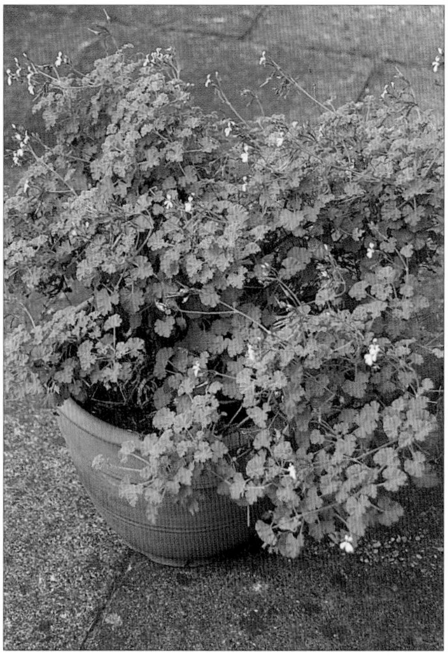

USES Culinary The pungency of the leaves makes them suitable as flavouring agents only – not to be eaten. Leaves of *P. graveolens* and *P. odoratissimum* are best for flavouring ice creams and cakes and fruit punches.

Aromatic Dried leaves and essential oil are added to potpourri and their strong scents make them effective in insect repellent or anti-moth sachets. "Geranium oil" is used as a commercial flavouring and perfume ingredient and used in aromatherapy.

Other name Scented pelargonium.

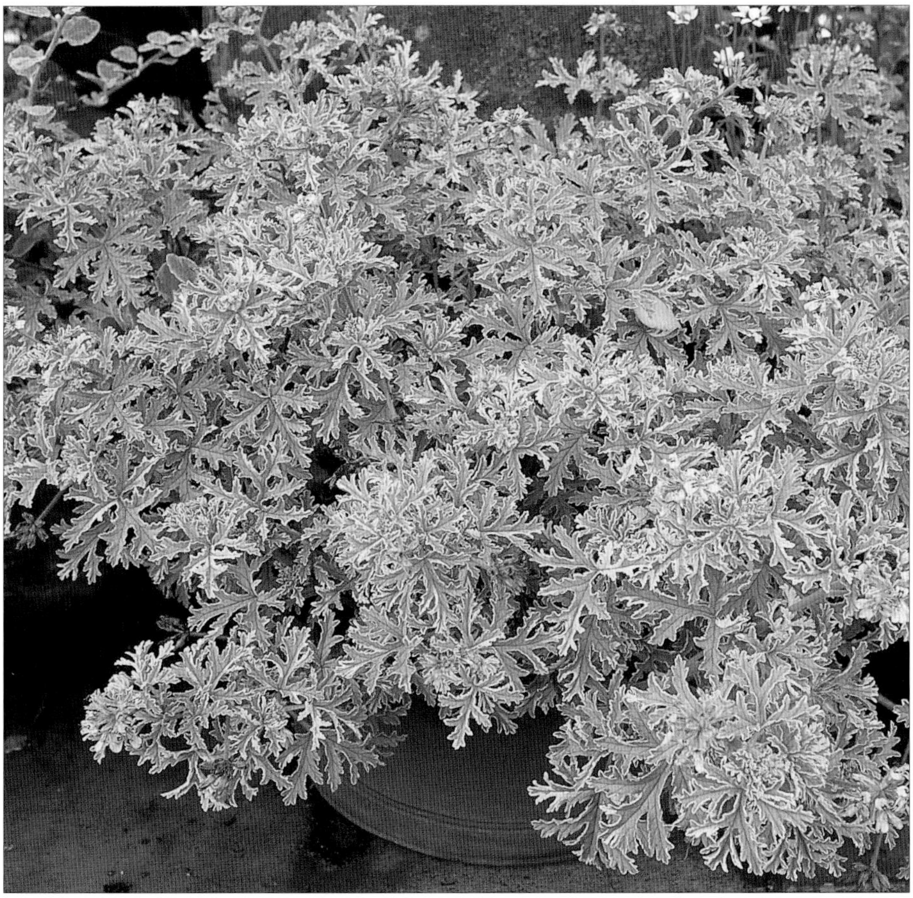

Opposite page, far left and top right Pelargonium graveolens; **below right** Pelargonium odoratissimum.

This page, clockwise from top to bottom Pelargonium tomentosum; Pelargonium *'Fragrans'*; Pelargonium *'Lady Plymouth'*; Pelargonium crispum.

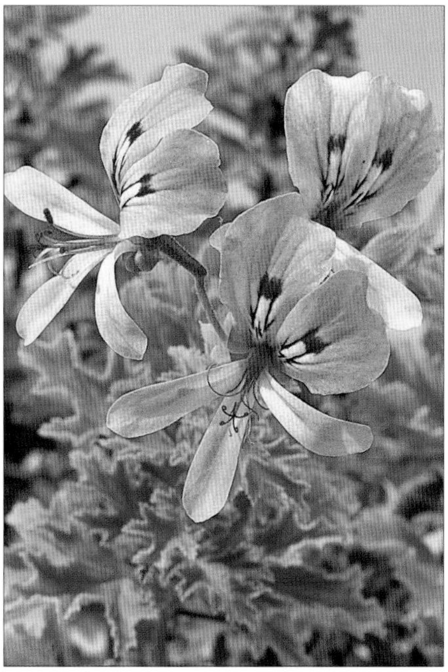

LABIATAE/LAMIACEAE

Perilla frutescens

Perilla

History and traditions In China, perilla has been a medicinal herb for centuries and it has long been cultivated in the East, from India to Japan, as a culinary herb and for its many economic uses. The leaves produce a sweet volatile oil, the seeds a pressed oil, which is used in similar ways to linseed oil. It has recently become increasingly popular in the West for its culinary uses and as an ornamental garden plant.
Description A half-hardy annual with broadly ovate, deeply-veined leaves, reddish stems and small spikes of white flowers in summer. There are both green and purple-leaved forms.
Related species *P. frutescens* 'Crispa' (pictured below) is a variety with curly-edged leaves.
Habitat/distribution Occurs from the Himalayas to East Asia, naturalized in parts of Europe and North America.
Growth Grows best in deep, rich, moist but well-drained soil, in sun or partial shade. Propagated by seed sown in spring, after frosts in cool temperate regions. Pinch out tips to encourage and maintain bushy plants.
Parts used Leaves – fresh for culinary use, dried for medicinal infusions and decoctions; seeds – dried for decoctions; volatile oil – from leaves; pressed oil – from seeds.

USES Medicinal Used in Chinese herbal medicine for colds and chest infections, nausea, stomach upsets and allergic reactions.
Culinary Leaves and seeds are a popular ingredient in Japanese cookery and add colour and an unusual spicy flavour to salads, seafood and stir-fry dishes.
General Volatile oil is added to commercial food, confectionery and dental products; oil from seeds is used to waterproof paper for umbrellas, in paints and printing inks.
Other names Beefsteak plant and shiso.

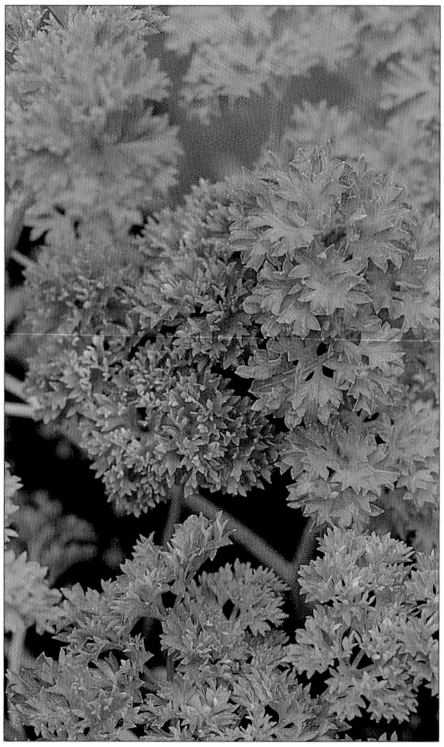

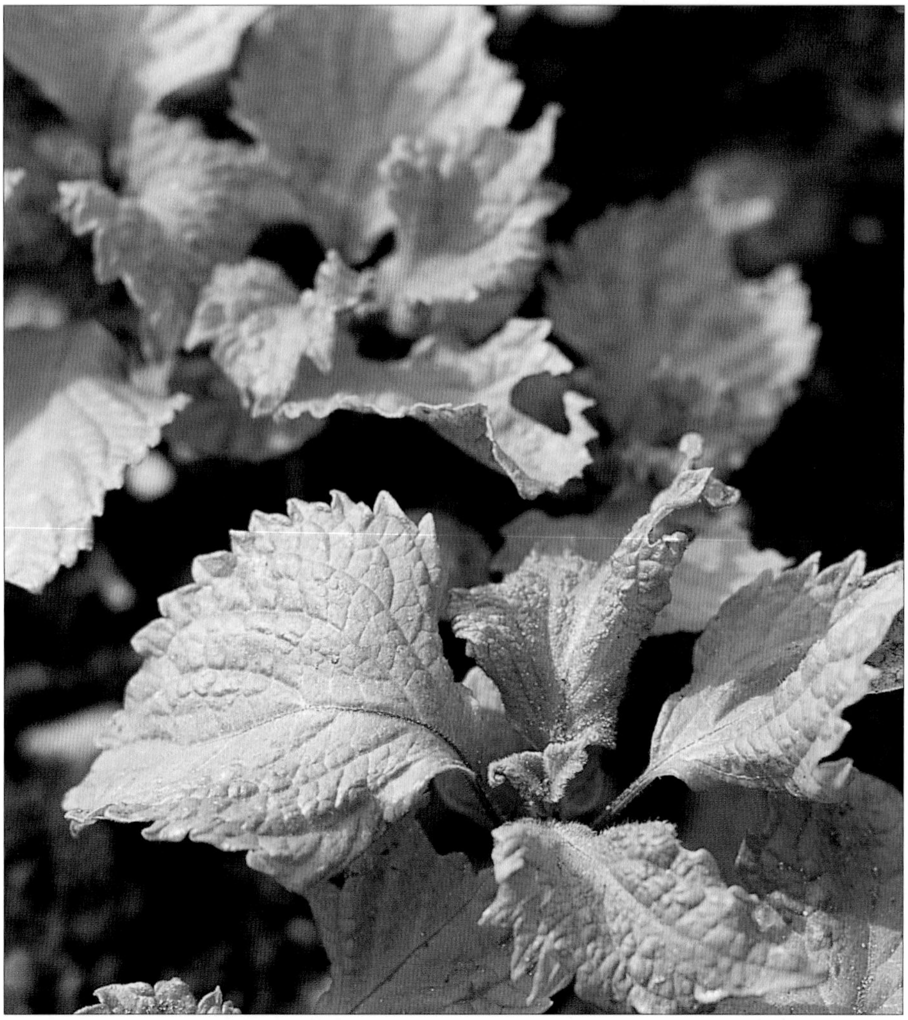

Above P. frutescens *'Crispa'*.

UMBELLIFERAE/APIACEAE

Petroselinum crispum

Parsley

History and traditions Petroselinum comes from the Greek name given to it by Dioscorides, *petros selinon*. In the Middle Ages this became corrupted to *petrocilium*, ending up in the anglicized version, by a process of "Chinese whispers" as parsley. The Greeks associated it with death and funerals and according to Homer fed it to their chariot horses, but it was the Romans who took to it as a major culinary herb. Pliny complained that every sauce and salad contained it, and it has remained ubiquitous as a sauce, salad and garnishing herb to this day. Parsley has attracted a mass of silly superstitions. Transplanting it, giving it away, picking it when in love and so on, all foretold disaster. Some said it flourished only where the "mistress is master", others that it would grow only for the wicked, or, conversely, for the honest. Its slowness to germinate when soil is cold led to tales that it had gone seven times to the devil and back, and should be sown on Good Friday to outwit him. *A Grete Herball,* 1539, has some ingenious ideas on how to ensure it is well "crisped" or curly: "Before the sowing of them, stuffe a tennis ball with the seedes and beat the same well against the ground, whereby the seedes may be a little bruised. Or when the

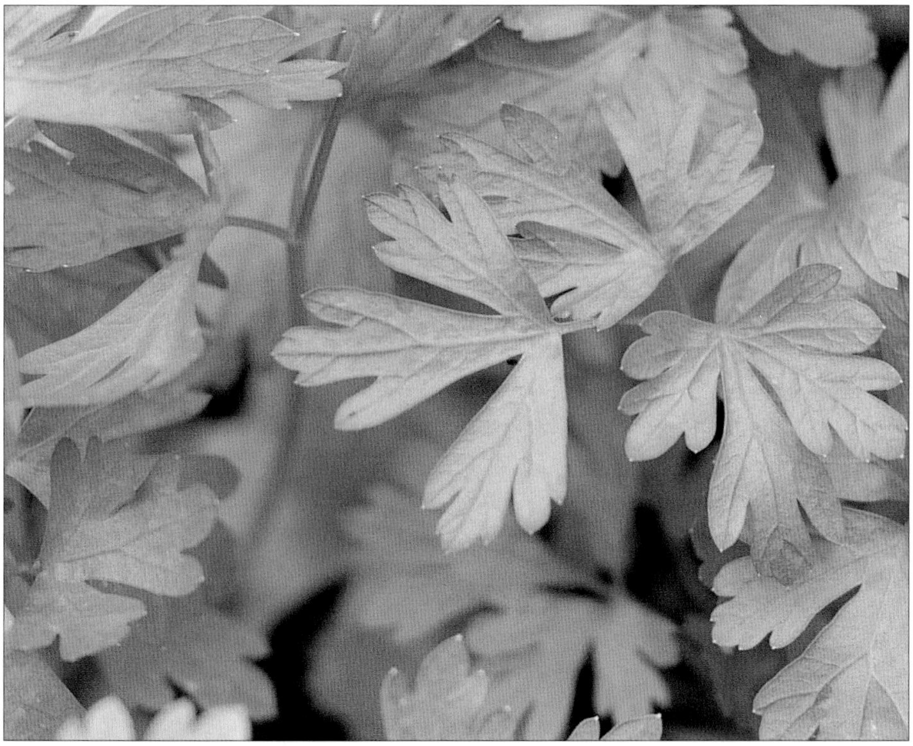

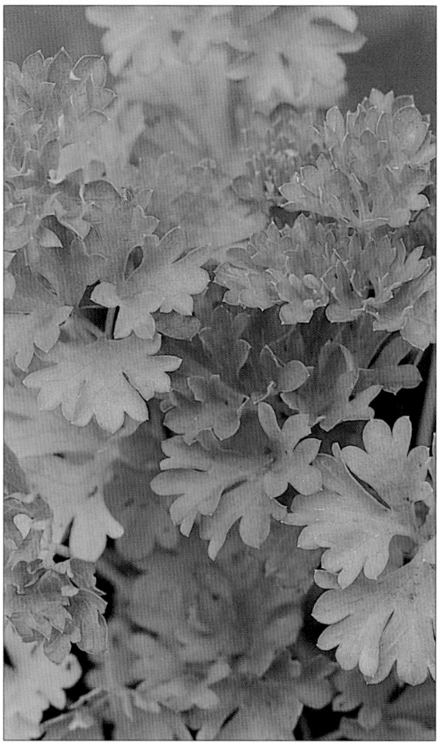

Above left *'Italian' or flat-leaved parsley.*

Above *Hamburg parsley.*

parcelye is well come up, go over the bed with a waighty roller whereby it may so presse the leaves down."

Description A frost-hardy biennial, growing on a short, stout taproot to 30–60cm/1–2ft, it has triangular, three-pinnate leaves, curled at the margin. Yellow-green flowers are borne in umbels in its second year.

Related species *Petroselinum crispum* 'Italian', also known as French or flat-leaved parsley, is a larger, hardier plant, growing to 80–90cm/32in–3ft and has smooth, uncurled three-pinnate leaves. *P. c.* var. *tuberosum,* Hamburg parsley, has small, flat leaves, with a celery-like flavour and is grown for its large roots, which are eaten as a vegetable.

Habitat/distribution The genus is native to the Mediterranean region of Europe, found in fields and on rocky slopes. *P. crispum* has been developed under cultivation and is widely grown as a crop in many countries.

Growth Parsley requires rich, moist but well-drained soil and a sunny position, or partial shade. As leaves coarsen in the second, flowering, year, it is often grown as an annual and is propagated by seed, sown in spring. If sown *in situ* before soil has warmed up, germination may be slow or erratic. For best results, sow in containers, maintaining a temperature of 18–21°C/64–70°F until seedlings appear. The young plants can then be hardened off to grow outside at lower temperatures.

Parts used Leaves, stems – best fresh or frozen for culinary use as flavour is lost with drying; roots – of 'Hamburg' variety; essential oil – distilled from leaves and seeds.

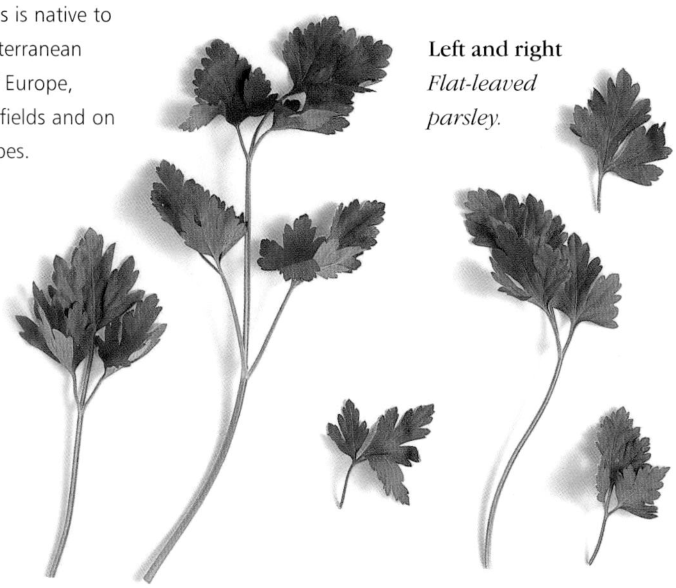

Left and right *Flat-leaved parsley.*

USES Medicinal Parsley is rich in vitamin A and C, and acts as an antioxidant. It also contains a flavonoid, apigenin, which is an anti-allergen. Although used in herbal medicine for a variety of complaints, including menstrual problems, kidney stones, urinary infections, rheumatism and arthritis, it is not for self-treatment. Tea can be made from leaves or roots used to treat jaundice and coughs.

Culinary The leaves of this herb are added to salads, sauces, salad dressings, butter, stuffings, snipped into meat, fish and vegetable dishes and used as a garnish. The stalks, which have a stronger flavour than the leaves, are essential to a *bouquet garni* for flavouring casseroles and cooked dishes. The roots of *P. tuberosum* are cooked as a vegetable. The essential oil is used in commercial food products.

CAUTION Although parsley is perfectly safe, used whole in culinary dishes, it is toxic in excess, particularly in the form of essential oil. Flat-leaved *Petroselinum* should not be confused with *Aethusa cynapium*, a highly poisonous wild plant. Should not be used medicinally if pregnant.

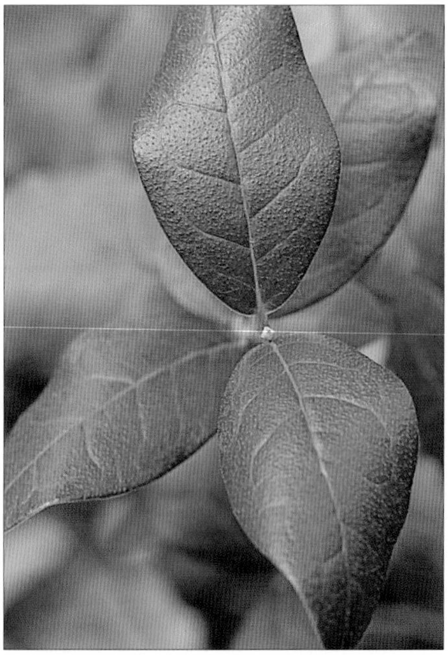

MONIMIACEAE

Peumus boldus

Boldo

History and traditions The medicinal properties of this small, shrubby tree from Chile were first investigated in Europe by a French doctor in 1869. It was discovered to be effective in stimulating the liver and expelling intestinal worms. In its country of origin it was formerly taken as a tonic tea and digestive, prescribed as a substitute for quinine and made into a powder to take as snuff.

Description An aromatic evergreen tree growing to 6–7m/19–23ft, it is the sole species of its genus. It has light to grey-green, leathery leaves, rich in a balsamic volatile oil. Greenish male and female flowers appear in late summer, borne on separate trees.

Habitat/distribution It is native to Chile, introduced elsewhere. Occurs on sunny slopes of the Andes mountains.

Growth It is frost-hardy, and grows best in sandy, acid soil in a sunny position. Propagated by semi-ripe cuttings in summer, may also be grown from seed sown in spring.

Parts used Leaves – dried for use in infusions and other medicinal preparations; bark – dried for extracts.

USES Medicinal It has mainly been used for liver complaints, urinary infections and to expel intestinal worms. Extracts are included in commercial and pharmaceutical products.

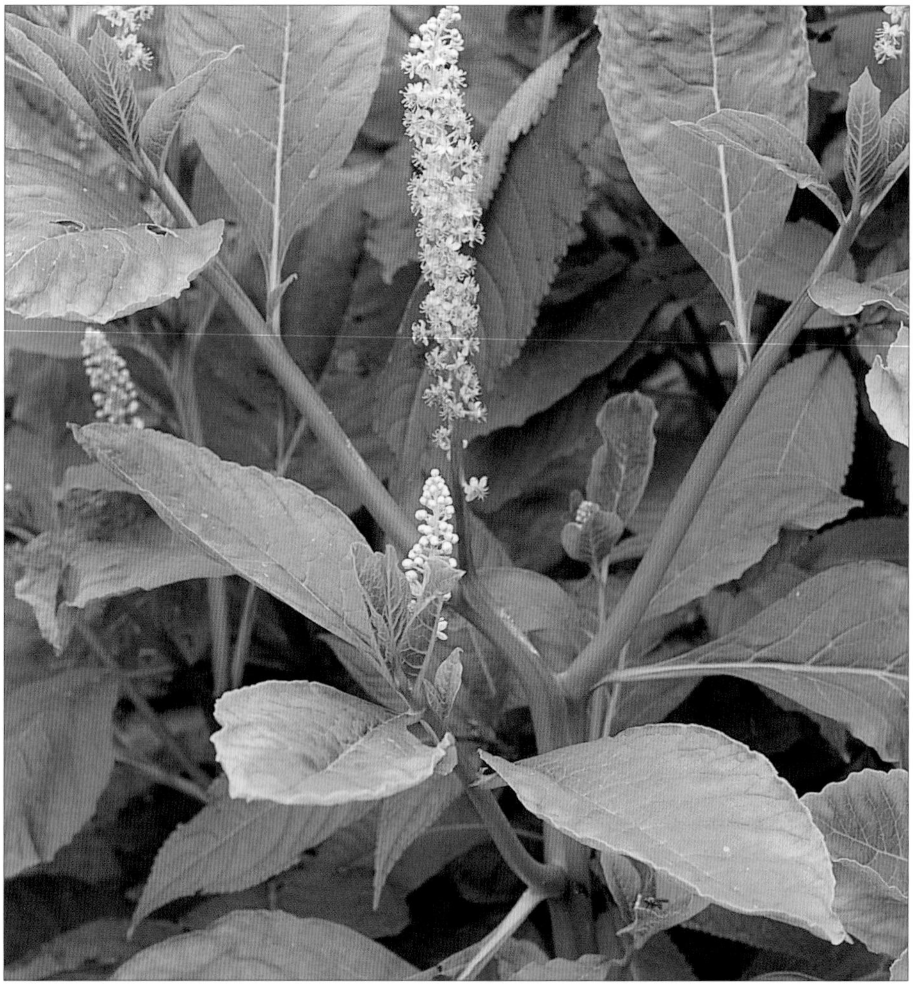

PHYTOLACCACEAE

Phytolacca americana

Pokeweed

History and traditions A poisonous plant, once used by Native Americans as a purgative and powerful treatment for various complaints. They knew it as *pocan*, which is where the name pokeweed comes from. It was adopted by European settlers as a treatment for venereal disease, and for its painkilling and anti-inflammatory properties. In modern times, its complex chemical structure has attracted much scientific interest. It contains compounds that affect cell division and it is currently being investigated as a potential source of drugs to combat AIDS-related diseases and cancers.

Description A large, frost-hardy perennial, 0.9–1.5m/3–5ft tall, with smooth, hollow, purplish stems and ovate to lanceolate leaves. It has racemes of white, sometimes pink-tinged flowers in late summer, followed by large drooping spikes of purple-black berries, which provide a dye to colour ink.

Habitat/distribution A North American native, it has been introduced elsewhere and widely grown in the Mediterranean region of Europe. Occurs in rich soils at field edges.

Growth Grow in rich, moist soil. Propagated by seed sown in spring or autumn or by division.

Parts used Roots and fruits (berries) – collected in autumn and dried for use in decoctions, tinctures and other medicinal preparations.

USES Medicinal Pokeweed has anti-inflammatory, antibacterial, antiviral, antifungal properties and is destructive to many parasitic disease-causing organisms. It is also capable of stimulating the immune and lymphatic systems. Used for many disorders, including auto-immune diseases, skin diseases, bronchitis and arthritis, but is for qualified practitioners only. Despite its toxicity, the leaves of this plant are sometimes boiled as a vegetable, the water being discarded.

CAUTION The whole plant is toxic if eaten, especially roots and berries.

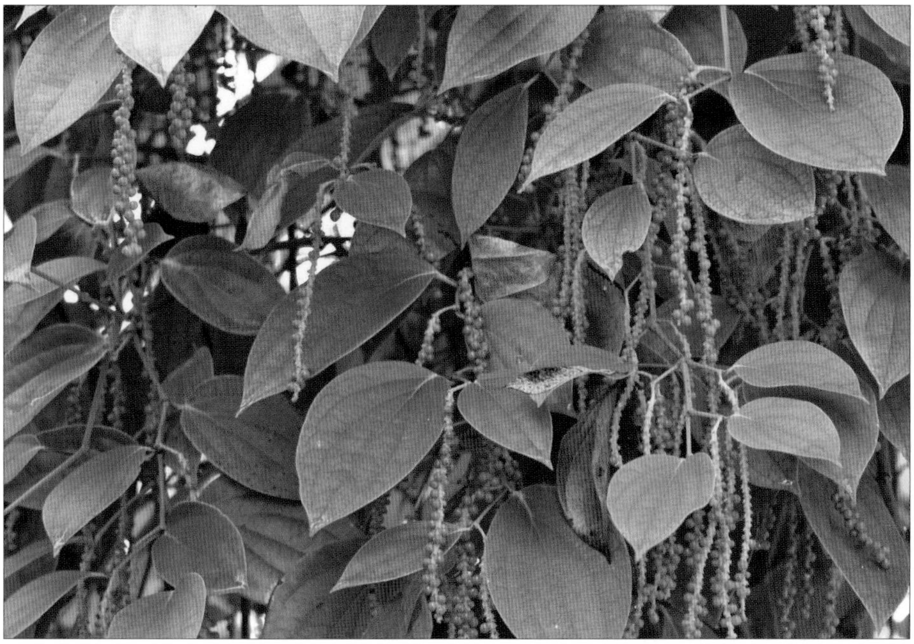

PIPERACEAE

Piper nigrum

Black pepper

History and traditions Black pepper has been a valuable trading commodity since Alaric I, King of the Visigoths, demanded 3,000lb of it as a ransom during his siege of Rome between 410–408BC. Its high price during the Middle Ages was a major incentive for the Portuguese to find a sea route to India, where it came from, although the price fell following the discovery of a passage round the Cape of Good Hope in 1498. As cultivation was extended into Malaysia, the Portuguese retained a lucrative trading monopoly in pepper into the 18th century, and much of the wealth of Venice and Genoa depended on its trade. In Britain it was heavily taxed from the 17th to the 19th centuries. Pepper's virtues as a digestive were early recognized in the West and it has a long tradition of medicinal use in Ayurvedic and Chinese systems of healing.

Description A perennial climber, growing to 6m/20ft, with a strong, woody stem and ovate, prominently-veined, dark green leaves.

It has drooping spikes of inconspicuous white flowers, followed by long clusters of spherical green fruits or berries, which redden as they mature. Black pepper is produced from whole fruits, picked and dried just as they start to go red; white pepper is from ripe fruits, with the outer layer removed, and green pepper is from unripe fruits, pickled to prevent it turning dark.

Habitat/distribution Native to southern India and Sri Lanka, introduced and cultivated in Indonesia, Malaysia, Brazil and many tropical regions. In the wild it grows in humus-rich, moist soil. It is cultivated by training it up trees or horizontally along frames.

Growth Pepper requires deep, rich, manured soil, plenty of water, a humid atmosphere and a shady position. It is sometimes grown as a pot plant in temperate climates.

Parts used Fruits (peppercorns).

USES Medicinal A pungent, stimulating digestive, which relieves flatulence. It is used in Ayurvedic medicine for coughs and colds and as a nerve tonic. It also has a reputation as an aphrodisiac.

Culinary Its chief use is as a condiment and flavouring in a wide range of dishes in the cookery of most countries. It is currently the most widely consumed spice in the world.

Below *Mixed peppercorns.*

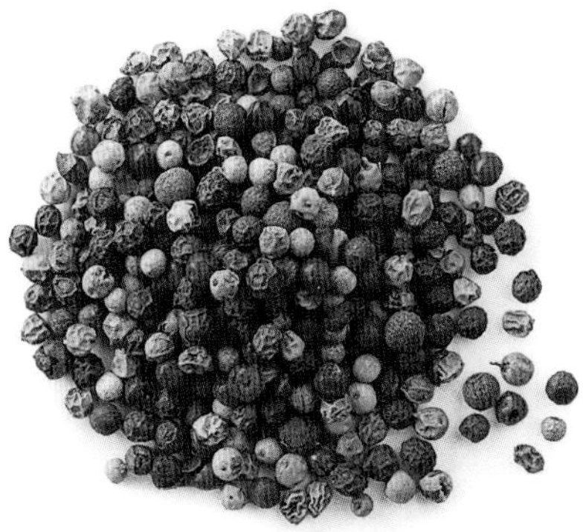

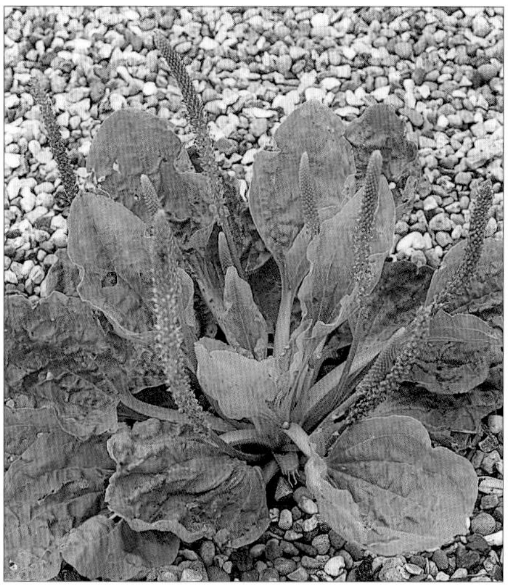

PLANTAGINACEAE

Plantago major

Plantain

History and traditions The Saxons called it *"waybroad"*, because it was so often found by the wayside. And the story goes that this plant was once a beautiful young girl, who was changed into plantain for refusing to leave the roadway where she expected her lover to appear. As a medicinal herb it was highly rated by Pliny, who attributed to it the ability to fuse together pieces of flesh cooking in a pot, and to cure the madness of dogs – or their bites. It was often recommended as an antidote to poison and in the US it was held to be a remedy for rattle-snake bite by native tribes.

Description A small, undistinguished perennial, 40cm/16in high, it has a basal rosette of ovate leaves and cylindrical spikes of inconspicuous brownish-green flowers.

Habitat/distribution Native to Europe and introduced in other temperate zones worldwide. Occurs widely in cultivated land, garden paths and lawns, fields, wastelands and roadsides.

Growth Said to prefer moist soil, but tolerates any conditions in sun or shade. Self-seeds freely.

Parts used Leaves – fresh or dried.

USES Medicinal Plantain is thought to promote healing and to have antibacterial properties. Mainly used as a poultice or in ointments to be applied externally to wounds, sores, ulcers, bites and stings. Greater plantain is generally considered to be most effective for topical use, whilst ribwort (*P. lanceolata*) is a gentle soothing expectorant used in irritated coughs and mild bronchitis.

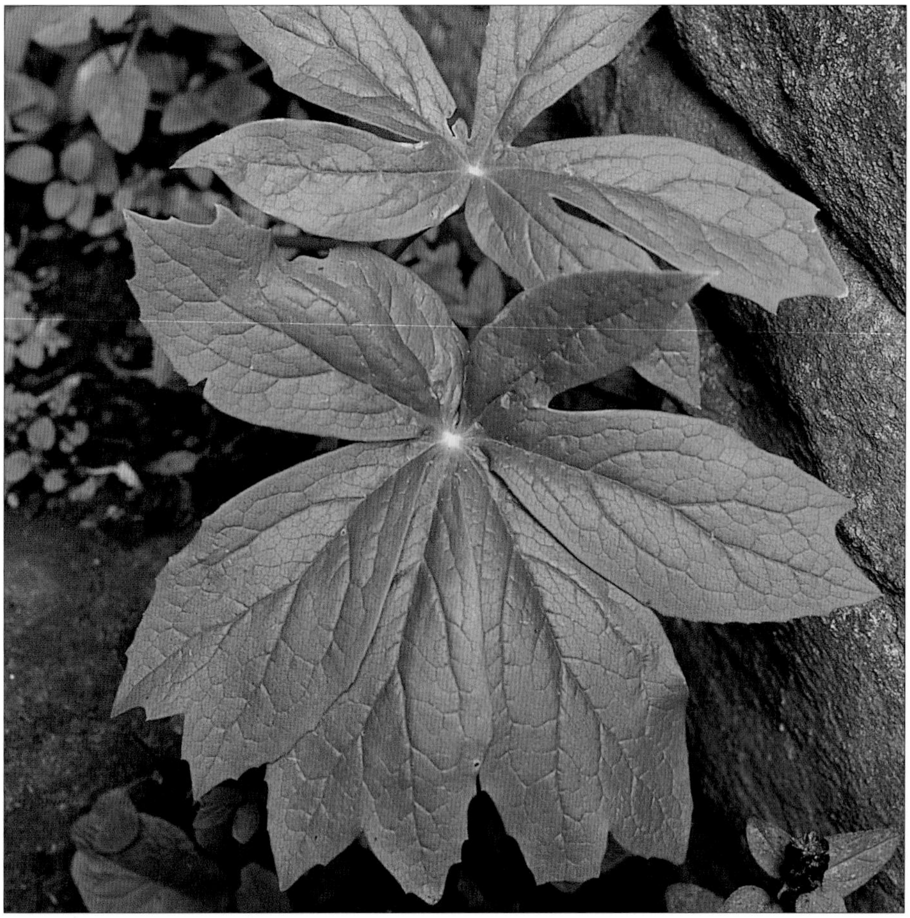

BERBERIDACEAE

Podophyllum peltatum

American mandrake

History and traditions A poisonous herb, *Podophyllum peltatum* was formerly used by Native Americans as a powerful purgative medicine, vermifuge and wart remover.
They also made it into an insecticide for potato crops and reputedly took it to commit suicide. It was introduced to Western medicine in the 1780s by a German doctor involved in the American War of Independence and by 1820 was listed in the United States *Pharmacopoeia*. It is called may apple for the juicy fruits, which were sometimes eaten, despite their relative toxicity. The generic name comes from the Greek for *podos*, a foot, and *phyllon*, a leaf, for its supposed resemblance to a bird's webbed foot. The specific term, *peltatum*, means shield-shaped. Despite being called mandrake it is not related to *Mandragora*. In recent years, the active ingredient, podophyllotoxin, has been isolated for use in anti-cancer drugs.
Description A hardy perennial with a creeping rhizome, and usually unbranched stems, it is 30–45cm/12–18in tall. The large leaves are deeply divided into 4–7 wedge-shaped segments, lobed at the tops. Small, drooping white flowers, with yellow centres, are followed by fleshy, lemon-shaped fruits. The whole plant has an unpleasant smell.
Related species *P. hexandrum* (Indian podophyllum) which grows in the Himalayas, has red fruits and is more poisonous, with a higher concentration of podophyllotoxin.
Habitat *P. peltatum* is native to North America, found in damp woods and meadows.
Growth Grow in humus-rich, moist soil in dappled shade. Propagated by division of runners.
Parts used Rhizomes – extracted for commercial drugs.

USES Medicinal It is a component of pharmaceutical drugs for treating certain cancers.
Other name May apple.

CAUTION Although once used in herbal treatments, it is very poisonous and should never be used for self-medication. Subject to legal restrictions in most countries.

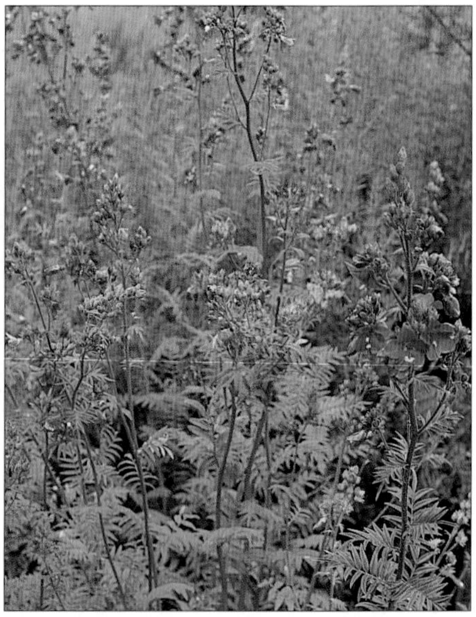

POLEMONIACEAE

Polemonium caeruleum

Jacob's ladder

History and traditions This is an ornamental plant, which retains its place in the herb garden through its ancient traditions and associations. Known to the Greeks, it was mentioned by Dioscorides, used for treating dysentery and thought to be effective against the bites of venomous beasts. It was still listed in various European pharmacopoeias into the 19th century. The whole flowering plant and roots were used and it was recommended for venereal disease and the bites of rabid dogs, but it is no longer considered to be of medicinal value. The name Jacob's ladder comes from the ladder-like arrangement of the leaves, and someone thought of associating it with the ladder to heaven of Jacob's dream in the biblical story (Genesis 28:12), with the sky represented by the blue flowers.
Description A hardy, clump-forming perennial, 30–90cm/1–3ft tall, it grows on a creeping rootstock, with pinnate leaves divided into lance-shaped leaflets. The lavender-blue, bell-shaped flowers are borne on erect stems in drooping panicles.
Habitat/distribution Occurs widely in northern and central Europe, North America, and Asia in damp areas and shady woodlands.
Growth Requires rich, moisture-retentive soil and a shady or partially shady position. Propagated by seed sown in spring or by division in autumn.
USES Medicinal Rarely used today.

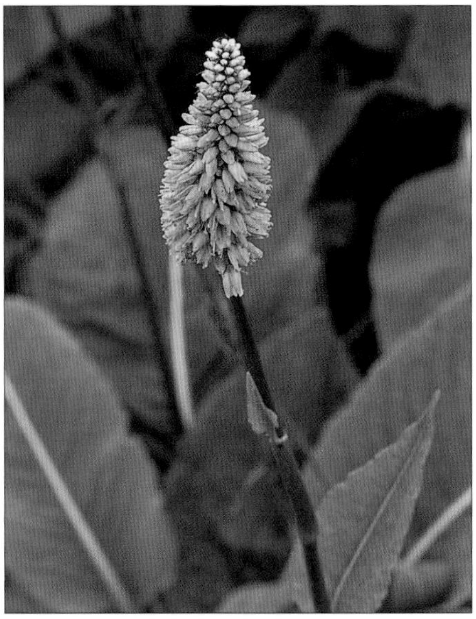

POLYGONACEAE

Polygonum bistorta

Bistort

History and traditions The generic name comes from the Greek *poly*, many, and *gonu*, knee, for the knotted shape of the stems of many polygonum species. Bistort became known as a medicinal plant in the 16th century, gaining a reputation as a wound-healing herb. It was cited in *The Universal Herbal*, 1832, as a treatment for "intermittent fever", and considered helpful for diabetes into the 20th century.
Description A hardy perennial with a stout, twisted rhizome, it has a clump of broad, ovate basal leaves, from which the pale pink, cylindrical flower spikes arise on erect "jointed" stems to about 50cm/20in.
Habitat/distribution Occurs throughout Europe and Asia, frequently found near streams and waterways in damp meadows, mixed woodlands and on high slopes.
Growth Grows best in rich, moist soil, in sun or partial shade. Easily propagated by division, it is an invasive plant, but can make useful ground cover in damp areas.
Parts used Rhizomes – dried for powders, extracts, decoctions and other medicinal preparations.

USES Medicinal High in tannins so has a strong astringent action. Said to reduce inflammation and promote healing, it is used as a gargle for gum disease, mouth ulcers and sore throats, applied externally to haemorrhoids, cuts and wounds and taken internally for diarrhoea.

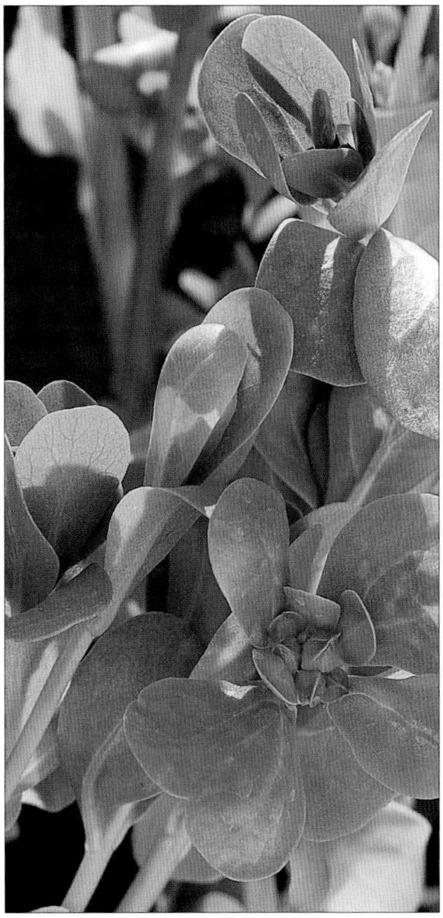

PORTULACACEAE

Portulaca oleracea

Purslane

History and traditions A herb of ancient origin, purslane was known to the Egyptians, and grown in India and China for thousands of years. The Romans ate it as a vegetable and it was cultivated in Europe from at least the beginning of the 16th century, though not introduced to Britain until 1582. An important remedy for scurvy, it was one of the herbs that the early settlers thought indispensable and took with them to North America. Although it had some medicinal applications in former times, especially in China, it has always been chiefly valued for its culinary uses. It is still appreciated in France and commercially cultivated there for this purpose.
Description A half-hardy annual, with pink, prostrate, much-branched stems and rounded, fleshy, bright green leaves, it grows to about 30cm/12in. It has very small, yellow flowers in late summer which soon fade to reveal the seed capsules with opening lids and filled with numerous black seeds.
Related species There is a golden-leafed variety, *P. oleracea* var. *aurea*, and the widely cultivated *P. oleracea* var. *sativa*.
Habitat/distribution Native to southern Europe, Asia and China, introduced elsewhere. Occurs on dry, sandy soils in sunny sites.
Growth Grow in light, well-drained soil, but provide plenty of water for good leaf development. Propagated from seed, sown after danger of frosts in cool temperate regions.
Parts used Leaves – fresh, picked before flowering for culinary use, fresh or dried for medicinal use.

USES Medicinal Recent scientific studies have found that *P. oleracea* contains omega-3 fatty acids, thought to be helpful in preventing heart disease and strengthening the immune system. The leaves are also a good source of Vitamin C and contain calcium, iron, carotene, thiamine, riboflavin and niacin. Purslane is also a diuretic and mildly laxative.
Culinary In 18th-century Britain it was a popular salad herb and is still eaten in the Middle East and India as a cooked vegetable and in salads. In France it is used in sorrel soup, helping to reduce the acidity of the sorrel.

Sorrel and purslane soup

Serves 4–6

15ml/1 tbsp olive oil
1 medium onion, chopped
2 cloves garlic, crushed
225g/8oz sorrel leaves
50g/2oz purslane leaves
225g/8oz potatoes, peeled and diced
1.2 litres/2 pints/5 cups water
salt and ground black pepper
a dash of grated nutmeg

Heat the oil in a pan, add the onion and garlic and cook gently for 5 minutes, until soft but not browned. Add the sorrel, purslane and potato and stir over a low heat for 2–3 minutes. Season, and add a little grated nutmeg. Pour in the water, bring to the boil then simmer for about 15 minutes until the potatoes are tender. Cool slightly, then liquidize the soup. Reheat before serving.

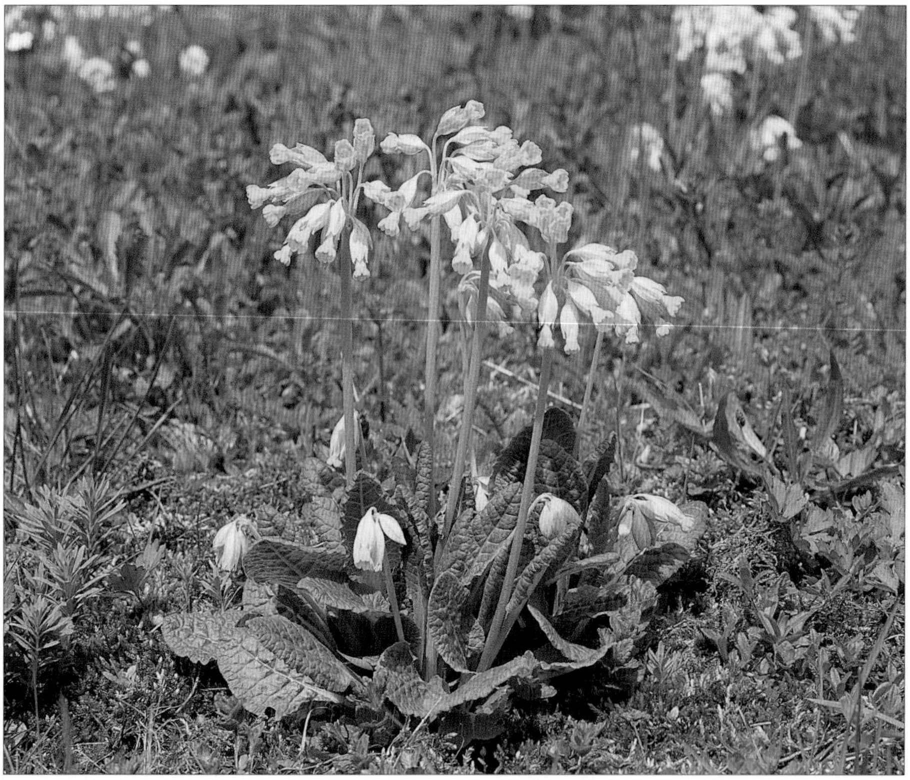

PRIMULACEAE

Primula veris

Cowslip

History and traditions Cowslips were sometimes known as "keyflowers", suggested by the shape of the flower clusters, which look like a little bunch of keys. In Norse mythology they were dedicated to Freya, giving access to her palace, but in the Christian era became "St Peter's Keys" or the "Keys to Heaven". The generic name, *Primula*, comes from *primus*, first, in recognition that they are among the earliest flowers of spring. At one time, when they were plentiful, they were gathered in vast quantities to make spring tonics and the gently soporific, pale yellow cowslip wine. Many medicinal uses were assigned to the flowers and distilled cowslip water was said to be good for the memory. The cosmetic applications were mentioned reprovingly by William Turner: "Some women we find, sprinkle ye floures of cowslip with whyte wine and after still it and wash their faces with that water to drive wrinkles away and to make them fayre in the eyes of the worlde rather than in the eyes of God, Whom they are not afrayd to offend" (*The New Herball*, 1551).

Description A perennial on a short rhizome with dense fibrous roots and a rosette of broadly ovate, rough-textured leaves. Flower stems rise above the basal leaves, 15–20cm/6–8in, and are topped by terminal umbels of fragrant, golden-yellow flowers, with tubular calyces.

Habitat/distribution Native to Europe and parts of Asia, introduced and sometimes naturalized elsewhere, found in meadows and pasture lands. A once common plant, it is now rare in the wild and a protected species in many European countries.

Growth Prefers deep, humus-rich, moist soil and partial shade. Propagated by seed sown in late summer in containers, left outside through the winter as a period of stratification, when they are exposed to frost, is necessary for germination. Easily propagated by division in autumn.

Parts used Flowers – fresh (but must not be picked from the wild, as they are quite rare).

USES Medicinal Cowslips have sedative, expectorant properties and contain salicylates (as in aspirin). They are mildly diuretic and are taken as a tea for insomnia, anxiety and respiratory tract infections.

Culinary Flowers may be added to salads.

> CAUTION Should not be taken medicinally during pregnancy or if sensitive to aspirin. May cause allergic skin irritations.

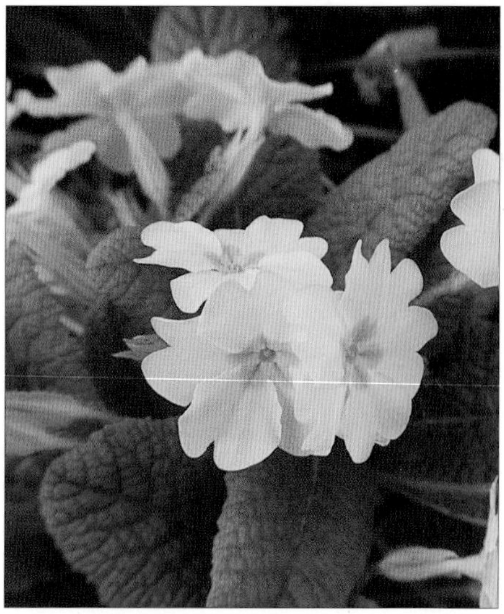

PRIMULACEAE

Primula vulgaris

Primrose

History and traditions The medicinal properties of the primrose, *P. vulgaris*, are similar to those of the cowslip (*P. veris*) and have been listed in old herbals, since Pliny's time, for similar complaints. The primrose was made into salves and ointments and considered an important remedy for paralysis, rheumatic pain and gout. Its value as a sedative was well known and Gerard remarks that primrose tea, drunk in the month of May, "is famous for curing the phrensie". It was popular in cookery.

Description A low-growing perennial, to 15cm/6in, with a rosette of deeply veined, softly hairy, broad ovate leaves and clusters of saucer-shaped, pale yellow, slightly fragrant flowers in early spring.

Habitat/distribution A European native, found in northern Asia, introduced elsewhere, found on rich, damp soils in shady woodlands and hedgerows. Now becoming rare in the wild, and a protected species in many countries.

Growth See *P. veris*.

Parts used Flowers (must not be picked from the wild, as they are becoming very rare).

USES Medicinal Taken as a tea to calm anxiety. They have similar properties to cowslips.

Culinary Flowers are added to salads and desserts or candied to decorate cakes.

> CAUTION Not be taken during pregnancy or if sensitive to aspirin.

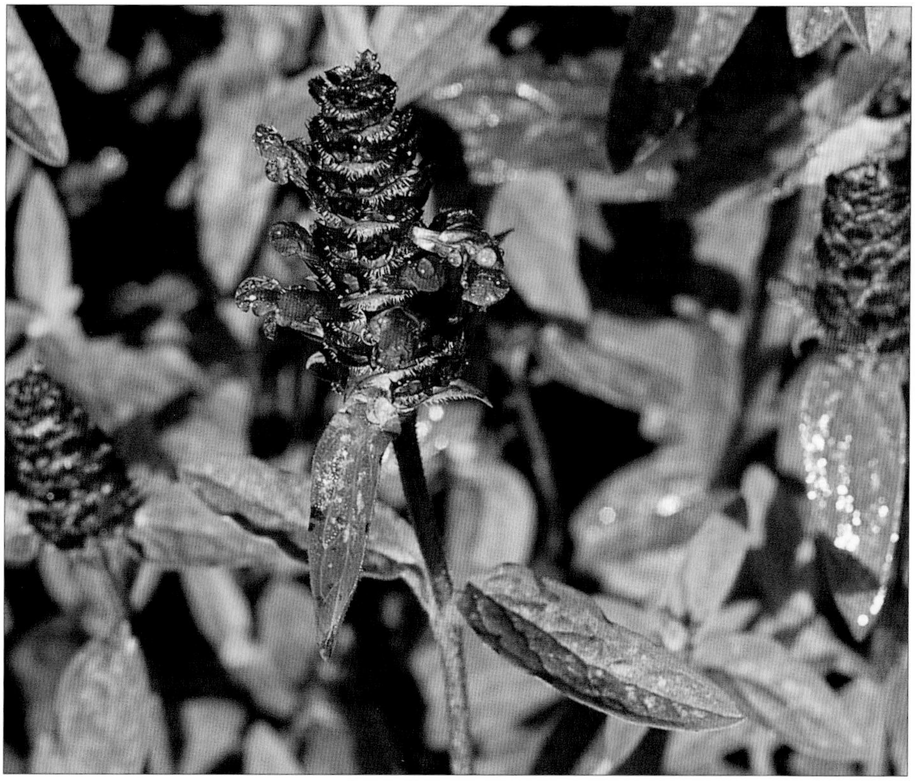

LABIATAE/LAMIACEAE

Prunella vulgaris

Selfheal

History and traditions A herb with an ancient history in Chinese herbalism, but apparently unknown to the ancient Greeks and Romans. *Prunella vulgaris* has featured in Chinese medical texts since the end of the previous millennium, where it is said to be mainly associated with "liver energy" disorders. In Europe its common names, "self-heal", "all-heal" and "hook-heal", all indicate its former use as a wound herb and activator of the body's defences, as explained by Culpeper: "Self-heal, whereby when you're hurt you heal yourself." It was held to be "a special remedy for inward and outward wounds" (Culpeper, *The English Physician*, 1653) and commonly taken to have the same virtues as *Ajuga reptans* (bugle). It was taken to North America by settlers, where it soon became established and known as "heart of the earth" and "blue curls". However, unlike *Ajuga* it still has a limited place in modern herbal medicine.

Description An aromatic perennial on a creeping rootstock, it is 50cm/20in in height. Leaves are linear to ovate, and compact spikes of violet, two-lipped florets are borne in the leaf axils from midsummer to mid-autumn.

Habitat/distribution Native to Europe, northern Africa and Asia, naturalized in North America, found on sunny banks, in dry grassland and open woodland.

Growth Grow in light soil in sun or dappled shade; tolerates most conditions. Propagated by seed sown in spring or by division in spring. It is inclined to be invasive.

Parts used Flowering stems – dried for use in infusions and medicinal preparations.

USES Medicinal It has antibacterial properties and is used externally to soothe burns, skin inflammations, bites and bruises, sore throats and inflamed gums.

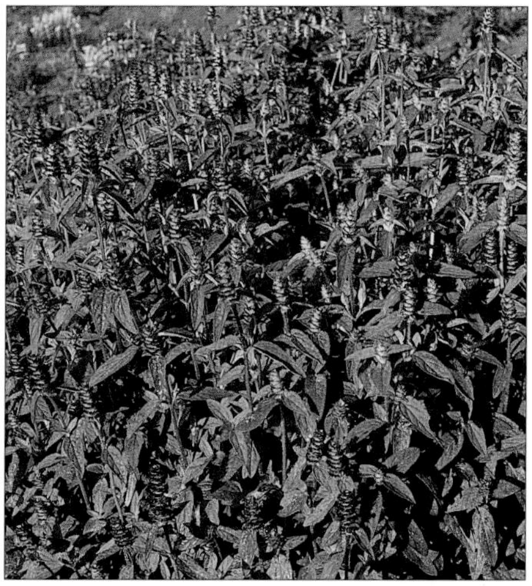

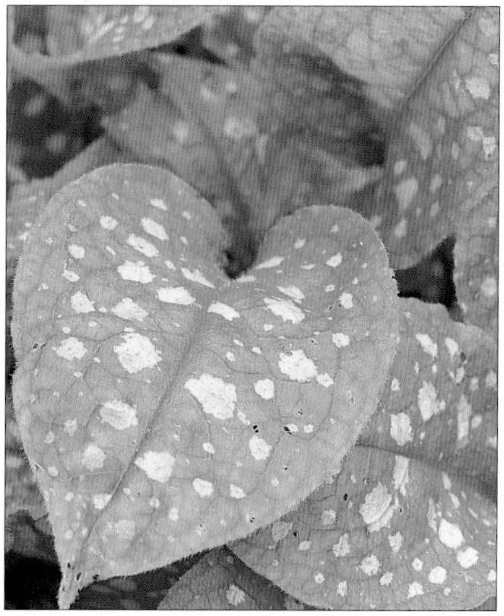

BORAGINACEAE

Pulmonaria officinalis

Lungwort

History and traditions Both the Latin and common names of this herb point to its principal former use in treating lung complaints. The spotted leaves were thought to resemble lungs and it is often cited as an example of the application of the Doctrine of Signatures, an influential Renaissance philosophy, which held that the medicinal uses of plants were indicated by their correspondence in appearance to the part of the human body affected. It is often grown in herb gardens for its historical associations and attractive foliage and habit.

Description A hardy perennial, growing to 30cm/12in, it has hairy stems and dark green leaves, blotched with creamy-white spots. The tubular flowers, borne in spring, are pink at first, then turn blue.

Habitat/distribution Occurs in Europe, parts of Asia and North America, in woodlands.

Growth Grows best in humus-rich, moist soil and a shady position. Propagated by division, in late spring after flowering, or in autumn. Although it self-seeds in the garden, collected seed seldom germinates satisfactorily.

Parts used Leaves – dried for use in infusions and extracts.

USES Medicinal The herb contains a soothing mucilage and has expectorant properties. It is still sometimes used for bronchial infections and coughs, but it is now thought that it may mirror some of the toxicity discovered in *Symphytum*, to which it is closely related.

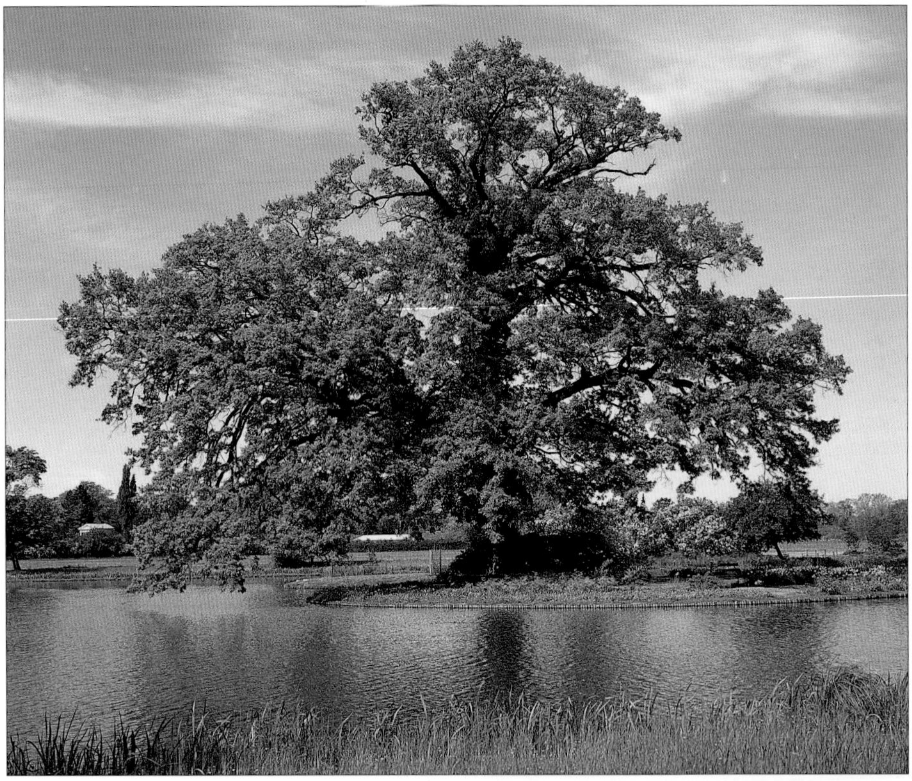

FAGACEAE

Quercus robur

Oak

History and traditions Few plants have been invested with as much magic, mystery and symbolic importance in Britain and much of Europe as the common oak. It was used in Druid ceremonies and thought to protect from lightning strikes – especially if planted near buildings to attract lightning away from them. Carrying an acorn was said to preserve youth, and dew gathered from beneath an oak was a potent ingredient in beauty lotions. They are exceptionally long-lived trees, and individual oaks were attributed characters of their own, complete with their own canon of folklore. They were also greatly valued for the durability of the wood, used in furniture, buildings and ships. The medicinal properties of the bark were well recognized by herbalists in former times. Culpeper lists many uses for it, declaring that it will "assuage inflammation and stop all manner of fluxes in man or woman".

Description A large deciduous tree, growing up to 25m/82ft in height. It has wide spreading branches, rugged grey-brown bark and small dark green ovate leaves, with deep rounded lobes. Male flowers are thin catkins; female flowers are borne in spikes in the leaf axils and followed by ovoid fruit, in little "cups" (acorns).

Related species The North American *Q. alba*, the white oak, also has a history of medicinal use, and was said to be effective against gangrene.

Habitat/distribution Native to Europe, occurs widely in the northern hemisphere in forests, open woodland and parkland, often found on clay soils.

Growth Grow in deep, fertile soil. May be propagated from seed, sown in containers in autumn. Very slow-growing.

Parts used Bark – stripped from mature trees and dried for use in decoctions and extracts.

USES Medicinal The oak has astringent, anti-inflammatory, antiseptic properties and is said to control bleeding. Applied externally to cuts, abrasions, ulcers, skin irritations, varicose veins and haemorrhoids. Sometimes recommended to be taken internally for haemorrhage, diarrhoea and gastric upsets. It was formerly used as a substitute for cinchona bark.

Other names Common oak and English oak.

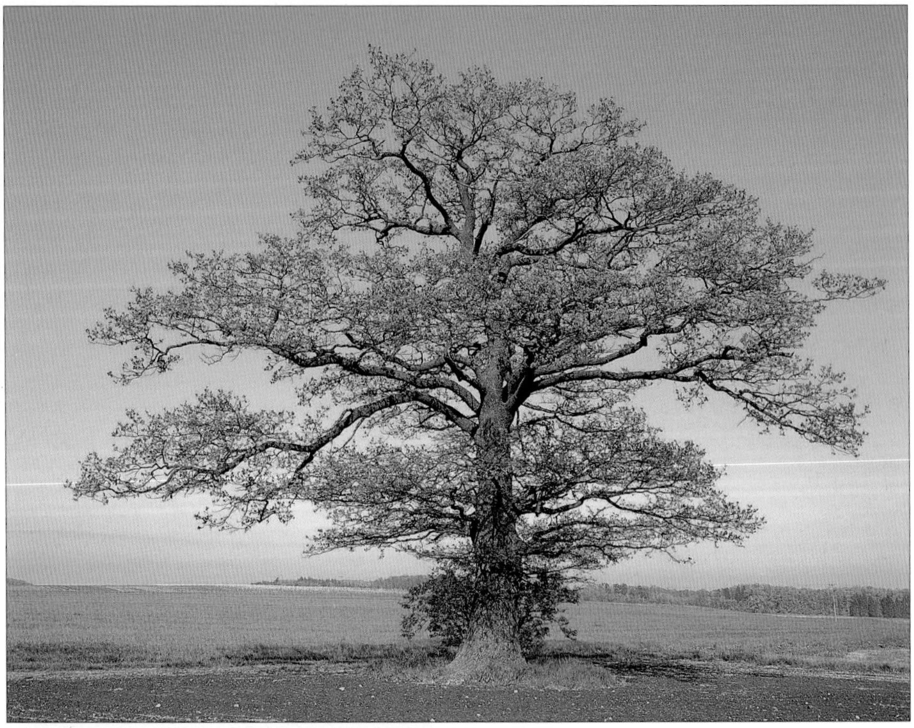

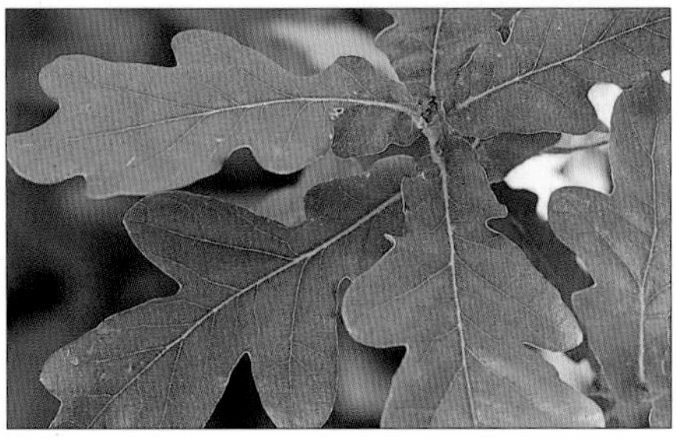

Top *An English oak,* Quercus robur, *growing in a park in Germany.*

Above *An oak tree.*

Left *The distinctive, lobed dark green leaves of the oak tree feature in decorative carvings through the centuries, as family emblems and on heraldic shields.*

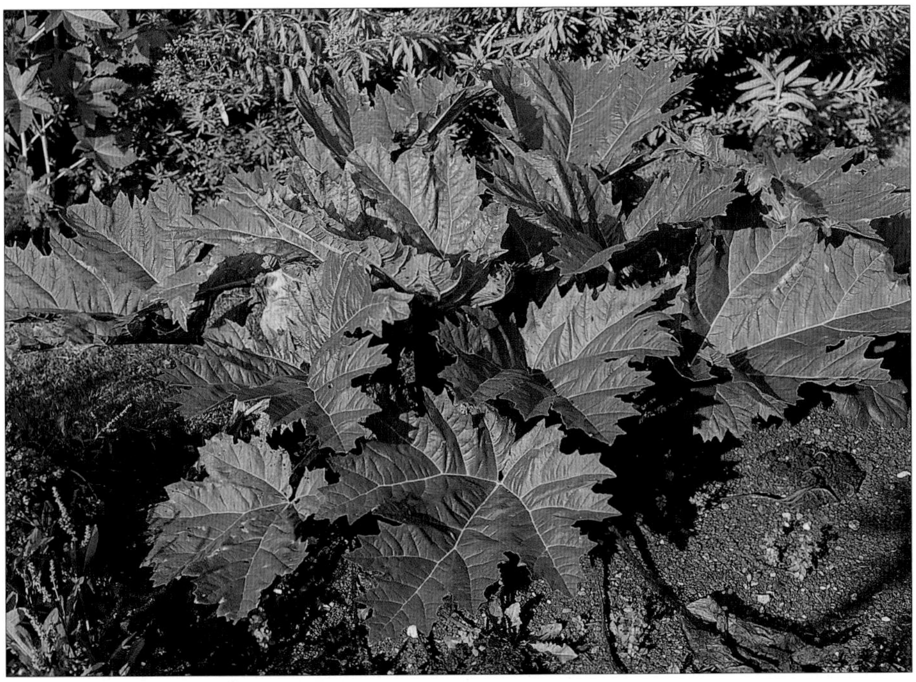

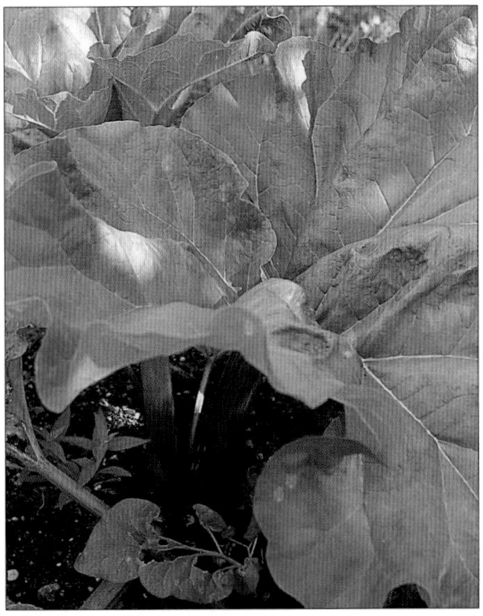

Left Rheum palmatum.

Above R. rhabarbarum.

POLYGONACEAE

Rheum palmatum

Rhubarb

History and traditions Rhubarb has been an important medicinal herb in China for many centuries. It is mentioned in the *Shen Nong Canon of Herbs*, dating from c.100BC, though claims exist that it has been recorded in much earlier Chinese texts, dating from 2700BC. Several species of rhubarb (there are 50 in the genus) were used, but *R. palmatum* is thought to be the main source of Chinese medicinal rhubarb. The plant was first grown in Europe in 1763. *R. officinale*, also medicinal and of Chinese origin, came to Europe, as a plant, in 1867. However, rhubarb in dried or powdered form had been known for centuries before that in the West. It was imported to ancient Greece, where they called it *rha-barbarum* because it was brought by traders from the barbaric regions beyond the river Rha (Volga). It reached Europe in the 13th century and was in demand as a purgative drug, which lacked the side effects of other more toxic products, remaining popular into the 20th century. Rhubarb powder was a major constituent of the 19th-century proprietary medicine, Gregory powder, named after the Scottish doctor who patented it. In an article in *The Lancet,* 1921, it is cited as a certain, even "magical", remedy for dysentery, when administered in small, strictly controlled amounts.

Description A large hardy perennial, to 2m/6ft, on a thick rhizome, with a basal clump of palmately lobed leaves. Spires of reddish-green flowers arise on long, hollow stems in summer.

Related species Edible garden rhubarb is from hybrids, developed during the 19th century, of *R. rhabarbarum* syn. *R. rhaponticum*, and there are now many cultivars. It is slightly laxative, but does not have medicinal properties.

Habitat/distribution Native to China and northeast Asia, found on deep, moist soils at altitudes of 3,000–4,000m. Introduced elsewhere in temperate zones.

Growth Requires rich, moist soil and a sunny situation. It is possible to propagate from seed, but division of roots in spring or autumn is the preferable method. Cultivars must be propagated by division.

Parts used Rhizomes – dried for use in decoctions, powders and medicinal preparations.

USES Medicinal Used in very small doses for diarrhoea and gastric upsets, and in larger doses for chronic constipation. Also given for liver and gall bladder complaints.

A 13th-century wonder drug

Rhubarb's reputation as a wonder drug is said to have been established in the 13th century after an Armenian monk staked his life (and won) that rhubarb would cure a lady of the court of the Mongol chieftain Mangu.

Medicinal dried rhubarb all came from China originally but was known by a variety of names after the route it took to reach its customers in Europe. "East India rhubarb" came down the Indus to the Persian Gulf, the Red Sea and Alexandria. "Turkey rhubarb" came overland, to the Turkish ports of Aleppo and Smyrna. "Chinese rhubarb" came via Moscow, and "Russian" or "Crown rhubarb" was the same product, so named once it had become a Russian monopoly, controlled from the early 18th century by the Kiachta Rhubarb Commission, set up on the Siberian/Mongolian border.

This organization maintained quality and price but prevented international trade until its eventual abolition in 1782. *R. rhabarbarum* (from which edible, garden rhubarb was later developed) comes from Siberia and was grown in the Padua Botanic Gardens from 1608.

CAUTION All rhubarb leaves are toxic. Medicinal rhubarb should not be taken during pregnancy or while breast-feeding.

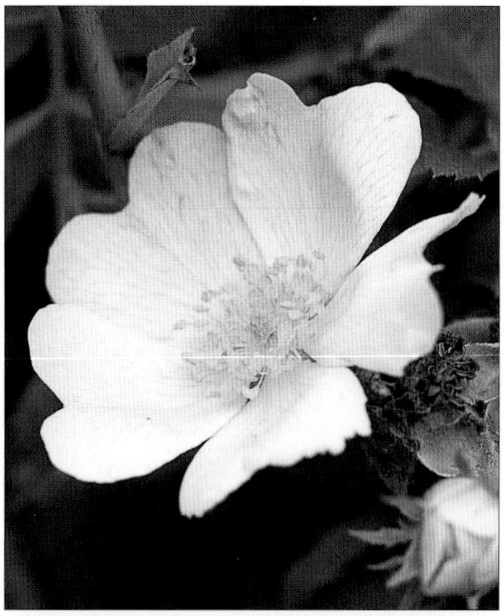

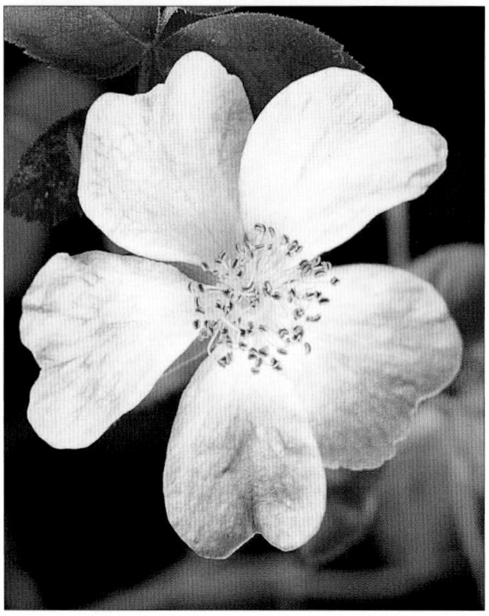

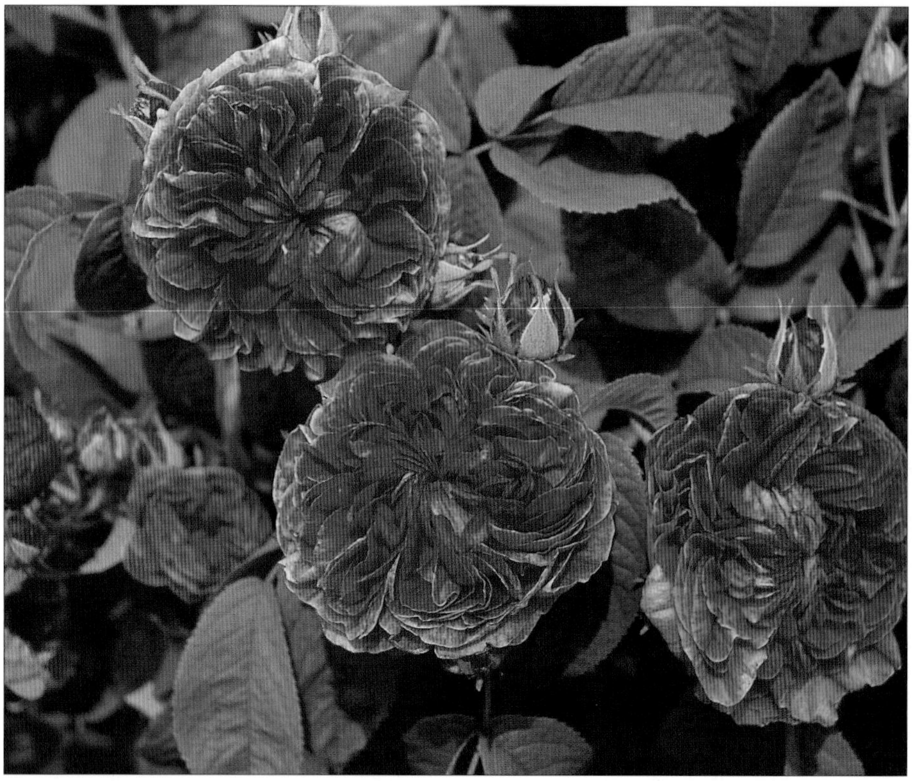

ROSACEAE

Rosa

History and traditions Roses have been cultivated for thousands of years and were once valued as much for their medicinal and culinary qualities as for their fragrance. Asian species of roses were used in ancient Chinese medicine and roses of Persian origin by the Greeks and Romans. The Greek poet Anacreon referred to their therapeutic value when he wrote, "The rose distils a healing balm, the beating pulse of pain to calm." In AD77 the Roman writer Pliny listed over 30 disorders as responding to treatment with preparations of rose. Medieval herbals contain many entries on the healing and restorative power of the rose, and in *The English Physician,* 1653, Culpeper gives pages of rose remedies for inflammation of the liver, venereal disease, sores in the mouth and throat, aching joints, "slippery bowels" and a host of other complaints. Red rose petals were listed in the British *Pharmacopoeia* as ingredients for pharmaceutical preparations until the 1930s. Their medicinal, culinary and fragrant uses are celebrated in all the old herbals and stillroom books with a huge range of recipes for ointments, lozenges, syrups, vinegars, conserves, cakes, candies and wafers. There are instructions for making rose water, rose oil and cosmetic lotions. Sir Hugh Platt, in *Delights for Ladies,* 1594, has at least three lengthy entries on different methods of drying rose "leaves" (petals) to best effect.

Description and species

R. canina **(Dog rose)** – This is the wild rose of English hedgerows, known as the dog rose for its supposed ability, according to Pliny, to cure the bites of mad dogs. Its succulent, but acidic, red hips were made into tarts in the 17th century, and came to be greatly valued in the 20th century for their high vitamin C content. It is a hardy, deciduous climber, 3 x 3m/10 x 10ft, with prickly stems and single flat, white, or pink-tinged flowers, followed by scarlet, ovoid hips.

R. rubiginosa **(Sweet briar**, or **Eglantine)** – A vigorous semi-climber, 2.5 x 2.5m/8 x 8ft, it has lovely apple-scented foliage and numerous single pink flowers, followed by rounded ovoid red hips. This is the rose which appears in the works of Chaucer and is described by Shakespeare as adorning Titania's bower:

With sweet musk roses and with eglantine
There sleeps Titania, sometime of the night
Lull'd in these flowers with dances and delight.

R. gallica var. ***officinalis*** **(Apothecary's rose)** – Probably the oldest of garden roses, it was widely grown in medieval times for its medicinal properties (though *R. damascena*, the damask rose, said to have been brought to Europe by the Crusaders in the 11th century, was almost as popular). A hardy deciduous, bushy shrub, 1.2 x 1.2m/4 x 4ft, it has large, very fragrant, semi-double, bright pink blooms and distinctive golden stamens.

R. gallica **'Versicolor'** Also known as Rosa Mundi, after the 'Fair Rosamund', mistress of King Henry IV of England, (1367–1413). A sport from *R. g. officinalis*, it has crimson-pink petals, splashed with cream.

Growth Fertile, moist soil and a sunny position are best for producing thriving rose plants with large flowers. However, *R. rubiginosa* does quite well on a poor, dry soil. The most suitable method of propagation is by hardwood cuttings in the autumn.

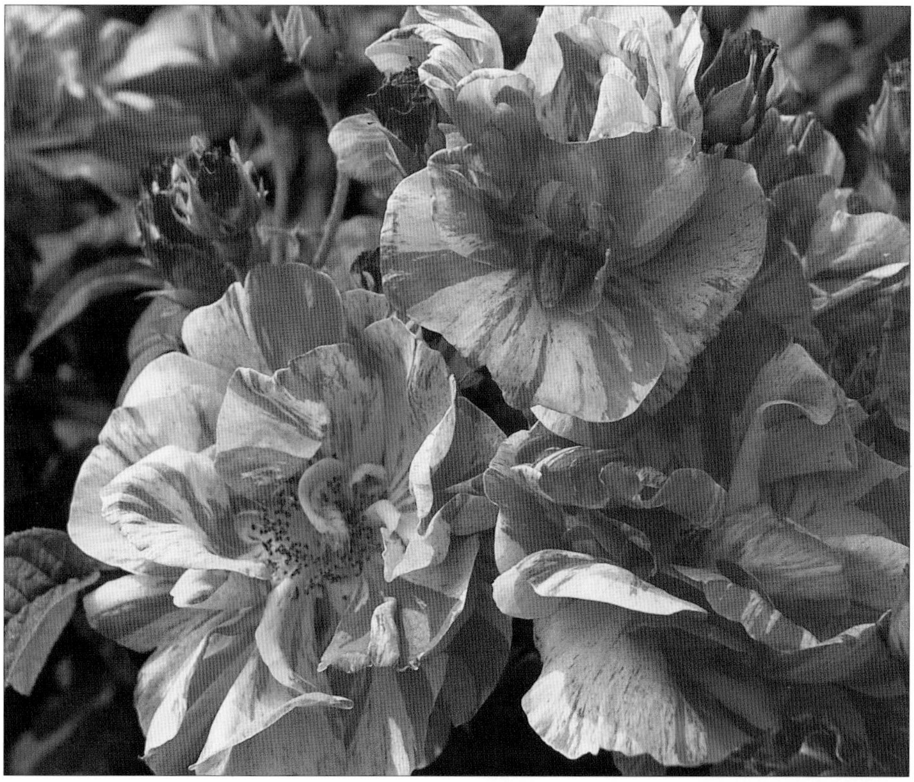

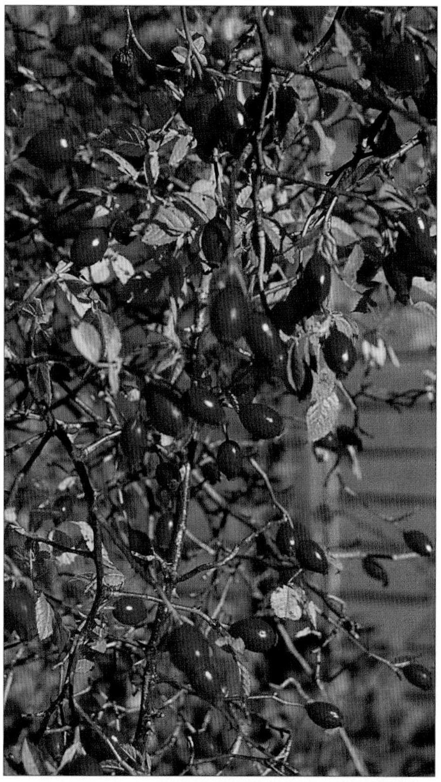

Parts used Flowers of *R. gallica*, hips of *R. canina*, essential oil, distilled rosewater from various rose species.

USES Medicinal Rose essential oil is used in aromatherapy for depression and nervous anxiety. In its purest form it is said to be the least toxic of the essential oils, safe to use undiluted. But many are adulterated, synthetic or semi-synthetic, and of no therapeutic value. Both hips and flowers are still sometimes recommended by herbalists to be taken internally in various preparations for colds, bronchial infections and gastric upsets and applied externally for sores and skin irritations. Rose hips are used nutritionally for their vitamin C content.
Culinary Hips are used for making vinegar, syrups, preserves and wines. Flower petals are added to salads and desserts, crystallized, made into jellies, jams and conserves. Distilled rose water is used to flavour confectionery and desserts, especially in Middle Eastern dishes.
Aromatic Dried petals and essential oil are added to potpourri, other fragrant articles for the home and beauty preparations, such as hand lotions and masks. Rosebuds and whole flowers are dried for decorative use. Dry roses in a warm, dry room but not in direct sunlight, which will bleach the petals.

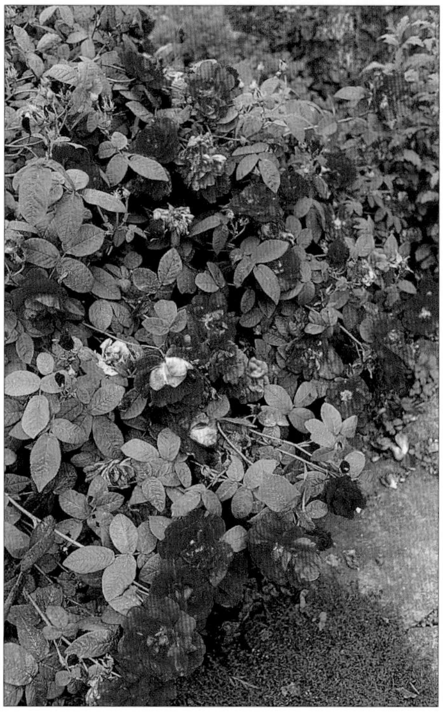

Opposite page, clockwise from lower left Rosa rubiginosa; Rosa canina; *and the superb double cultivar* Rosa *'Charles de Mills'.*

This page, clockwise from top left Rosa gallica *'Versicolor'; the hips of* Rosa canina*; a single flower of* Rosa gallica *var.* officinalis – *the famed Apothecary's rose; and the massed blooms of the Apothecary's rose on a bush.*

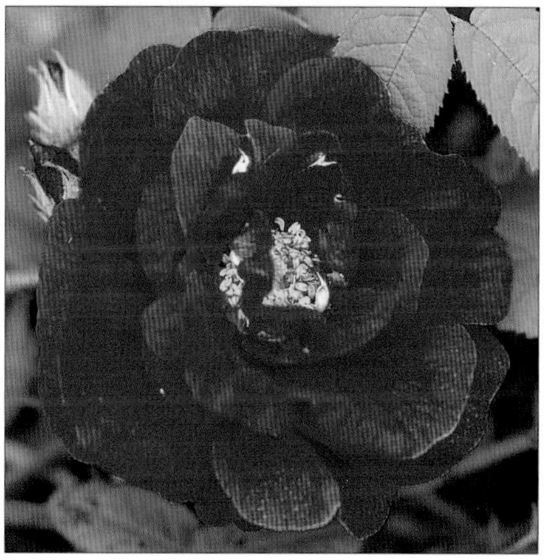

Rose-petal skin freshener

40g/1½oz fragrant fresh red rose petals
600ml/1 pint/2½ cups boiling distilled water
15ml/1 tbsp cider vinegar

Put the rose petals in a bowl, pour over the boiling water and add the vinegar. Cover and leave to stand for 2 hours, then strain into a clean bottle. Apply to the face with cotton wool (cotton balls) to tone the skin. Keep chilled or in a refrigerator and use up within 2–3 days.

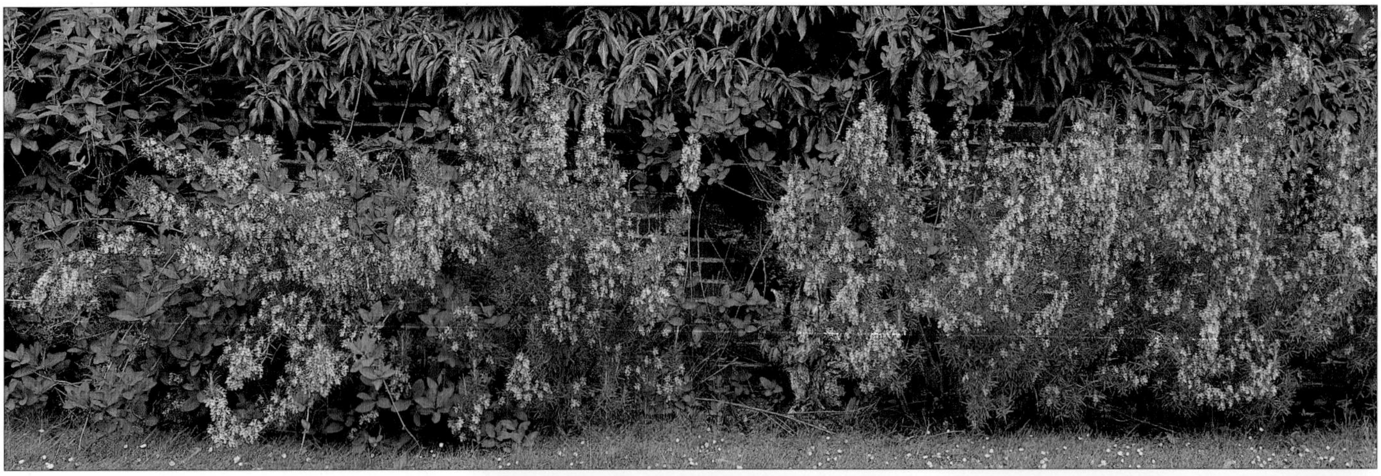

LABIATAE/LAMIACEAE

Rosmarinus officinalis

Rosemary

History and traditions Rosemary was well known in ancient Greece and Rome and the Latin generic name, *Rosmarinus*, means "dew of the sea", from its coastal habitat and the appearance of its flowers. It gained an early reputation for improving memory and uplifting the spirits, which is referred to in many herbals. *Bancke's Herbal*, 1525, includes a long list of remedies, practical suggestions and superstitions regarding rosemary, including putting it under the bed to "be delivered of all evill dreames", boiling it in wine as a cosmetic face wash, binding it round the legs against gout, and drinking it in wine for a cough or for lost appetite. It was also a major ingredient of Hungary Water, said to be invented by a hermit for Queen Elizabeth of Hungary, who was cured of paralysis after rubbing it on daily. A symbol of remembrance, it found a place at weddings, funerals and in Christmas decorations, when it was often gilded. In Spanish folklore rosemary is believed to give protection from the evil eye and to have sheltered the Virgin Mary, during the flight into Egypt, when the once white flowers took on the celestial blue of her cloak.

Description A variable evergreen shrub, to 2m/6ft, it has woody branches and strongly aromatic, needle-like foliage. A dense covering of small, tubular, two-lipped flowers, usually pale blue (but there are dark blue and occasionally pink variants) appear in spring.

Habitat/distribution Native to the Mediterranean coast, found on sunny hillsides and in open situations. It is introduced and widely grown elsewhere.

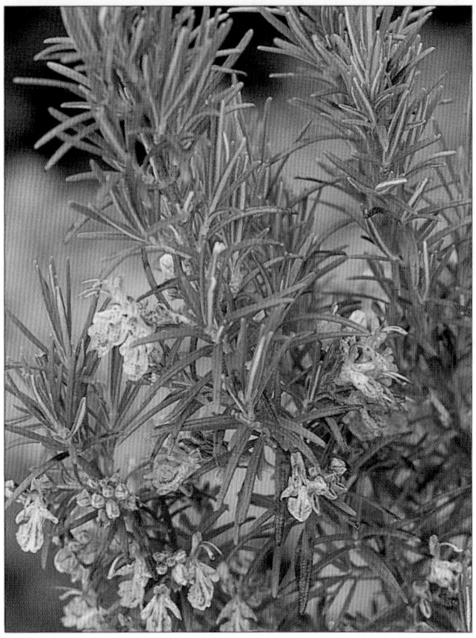

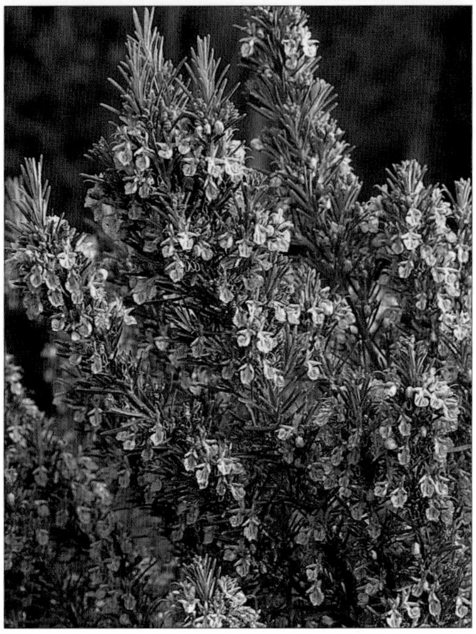

Growth Thrives on sharply drained, stony soils and requires little moisture. Although *R. officinalis* is frost hardy (not all species are), it needs a sunny, sheltered position and protection in cold winters and periods of prolonged frost. Easily propagated from semi-ripe cuttings taken in summer. It becomes straggly unless pruned hard in summer, after flowering, but must not be cut back to old wood.

Parts used The leaves and flowering tops are used fresh or dried for cookery and in medicinal preparations; essential oil distilled from leaves.

USES Medicinal A restorative, tonic herb, with antiseptic and antibacterial properties. It is taken internally as an infusion for colds, influenza, fatigue and headaches, or as a tincture for depression and nervous tension; and applied externally in massage oil for rheumatic and muscular pain. The essential oil is added to bath water for aching joints and tiredness.

Above left *Flowers of* Rosmarinus officinalis.

Above Rosmarinus officinalis *'Miss Jessopp's Upright'.*

Culinary A classic flavouring for lamb, stews and casseroles, and added to marinades, vinegar, oil and dressings.

Cosmetic Infusions are used as rinses for dry hair and dandruff and added to bath lotions and beauty preparations. Essential oil is used in perfumery and cosmetic industries.

Aromatic Dried leaves add fragrance to potpourri and insect-repellent sachets.

CAUTION Not suitable to be taken internally in medicinal doses when pregnant, especially in the form of essential oil, as excess may cause miscarriage. Safe for normal culinary use.

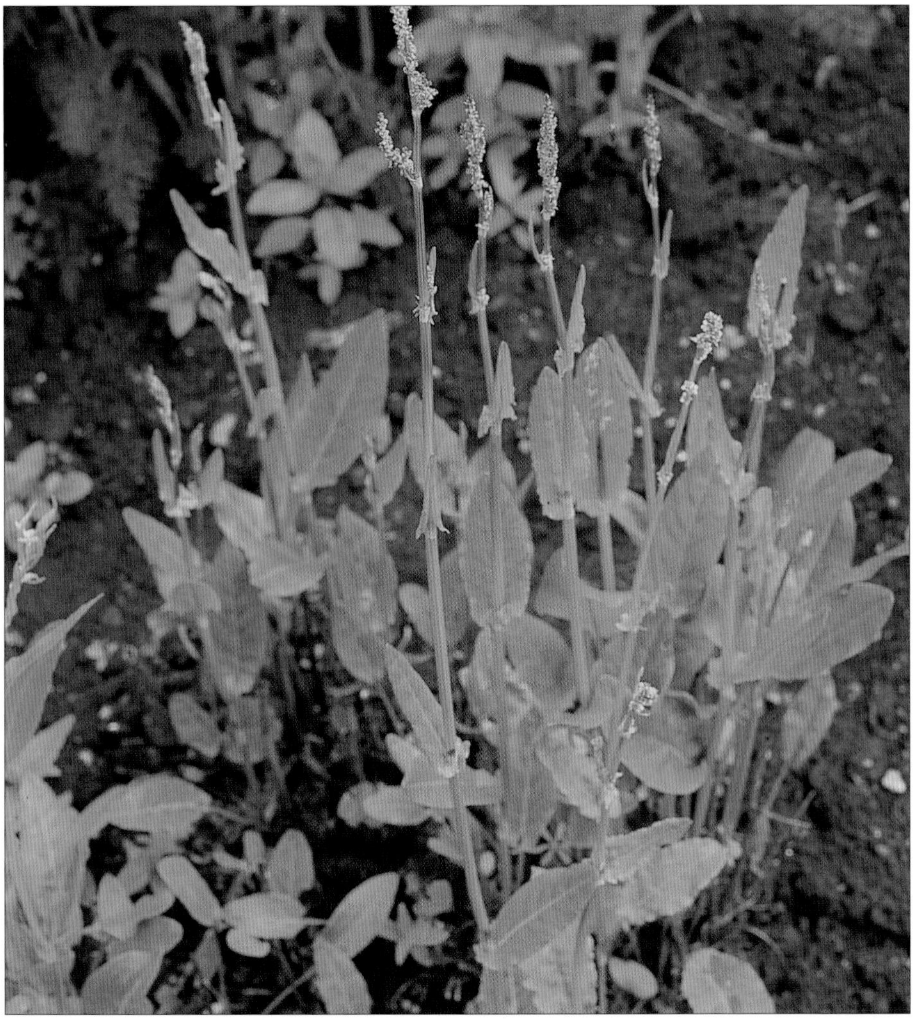

Description A hardy perennial, growing up to 1.2m/4ft, with large, pale green, oblong to lanceolate leaves, and large terminal spikes of small disc-shaped reddish-brown flowers on long stalks.

Related species *R. scutatus*, Buckler-leaved, or French Sorrel, is a lower-growing plant, with shield-shaped leaves and less acidity, and is favoured for culinary uses in France.

Habitat/distribution Occurs in Europe and North Asia in grasslands and is frequently found on nitrogen-rich soils.

Growth Grows best and runs to seed less quickly in rich, moist soil, in a sunny or partially shady position. Propagated by seed sown in spring or by division in spring or autumn.

Parts used Leaves – when fresh and young.

USES Culinary Sorrel adds a pleasant, lemony flavour to soups, sauces, salads, egg and cheese dishes. But it is acidic and not recommended for rheumatism and arthritis sufferers. The leaves have the best flavour and texture in spring, before they become coarse and fibrous.

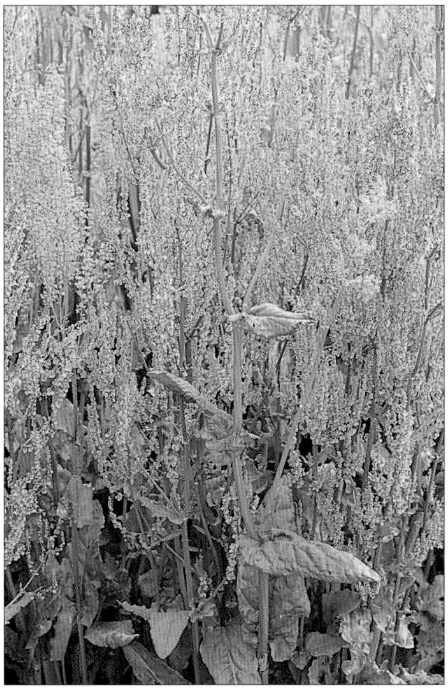

Right Rumex scutatus, *French sorrel.*

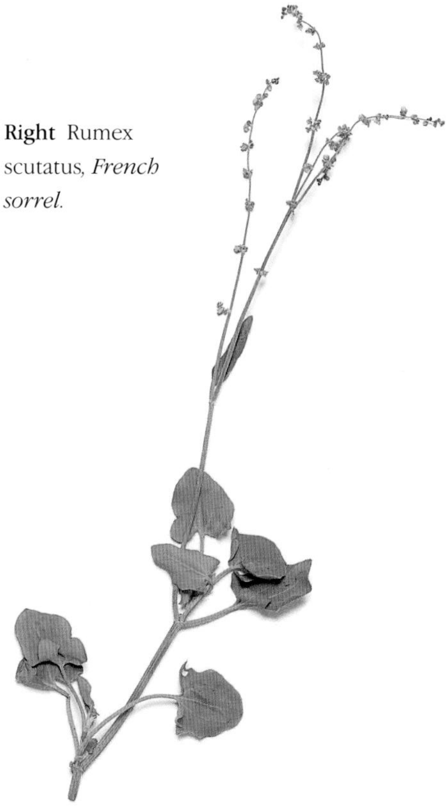

POLYGONACEAE

Rumex acetosa

Sorrel

History and traditions Various species of sorrel were used medicinally from at least the 14th century, but it was always chiefly valued as a culinary herb, especially in France and Belgium, where it was even potted as a preserve for winter use. Recipe books of the 17th and 18th centuries reveal that sorrel was not just made into soup, but frequently served with eggs, put into a sweet tart with orange flowers and cinnamon, as well as being cooked as a spinach-like vegetable. John Evelyn considered that it should never be left out of a salad, lending it sharpness, as a useful substitute for lemons and oranges when they were scarce. He also wrote that it "sharpens appetite ... cools the liver and strengthens the heart" (*Acetaria*, 1719). Culpeper recommended it for many medicinal purposes, including the breaking of plague sores and boils.

Above left Rumex acetosa – *the leaves are high in vitamin C.*

Above *Sorrel in flower.*

CAUTION Sorrel contains oxalates, also found in spinach and rhubarb, which are toxic in excess.

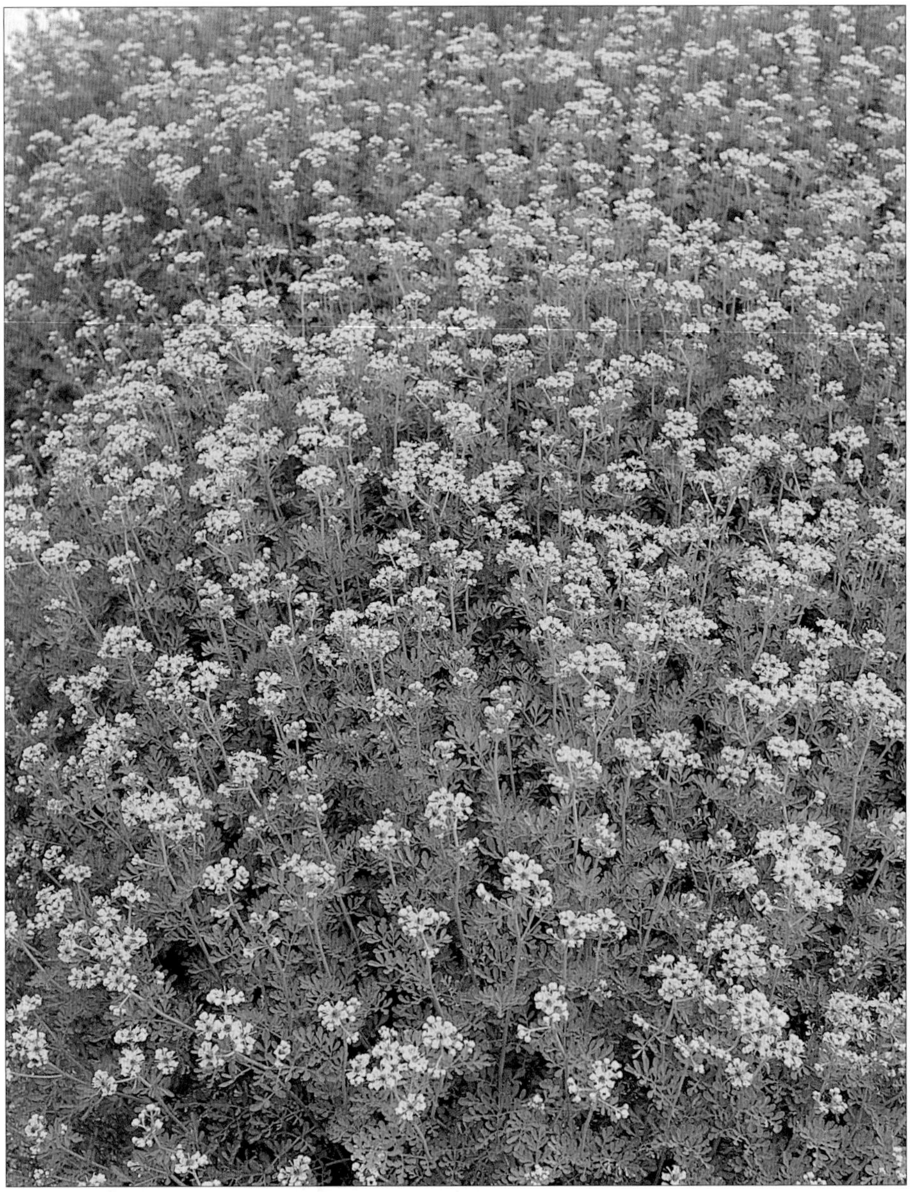

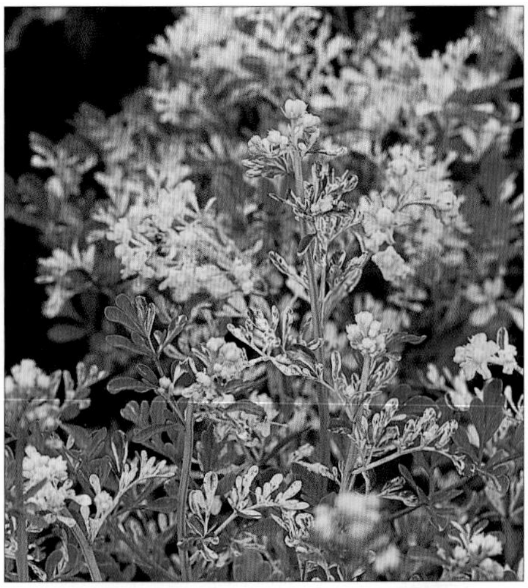

Above Ruta graveolens *'Variegata'*.

Left Ruta graveolens *in flower.*

RUTACEAE

Ruta graveolens

Rue

History and traditions Rue has a long tradition as an antidote to poison and defence against disease. The Greek physician Galen (*c.* AD130–201) took rue and coriander (cilantro), mixed with oil and salt, as a protection against infection, and Dioscorides (*c.* AD40–90) recommended it against every kind of venom. Most 17th-century herbalists continued the anti-venom theme, as illustrated by William Coles: "The weasell when she is to encounter the serpent arms herselfe with eating of rue" (*The Art of Simpling*, 1656). Rue was an ingredient of the celebrated anti-plague concoction, Four Thieves Vinegar, and always included in the judge's posy, placed in the courtroom to protect him from diseased prisoners and the dreaded jail-fever. The name "herb of grace" is said by some to originate from the practice of sprinkling holy water with a sprig of rue at Sunday mass. Its potent smell and protective attributes ensured its place as a powerful anti-witchcraft and spells herb. Although it is an attractive plant and widely grown in herb gardens, it has few herbal uses today. Far from being a protective, it is now recognized as a toxic irritant.

Description An evergreen, or semi-evergreen, shrubby perennial to 60cm/2ft, it has deeply divided blue-green leaves, with rounded spatulate leaf segments and a mass of small yellow, four-petalled flowers in midsummer.

Related species *R. graveolens* 'Jackman's Blue' is a widely grown cultivar with steel-blue foliage. There is also a variegated cultivar with cream and grey-green leaves.

Habitat/distribution Native to southern Europe on dry rocky soils, introduced and often naturalized throughout Europe, North America and Australia.

Growth Prefers light, well-drained soil and, although reasonably hardy, requires a sunny, sheltered position in cooler regions. Variegated cultivars are slightly less hardy. Propagated from seed (not cultivars) sown in spring, or from cuttings taken in spring (always wear gloves to handle). Prune in spring, or just after flowering in summer, to maintain a neat shape, but do not cut into old woody stems. It should not be planted at the front of a border where it can be brushed against.

Parts used Leaves.

USES Medicinal Although recommended by some herbalists for various complaints, including painful menstruation, it is a dangerous, toxic herb and there are safer alternative remedies for such conditions.

Aromatic It has insect-repellent properties and leaves may be dried for adding to potpourri.

CAUTION For practitioner use only. Rue is a skin irritant, especially in full sun, and causes severe blistering. Gloves should be worn when handling. Toxic if taken internally in excess, it affects the central nervous system and may be fatal. It is also an abortifacient.

SALICACEAE

Salix alba

Willow

History and traditions The willow contains salicylic acid and is the origin of aspirin (acetylsalicylic acid), which was synthesized from it as early as 1853. The bark had been used in Europe for centuries to reduce pain and fever, and in Native American traditional medicine several willow species were used for the same purposes. Willow branches were popular church decorations in Britain and used as substitute palms (which were not readily available) on Palm Sunday. In Russia, the week leading up to Easter was often called "willow week". The tree was always an emblem of sadness (it was a willow beneath which the "children of Israel" sat down and wept) and garlands of it were worn by the forsaken in love.

Description A spreading, fast-growing deciduous tree, up to 25m/82ft, it has greyish, fissured bark, arching branches and silvery-green, slender lanceolate leaves. Stalkless, yellow male and female catkins are borne in spring.

Related species There are several species of willow with medicinal properties in this large genus, including the North American *S. myrsinifolia* or black willow.

Habitat/distribution *S. alba* occurs widely in Europe and Asia, most often near rivers, streams and waterways.

Growth Requires damp soil and even does well on heavy clay, but dislikes chalk. Propagated by greenwood cuttings in spring, or by hardwood cuttings in winter.

Parts used Bark – collected from 2–3-year-old trees and dried for use in decoctions and other preparations; leaves – are also occasionally used in infusions.

USES Medicinal The salicylic compounds it contains give willow fever-reducing, analgesic, anti-rheumatic properties. Although it has been completely replaced by synthetics in pharmaceutical preparations it is still sometimes used in herbal medicine in baths for rheumatic pain and in ointments and compresses for cuts, burns and skin complaints.

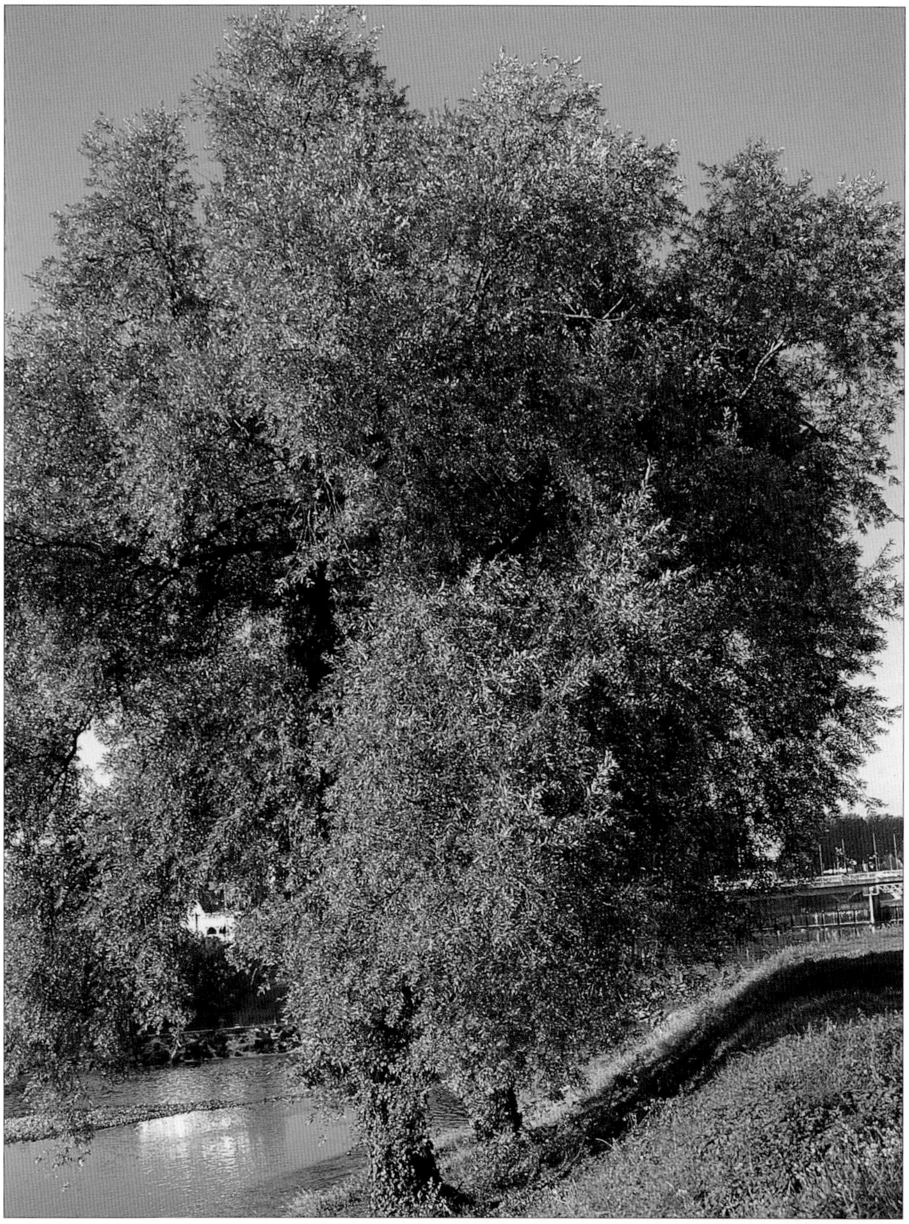

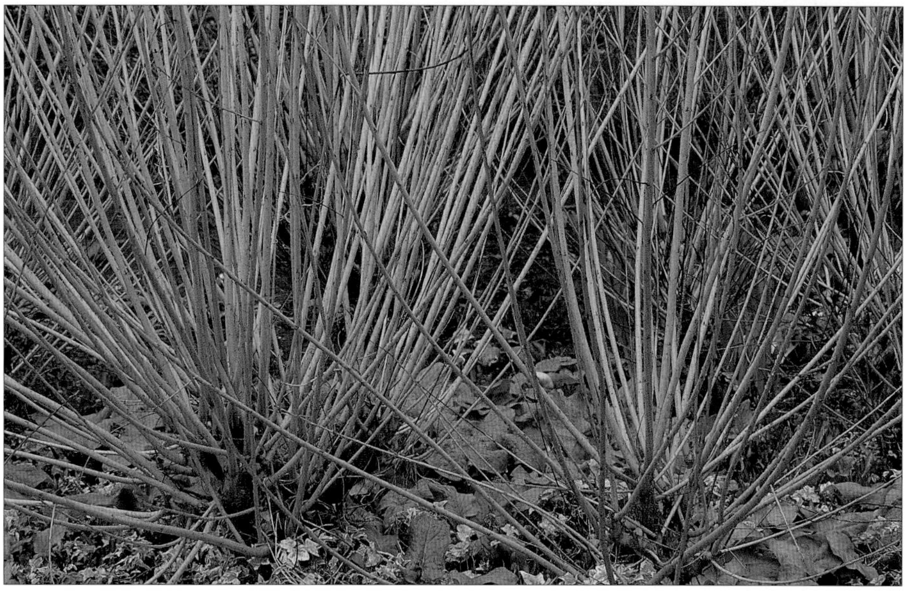

Above right Salix alba *(white willow).*

Right Salix alba *subsp.* vitellina, *coppiced to maintain its ornamental stems.*

LABIATAE/LAMIACEAE

Salvia

Salvia officinalis
Sage

History and traditions The Latin name comes from *salvere*, to save or heal, and this herb has always been connected with good health and a long life – even immortality. An old Arabian proverb asks, "How can a man die who has sage in his garden?" and John Evelyn wrote, 'Tis a plant, indeed, with so many and wonderful properties as that the assiduous use of it is said to render men immortal", (*Acetaria*, 1719). And Sir John Hill in *The Virtues of British Herbs,* 1772, has many anecdotes of people living to improbable ages through regular intake of sage. It is another plant, like rosemary, which is said to thrive where the woman rules the household: "If the sage tree thrives and grows/The master's not master and he knows."
Description An evergreen, highly aromatic, shrubby perennial, growing to 60cm/2ft, it has downy, rough-textured, grey-green, ovate leaves and spikes of tubular, violet-blue flowers in early summer. *S. officinalis* is one of the few hardy plants in this huge genus of around 900 species worldwide.
Related species *S. o.* 'Icterina' (golden sage) has gold and green variegated leaves. It seldom flowers in cool climates, but in warmer regions sometimes has pale mauve blooms. Although it may be used as a culinary herb it does not have such a good flavour as the species, or as the purple sages. But it does add colour when used in salads. It is reliably variegated, not as prone to revert as many and makes an attractive contrasting foliage plant for the border. *S. o.* Purpurascens Group (purple sage, or red sage) has striking purple, grey and green foliage. Some of its variants produce blue flower spikes. It has a strong flavour, is often used as a culinary herb and widely cultivated for its ornamental value. *S. elegans* (pineapple sage) is a half-hardy perennial with green, soft, ovate leaves, scented with pineapple, and scarlet, tubular flowers in winter.
Habitat/distribution Sage is native to southern Europe, found on dry, sunny slopes, introduced in cool temperate regions.
Growth Grow in light, well-drained soil in full sun. Although *S. officinalis* is hardy, it does not always withstand prolonged cold below -10°C/14°F, especially in wet conditions. The cultivars are slightly less hardy than the species. *S. officinalis* may be propagated from seed; cultivars must be propagated from cuttings or by layering. Prune sage in the spring to keep it

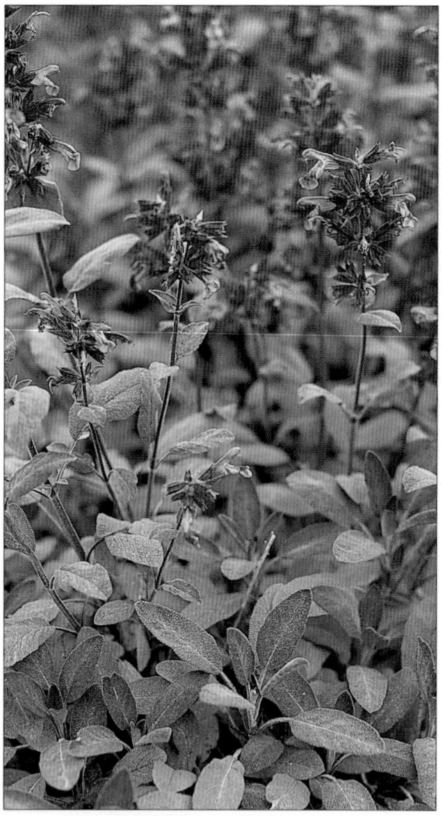

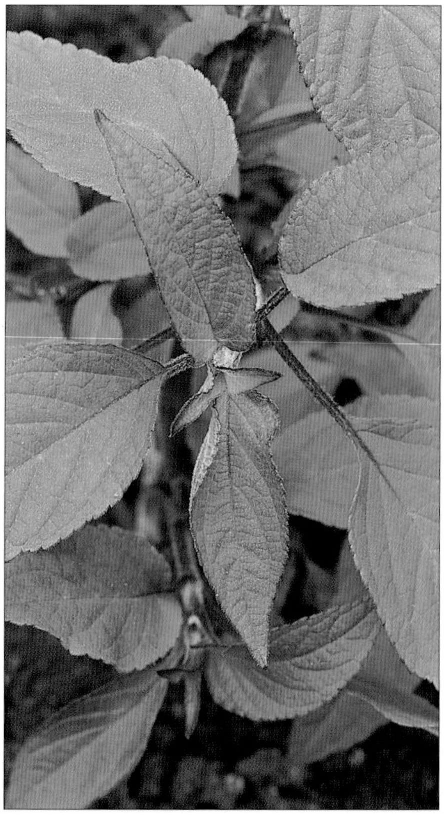

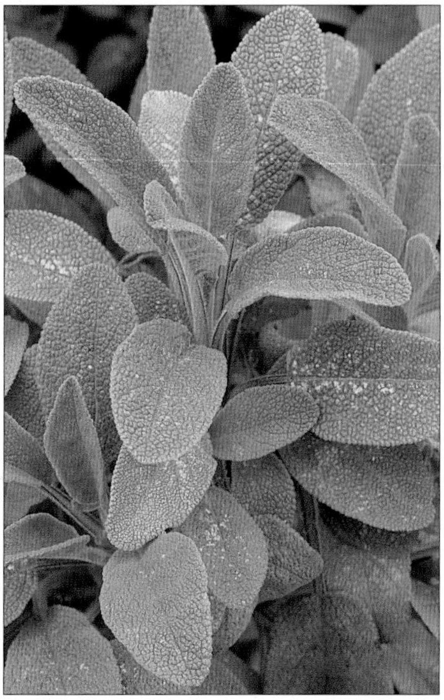

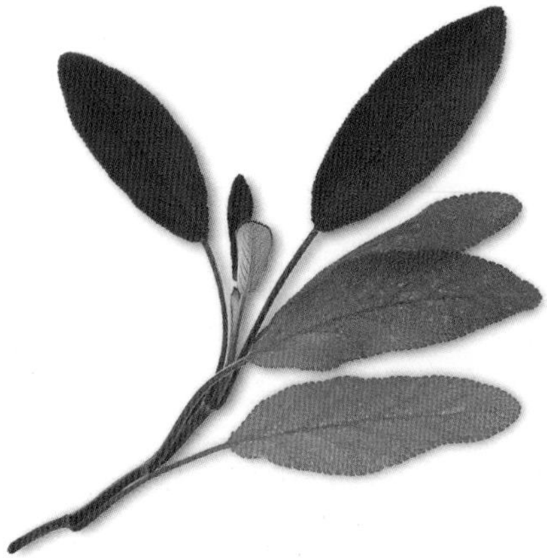

Above Salvia officinalis *Purpurascens Group.*

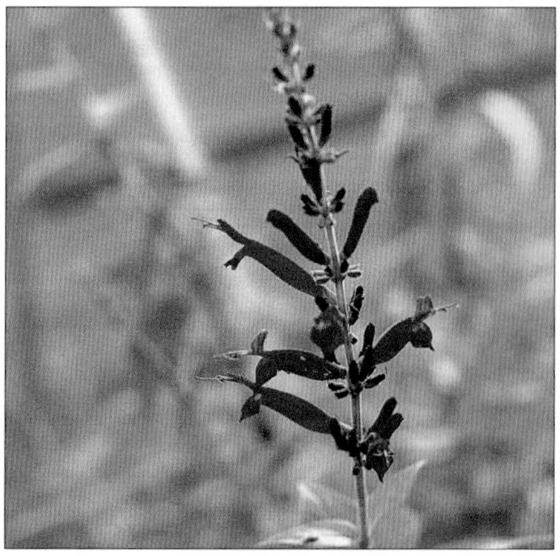

Above Salvia elegans *in flower.*

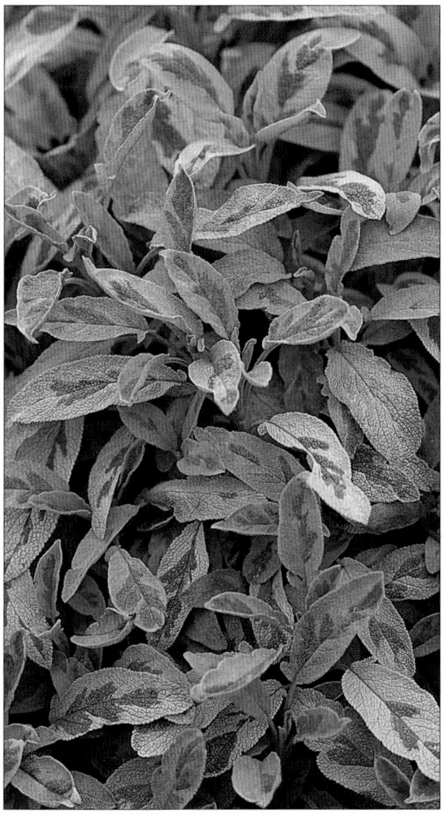

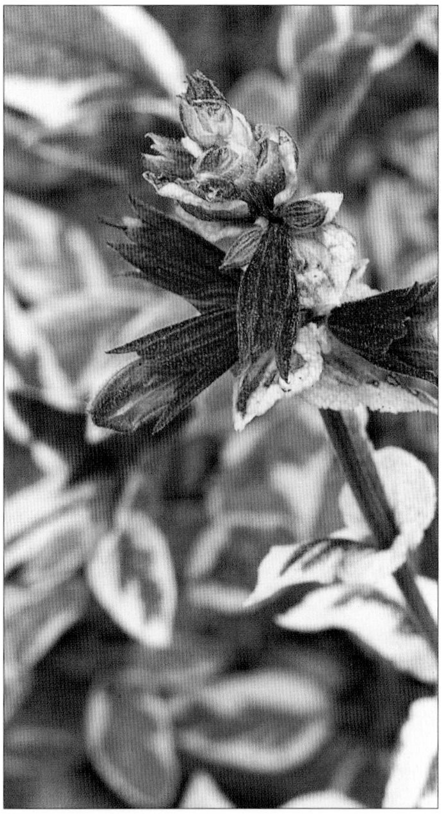

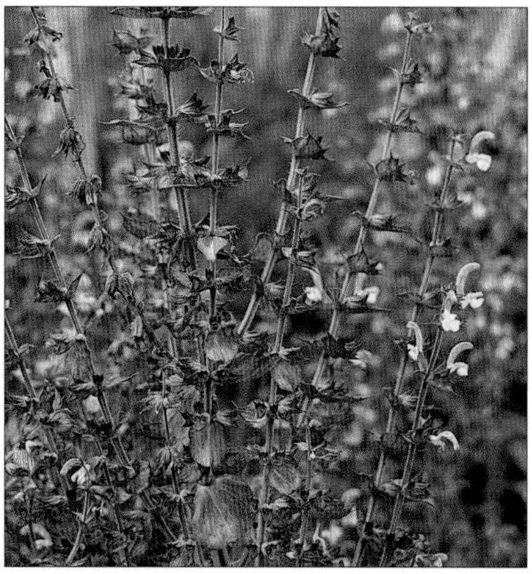

in good shape, or just after flowering, but do not cut into old wood. After a few years, sages can become straggly and need to be replaced. Pineapple sage must be protected from frost and kept under cover during the winter.
Grow in moist soil, and if container-grown, keep the compost (soil mix) damp. It is very easy to propagate from softwood cuttings taken throughout the summer.
Parts used Leaves – fresh or dried, essential oil.

USES Medicinal An astringent, antiseptic, antibacterial herb, infusions of the leaves are used as a gargle or mouthwash for sore throats, mouth ulcers, gum disease, laryngitis and tonsillitis. Infusions are taken internally as tonics, to aid digestion and for menopausal problems, and applied externally as compresses to help heal wounds.
Culinary Leaves are used to flavour Mediterranean dishes, cheese, sausages, goose, pork and other fatty meat. In Italy it is added to liver dishes. It is also made into stuffings, a classic combination is sage and onion. Leaves of pineapple sage may be floated in drinks.
Aromatic/cosmetic An infusion of the leaves makes a rinse for dark hair and to treat dandruff. The essential oil is used in the perfume and cosmetic industries.

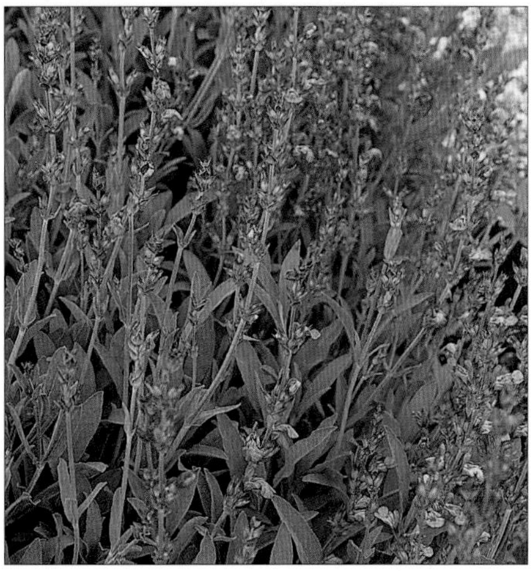

Above Salvia officinalis *in flower.*

Opposite page, bottom left Salvia officinalis; top left *A flowering form of* S. o. *Purpurascens Group;* top right S. elegans *in leaf.*

This page, top left S. o. *'Icterina';* top centre S. o. *'Tricolor'.*

CAUTION Sage, especially the essential oil, is toxic in excess doses, and should not be taken medicinally over long periods, by pregnant or breast-feeding women or by epileptics (the thujone content may trigger fits). It is safe in small amounts in cookery.

Salvia sclarea
Clary sage

History and traditions The specific name, *sclarea*, comes from *clarus*, meaning clear, and is the origin of the common name clary, a corruption of "clear eye" which refers to an old use of clary sage as a lotion for eye inflammations. It has long been a flavouring for alcohol and clary wine is said to have been a 16th-century aphrodisiac. In the 19th century it was sometimes used as a hop substitute, to make beer heady and intoxicating. With elderflowers, it provided German wine producers with a way of adding a muscatel flavour to Rhenish wine.
Description A biennial, up to 1.2m/4ft tall, it has a large basal clump of broadly ovate grey-green leaves, and in its second year a tall, branched, flower spike of silvery, lilac-blue and pink two-lipped florets. The whole plant has an unpleasantly overpowering scent, but it is showy and decorative in the border.
Habitat/distribution Native to southern Europe, found on dry, sandy soils.
Growth Grow in free-draining, but reasonably moist and fertile soil. Propagated by seed sown in spring or autumn. Often self-seeds.
Parts used Leaves – fresh or dried, essential oil.

USES Medicinal Infusions of the leaves are used as lotions for cuts and abrasions, and as a gargle for mouth ulcers. Sometimes recommended to be taken internally in small doses for promoting appetite. The essential oil is used in aromatherapy to treat a range of actions including cystitis and anxiety.
Aromatic Essential oil is used to flavour vermouth and liqueurs, and widely used in commercial soaps, scents and eau-de-Cologne.

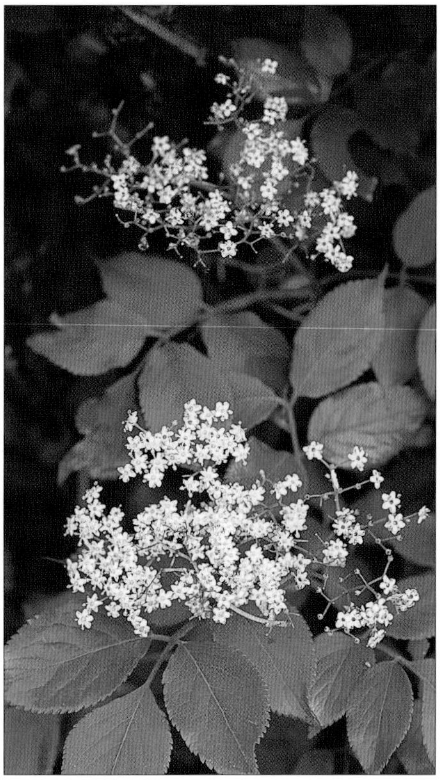

CAPRIFOLIACEAE

Sambucus nigra

Elder

History and traditions The elder has been associated since earliest times with myth and magic, witchcraft and spells. At the same time it was always valued for its many practical uses, medicinal, household, culinary and cosmetic. In Norse mythology, hauntings, deaths and harmed babies were the result of upsetting the Elder-Mother and guardian spirit, by not obtaining her permission before cutting down a tree to make furniture or cradles. Christian legends, referred to in English literature from the 14th-century *Piers Plowman* by William Langland to Spenser and Shakespeare, included the story that Judas hanged himself on an elder tree, and that it was the wood used to make the cross of Calvary. From this it became a symbol of sorrow and death and was planted in graveyards.
The idea that elders provided protection from witchcraft and evil spirits has ancient roots, and it is cited in Coles's *The Art of Simpling,* 1656, as being planted near cottages and fixed to doors and windows on the last day of April for this purpose. Some years earlier, in 1644, *The Anatomie of the Elder* was published, which celebrated its medicinal properties and asserted its capability of curing all known ills. Old herbals are full of culinary recipes, too, for the flowers, shoots, buds and berries, and the distilled water was said to ensure a fair complexion. The timber was valued for making fences, skewers, pegs and small household articles and the easily removable core of soft pith made elder prime material for pop-guns (as referred to by Culpeper), penny whistles and musical pipes, a use it has been put to since classical times.
The generic name, *Sambucus*, is from the Greek for a musical instrument.

Description A small deciduous tree, up to 10m/33ft tall, it has dull green, pinnate leaves, divided into five elliptic leaflets. Flat umbels of creamy, musk-scented flowers in early summer are followed by pendulous clusters of spherical black fruits on red stalks in early autumn.

Related species There are a few ornamental cultivars which make attractive subjects for the garden but have no medicinal or culinary value.

Habitat/distribution Native to Europe, western Asia and northern Africa. Occurs widely in temperate and subtropical regions in hedgerows, woodlands and roadsides.

Growth Prefers moist but well-drained, humus-rich soil in sun or partial shade. Propagation by suckers or semi-ripe cuttings in summer are the easiest methods. The species, but not cultivars, can also be grown from seed. Elders often self-seed prolifically.

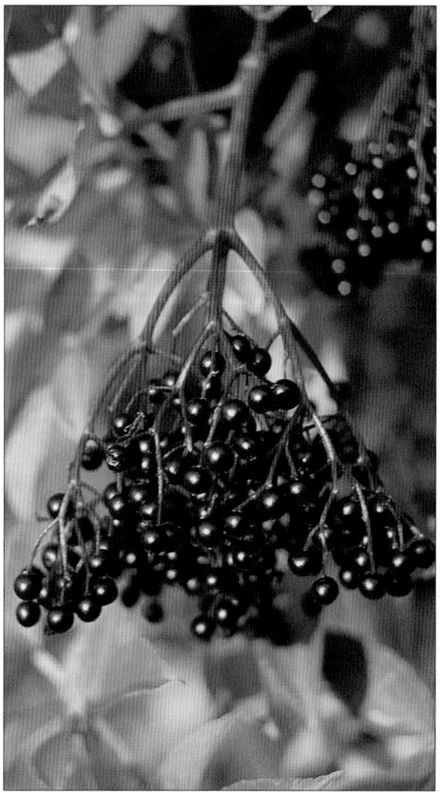

Parts used Leaves – fresh; flowers – fresh or dried; fruits – fresh.

USES Medicinal Has anticatarrhal and anti-inflammatory properties. Infusions of the flowers are taken for colds, sinusitis, influenza and feverish illnesses, and are said to be soothing for hayfever. The fruits (berries) are made into syrups, or "elderberry rob", also for colds.

Culinary Fresh flower heads in batter make elderflower fritters; fresh or dried flowers give a muscatel flavour to gooseberries and stewed fruits, and are added to desserts and sorbets. Flowers and berries are used to make vinegars, cordials and wines.

Cosmetic Fresh or dried flowers are used in skin toners, face creams and other home-made beauty preparations.

General The leaves have insecticidal properties and are boiled in water to make sprays against aphids and garden pests.

Elderflower

To take away the freckles in the face
Wash your face, in the wane of the Moone, with a sponge, morning and evening, with the distilled water of Elder-leaves, letting the same dry into the skinne. Your water must be distilled in May. This from a Traveller, who hath cured himselfe thereby.

Delights for Ladies, 1659

Elderflower skin freshener
A soothing and refreshing lotion for sensitive or sunburned skin. Pour 600ml/1 pint/2½ cups boiling distilled water over 25g/1oz dried elderflowers. Leave to cool, strain off the flowers and apply to the skin on cotton wool (cotton balls). Keep the lotion refrigerated and use within 2–3 days.

CAUTION Leaves contain toxic cyanogenic glycosides and should not be eaten. Berries are harmful if eaten raw.

Top left Sambucus nigra *in flower.*

Left *Elderberries.*

ROSACEAE

Sanguisorba minor

Salad burnet

History and traditions This is a traditional herb-garden plant recommended by Francis Bacon in his essay on the ideal garden (1625), to be planted in "alleys", or walks, along with thyme and water mints, for the pleasant perfume when crushed. The common name is a reference to the fact that this herb often lasted through the winter, providing welcome edible greenery when little else was available. It was also added to wine cups or ale for the cooling effect of the leaves. The generic name, *Sanguisorba*, comes from the Latin for *sanguis*, blood, and *sorbere*, to absorb, as it was formerly used medicinally as a wound herb interchangeably with *S. officinalis*, greater burnet.
Description A clump-forming perennial, 15–40cm/6–16in in height, it has pinnate leaves with numerous pairs of oval, serrated-edged leaflets and long stalks topped by rounded crimson flower heads.
Habitat/distribution It is native to Europe and Asia, naturalized in North America. It is found on chalky soils in grassy meadows and roadsides.
Growth Thrives on chalk (alkaline). Requires reasonably rich, moist soil for good leaf production and a sunny or partially shady position. Propagated by seed sown in spring. Cut it back as soon as the flower buds appear in order to ensure a continuous supply of leaves.
Parts used Leaves – fresh.

USES Culinary The leaves have a mild, cucumber flavour, make a pleasant addition to salads and are floated in drinks or wine punch.

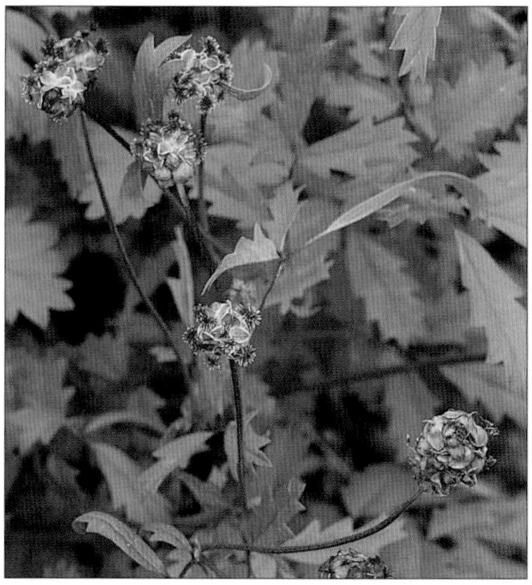

COMPOSITAE/ASTERACEAE

Santolina chamaecyparissus

Cotton lavender

History and traditions Cotton lavender is a native of southern Europe and was well known to the ancient Greeks and Romans and has long been valued as a vermifuge and for its insect-repellent properties. Culpeper recommended it also against poisonous bites and skin irritations (*The English Physician*, 1653). The neat, silvery foliage responds well to close clipping and it was introduced to Britain and northern Europe in the 16th century as hedging for knot gardens.
Description A small highly aromatic shrub, growing to about 60cm/2ft, it has silvery-grey, finely divided, woolly foliage and bright yellow, globular button-shaped flowers.
Related species *S. rosmarinifolia* subsp. *rosmarinifolia* syn. *S. viridis* has bright green foliage and makes an interesting contrast in knot garden work.
Habitat/distribution Cotton lavender is native to the Mediterranean region, introduced and widely cultivated worldwide. Found in fields and wastelands on calcareous soil.
Growth Grow in light, sandy soil and a sunny position. Tolerates drought. Propagated by semi-ripe cuttings in summer. Prune hard in spring to maintain a neat, clipped shape. It will regenerate if cut back to old wood.
Parts used Leaves – dried.

USES Medicinal Formerly used to expel intestinal worms. It is said to have anti-inflammatory properties and is sometimes made into an infusion as a lotion for skin irritations and insect bites, but in general it is little used in herbal medicine today.
Aromatic Dried leaves are added to potpourri and insect-repellent sachets.

Other name Lavender cotton in the US.

Below Santolina chamaecyparissus.

Bottom Santolina rosmarinifolia *subsp.* rosmarinifolia *syn.* S. viridis.

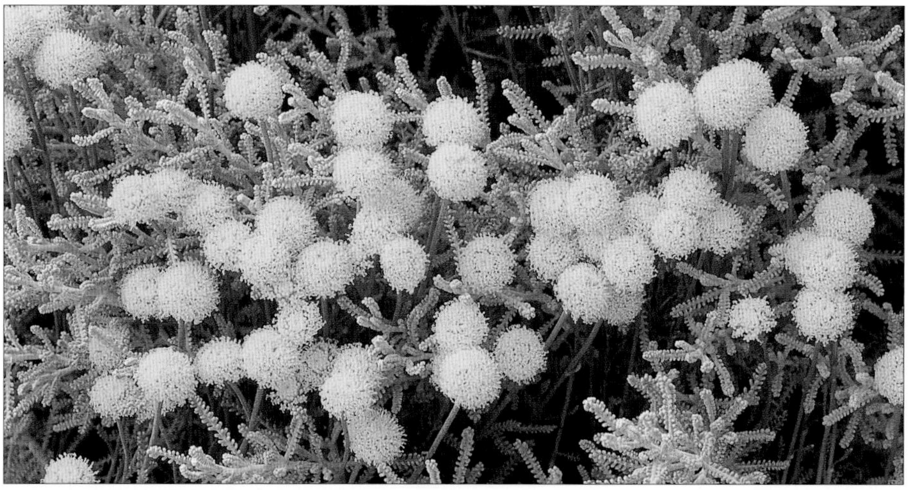

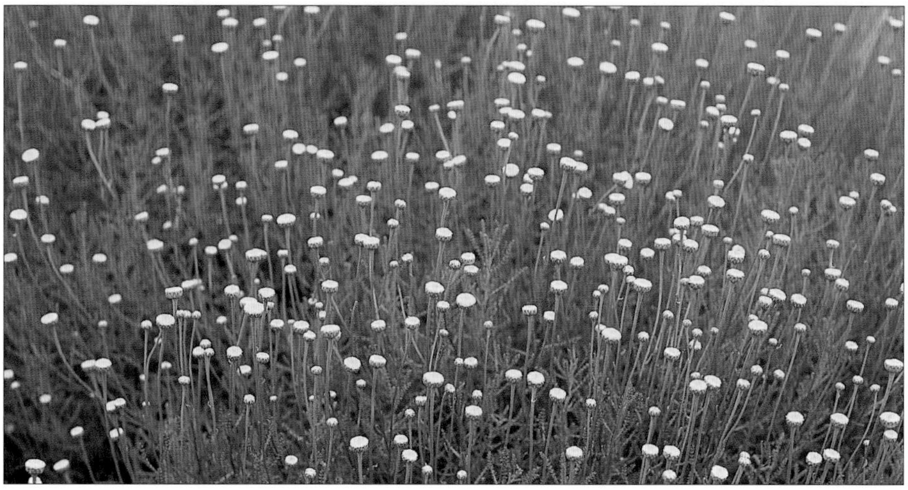

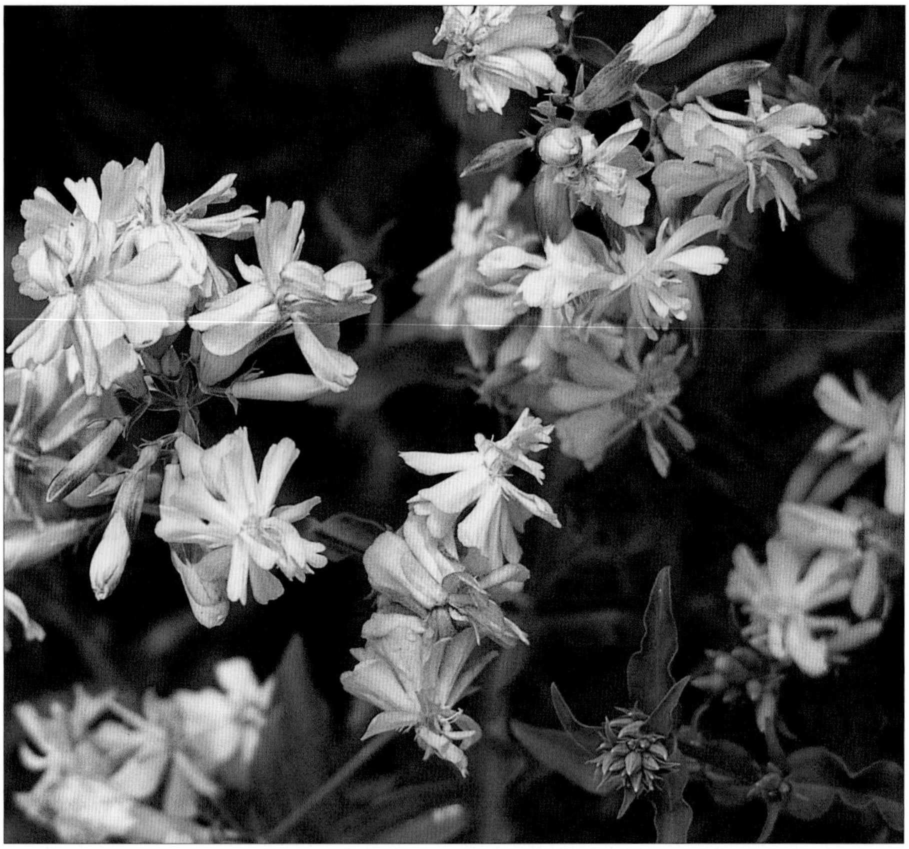

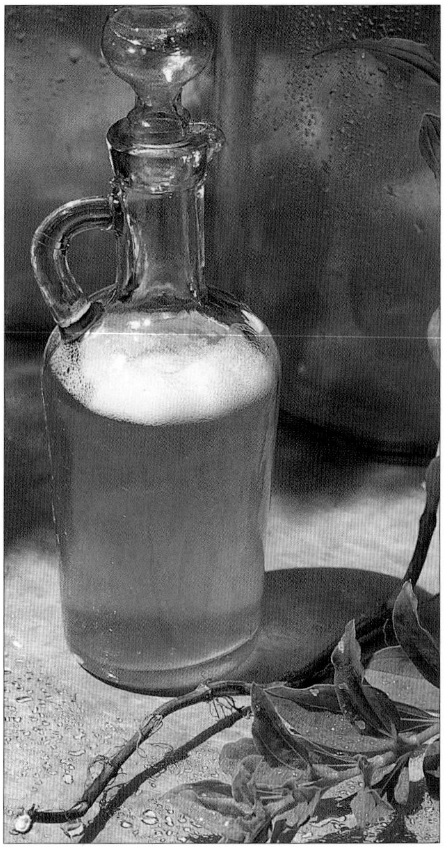

CARYOPHYLLACEAE

Saponaria officinalis

Soapwort

History and traditions Soapwort is indigenous to Europe and the Middle East and has been used there for its cleansing properties for many centuries. Some authorities claim that it was even known to the Assyrians around the 8th century BC. The name *Saponaria* comes from *sapo*, the Latin for soap, and, because of the high saponin content, soapwort roots produce a foamy lather when mixed with water. In Syria it was used for washing woollens, in Switzerland for washing sheep before shearing, and the medieval fullers, who "finished" cloth, used soapwort in the process. The common name, bouncing Bet, is a reference to the activity of plump washerwomen. It had its medicinal uses too. A decoction of the roots was formerly used for a variety of ailments from rheumatism to syphilis. Soapwort has been used until very recently by museums and by the National Trust in Britain, as it was found to be more suitable for cleaning delicate old tapestries and fabrics than most modern detergents.

Description A spreading, hardy perennial, on a creeping rhizomatous rootstock, 60–90cm/2–3ft tall, it has bright green, fleshy, ovate to elliptical leaves, and clusters of pale pink flowers in mid- to late summer.

Habitat/distribution Native to Europe, the Middle East and western Asia, naturalized in North America and widely grown in temperate regions. Found near streams and in wastelands, often as an escapee from gardens.

Growth Prefers moist, loamy soil, but tolerates most conditions and can become invasive. The easiest method of propagation is by division of the runners in spring. It can also be grown successfully from seed.

Parts used Roots, leafy stems – fresh or dried.

USES Medicinal It is seldom used in herbal medicine today.

Cosmetic An infusion or decoction of the roots and leafy stems makes shampoo – the addition of eau-de-Cologne improves the slightly unpleasant smell.

Household Used for cleaning delicate fabrics.

Other name Bouncing Bet.

Above left Saponaria officinalis.

Above right *A decoction of the whole plant makes a gentle shampoo.*

Soapwort shampoo

The gentle cleansing properties of soapwort shampoo are beneficial if you suffer from an itchy scalp or dandruff.

25g/1oz fresh soapwort root, leaves and stem or 15g/½ oz dried soapwort root
750ml/1¼ pints/3 cups water
lavender water or eau-de-Cologne

Break up the soapwort stems, roughly chop the root and put the whole lot into a pan with the water. Bring to the boil and simmer for 20 minutes. Strain off the herbs and add a dash of lavender water or eau-de-Cologne, as soapwort has a slightly unpleasant scent.

Use like shampoo, rubbing well into the scalp and rinsing.

CAUTION Soapwort should not be taken internally as it can be upsetting to the digestive system and is capable of destroying red blood cells if taken in large quantities.

LABIATAE/LAMIACEAE

Satureja

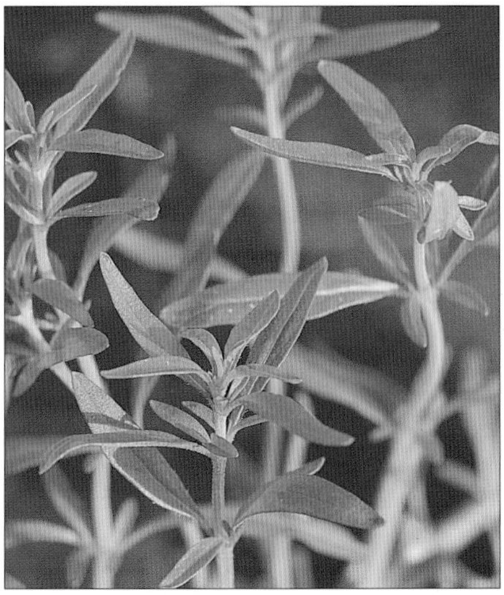

Satureja hortensis

Summer savory

History and traditions Both summer and winter savory are Mediterranean herbs that were appreciated by the Romans and commonly used in their cuisine. The poet Virgil, 70–19BC, celebrated them as being among the most fragrant of plants suitable for growing near beehives. Shakespeare too, writes of the scent of savory and it is included in Perdita's herbal gift to Polixenes in *The Winter's Tale.* The savories were among the herbs listed by John Josselyn which were taken to North America by early settlers to remind them of their English gardens. Culpeper promotes both herbs to ease a range of ailments, including asthma, and for expelling "tough phlegm from the chest", with summer savory especially suitable for drying to make conserves and syrups. It has been established by modern scientific studies (carried out in the 1980s) that the savories do have strong antibacterial properties. However, the subtle, spicy flavour (like marjoram, with a hint of thyme) ensures that both summer and winter savory remain first and foremost culinary herbs.

Description A small, bushy, hardy annual, to 38cm/15in high, it has woody, much-branched stems and small, leathery, dark green, linear-lanceolate leaves. Tiny white or pale lilac flowers appear in summer.

Habitat/distribution Mediterranean in origin, introduced and widely grown in warm and temperate regions elsewhere. Occurs on chalky soils (alkaline) and rocky hillsides.

Growth Grow in well-drained soil in full sun. Propagated from seed sown in containers, or *in situ,* in early spring. It may help reduce the incidence of blackfly when grown near beans.

Parts used Leaves, flowering tops – used fresh or dried.

USES Medicinal Has antiseptic, antibacterial properties and is said to improve digestion.

Culinary Summer savory has an affinity with beans and adds a spicy flavour to dried herb mixtures, stuffings, pulses, pâtés and meat dishes. Extracts and essential oil are used in commercial products in the food industry.

CAUTION The savories stimulate the uterus and are not to be given to pregnant women in medicinal doses.

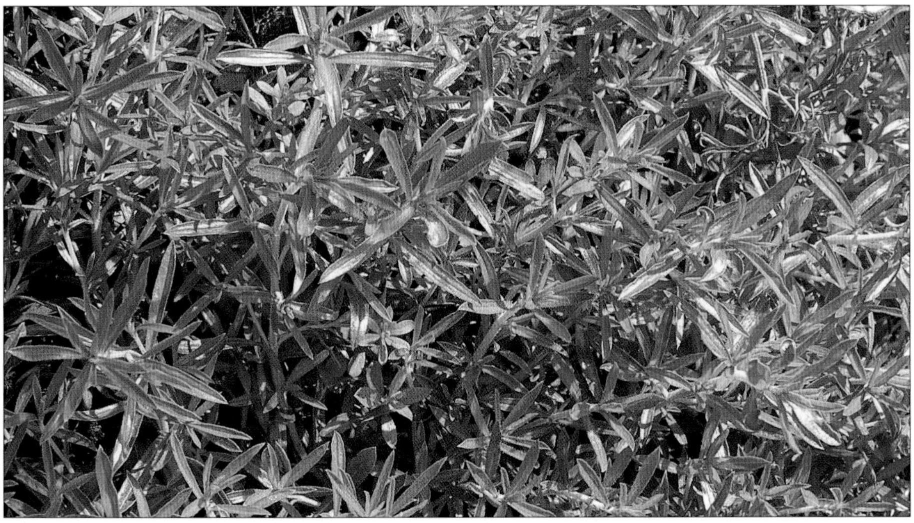

Below *The leaves have a mildly spicy flavour.*

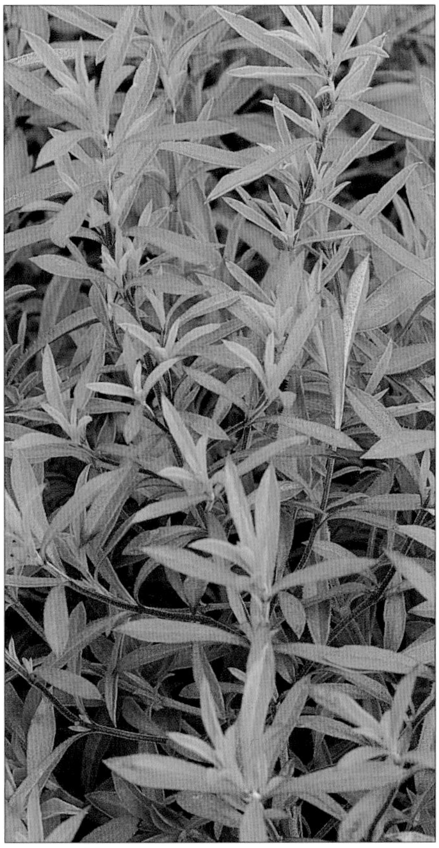

Satureja montana

Winter savory

Description A clump-forming, hardy perennial, to 38cm/15in tall, it is semi-evergreen (does not keep all its leaves in cool temperate regions through the winter, especially if frosts are prolonged). It has dark green, linear-lanceolate, pointed leaves and dense whorls of small white flowers in summer. It has a stronger, coarser fragrance than summer savory, due to the higher proportion of thymol it contains.

Growth Grow in well-drained soil, in full sun. Propagated by seed, by division in spring, or by cuttings in summer. Prune lightly in early summer, after flowering, to maintain a neat shape.

USES It has the same uses as summer savory, but to most tastes has a less refined flavour for culinary purposes.

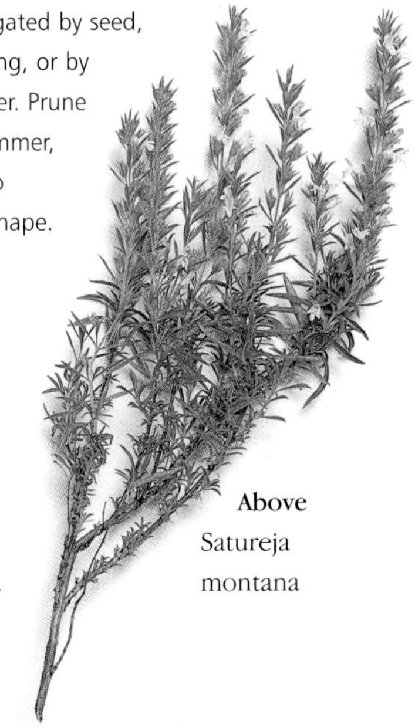

Above Satureja montana

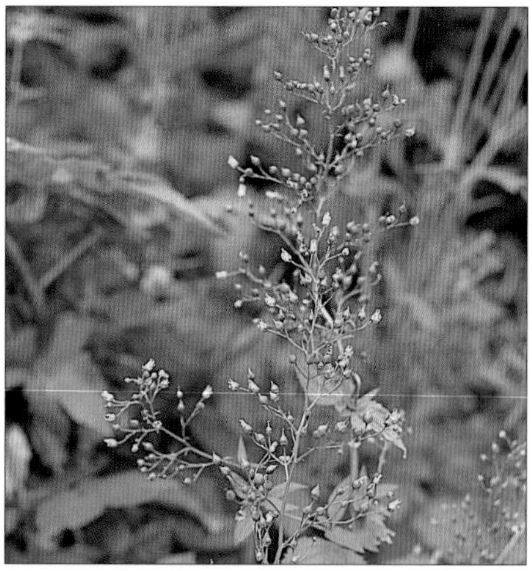

SCROPHULARIACEAE

Scrophularia nodosa

Figwort

History and traditions This herb was used in the past to treat scrofula or "the king's evil", a disease which affected the lymph glands in the neck. It conformed to the Doctrine of Signatures theory because the knots on the rhizome were thought to resemble swollen glands. Culpeper, writing in 1653, called it "Throatwort", adding that "it taketh away all redness, spots and freckles in the face, as also the scurf and any foul deformity therein".

Description A strong-smelling perennial on a stout, knotted rhizome, 40–80cm/16–32in in height, it has ovate to lanceolate leaves and terminal spikes of small, dull pink flowers.

Habitat/distribution Native to Europe and temperate parts of Asia, naturalized in North America. Found in woods and hedgerows.

Growth Grow in very damp soil, in sun or partial shade. Propagated by division in spring, or by seed sown in spring or autumn.

Parts used Rhizomes – dried for use in decoctions and other medicinal preparations; leaves and flowering stems – fresh or dried.

USES Medicinal This has cleansing properties. Infusions of the leaves are taken internally or applied externally in washes or compresses for skin disorders and inflammations. Decoctions of the root are taken internally for throat infections, swollen glands and feverish illnesses.

CAUTION This herb has a stimulating effect on the heart and is not given to patients with heart diseases.

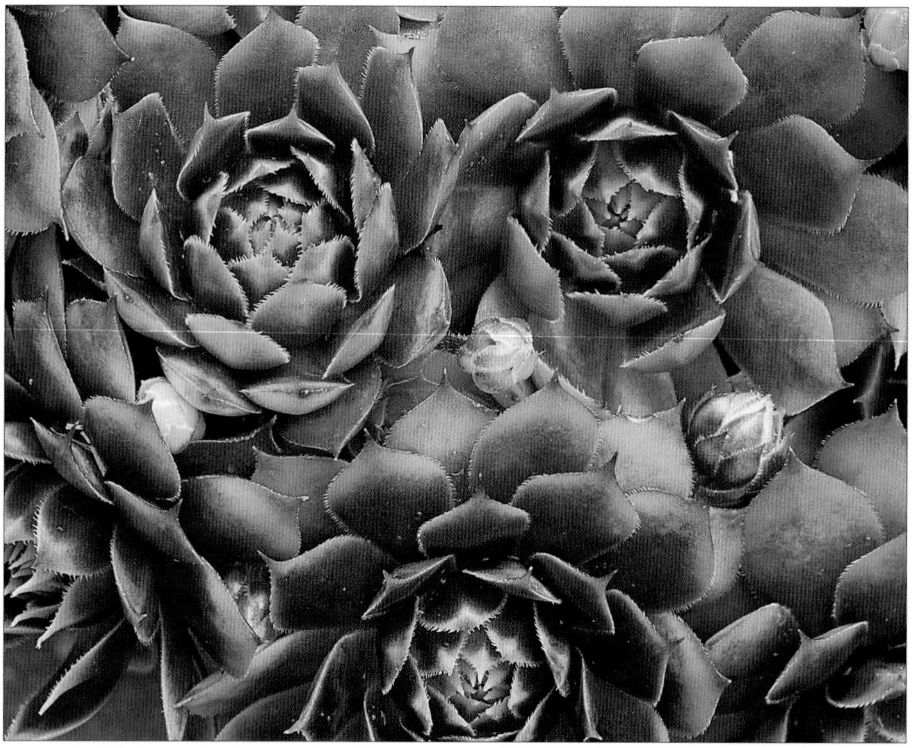

CRASSULACEAE

Sempervivum tectorum

Houseleek

History and traditions In the folklore of most European countries, houseleek is dedicated to Jupiter or Thor and was deemed to provide protection from lightning. It has been planted on thatched roofs or in the crevices of roof tiles ever since the Emperor Charlemagne, 747–814AD, decreed to this effect. The second part of the common name, houseleek, is from the Anglo-Saxon word for plant, *leac*. Its Latin name refers to its ability to withstand any conditions, and comes from *semper*, always, and *vivum*, living or alive. The specific name *tectorum* is a reference to its roof use.
This herb has been used since the time of Dioscorides and Pliny as a soothing agent for skin complaints. And Culpeper, writing in the 17th century, suggests a first-aid measure, which is equally valid today: "the leaves being gently rubbed on any place stung with nettles or bees, doth quickly take away the pain".

Description A mat-forming hardy succulent, it has blue-green, rounded leaves with pointed spiny tips, arranged in rosettes. Erect, hairy stems, to a height of 30cm/12in, bear pinkish-red star-shaped flowers in summer.

Habitat/distribution Native to southern Europe and western Asia, found on rocky slopes and in mountainous areas. Introduced and widely grown elsewhere.

Growth Thrives in gritty or stony, sharply drained soil and withstands drought. The easiest method of propagation is by separating and replanting offsets in spring.

Parts used Leaves – fresh.

USES Medicinal The leaves are made into infusions, compresses, lotions and ointments, or cut open to release the sap and applied directly to insect bites and stings, sunburn, skin irritations, warts and corns.

Above *A cultivar of* Sempervivum tectorum *with red-suffused leaves.*

Below *Break open leaves to release the sap.*

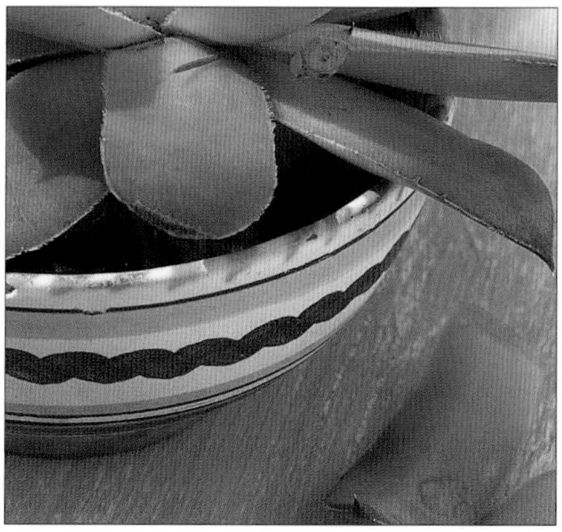

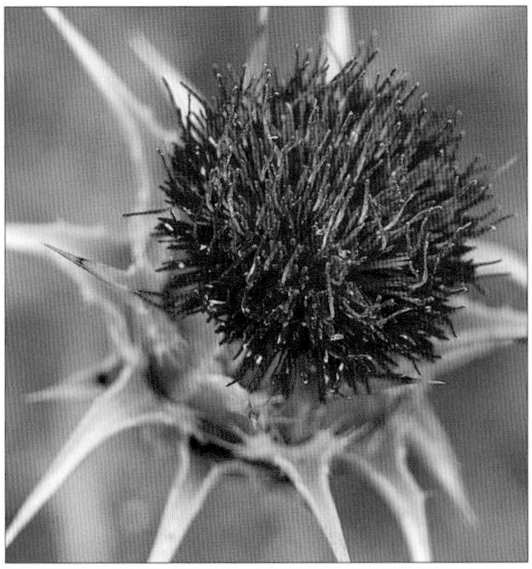

COMPOSITAE/ASTERACEAE

Silybum marianum

Milk thistle

History and traditions It is called milk thistle for its milky-white veins, from which it earned its reputation, under the Doctrine of Signatures, as improving the milk supply of nursing mothers. The Latin specific name, *marianum*, associates it with the Virgin Mary, from the tradition that her milk once fell upon its leaves, and the genus name is a corruption of *silybon*, which was Dioscorides' term for this herb. .

Description A tall annual or biennial, up to 1.2m/4ft in height, it has large, deeply lobed, spiny leaves with white veins and purple thistle flowers in summer.

Habitat/distribution Native to Europe, introduced elsewhere and naturalized in North America and other countries. Found on dry, stony soils, in fields and roadsides.

Growth Grows in any well-drained soil in a sunny position. Propagation is by seed, sown in spring or autumn, and it self-seeds prolifically.

Parts used Leaves and flowering stems – dried for use in infusions or for extractions of the active principle silymarin.

USES Medicinal Recent research demonstrates that milk thistle is a valuable protective liver herb, promoting the regeneration of diseased liver cells. It is used in chronic liver disease, particularly those due to alcohol, drug or dietary abuve. It will also aid in gall bladder problems. It will increase the production of milk and is safe to use by all breastfeeding mothers.

Other name Marian thistle.

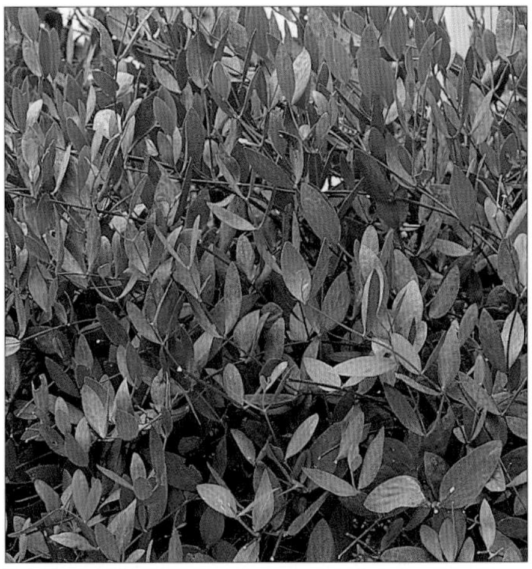

SIMMONDSIACIAE

Simmondsia chinensis

Jojoba

History and traditions The oil from the seeds of this herb was used by Native Americans as a cosmetic and for softening garments made from animal skins. In the 1970s jojoba was discovered to be a valuable replacement for sperm whale oil and large commercial plantations have since been established in Arizona and across wide areas of semi-arid grassland in the United States.

Description A half-hardy shrub, up to 2m/6ft in height, with leathery, ovate leaves, it is the only species in the genus. Pale yellow flowers appear in axillary clusters on male plants, the greenish female flowers are usually solitary and followed by ovoid seed capsules.

Habitat/distribution It is native to south-western North America and Mexico, and is widely grown as a crop in the United States and the Middle East.

Growth Tolerant of drought, it thrives in dry, gravelly soil. A half-hardy plant, it is propagated by seed sown in spring, or by heel cuttings taken in autumn.

Parts used Oil – expressed straight from the ripe seeds.

USES Medicinal Jojoba oil has exceptionally soothing and softening properties and is used in pharmaceutical ointments for dry skins, psoriasis and eczema.

Cosmetic It is also an important ingredient of moisturisers, body lotions and sunscreens.

General The oil is used as an engine lubricant. The shrubs are planted to prevent further encroachment of total desert in arid areas.

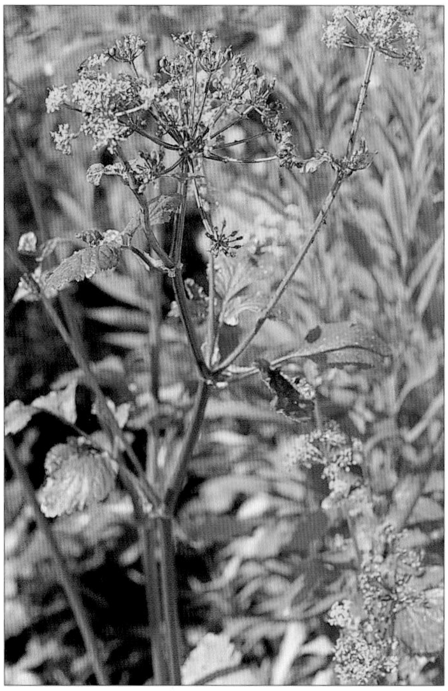

APIACEAE

Smyrnium olusatrum

Alexanders

History and traditions Alexanders was valued chiefly as a culinary herb from the days of the ancient Greeks until well into the 19th century. It is high in vitamin C and at one time was recognised as a useful aid against scurvy. It was also thought to have some medicinal properties, chiefly as a diuretic and stomachic. It was taken for asthma and to help menstrual flow, but it is no longer used in herbal medicine.

Description A large perennial, it grows up to 1.5m/5ft tall, with thick ridged stems, dark green, shiny leaves and domed umbels of greenish-yellow flowers, followed by black seeds. It is sometimes confused with angelica, of which it is taken to be a wild species.

Habitat/distribution Native to Europe and the Mediterranean, frequently found on coastal sites.

Growth It grows best in sandy, but moist and reasonably fertile soil, and is propagated by seed sown in spring.

Parts used Leaves, young stems, flower buds, seeds, roots.

USES Culinary The whole plant is edible. Leaves and young stems may be used like celery, the roots cooked as parsnips, the flower buds added to salads and the seeds lightly crushed or ground as a seasoning.

Other name Black lovage.

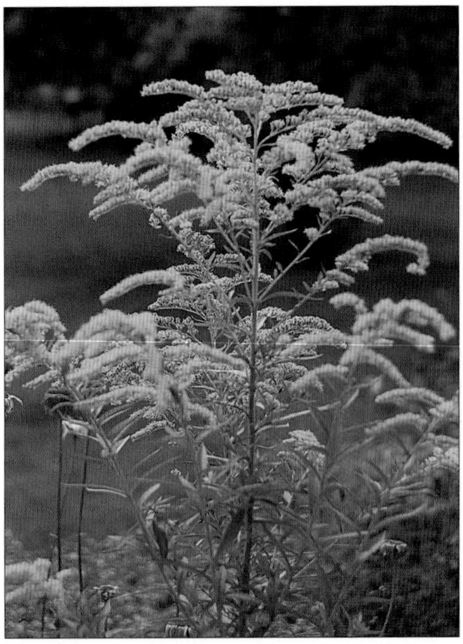

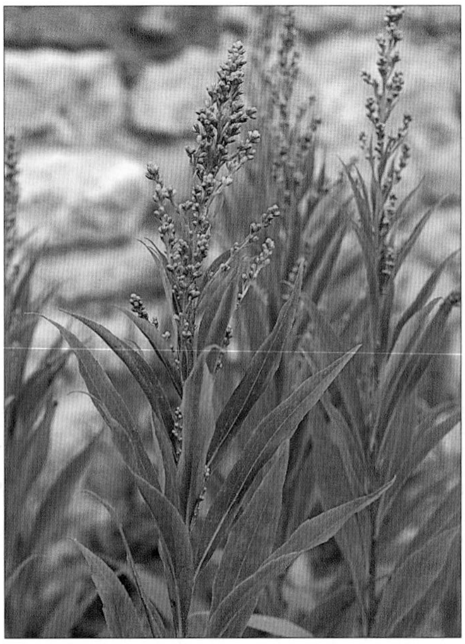

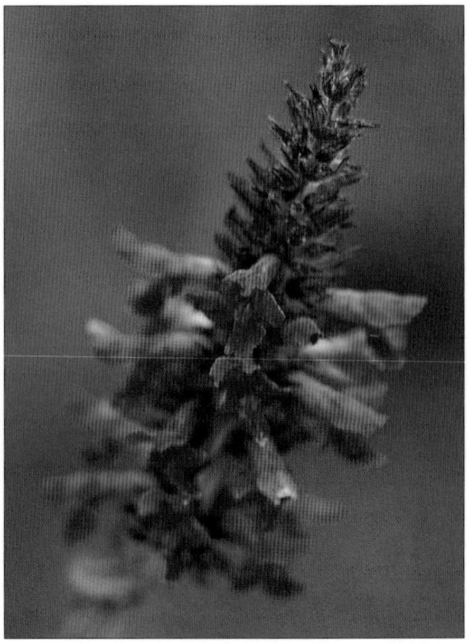

COMPOSITAE/ASTERACEAE

Solidago virgaurea

Golden rod

History and traditions Most of the nearly 100 species of *Solidago* came from North America, where a number of them were used in the traditional Native American medicine for healing wounds, sores, insect bites and stings. In the 17th century the dried herb was imported and sold on the London market for high prices as an exotic cure-all, until one day someone noticed golden rod growing wild on Hampstead Heath in London and the bottom dropped out of the market. As Thomas Fuller put it in his *History of the Worthies of England,* 1662, "When golden rod was brought at great expense from foreign countries, it was highly valued; but it was no sooner discovered to be a native plant, than it was discarded." However, by the 19th century, in Britain, it was firmly established as a popular ornamental, causing William Cobbett to complain in *The American Gardener,* 1816, "A yellow flower called the 'Plain-weed', which is the torment of the neighbouring farmer, has been above all the plants in this world, chosen as the most conspicuous ornament of the front of the King of England's grandest palace, that of Hampton Court."

Description A vigorous hardy perennial, growing to 1m/3ft in height. It has branched stems, lanceolate, finely toothed leaves and terminal panicles of golden-yellow flowers in late summer. It is an invasive plant and spreads very rapidly.

Related species *S. canadensis*, native to Canada and North America, is a taller plant, growing to 1.5m/5ft, often seen in gardens, and also has medicinal properties. Most garden varieties of golden rod are hybrids.

Habitat/distribution *S. virgaurea* is the only native European species, and is found in woodland and grassland on acid and calcareous (alkaline) soils. Many closely-related species are native to North America.

Growth Prefers not too rich soil and an open, sunny position. Propagated by seed sown in spring, or by division in spring and autumn.

Parts used Leaves, flowering tops – dried for use in infusions, powders, ointments and other medicinal preparations.

USES Medicinal Golden rod has antifungal, anti-inflammatory and antiseptic properties. It is applied externally in lotions, ointments and poultices to help heal wounds, skin irritations, bites, stings and ulcers. Used traditionally to treat chronic catarrh.

Above left *A garden hybrid of* Solidago canadensis *and* S. virgaurea *in flower, and in bud (*above*).*

Golden rod superstitions

- Where golden rod grows, secret treasure is buried.
- When it springs up near the door of a house, it brings good fortune.

LABIATAE/LAMIACEAE

Stachys officinalis

Betony

History and traditions Betony was highly prized as a medicinal herb in Roman times, when Antonius Musa, physician to the Emperor Augustus, wrote a treatise on its virtues, assigning 47 remedies to it. It was of great importance to the Anglo-Saxons for its magical as well as its medicinal properties and is mentioned in the 10th-century manuscript herbal, the *Lacnunga*. It was made into amulets to be worn against evil spirits, planted in churchyards and held to be capable of driving away despair. *The Herbal of Apuleius* (*c.* AD400) describes betony as "good for a man's soul or his body". Betony was much valued throughout Europe, and inspired the Italian proverb "sell your coat and buy betony". It was always associated with treatments for maladies of the head and said to be a certain cure for headaches – a use that it retains today in modern herbal practice. The name betony derives from *vettonica*, as the Romans knew it, which became *betonica* (as it was until recently classified). *Stachys* is from the Greek for a spike or ear of corn and refers to the shape of the flower cluster.

Description A mat-forming, hairy, hardy perennial, it has a basal rosette of wrinkled, ovate leaves with dentate margins. Flower stems rise to 60cm/2ft with smaller opposite leaves and dense, terminal spikes of magenta-pink two-lipped flowers borne in summer.

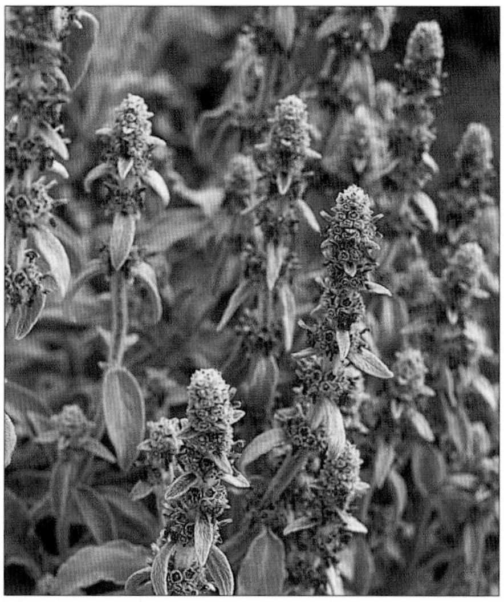

Above S. byzantina *syn* S. lanata.

Related species *S. byzantina* syn. *S. lanata* is popularly known as "lambs' ears", "lambs' lugs", "lambs' tails" or "lambs' tongues" for its white, woolly foliage. It forms a mat of whitish-green, soft, downy, wrinkled leaves with short mauve flower spikes to 45cm/18in tall. It is grown as a herb garden ornamental.
Habitat/distribution Native to Europe, grows on sandy loam in open woods and grassland.
Growth Grow in ordinary, dry soil in sun or partial shade. Propagated by seed sown in spring or by division during dormancy.
Parts used Leaves, flowering stems – fresh or dried for infusions, ointments and lotions.

USES Medicinal Infusions are taken for headaches, especially if associated with anxiety and nervous tension, often combined with *Hypericum perforatum* and *Lavandula*. Made into lotions or ointments (often in combination with other herbs) for applying to cuts, abrasions and bruises.

Conserve of betony

Betony new and tender one pound, the best sugar three pound, beat them very small in a stone mortar, let the sugar be boyled with two quarts of betony water to the consistency of a syrup, then mix them together by little and little over a small Fire, and so make it into a Conserve and keep it in Glasses [bottles].

The Queen's Closet Opened by W. M., cook to Queen Henrietta Maria, 1655.

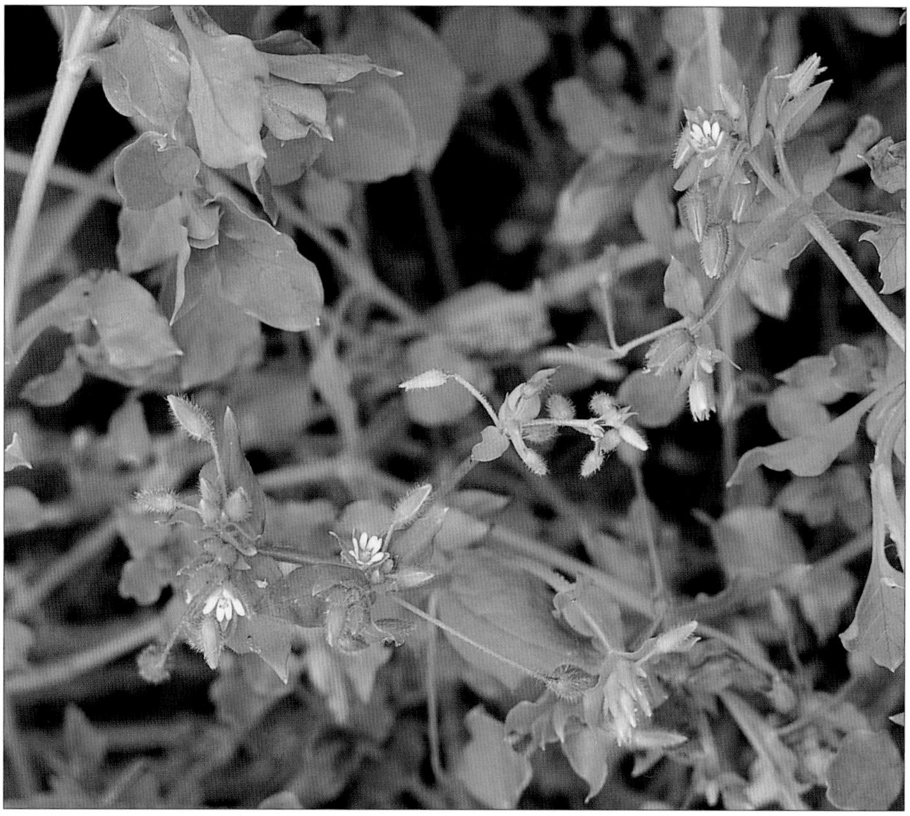

CARYOPHYLLACEAE

Stellaria media

Chickweed

History and traditions The common name, chickweed, and the popular names in several other European languages refer to this herb's former usefulness as bird feed. It provided a source of fresh greens and seeds during the winter when other foods were scarce. For the same reason it was much valued as a culinary herb in broths and salads. Although it does not seem to have made its mark in the classical world, it appears in herbals from medieval times usually as an ingredient in a mixed green ointment based on lard, for rubbing on sores and swellings. The Latin name of the genus is from *stella*, a star, for the shape of the flowers.
Description A spreading, mat-forming annual, the much-branched stems grow up to 40cm/16in long, but most are decumbent and creep along the ground. It has small ovate leaves and tiny, white, star-shaped flowers. It propagates quickly, reappearing throughout the year, and is often seen in the winter months.
Habitat/distribution Chickweed is native to Europe but naturalized in many countries throughout the world. Found on moist cultivated land and field edges.
Growth Grows in any reasonably moist soil in sun or partial shade. Self-seeds.
Parts used Leaves – fresh.

USES Medicinal It is rich in mineral salts, including calcium and potassium, and has anti-rheumatic properties when taken internally as a juice or infusion. Applied as a poultice or ointment for eczema, skin irritations and other skin complaints.
Culinary A pleasantly neutral-tasting herb for inclusion in salads or for cooking as a vegetable. It combines well with parsley to make a dip.

Chickweed and parsley dip

25g/1oz fresh chickweed
25g/1oz flat-leaved parsley
225g/8oz fromage frais
15ml/1 tbsp mayonnaise
Salt and ground black pepper

Rinse and pick over the chickweed, and chop it finely with the parsley. Mix well with the fromage frais and mayonnaise. Season to taste.

Serve as a dip with raw carrots, celery, cucumber and peppers.

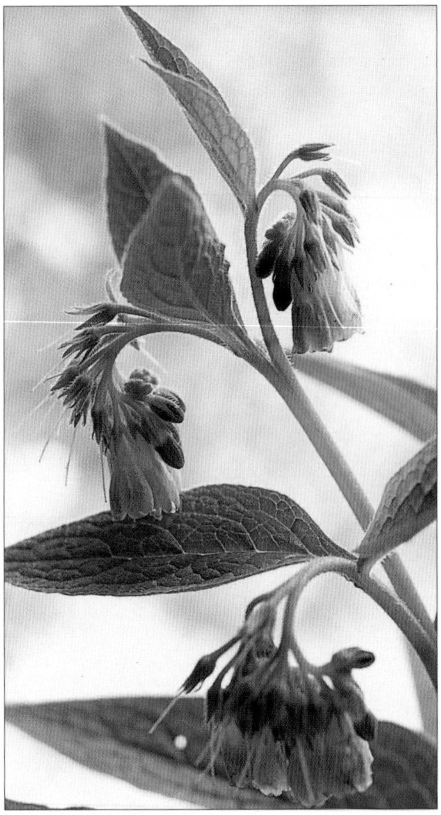

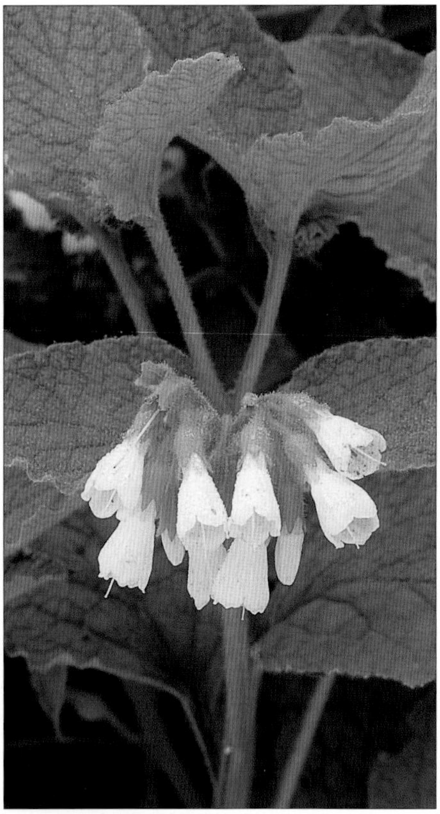

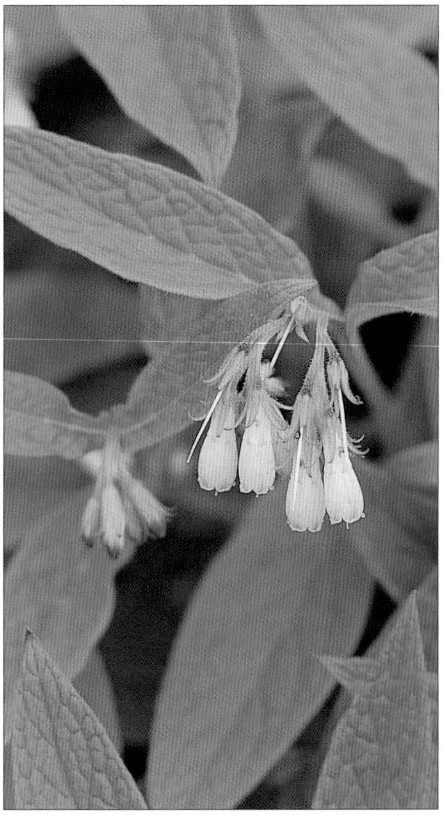

BORAGINACEAE

Symphytum officinale

Comfrey

History and traditions Comfrey has been known since at least the Middle Ages as a healing agent for fractures. The generic name, *Symphytum*, is from the Greek, *sympho*, "growing together", and *phyton*, a plant. The common English name, comfrey, is derived from the medieval Latin, *confervia*, meaning to heal or "boil together". Gerard wrote that "a salve concocted from the fresh herb will certainly tend to promote the healing of bruised and broken parts" (*The Herball*, 1597), and he and other herbalists of his time advised taking it internally for "inward hurts" as well. The modern history of this herb is a chequered one. In about 1910 it was established that it contained allantoin, a cell-proliferant substance, which promotes healing of bone and bodily tissues. By the 1960s Russian comfrey, *S.* x *uplandicum*, was being promoted as a herbal wonder cure. However, scientific studies of the late 1970s and 1980s, mostly carried out in Australia and Japan, revealed that comfrey also contains pyrrolizidine alkaloids (plant toxins that are most associated with disease in humans and in animals). Levels are higher in the roots than the leaves. These toxins were shown to cause liver damage and tumours in laboratory animals when extracts were injected in large quantities. This has led to a ban on comfrey in many countries, including Australia, New Zealand, Canada and the United States.

Description A vigorous perennial, growing on thick taproots, 0.6–1.2m/2–4ft in height, it has oval, lanceolate leaves, with a rough, hairy texture. Pinkish-purple to violet, tubular flowers are borne in drooping clusters in early to midsummer.

Related species *S.* x *uplandicum* (Russian comfrey) is a larger – to 2m/6ft – and more vigorous hybrid.

Habitat/distribution Native to Europe and the Mediterranean, and also from Siberia to Asia, introduced and naturalized elsewhere. Found in damp meadows, near rivers and streams.

Growth Although it favours damp soil in the wild, comfrey is a vigorous plant, which flourishes under any conditions and grows happily when planted in dry soil, in sun or partial shade. It is easily propagated by division of roots in spring, but is invasive and almost impossible to eradicate once established.

Parts used Leaves – fresh.

USES Medicinal The leaves are made into poultices, compresses and ointments and applied externally to bruises, varicose veins, inflamed muscles and tendons. While external use of the whole leaf is considered safe, it is inadvisable to take comfrey internally.

Horticultural The leaves are high in potash and make a good garden fertilizer, mulch and compost activator.

Other name Knitbone.

Top, from left to right *The flowers of* Symphytum officinale *are usually pink or blue, but there are forms with white or yellow flowers too.*

CAUTION Comfrey is subject to legal restrictions in some countries. Do not use the root internally due to the high levels of pyrryolizidine alkaloids in the plant, which are known to be toxic to the liver.

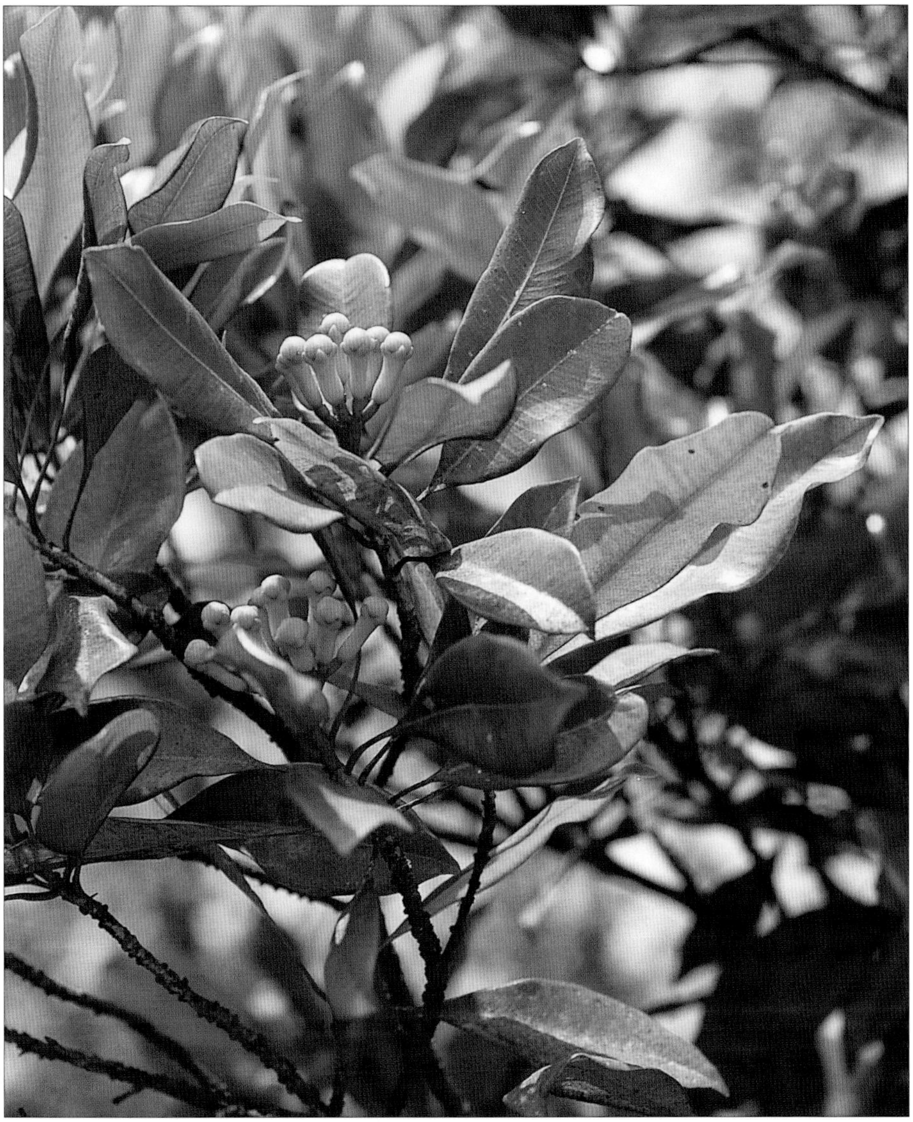

MYRTACEAE

Syzygium aromaticum

Clove tree

History and traditions The medicinal use of cloves is first mentioned in ancient Chinese texts, and it was a custom during the Han dynasty (266BC–AD220) to keep a clove in the mouth when addressing the emperor. Cloves originally came from the Molucca Islands, a group of islands in Indonesia, and were brought to the Mediterranean by Persian and Arab traders. They are mentioned in the writings of Pliny under the name *caryophyllon*, and were widely used in Europe by the 4th century, when their strong fragrance made them popular as ingredients of pomanders and as prevention against plague and infection. During the 17th century there was rivalry between the Dutch and the Portuguese over establishing a trading monopoly in this valuable spice. But by 1770 the French were growing their own crops in Mauritius, and they were subsequently cultivated in Guiana, Brazil, the West Indies and Zanzibar. The name cloves comes from the French word for nail, *clou*, which they are supposed to resemble.

Description An evergreen tree, 20m/65ft in height, it has soft, grey bark and dark green, ovate leaves, with a shiny, leathery texture. At the beginning of the rainy season, fragrant green buds (cloves) appear at the ends of the branches. They gradually turn red and, if left unpicked, develop into pink or crimson flowers.

Habitat/distribution Native to the Moluccas, introduced and cultivated in other tropical zones.

Growth Tender, tropical trees, grown in fertile soil and requiring high humidity and minimum temperatures of 15–18°C/59–64°F. Propagated by seed or cuttings. The cloves (the unopened flower buds) are harvested when the tree is 6–8 years old. The crop can be sporadic: one year heavy and the next light. Cloves are usually hand picked to avoid damage to the branches which would jeopardize subsequent crops.

Parts used Unripe flower buds – sun-dried; essential oil.

USES Medicinal Cloves have digestive properties, help relieve nausea, control vomiting and prevent intestinal worms and parasites. Oil of cloves is still used as a dental antiseptic and analgesic. A cotton bud (cotton swab) soaked in oil of cloves and applied directly to the tooth will ease toothache.

Culinary Widely used as a spice in whole or ground form to add flavour to curries, pickles, preserves, chutneys and meat dishes – especially baked ham. It is also used in baked apples and apple pie, desserts and cakes, and for making mulled wine.

Aromatic Added whole or ground to potpourri and used to make pomanders. Essential oil is used in perfumery, and added to toothpastes, mouthwashes and gargles.

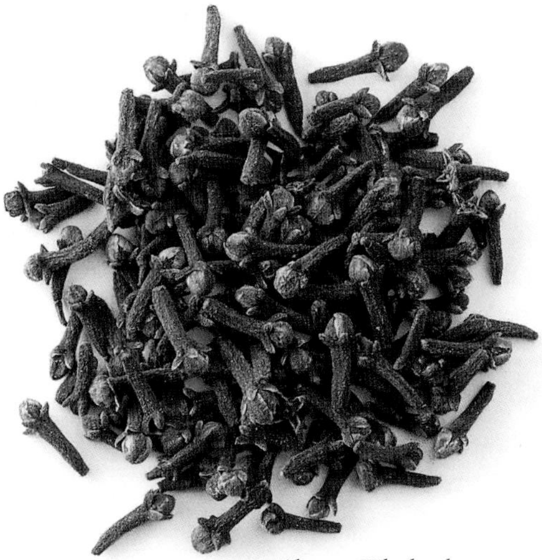

Above *Whole cloves.*

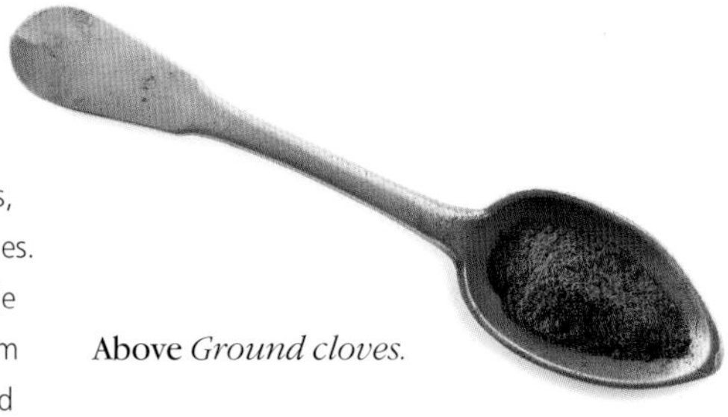

Above *Ground cloves.*

COMPOSITAE/ASTERACEAE

Tanacetum

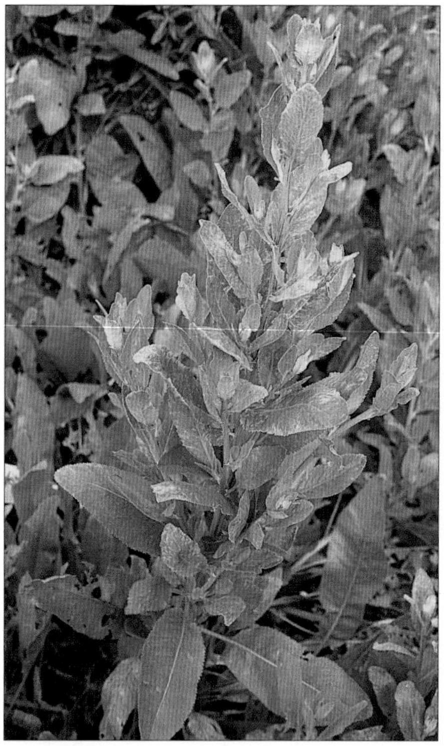

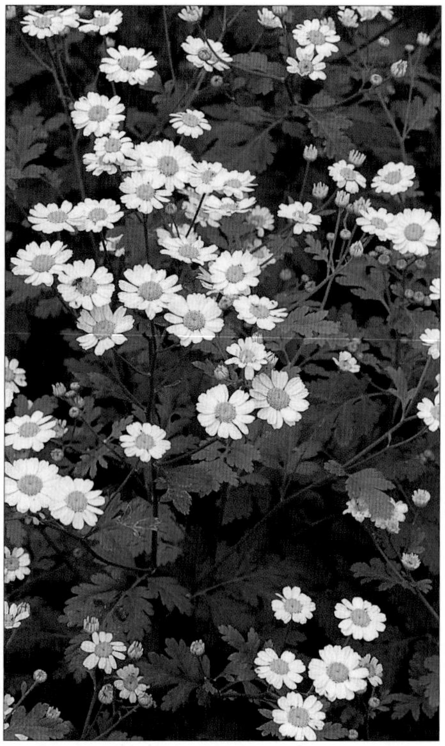

Tanacetum balsamita

Alecost

History and traditions Alecost came to Europe from the Middle East during the 16th century and soon became popular for its pleasant balsam fragrance. As Culpeper wrote a century later, "This is so frequently known to be an inhabitant in almost every garden, that I suppose it is needless to write a description thereof." As its common name suggests, it was used to flavour ale, the second syllable "cost" is from a Greek word, *kostos*, meaning fragrant or spicy. In the 17th century it was taken to America by settlers, where it became known as Bible-leaf from the custom of using it as a Bible bookmark and sniffing its revivifying scent during long sermons. As a medicinal herb it was frequently recommended for disorders of the stomach and head, and Culpeper gives instructions for making it into a salve with olive oil, thickened with wax, rosin and turpentine. It is now little used as a medicinal herb.

Description A hardy perennial, up to 1m/3ft tall, it has a creeping rhizome and oval, silvery-green, soft-textured leaves, with a minty balsamic fragrance. Small, daisy-like flowers are borne in mid- to late summer. Formerly classified in the *Chrysanthemum* genus.

Habitat/distribution Native to western Asia, naturalized in Europe and North America.

Growth Prefers a moisture-retentive but well-drained soil and a sunny position. Most easily propagated by division or cuttings in spring, but can also be grown from seed.

Parts used Leaves – fresh or dried.

USES Medicinal An infusion of the leaves helps reduce the pain of insect bites and stings, and a fresh leaf may be applied directly to the spot as "first aid".

Culinary Fresh leaves may be added to fruit cups and drinks; fresh or dried leaves make an aromatic tea.

Aromatic The dried leaves are added to potpourri and make fragrant bookmarks.

Other names Costmary and Bible-leaf.

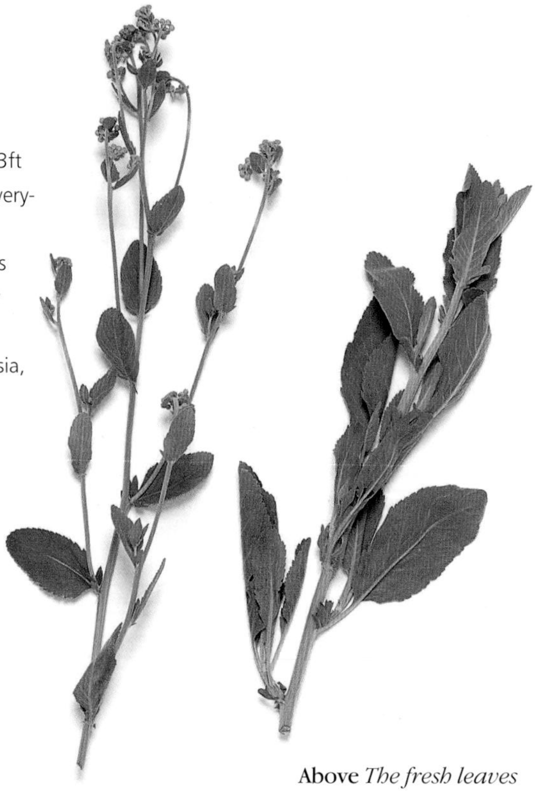

Above *The fresh leaves of* Tanacetum balsamita *have a pleasant minty fragrance.*

Tanacetum parthenium

Feverfew

History and traditions The medicinal properties of feverfew have long been recognized. The Greek philosopher, Plutarch, writing in 1st-century Athens, says that the plant was named *parthenium* after treatment with feverfew saved the life of a workman who fell from the Parthenon. The common name comes from the Latin *febris*, fever, and *fugure*, to chase away. In the centuries that followed, herbalists recommended this herb, usually in a mixture of honey or sweet wine to disguise its bitterness, for a range of ills. *Bancke's Herbal*, 1525, advocates it for stomach disorders, toothache and insect bites, Culpeper recommends it for 'women's troubles' and as an antidote to a liberal intake of opium (*The English Physician*, 1653). But others evidently recognized its value for the relief of headaches and migraine. Gerard wrote, "it is very good for them that are giddie in the head, or which have the turning called Vertigo, that is, swimming and turning in the head" (*The Herball*, 1597). And Sir John Hill, in his *Family Herbal*, 1772, states clearly, "in the worst headaches, this herb exceeds whatever else is known." Feverfew came to prominence in modern times after a Welsh doctor's wife found relief in 1974 from both chronic migraine and rheumatism by

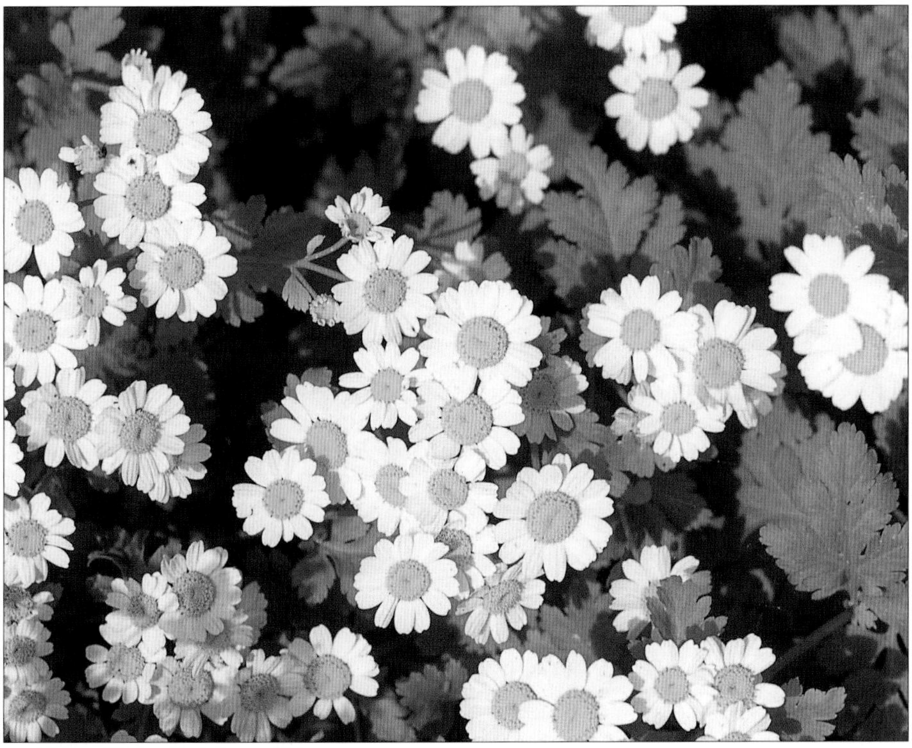

eating feverfew leaves. Since then this herb has undergone much scientific study and has been found to be a relatively effective and safe remedy for these complaints.

Description A bushy, hardy perennial, to 1m/3ft, with bright green, pungently aromatic, pinnately-lobed leaves and a mass of white daisy-like flowers, with yellow centres, in early to midsummer.

Related species There are a number of cultivars, including some with golden foliage (as above), or double flowers, which make attractive ornamentals, but do not have the same medicinal properties.

Habitat/distribution It is native to southern Europe, widely introduced elsewhere. Found on dry, stony soils.

Growth Grows in any poor, free-draining soil and tolerates drought. Propagate by seed sown in spring, or by cuttings or division in spring. Self-seeds prolifically.

Parts used Leaves, flowering tops – for eating fresh, or dried for use in tablets and pharmaceutical products.

USES Medicinal Feverfew lowers fever and dilates blood vessels. Fresh leaves are sometimes eaten (usually sweetened with honey, as they are very bitter) to reduce the effects of migraine headaches. It is also taken in tablet form for migraine, rheumatism and menstrual problems.

Above *Golden feverfew does not have the medicinal properties of the species.*

CAUTION Only to be taken on medical advice if on other medication. Can interact with anti-coagulant and other pharmaceutical drugs. Not to be taken in pregnancy or while breast-feeding. Can cause dermatitis, allergic reactions, mouth ulcers and gastric upsets.

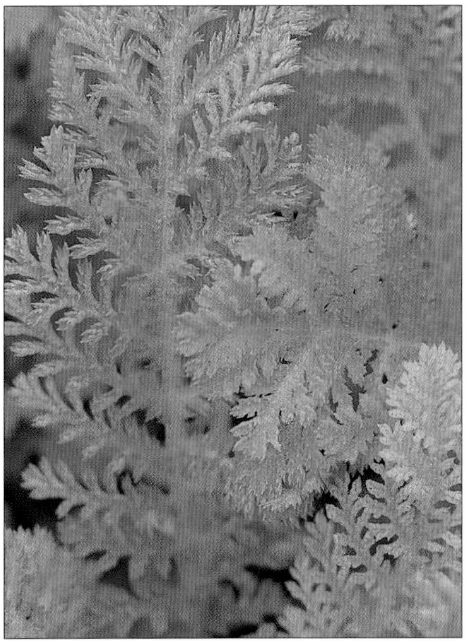

Above Tanacetum vulgare.

Tanacetum vulgare
Tansy

History and traditions Tansy is one of the essential strewing herbs, listed by Thomas Tusser in *One Hundred Points of Good Husbandry,* 1577, doubtless chosen for its insect-repellent properties. Despite the bitter flavour, there is evidence that it was widely used for culinary purposes in the past. It was a popular ingredient of cakes and puddings, made with eggs and cream, traditionally served on Easter Day. William Coles, in *The Art of Simpling,* 1656, refers to the effect of tansy on the constitution after a Lenten diet of salt-fish. Tansy was also a popular substitute for mint in a sauce to accompany lamb. One authority refers to its cosmetic application. "I have heard that if maids will take wild Tansy and lay it to soake in Buttermilk for the space of nine days and wash their faces therewith, it will make them look very faire" (Jerome Braunschwyke, *The Virtuose Boke of Distyllacion*, 1527).

Description A spreading rhizomatous perennial, to 1.2m/4ft in height, it has dark green, feathery, pinnately-divided leaves, which are pungently aromatic, and terminal clusters of button-like bright yellow flowers in summer.

Related species *T. vulgare* var. *crispum* is a more compact plant, with attractive, curly, fern-like leaves.

Growth Grows well in dry, stony soil and prefers a sunny position. Propagated by seed, division or cuttings in spring.

Parts used Leaves.

USES Medicinal This herb is said to have been used in enemas for expelling intestinal worms, but is seldom used in herbal medicine today.

Culinary Despite the wealth of recipes in old books, Tansy is not recommended as a pudding ingredient as it has an unpleasantly bitter taste, although the leaves used to be added to lamb dishes and spring puddings.

Horticultural Tansy is supposed to be an insect repellent and ward off aphids in companion planting.

CAUTION It is unsafe to take internally as a medicinal herb. The volatile oil is extremely toxic and should be avoided. Do not take during pregnancy or while breast-feeding.

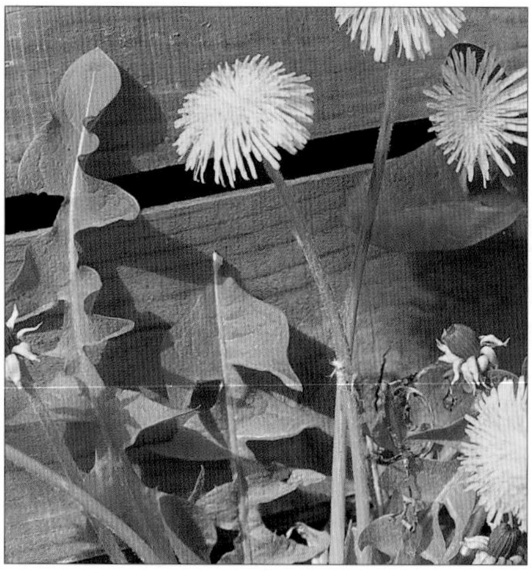

COMPOSITAE/ASTERACEAE

Taraxacum officinale

Dandelion

History and traditions Although known much earlier in Chinese medicine, the dandelion was first recognized in Europe in the 10th or 11th century, through the influence of the Arabian physicians, then prominent as medical authorities. The name, dandelion, comes from the French *dents de lion*, lion's tooth.

Description A perennial which grows on a stout taproot to 30cm/1ft long, it has a basal rosette of leaves and yellow, solitary flowers followed by spherical, fluffy seed heads.

Habitat/distribution Native to Europe and Asia, and occurs widely in temperate regions of the world, often found on nitrogen-rich soils.

Growth Grows in profusion in the wild and self-seeds. Cultivated dandelions are grown in moist, fertile soil. Propagated from seed.

Parts used Leaves, flowers – fresh for culinary use, fresh or dried for medicinal preparations; roots – dried.

USES Medicinal An effective diuretic, it is taken internally for urinary infections and diseases of the liver and gall bladder. Considered beneficial for rheumatic complaints and gout. Also said to improve appetite and digestion. Of great benefit nutritionally, high in vitamins A and C and a rich source of iron, magnesium, potassium and calcium.

Culinary Young leaves of dandelions are added to salads, often blanched first to reduce bitterness, or cooked, like spinach, as a vegetable. Flowers are made into wine.
The roasted root makes a palatable, soothing, caffeine-free substitute for coffee.

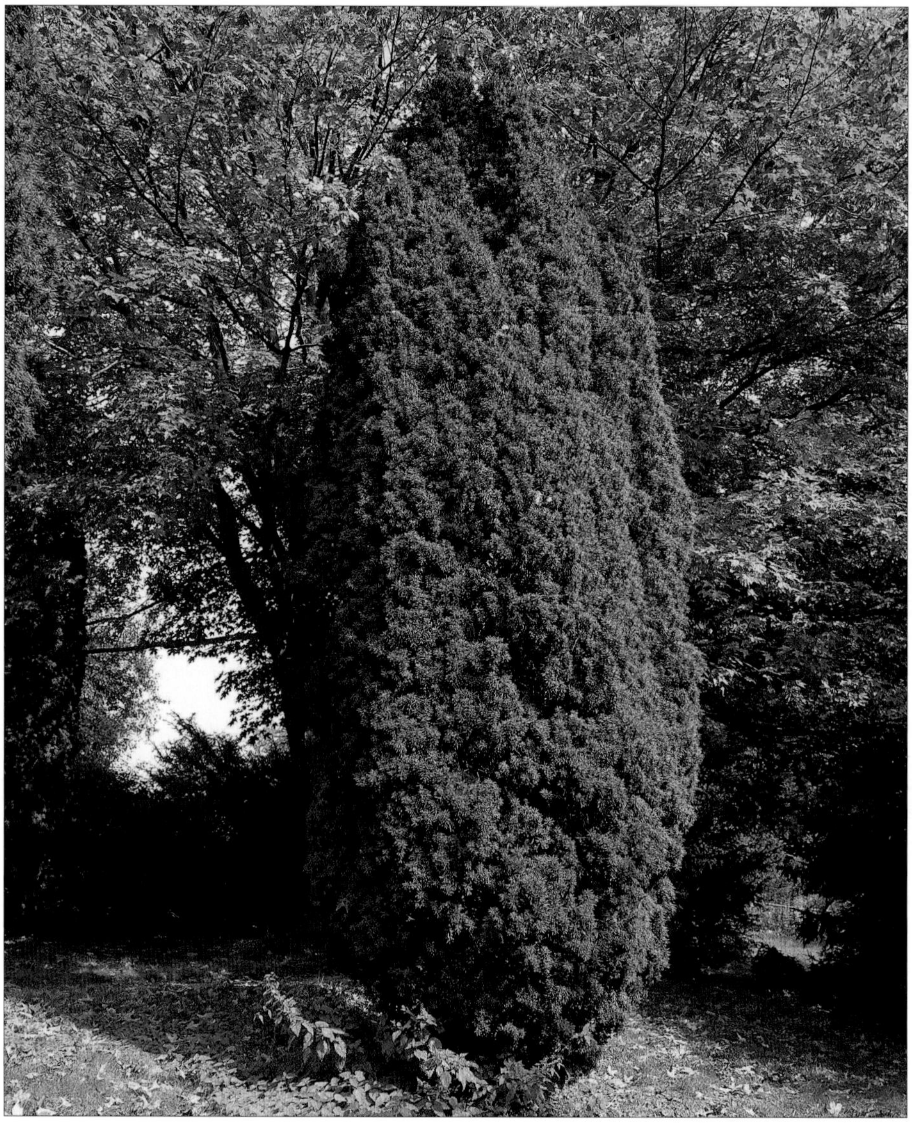

TAXACEAE

Taxus baccata

Yew

History and traditions Yews were sacred to the Druids and used in their ceremonies. They have also been grown in churchyards from the beginning of the Christian era. As evergreens and exceptionally long-lived trees (1,000–2,000 years), they were a life symbol and often used to decorate the church or to scatter in graves. *Taxus* is from the Greek word *taxon*, a bow, and the flexible, close-grained wood was the traditional material for longbows. Yew is from the Anglo-Saxon name for the tree. There are rare references to its former medicinal uses, in treating snakebite and rabies for example, but its poisonous nature was always recognized and it was known to kill cattle at a stroke. It has sometimes been used in homeopathy. In recent times yews have come to prominence as a source of taxol, used in the treatment of ovarian cancer.

Description *T. baccata* is a spreading, evergreen tree, growing to about 15m/50ft, with a rounded crown and reddish-brown scaly bark. The leaves are dark green, flattened needles, arranged alternately. It is a dioecious tree, and the male flowers are small globular cones, which release clouds of pollen in very early spring; the female flower is a small green bud, followed by the fruit, a highly poisonous seed, partially enclosed in a fleshy, red, non-poisonous aril.

Related species *T. brevifolia*, the Pacific yew, has the highest taxol content, mostly in the bark, and is the main source of the drug, but six trees are needed to make one dose and wild stocks have been grossly over-exploited. *T. baccata*, the common yew, contains less significant levels of taxol-yielding compounds, found in the leaves, but is now used in taxol synthesis.

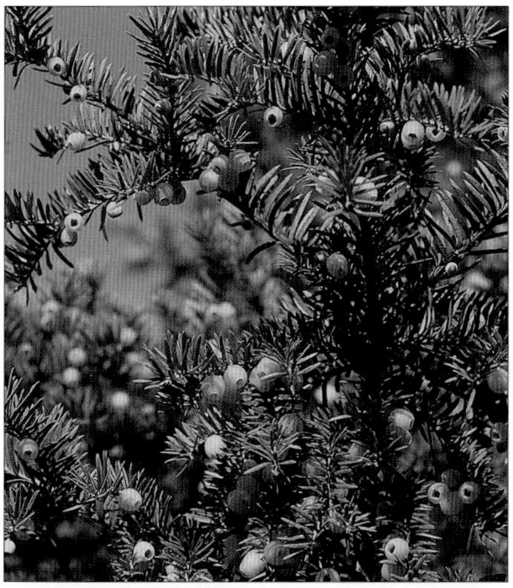

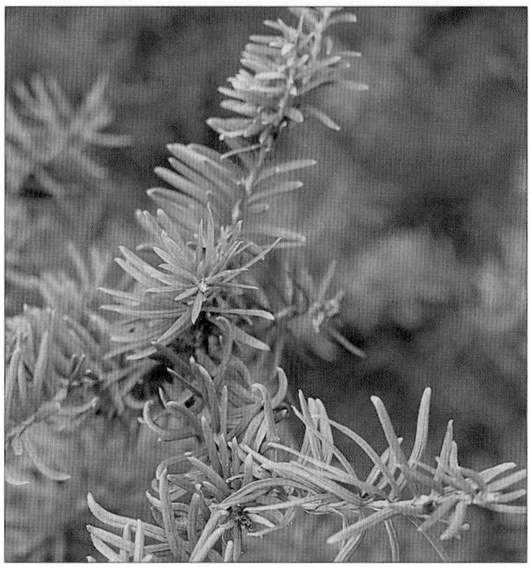

Above *Taxus brevifolia.*

Top *Taxus baccata 'Fruco-luteo', a cultivar with yellow fruits.*

Left *Taxus baccata 'Fastigiata', the Irish yew.*

Habitat/distribution *T. baccata* is native to Europe, Asia and northern Africa and *T. brevifolia* is found in north-western North America to the south-west of Canada.
Growth Yews will grow in any soil, including chalk. Propagated by seed, sown in early spring, or by cuttings in September. *T. baccata* responds well to close clipping and is frequently used as a hedge, or in topiary work.
Parts used Leaves, bark – for extraction of taxol.

USES Medicinal Extracts of yew are used in drugs for treatment of cancers, mainly ovarian, breast and lung cancer.

CAUTION All parts of yew are poisonous and it should never be used for self-medication.

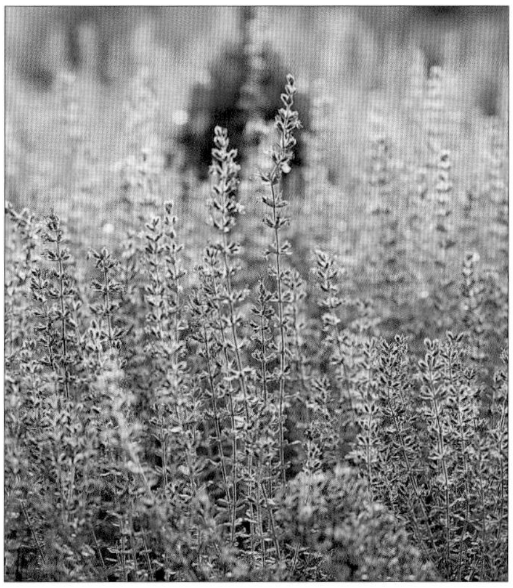

LABIATAE/LAMIACEAE

Teucrium chamaedrys

Wall germander

History and traditions *T. chamaedrys* is said to be named after Teucer, son of Scamander, King of Troy, who, according to Greek mythology, was the first to recognize the medicinal properties of this herb. It is mentioned in the works of Dioscorides and developed a reputation over the centuries for being an effective treatment for gout. It was also taken in powdered form for catarrh and as a herbal snuff. Germander comes from the Latin form, *gamandrea*, of the Greek *khamaidrys*, and means "ground-oak", from *khamai*, on the ground, and *drus*, oak, a reference to the shape of the leaves.
Description A shrubby, evergreen perennial, 10–30cm/4–12in in height, it has creeping roots and dark green, glossy foliage, shaped like miniature oak leaves. Tubular, rose-purple flowers are borne in dense terminal spikes.
Habitat/distribution It is native to Europe and western Asia, widely introduced elsewhere and found in rocky areas, on old walls and in dry woodlands.
Growth Flourishes in light, dry, stony soils. Easily propagated by semi-ripe cuttings taken in early summer. Although the branches are erect to start with, it is inclined to sprawl, especially if allowed to flower. Clip hard in late spring or early autumn to maintain a neat shape.
Parts used Leaves, flowering stems.

USES Medicinal Although it is said to have some medicinal uses and digestive properties, it may cause liver damage and is best avoided.

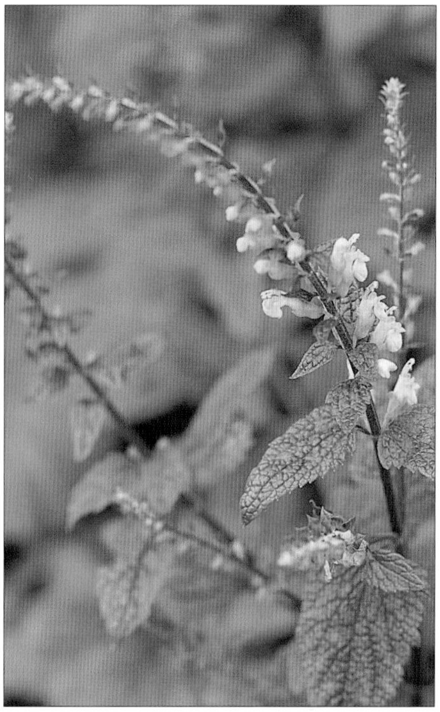

LABIATAE/LAMIACEAE

Teucrium scorodonia

Wood sage

History and traditions A bitter-tasting herb, wood sage is one of the many plants said to have been used at one time for flavouring beer before hops became common for this purpose. One old story tells that hinds, wounded in the chase, sought it out for its healing properties. In past times it was used, like *Teucrium chamaedrys*, to treat gout and rheumatism and as a poultice or lotion for "moist ulcers and sores" (Culpeper). Its specific name, *scorodonia*, is from a Greek word for garlic, and if the leaves are crushed, it is possible with a little imagination, to detect a faint garlic odour.
Description: A hardy perennial, 30–60cm/1–2ft tall, it has ovate to heart-shaped, pale green, soft-textured leaves and inconspicuous greenish-yellow flowers in summer. *T. scorodonia* 'Crispum' has attractive, curly-edged foliage.
Habitat/distribution Native to Europe, naturalized in many northern temperate regions. Found in dry, shady woodland areas.
Growth It will grow in most conditions, but prefers a light, gravelly soil and partial shade.
Parts used Leaves (formerly).

USES Its herbal uses are now obsolete, but it makes an attractive traditional herb-garden plant – especially the curly-leaved form.

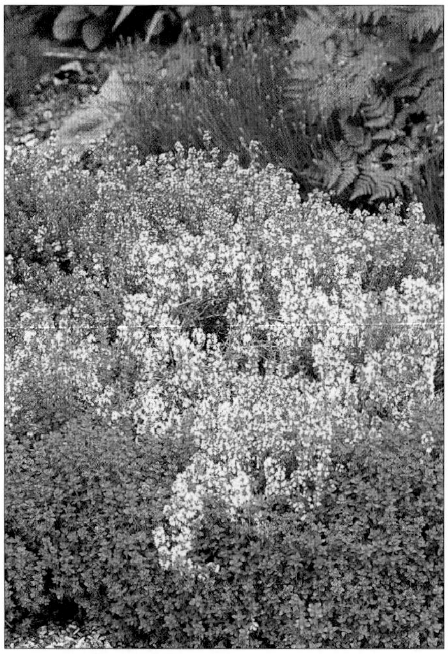

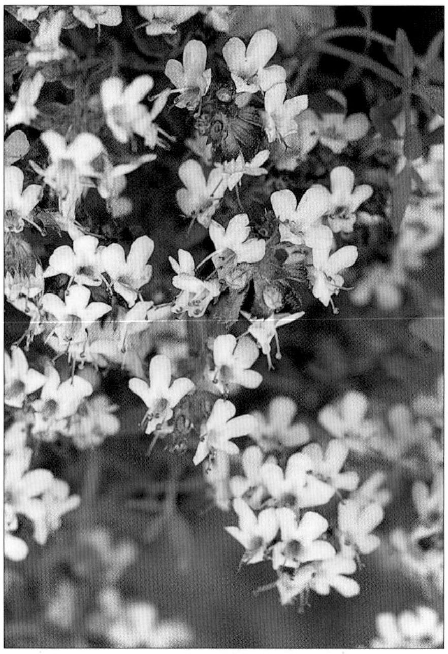

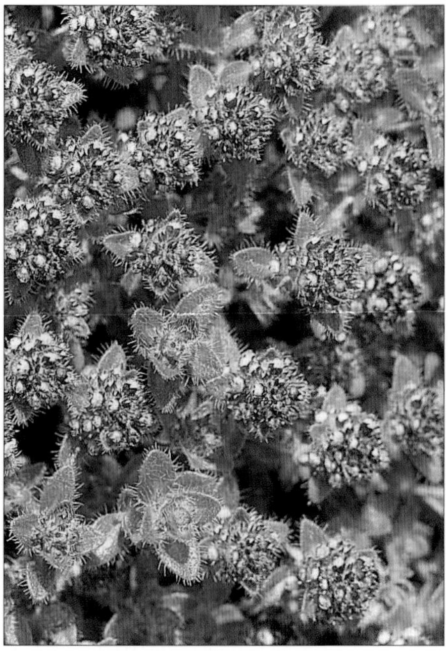

LABIATAE/LAMIACEAE

Thymus

History and traditions To the Greeks, thyme was an emblem of courage, to the Romans a remedy for melancholy, and appreciated by both for its scent. To tell someone they smelled of thyme was a compliment in ancient Greece, and Gerard refers to a description by the 3rd-century Roman writer, Aelianus, of the houses of a newly taken city being strewn with roses and thyme to sweeten them. *Thymus* is the original Greek name, used by Dioscorides. The scent of thyme is irresistible to bees, and the finest-flavoured honey comes from its nectar. The image of bees hovering over thyme was a frequent embroidery motif in former times. Its medicinal virtues were well known to the 16th- and 17th-century herbalists. Gerard recommended it to treat "the bitings of any venomous beast, either taken in drinke, or outwardly applied" and for Culpeper it was "a noble strengthener of the lungs".
In modern times its antiseptic, antibacterial credentials have been fully established.

Description and species There are some 350 species of thyme, many hybrids and cultivars. The classification of them is complex and there are many synonyms and invalid names. For medicinal purposes, *T. vulgaris* and *T. serpyllum* are the main ones. For cookery, *T. vulgaris* and *T.* x *citriodorus* have the best flavour, though most of the others may also be used.

T. serpyllum (wild thyme) – Also sometimes called the "mother of thyme" and "creeping thyme", has a prostrate habit, growing to about 7.5cm/3in, and has tiny, ovate leaves and clusters of mauve to pink flowers in early summer, but is very variable in form. It is found throughout Europe and Asia on well-drained, stony or sandy soils and on sunny slopes.

T. vulgaris (common thyme) – Is a variable sub-shrub, 30–45cm/12–18in tall, with gnarled, woody stems, dark green to grey-green leaves and white, sometimes mauve, flowers. Native to southern Europe and the Mediterranean region, introduced elsewhere.

T. x *citriodorus* (lemon thyme) – A variable hybrid, 25–30cm/10–12in tall, with bright green, ovate to lanceolate, lemon-scented leaves and pale mauve flowers in early summer. Cultivated worldwide.

T. x *citriodorus* 'Aureus' (golden lemon thyme) – Is a cultivar with golden foliage, which may be used interchangeably with *T.* x *citriodorus.*

Of the many ornamental thymes, these are some of the most attractive:

T. serpyllum 'Pink Chintz' – Is a creeping thyme with grey-green woolly foliage and striking, bright pink flowers. First selected as a cultivar, at the Royal Horticultural Society gardens at Wisley in 1939.

T. serpyllum 'Coccineus' – Is a favourite prostrate variety for the depth of colour of its crimson-pink flowers and the attractive form of dark green foliage.

Above far left Thymus vulgaris *in flower with* T. x citriodorus; **above left** Thymus serpyllum.

Above Thymus serpyllum *'Pink Chintz'.*

Below Thymus serpyllum *var. 'Coccineus'.*

T. vulgaris, 'Silver Posie', and *T.* x *citriodorus*, 'Silver Queen' – Are grown for their variegated silver foliage, useful for giving contrast to an ornamental scheme.

T. pseudolanuginosus (woolly thyme) – Is a prostrate form with grey-green woolly leaves and pale pink flowers.

Growth All thymes require very free-draining, gritty soil and a sunny position. Though the

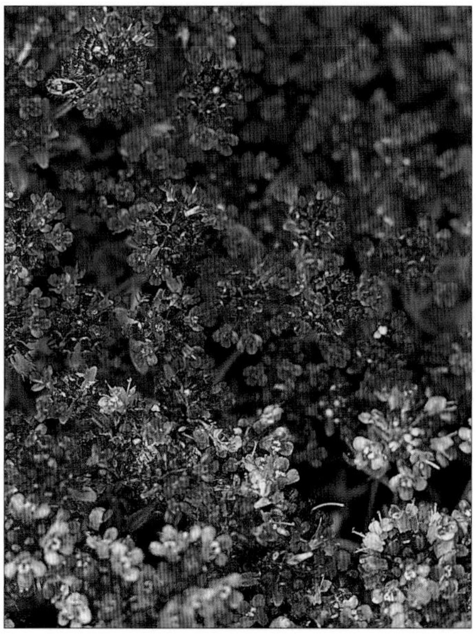

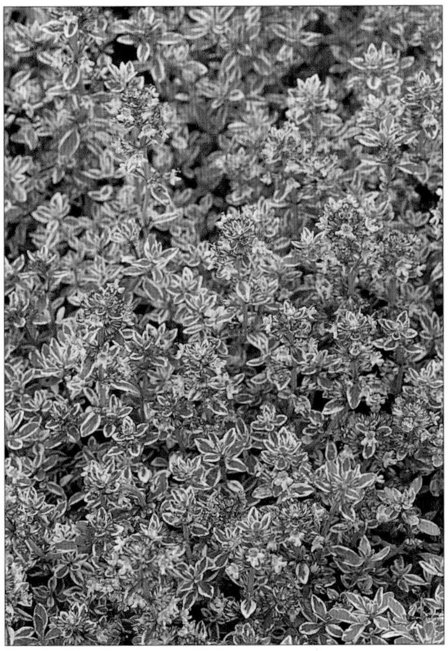

Thyme and the ageing process

Research carried out by Dr Stanley Deans at the Scottish Agricultural College, Ayr, during the 1990s, in conjunction with Semmelweiss Medical University in Budapest, has found that laboratory animals fed with thyme oil aged much slower than animals that did not receive it. Thyme oil apparently delayed the onset of age-related conditions such as deterioration of the retina, loss of brain function and wasted muscles.

A key factor was the high level of antioxidants present in thyme oil, which helped prevent a decline in PUFAs (polyunsaturated fatty acids), important components of every living cell which help keep cell membranes fluid and strong.

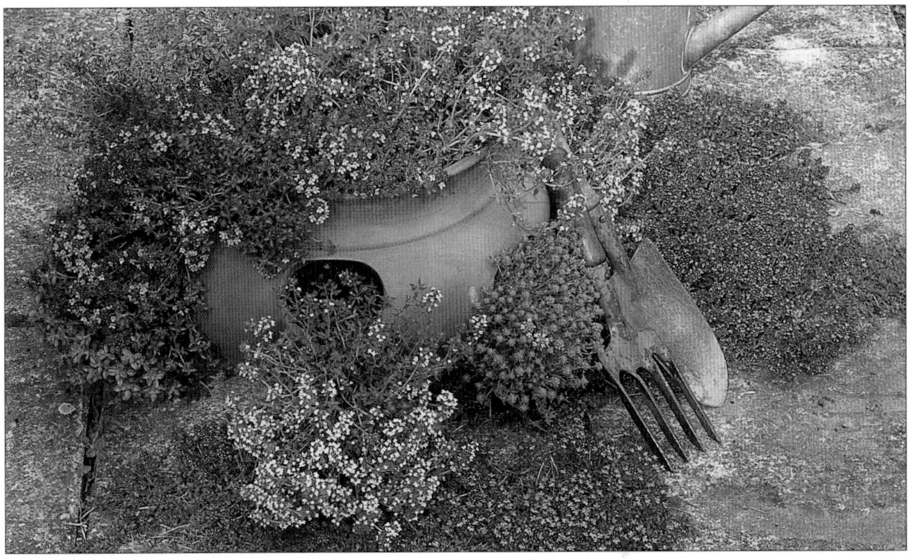

Above Thymus x citriodorus *'Silver Queen'.*

Right A decorative thyme pot.

Below left Thymus pulegioides *'Broad-leafed thyme'*; **below right** Thymus pseudolanuginosus.

ones mentioned are hardy to at least -10°C/14°F, in cool temperate climates they may need some protection in winter, as they are vulnerable to cold winds, especially if soil becomes too wet. Propagated by layering in spring, or by cuttings in summer. *T. vulgaris* and *T. serpyllum* can be propagated by seed sown in spring.

Parts used Leaves – fresh or dry for culinary use; leaves, flowering tops – fresh or dried for infusions and medicinal preparations; essential oil – distilled from leaves and flowering tops.

USES Medicinal A strongly antiseptic, anti-bacterial and antifungal herb. Infusions are taken for coughs, colds, chest infections and digestive upsets. Made into syrups for coughs, and gargles for sore throats. The diluted essential oil is used as as a rub for chest infections, as a massage oil for rheumatic pain and has been found to be effective against head lice.

Culinary Widely used as a culinary flavouring in marinades, meat, soups, stews and casseroles.

CAUTION Avoid medicinal doses of thyme, and especially of thyme oil during pregnancy, as it is a uterine stimulant.

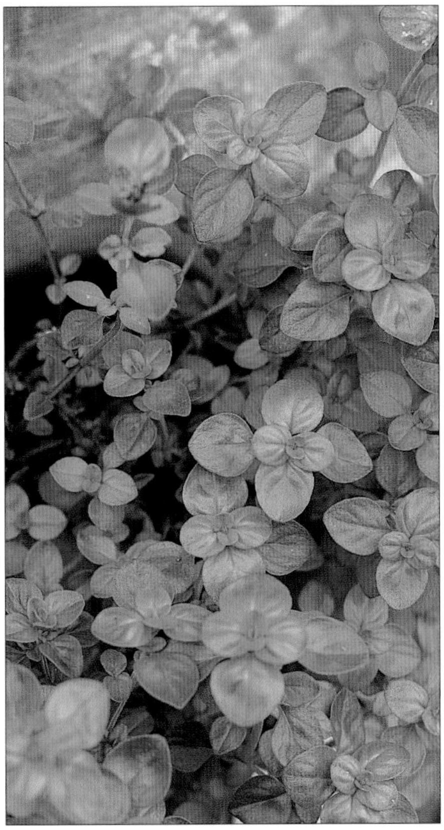

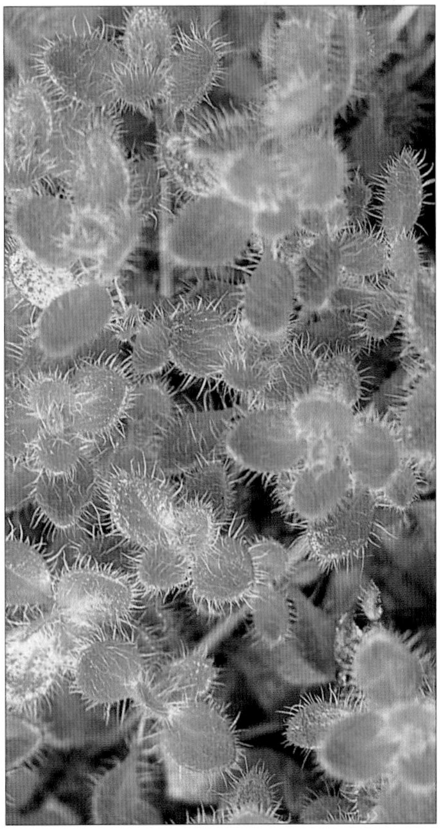

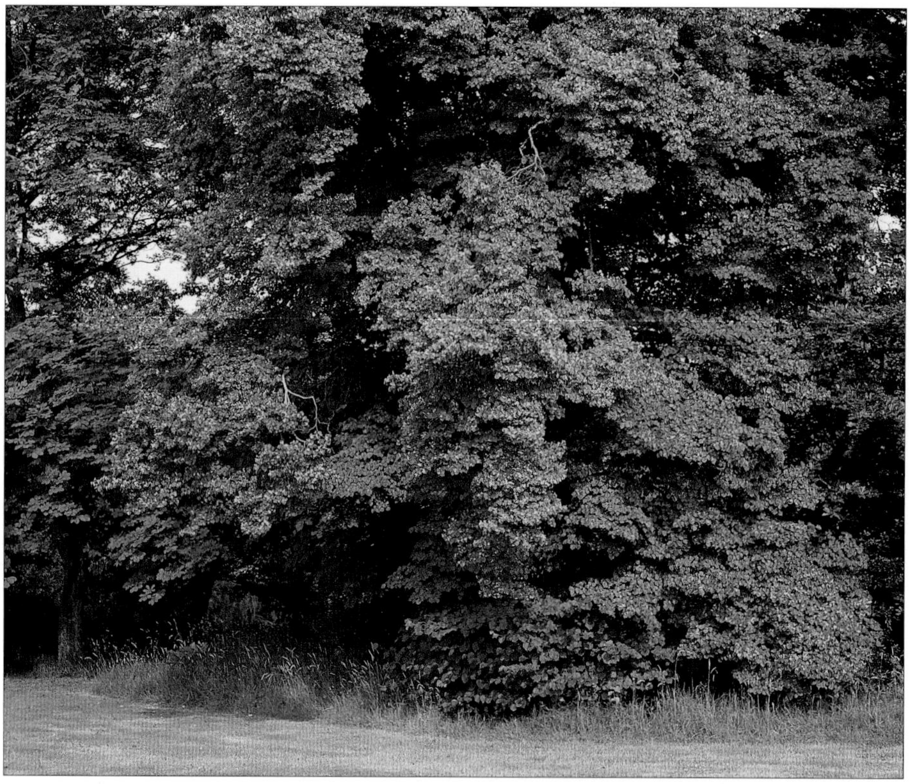

TILIACEAE

Tilia cordata

Lime

History and traditions Linden tea, made from the flowers of *T. cordata*, has always been popular in Europe, especially in France, where it is called "tilleul" – as a soothing drink and for its medicinal properties. An infusion of the leaves as a complexion wash is an old prescription for a "fair" skin. The tree has been valued over the centuries for its many economic uses. The white, close-grained wood was used to make household articles, piano keys and carvings (notably by Grinling Gibbons, 1648–1721, at Windsor Castle and Chatsworth House, England). The inner bark produced fibre for matting and baskets; the sap provided a sweetener and the foliage animal fodder.

Description A hardy, deciduous tree, to 25m/82ft in height, with a large rounded crown, it has smooth, silver-grey bark and heart-shaped leaves, dark green above and greyish below. The five-petalled, fluffy, pale yellow flowers have a honey scent and appear in clusters in midsummer, followed by globe-shaped fruits.

Related species *T. cordata* is the small-leaved lime. Flowers of *T. platyphyllos*, the large-leaved lime, and of hybrids, such as *T.* x *europaea*, are also collected for tea. *T. tomentosa* (silver lime) and *T. americana* (American lime) do not have the same concentrations of active principles.

Habitat/distribution *T. cordata* occurs in Europe and western Asia.

Growth Prefers moist, well-drained soil in full sun or partial shade. Propagated from seed, which needs a long period of stratification (at least three months) to germinate.

Parts used Flowers – collected when they first open and dried for teas.

USES Medicinal A soothing herb, which increases perspiration and is said to help lower blood pressure, the flowers are taken as an infusion, often sweetened with honey and flavoured with lemon, for colds, catarrh and feverish illnesses, for anxiety and as a digestive.

Other name Linden.

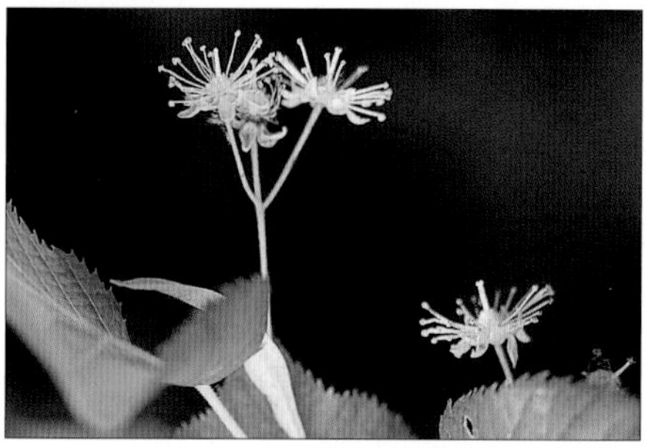

Above *The flowers of* Tilia cordata, *the small-leaved lime, are collected for tea.*

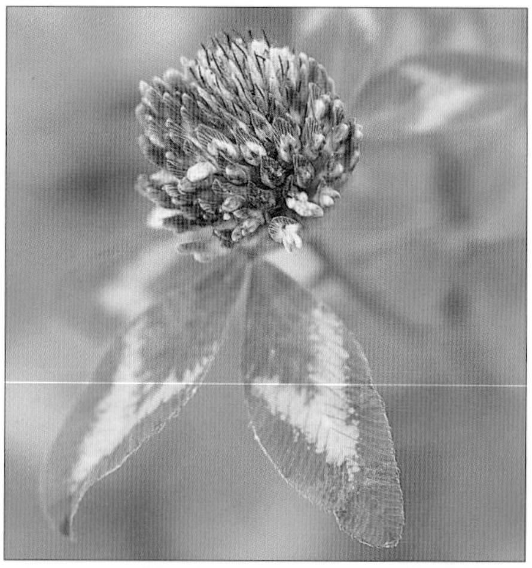

LEGUMINOSAE/PAPILIONACEAE

Trifolium pratense

Red clover

History and traditions Red clover has been an important agricultural and animal fodder crop since ancient times. But it was seldom used medicinally until its early introduction to the United States, where Native American tribes discovered its therapeutic properties. They used it to treat cancerous tumours and skin complaints, took it during pregnancy and childbirth and as a general purification for bodily systems. It found its way into British herbal medicine sometime during the 19th century.

Description A short-lived perennial, it is decumbent to erect, 20–60cm/8in–2ft in height. The leaves are trifoliate and the flowers rose purple to white.

Habitat/distribution It is native to Europe, found across Asia to Afghanistan, and naturalized in North America and Australia.

Growth It requires moist, well-drained soil and is propagated from seed.

Parts used Flowering tops.

USES Medicinal Red clover blossoms are taken internally for skin complaints such as eczema and psoriasis, and applied externally for ulcers, sores and burns. Infusions were at one time thought to be helpful for bronchial complaints and the herb is also said to be effective in balancing blood sugar levels. Clinical research shows red clover can be as effective as HRT for some individuals.

CAUTION Not to be taken in pregnancy or while breast-feeding. Can cause allergy.

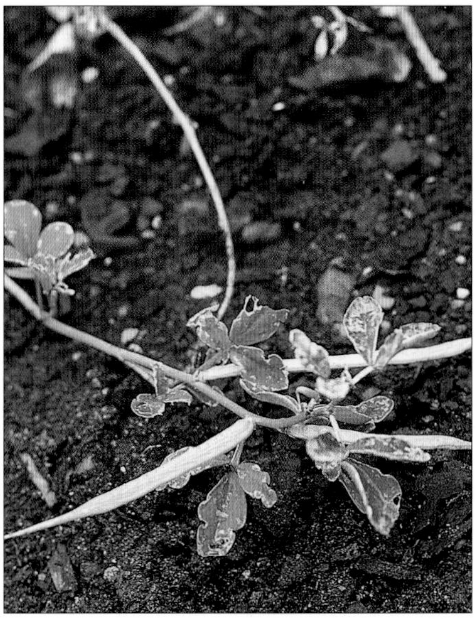

LEGUMINOSAE/PAPILIONACEAE

Trigonella foenum-graecum

Fenugreek

History and traditions A herb with an ancient history, fenugreek has been cultivated since the time of the Assyrians and its seeds were found in Tutankhamun's tomb, c.1325BC. In Europe it was one of the many herbs promoted by the Emperor Charlemagne, c. AD742–814, and the seeds were sold for medicinal uses by the 16th- and 17th-century druggists and apothecaries. In Chinese medicine they have a history as a tonic and in Ayurvedic medicine are renowned for their exceptional ability to cleanse the system of impurities. They also have a reputation as an aphrodisiac. *Trigonella*, meaning triangle, refers to the leaf shape and the specific name, *foenum-graecum*, translates as "Greek hay", a reference to its long use as horse fodder. In recent times it has aroused interest for components of the seeds: the alkaloid, trigonelline, for its anti-cancer potential and a steroidal saponin diosgenin for its contraceptive effects.

Description A hardy annual, 60cm/2ft tall, it has an erect, branched stem and trifoliate leaves. Pale yellow pea-flowers appear in the upper leaf axils in summer followed by the fruit, a curved pod with a pointed "beak", containing up to 20 light brown, aromatic seeds.

Habitat/distribution Native to southern Europe and Asia, widely cultivated in the Middle East, India and northern Africa.

Growth Grow fenugreek in well-drained, fertile soil in a sunny position. Propagated by seed, sown in spring.

Parts used Leaves – fresh for culinary use; seeds – dried for cookery or for making infusions, decoctions, powders or extracts.

USES Medicinal The seeds are rich in a softening mucilage and are used in compresses or ointments to ease swellings, inflammations, ulcers and boils. They are taken in infusions to reduce fevers, have digestive properties and are said to rid the body of toxins, dispelling bad breath and body odour. Fenugreek is also thought to control blood sugar levels in cases of diabetes.

Culinary Leaves, which have a high vitamin, mineral and iron content, are cooked as vegetables, mainly in India. Seeds are sprouted as salad vegetables, and used as a flavouring and condiment in northern African, Ethiopian, Middle Eastern, Egyptian and Indian cookery.

CAUTION Only to be taken on medical advice if taking other medication. Can interact with anti-coagulant and diabetes medicines. Can cause gastric upsets.

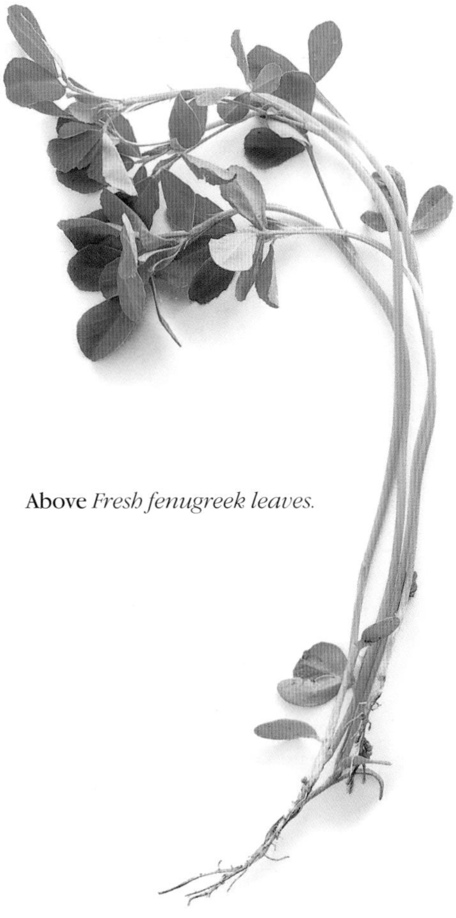

Above *Fresh fenugreek leaves.*

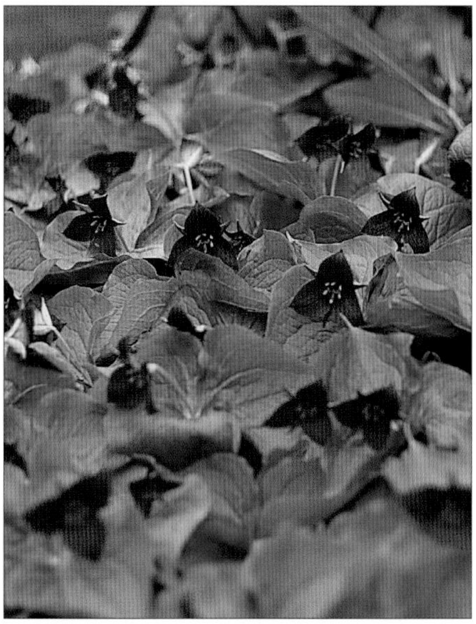

TRILLIACEAE

Trillium erectum

Bethroot

History and traditions Bethroot – the name is a corruption of birthroot – was traditionally used by Native Americans to control bleeding after childbirth and for soothing the sore nipples of nursing mothers. It was taken up by the Shaker community for the same purposes, for easing excessive menstruation and for haemorrhages in general. Sniffing the unpleasant smell of the flowers, which has been likened to rotting meat, was said to stop a nosebleed. The generic name comes from the triple arrangement of all its parts.

Description A variable perennial, 25–38cm/10–15in tall, it has broadly rhomboid three-sectioned leaves and solitary three-petalled flowers, ranging from crimson purple to white.

Habitat/distribution Native to north-eastern North America and the Himalayan region of Asia and found in damp, shady woodland.

Growth Trilliums require moist, humus-rich soil and partial shade. Propagation by division in the dormant period is the easiest method, as growing from seed is slow and erratic.

Parts used Rhizomes – dried for use in decoctions and extracts.

USES Medicinal An antiseptic, astringent herb, it is said to be helpful to the female reproductive system and to control bleeding. Poultices are applied for skin diseases and the roots were at one time boiled in milk to be taken for diarrhoea and dysentery.

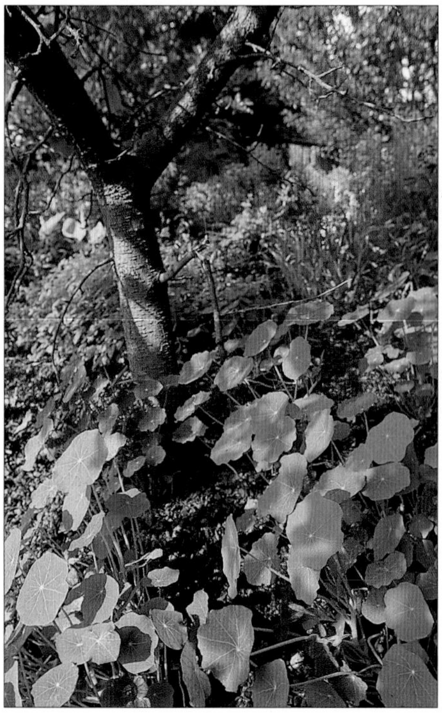

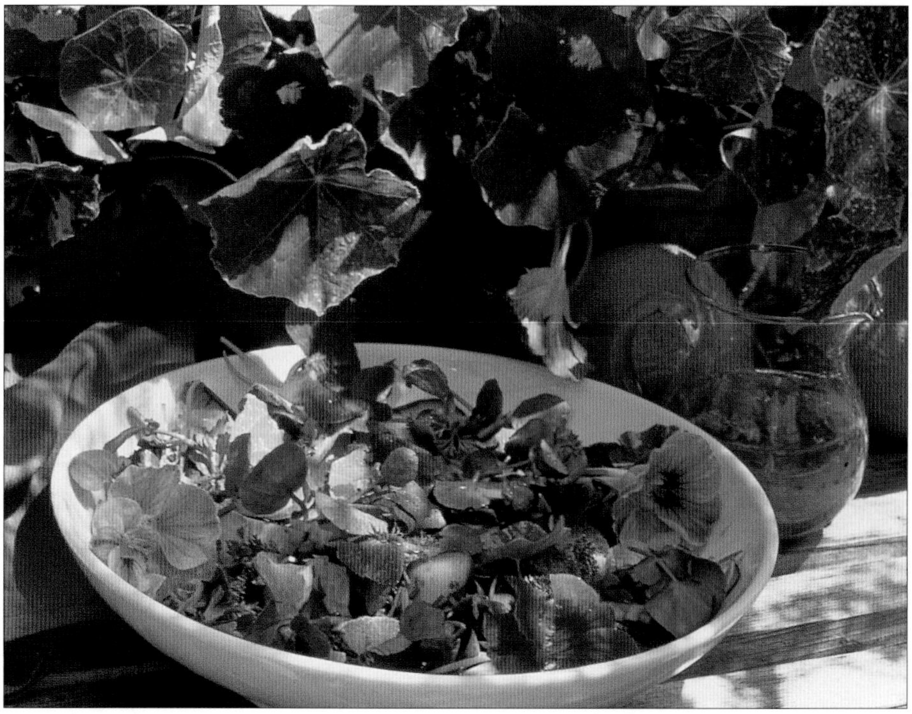

TROPAEOLACEAE

Tropaeolum majus

Nasturtium

History and traditions The garden nasturtium comes from South America. It was introduced to Spain, from Peru, in the 16th century and originally known as *Nasturtium indicum*, or Indian cress, for the spicy flavour of its leaves. Leaves and flowers were popular 17th-century salad ingredients. As nasturtiums are high in vitamin C, they were useful for preventing scurvy. The generic name *Tropaeolum* comes from *tropalon*, the Greek word for a trophy, as the round leaves were thought to resemble the trophy-bearing shields of the classical world.

Description In South America it is a perennial, but in Europe and cool temperate regions it is a half-hardy annual. It has trailing stems, to about 3m/10ft, and circular leaves with a radiating pattern of veins. The yellow or orange flowers grow on stalks arising singly from the leaf axils, and have prominently spurred calyces. They are followed by the globular fruits. There are many low-growing and climbing cultivars.

Habitat/distribution Native to South America, now widely grown throughout the world.

Growth Grow in relatively poor soil for the best production of flowers, but supply plenty of moisture. Easily propagated from seed sown in containers, or *in situ*, in spring.

Parts used Leaves, flowers, seeds – used fresh.

USES Medicinal The seeds have antiseptic, antibacterial properties and are taken in infusions for urinary and upper respiratory tract infections.

Culinary The leaves are added to salads for their peppery taste and the flowers for their colour. Flowers are also used as a flavouring for vinegar. Seeds, when still green, are pickled as a substitute for capers.

Other name Indian cress.

Above *The flowers and leaves make colourful and nutritious additions to a summer salad.*

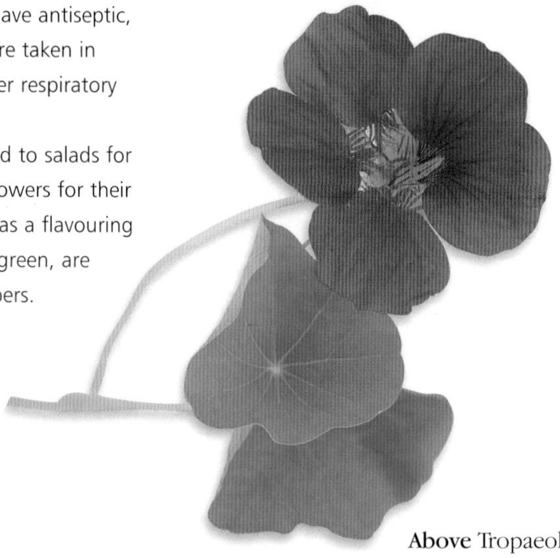

Above Tropaeolum majus

An old recipe for pickled nasturtium seeds

Gather your little knobs quickly after your blossoms are off; put them in cold water and salt for three days, shifting them once a day; then make a pickle (but do not boil it at all) of some white wine, shallot, horse-radish, pepper, salt, cloves, and mace whole and nutmeg quartered; then put in your seeds and stop them close; they are to be eaten as capers.

The Complete Housewife, 1736.

A simple modern version

Collect the nasturtium seeds while they are still green, until you have about 50g/2oz. Stir 25g/1oz salt into 300ml/½ pint/1¼ cups water, add the nasturtium seeds and leave for 24 hours. Then strain them and rinse well in fresh water. Put the seeds into a jar with a muslin bag filled with mixed pickling spice, top up with malt vinegar and seal with an airtight lid. Leave for 3–4 weeks before eating.

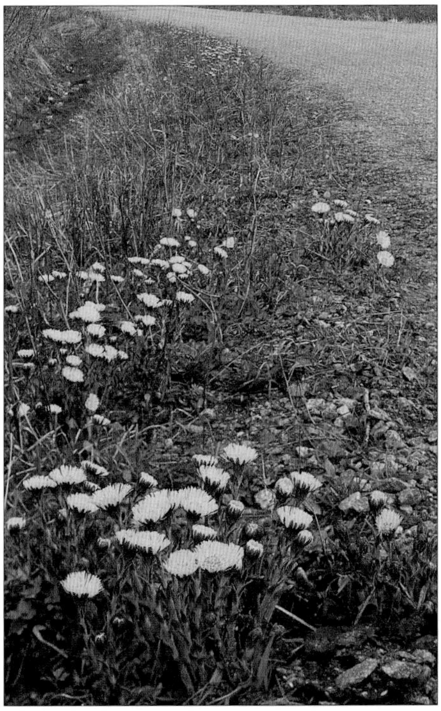

COMPOSITAE/ASTERACEAE

Tussilago farfara

Coltsfoot

History and traditions Known since the days of Dioscorides and Pliny as a herb to relieve coughs, often taken in the form of a smoking mixture, it is still a basic ingredient of herbal tobaccos. The generic name comes from *tussis*, a cough (from which we get the word tussive), and *agere*, to take away. In the Middle Ages it was sometimes known as *Filius ante patrem* (son before father), because the flowers appear before the leaves. Although still used in herbal medicine for cough remedies, recent tests have revealed that it contains low quantities of pyrrolizidine alkaloids, which are carcinogenic in high doses. (Also found in *Symphytum officinale* – comfrey).
Description A small perennial, on a creeping rhizome, 15–20cm/6–8in in height. The bright yellow, dandelion-like flowers, borne singly, appear before the rosette of toothed heart-shaped leaves.
Habitat/distribution Native to Europe, western Asia and northern Africa, introduced elsewhere including North America. Found on roadsides, wastelands, fields and hedgerows, in moist, loamy soil.
Growth It is an invasive plant that needs no cultivation. Propagated from seed or by division.
Parts used Leaves, flowers – fresh or dried.

USES Medicinal Coltsfoot is said to have tonic effects and contain mucilage, which is soothing to the mucous membranes. It is still recommended by herbalists to be taken in infusions for coughs and applied externally as a wash or compress, or as fresh leaves mixed in a paste of honey, for sores, ulcers, skin inflammation and insect bites.
Culinary Traditionally, leaves were added to springtime salads and soups.

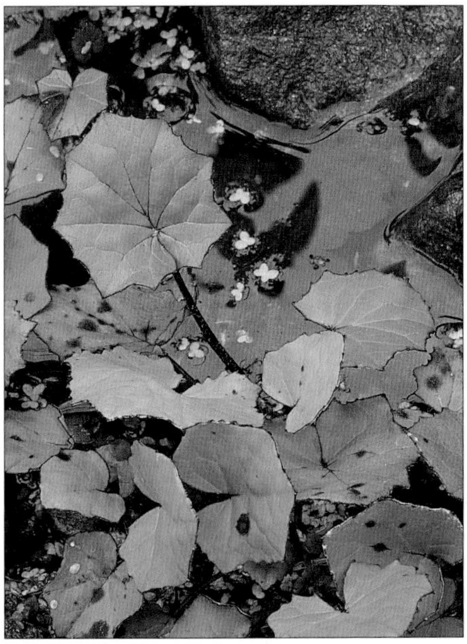

Above *The leaves of* Tussilago farfara *appear after the flowers have faded.*

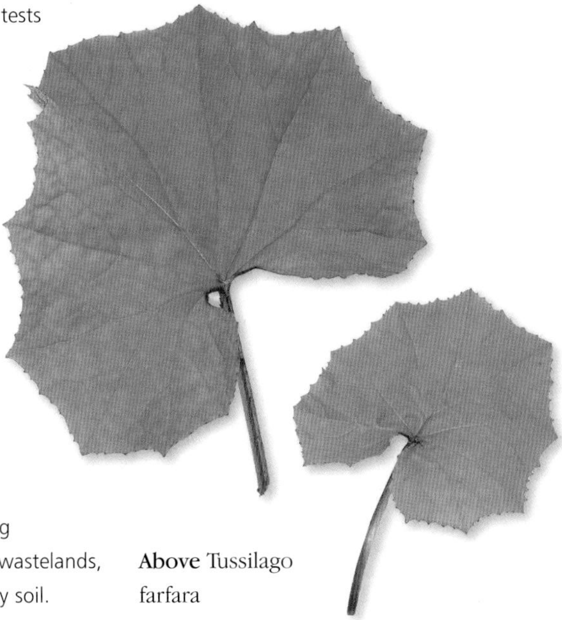

Above Tussilago farfara

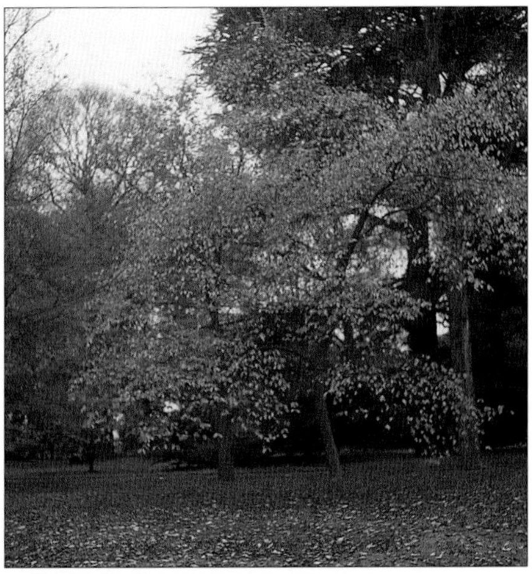

ULMACEAE

Ulmus rubra syn. *Ulmus fulva*

Slippery elm

History and traditions The common name is taken from the slippery texture of the inner bark when moistened. It was a traditional medicine of Native Americans, used mainly for gastric problems and for healing wounds, and was taken up by early settlers, who made the powdered bark into a nutritious gruel for invalids with weak digestions.
Description A deciduous tree 15–20m/50–65ft in height, it has dark brown, rough bark, and obovate, toothed, deeply-veined leaves. Inconspicuous clusters of red-stamened flowers are followed by reddish-brown, winged fruits.
Habitat/distribution Native to eastern and central North America and eastern Canada. It is found in moist woodlands.
Growth This tree grows well in poorish soil and is propagated by seed or cuttings.
Parts used Inner bark – dried and ground into powder. (Bark should not be stripped from wild trees, which are becoming rare, only from those cultivated for the purpose.)
USES Medicinal Rich in mucilage, slippery elm powder is taken for stomach and bowel disorders, gastric ulcers, cystitis and urinary complaints. It is soothing to sore throats and applied in poultices for skin inflammations, boils, abscesses and ulcers and to encourage the healing of wounds.
Other name Red elm.

CAUTION Subject to legal restrictions in some countries. It is now threatened in the wild so only buy from responsible sources.

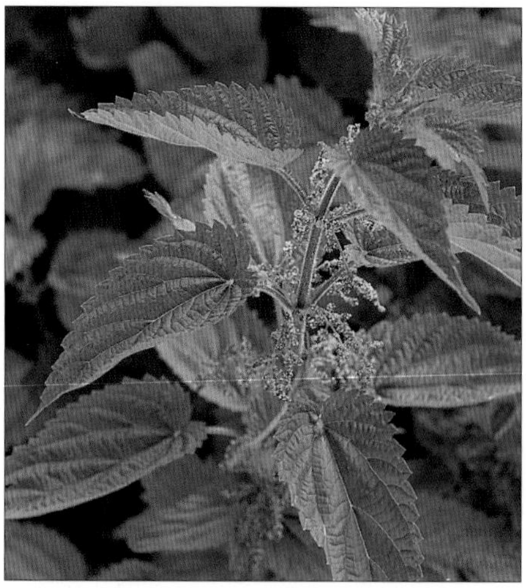

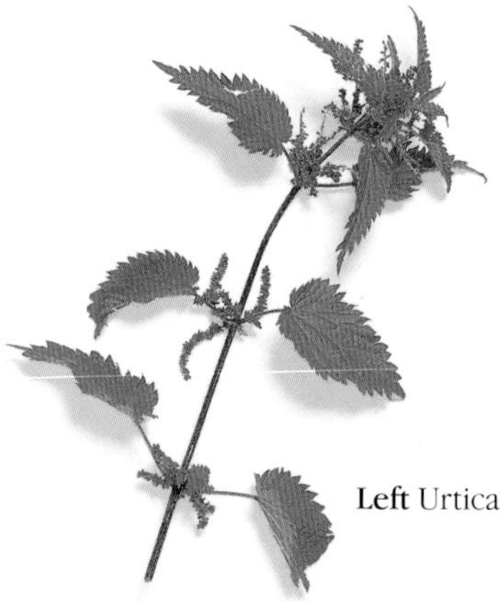

Left Urtica dioica

URTICACEAE

Urtica dioica

Stinging nettle

History and traditions The common stinging nettle may be an unpopular weed, but over the centuries it has been put to many practical uses, remaining an important nutritious and medicinal herb. It was named *Urtica* by Pliny, from *urere*, to burn. Roman legionaries are said to have flailed themselves with nettles against the bone-chilling cold of a northern British winter. They even brought their own seeds, in case no plants grew locally. Whipping with nettles later became an established cure for rheumatism. The nettle was a common source of fibre (similar to that of flax and hemp) in many northern European nations. One of Hans Andersen's fairy-tales tells of the Princess who wove nettle coats for her brothers. Above all, in former times, it made a valuable springtime pot-herb, tonic and antiscorbutic after the deprivations of winter and was made into all manner of soups, puddings and porridges, as well as nettle beer.

Description A tough, spreading perennial, the erect stems grow to 1.5m/5ft tall, on creeping roots. The stems and ovate, toothed, dull green leaves are covered in stinging hairs. Inconspicuous greenish-yellow flowers (male and female on separate plants) appear in mid to late summer.

Related species *U. urens* is a small, annual nettle, found in cool, northern temperate regions. *U. pilulifera* (Roman nettle) originates in southern Europe.

Habitat/distribution Found in waste ground, grassland, field edges, gardens, near human habitation or ruins, in nitrogen-rich soil.

Growth Cultivation is usually unnecessary for domestic use as nettles are plentiful in wild and semi-wild areas and can be invasive in the garden. Grown as a crop they require moist, nitrogen-rich soil. Cut back before flowering to ensure a second crop of young leaves.

Parts used Leaves – harvest in spring, before flowering, fresh for cookery, fresh or dried for infusions, extracts, lotions and ointments. Roots – fresh or dried for decoctions for hair use. Seeds – fresh or dried as a nutritionally dense snack or food seasoning.

USES Medicinal Constituents include histamine and formic acid, which causes the sting. The leaf is rich in vitamins A, B, C, K, iron and other minerals. The high vitamin C content ensures proper absorption of iron and the juice is taken for anaemia. Its diuretic properties help rid the body of uric acid and it is taken as an infusion for rheumatism, arthritis and gout and can help lower blood pressure. It can be helpful in gynaecological issues to support fatigue from low iron and reduce heavy menstrual bleeding. Nettle leaves can be applied as a compress to help ease pain. Decoctions of the root and leaves are applied for dry scalp, dandruff and eczema. Nettle root is indicated to support enlarged prostate conditions in men.

Culinary Only fresh young leaves should be used, cooked as a spinach-like vegetable or made into soup. Leaves should not be eaten raw as they are highly irritating in this state.

CAUTION May cause hypersensitivity or allergy response in some individuals. Start using in small dosages if you are susceptible to allergies.

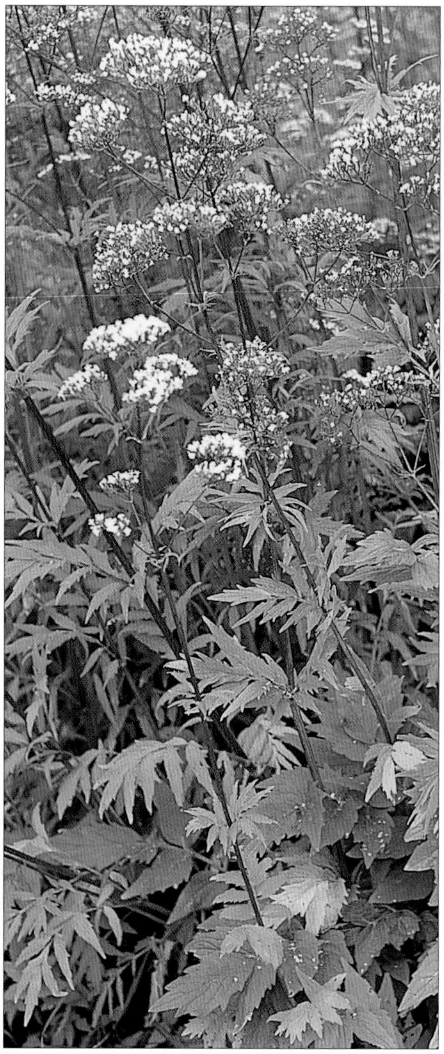

VALERIANACEAE

Valeriana officinalis

Valerian

History and traditions This is thought to be the same plant known to the medical authorities of ancient Greece as *phu*, for the offensive odour of its roots, and recommended by them for its diuretic properties. The name *Valeriana* dates from about the 10th century and is said to be from the Latin *valere*, to be in good health. It was promoted by the Arabian physicians of this era, appears in Anglo-Saxon leech-books of the 11th century and became known in medieval Europe as "All-heal" for its supposed therapeutic powers. It was appreciated as a perfume in the 16th century and Turner's *Herbal*, 1568, describes laying the aromatic dried roots among linen. In fact it has a musky scent, similar to *Nardostachys jatamansi* (once classified as a valerian), and the essential oil is a perfumery ingredient to this day. It is

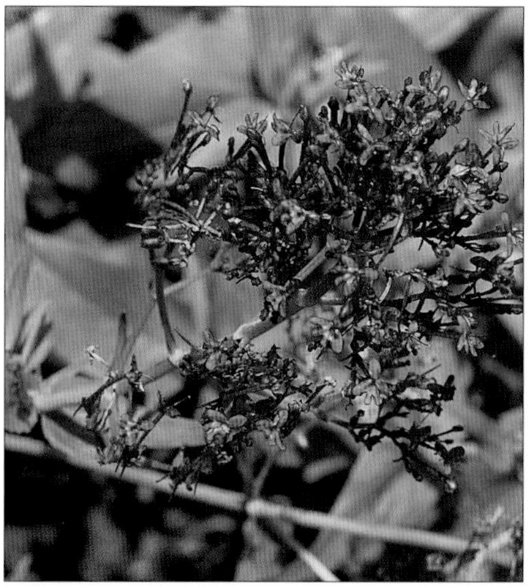

Above *Flowers of* Centranthus ruber.

also attractive to cats and rats.
Description A tall, hardy perennial, growing to 1.5m/5ft, it has grooved stems and pinnate leaves with lanceolate, toothed leaflets. The white, sometimes pinkish, flowers are borne in terminal clusters in summer. *V. officinalis* should not be confused with red valerian, *Centranthus ruber*, which has no medicinal value, but is grown as a herb garden ornamental.
Habitat/distribution Native to Europe and western Asia, introduced to many temperate regions and naturalized in North America. Found in damp meadows and ditches, often near streams.
Growth Grow in damp, fertile soil in a sunny position. Propagated by seed sown in spring, or by division in spring or autumn. It is inclined to be invasive.
Parts used Roots – dried for use in decoctions, medicinal preparations and extracts; essential oil – distilled from roots.

USES Medicinal It has sedative properties and is taken as a tea for insomnia, nervous tension, anxiety, headaches and indigestion. Also said to lower blood pressure.
Aromatic The essential oil is used in perfumery, and extracts as a flavouring in the food industry.

> **CAUTION** Only to be taken on medical advice if on other medication. Can interact with epilepsy drugs. Excess doses are harmful and may cause headaches or a racing heart. Should not be taken long term or where there is liver disease.

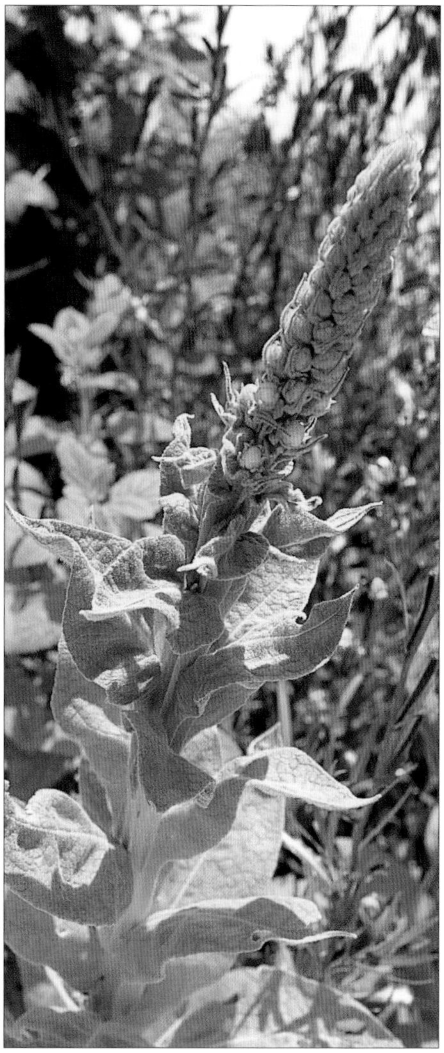

SCROPHULARIACEAE

Verbascum thapsus

Mullein

History and traditions "Candlewick plant" and "hag's taper" are two of the many country names for this plant and refer to its former use, when dried, as a lamp wick or taper. The tall flower spires also look like giant candles, as described by Henry Lyte: "the whole toppe, with its pleasant yellow floures sheweth like to a wax candle or taper cunningly wrought" (*The Niewe Herball*, 1578). As a medicinal herb, it was taken for colds, in the form of "mullein tea", as indeed it still is, and was sometimes smoked as a tobacco for coughs and asthma (which must have made things worse). It also made a yellow hair dye. Throughout Europe and Asia mullein had an ancient reputation as a magic plant, capable of driving away evil spirits.
Description A tall, hardy biennial, growing to 2m/6ft, it has a basal rosette of soft, downy, blue-grey leaves, broadly ovate in shape, in the first year. Yellow flowers are borne on tall spikes in the second year.
Habitat/distribution Native to Europe, Asia and northern Africa, found on shallow, stony soils in grassland and wasteland.
Growth Thrives in dry, stony or gravelly soil and a sunny position. Propagated by seed sown in autumn. Often self-seeds.
Parts used Leaves – dried for use in infusions and liquid extracts; flowers – fresh or dried for infusions. Preparations must be carefully strained to eliminate irritating fine particles.
USES Medicinal It has antiseptic properties and is rich in soothing mucilage. Its main use is for coughs, colds, influenza and respiratory infections, when it is taken as an infusion.
It is sometimes recommended for colic, digestive upsets, nervous tension and insomnia. An infused oil, made of the flowers, has been applied to sores, chapped skin and to relieve earache.
Other name Aaron's rod.

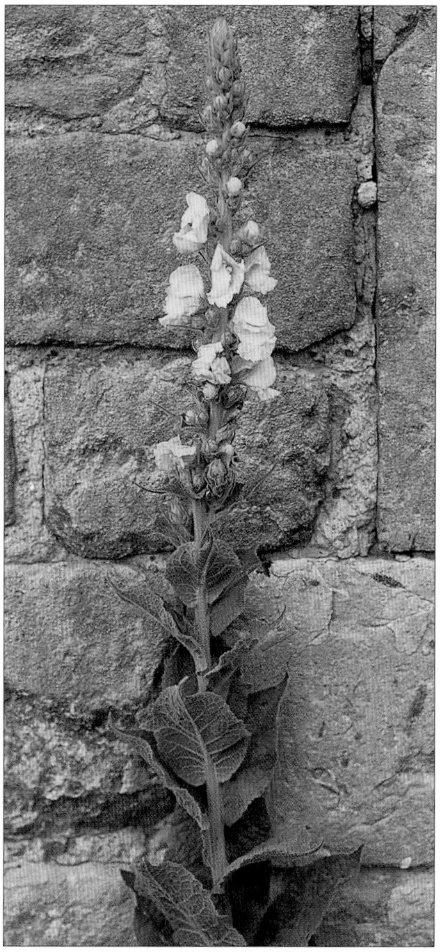

Above *The tall flower spikes of* Verbascum thapsus *appear in the second year.*

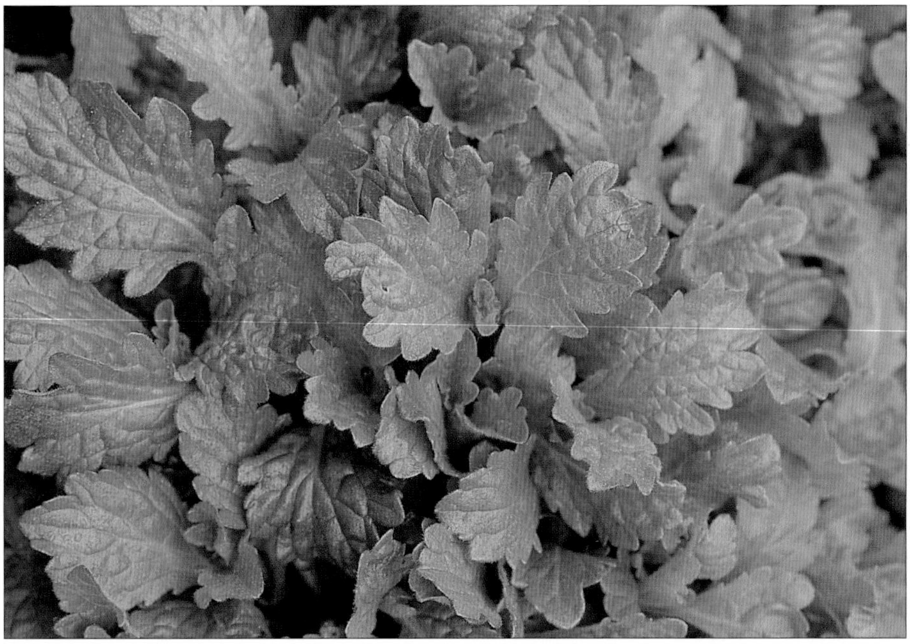

VERBENACEAE

Verbena officinalis

Vervain

History and traditions This unspectacular plant has a long history as a magical herb of exceptional powers and features widely in the folklore of Celtic and northern European cultures. It was venerated by the Romans, who scattered it on their temple altars and whose soldiers carried sprigs to protect them. A story began that it grew at the site of Christ's crucifixion and was used to staunch his wounds on the cross. It was called *herba sacra*, a holy herb, when used in religious ceremonies, and *herba veneris* for its supposed aphrodisiac powers. In Anglo-Saxon and medieval times it was worn as an amulet to protect against plague, snakebites and evil in general. And, with so much going for it, by the 16th century it became an "official" herb of the apothecaries, used for at least 30 complaints. Although it had largely fallen from favour by the early 19th century, it does have a place in herbal medicine today and in traditional Chinese medicine.
Related species Many of the ornamental verbenas grown in gardens come from Brazil and South America. Others with medicinal properties include a West Indian species and *V. hastata*, with blue flowers, which is indigenous to eastern North America.
Description A hardy, rather straggly perennial, with an erect, branched stem, it has ovate, deeply lobed, sometimes pinnate, leaves, which are dull green and slightly hairy. Small, pale lilac flowers are sparsely arranged in terminal spikes.
Habitat/distribution Native to Europe, western Asia and northern Africa, found in waste places and roadsides, usually in a sheltered, sunny position.
Growth Grow in well-drained but moist soil in full sun. Propagated by seed sown in spring.
Parts used Leaves, flowering stems – dried for use in infusions, ointments, liquid extracts and other medicinal preparations.

USES Medicinal Not to be taken internally without medical advice. Vervain has mildly sedative properties and is taken as infusions for nervous exhaustion, anxiety, insomnia, tension headaches and migraine. Also for disorders associated with the stomach, kidneys, liver and gall bladder. Externally it is used in compresses and lotions for skin complaints and as a gargle for sore gums and mouth ulcers.

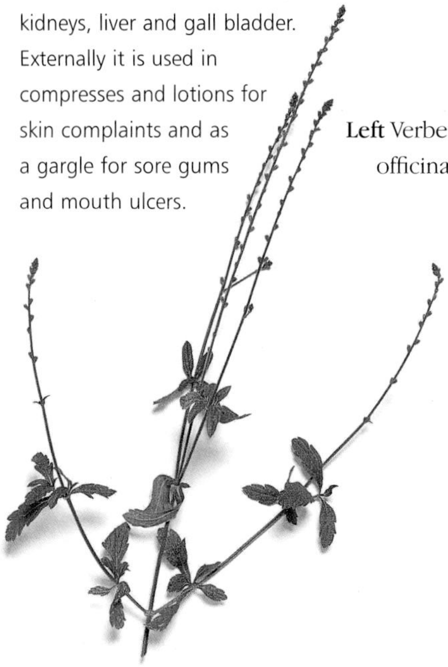

Left *Verbena officinalis*

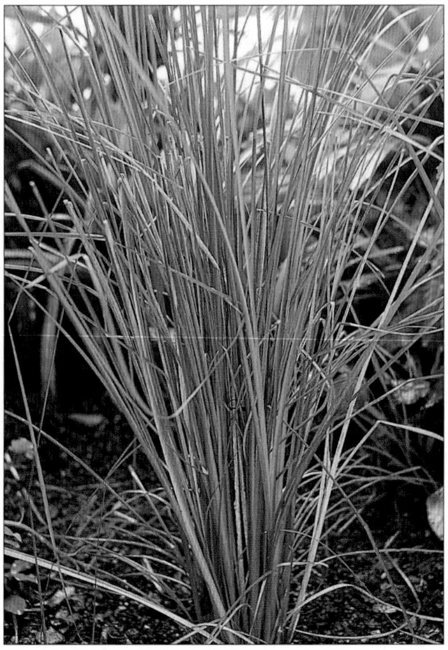

GRAMINEAE/POACEAE

Vetiveria zizanioides

Vetiver

History and traditions A large coarse grass with many economic uses in the East, it was at one time planted on Sri Lankan tea estates to control erosion. An Indian name for it is *khus-khus*, and it has been used since the time of the Moghul Emperors to make scented screens, popularly known as "*khus-khus* tatties" which were sprinkled with water to keep buildings cool before the days of air conditioning, and which deterred insects as well. It is now widely cultivated for the volatile oil contained in its roots, especially in Réunion, which produces more than 35 tons annually.
Description A clump-forming grass, which grows to about 1.5m/5ft, with aromatic, rhizomatous roots, it has linear spears of leaves and brownish flowers produced on long stalks.
Habitat/distribution Grows wild in tropical Asia, eastern Africa and Central America and is widely cultivated there as well; also in Java, Réunion, the Seychelles, New Guinea and Brazil.
Growth A tender, tropical plant. Propagated by division or layering.
Parts used Roots – distilled for essential oil.

USES Aromatic The essential oil has a woody, musky odour, is strongly insect-repellent and antiseptic, and has sedative properties. It is used as a fixative for perfumes and as an ingredient of soaps and cosmetics.

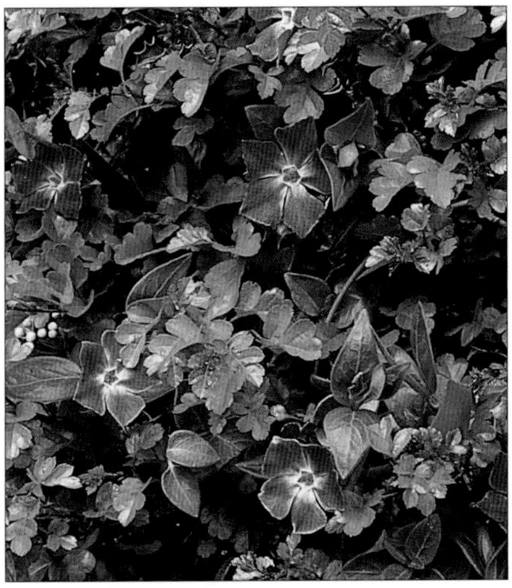

Left Vinca major *produces bright blue flowers in early spring.*

Right Viola tricolor *(heartsease or wild pansy) has some medicinal value, but the flowers are not scented.*

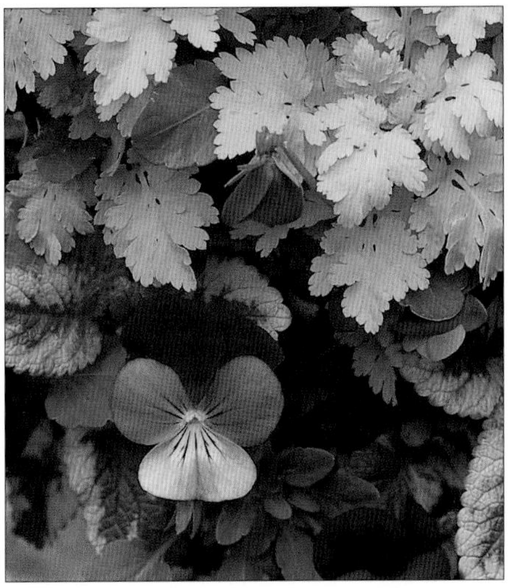

APOCYNACEAE

Vinca major

Greater periwinkle

History and traditions The periwinkle was woven into garlands in ancient Greece and Rome to decorate rooms, or to wear at celebratory banquets. An old name for it is "sorcerer's violet" and it has a long tradition in early herbal literature as an anti-witchcraft herb. *Macer's Herbal*, dating from the 11th century, writes of its power against "wykked spirits", and the *Herbal of Apuleius* recommends it "against devil sickness and demoniacal possession". The always imaginative 14th-century *Boke of Secrets of Albertus Magnus* tells of a recipe for wrapping it in earthworms, reducing it to a powder and mixing it with houseleek, to be eaten with a meal for inducing love. In European cultures it has variously been seen as a flower of death, of immortality and of friendship. The generic term *Vinca* is from the Latin, *vincire*, to bind, a reference to the plant's twining stems. The name periwinkle is derived from the full Latin version of the name, *pervinca*.

Description A trailing evergreen perennial, to 45cm/18in, it has prostrate stems which root at the nodes, and glossy, ovate, dark green leaves. Five-petalled, violet-blue flowers appear in the axils of the upper leaves in summer.

Related species *V. minor* is quite similar in appearance, but lower-growing and with smaller flowers; it also has similar medicinal properties. The Madagascan periwinkle, *Catharanthus roseus*, formerly *Vinca rosea*, contains the toxic alkaloids vincristine and vinblastine. These are isolated to make drugs used in the treatment of certain cancers.

Habitat/distribution Periwinkle is native to Europe, found on loamy calcareous (alkaline) soils, often in woodland.

Growth Tolerates dry conditions, but prefers moist soil and shade or partial shade. .

Parts used Leaves, flowering stems – processed for extraction of alkaloids.

USES Medicinal Both *V. major* and *V. minor* contain the alkaloid vincamine, which dilates blood vessels and reduces blood pressure, and is used in pharmaceutical preparations for cardiovascular disorders. Periwinkle has a long tradition in herbal medicine, particularly in the treatment of diabetes. Today, it is used more of a cerebral tonic and is often combined with ginkgo and rosemary for poor memory and/or disordered thinking.

CAUTION All parts of the plant are poisonous if eaten. Do not take internally or use for self-treatment.

VIOLACEAE

Viola odorata

Sweet violet

History and traditions The Greek word for violet is *io* and in Greek mythology Io, daughter of the King of Argos, was ravished by Zeus and then turned into a heifer so that his wife Hera wouldn't find him out. Violet was the favourite perfume of Josephine and the flowers became the emblem of the Bonapartes after Napoleon became sentimentally attached to them. The violet has long been an emblem of constancy. Many medicinal uses are listed in old herbals and syrup of violets was a gentle laxative.

Description A low-growing, hardy perennial, 15cm/6in tall, with a short rhizome and creeping stolons that root at the tips. The toothed, heart-shaped leaves form a basal rosette from which the solitary, drooping, purple or white flowers arise on long stalks, in spring.

Related species *V. tricolor*, heartsease, or wild pansy, is a hardy annual or perennial, which has branched stems and alternately arranged, lobed or toothed, ovate to lanceolate leaves. The flowers, like small pansies, are in combinations of yellow, white, purple or mauve borne on leafless stems sprouting from the leaf axils. Medicinal uses are similar to those of *V. odorata.* Strong doses may cause vomiting and allergic skin reactions. The common dog violet and wood violets are unscented and have no herbal value.

Habitat/distribution Native to Europe, Asia and northern Africa, introduced elsewhere.

Growth Grow in humus-rich, moist but well-drained soil, in sun or partial shade. The easiest method of propagation is by division in autumn. Also grown from seed sown in spring or autumn.

Parts used Flowers – fresh for culinary use; leaves, flowers, rhizomes – fresh or dried for use in infusions and medicinal preparations; essential oil – extracted from flowers.

USES Medicinal A healing, anti-inflammatory herb with expectorant, diuretic properties, it is taken internally as a tea for coughs, colds and rheumatism. Applied externally in compresses and lotions for skin complaints, swellings and ulcers and in gargles for mouth and throat infections. The essential oil is used in aromatherapy. *V. tricolor* is known to be a heart tonic, used to treat high blood pressure, colds and indigestion.

Culinary The flowers are candied, made into jellies, jams, conserves and vinegars, or added fresh to salads and desserts.

Aromatic The essential oil is used in perfumery.

CAUTION Not to be taken in pregnancy. *Viola tricolor* is toxic in high doses.

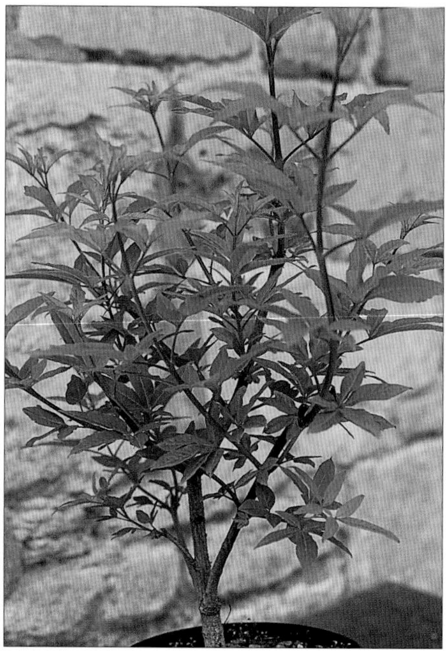

VERBENACEAE

Vitex agnus-castus

Chaste tree

History and traditions The association of this tree with chastity probably stems from its former use as a pepper substitute (made from the dried, powdered fruits) said to have been served in monasteries to suppress libido. It was used in earlier times to relieve aches and pains.
Description A hardy deciduous shrub or small tree, to 5m/16ft tall, it has palmate leaves, dull green on the upper surfaces, downy and greyish beneath, with long spikes of fragrant lilac flowers in summer, followed by small black fruits.
Habitat/distribution Originates in southern Europe and western Asia, also found in North and South America. Found on dry coastal sites.
Growth Grows in most soils and tolerates dry conditions. Propagated by seed or by semi-ripe cuttings taken in summer.
Parts used Fruits.

USES Medicinal Traditionally used for gynaecological complaints, chaste tree has also been researched for treating menstrual problems.

CAUTION Only to be taken on medical advice if on other medication. Can interact with other drugs, especially the contraceptive pill, HRT and fertility treatment. Not to be taken in pregnancy. May cause headaches, dizziness and gastric upsets.

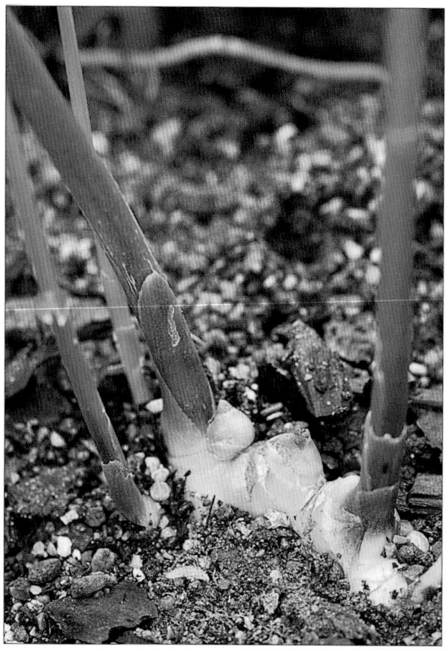

ZINGIBERACEAE

Zingiber officinale

Ginger

History and traditions Ginger has been known in China and India since earliest times, valued for its medicinal properties and as a potent culinary flavouring. It was imported by the Greeks and Romans from the East. During the Middle Ages it was an important trading commodity, appearing on import-duty tariffs at European ports from 1170 onwards. It is frequently referred to in Anglo-Saxon leech-books, and in the 13th and 14th centuries it was second only to pepper as an imported spice. At the start of the 16th century, ginger was taken by the Spaniards from the East Indies to the Americas and West Indies, where it soon became established and was exported to Europe in large quantities. Ginger is one of the most popular culinary flavourings worldwide. It is an important ingredient in Chinese and Ayurvedic medicine, known in the latter as *maha-aushadi*, "the great medicine", and has an eastern tradition as an aphrodisiac, probably because it stimulates circulation and increases blood flow.
Description A perennial reed-like plant, it has thick, branching rhizomes and grows 1–1.2m/3–4ft tall, with bright green, lanceolate, alternately arranged leaves, on short, sheathed stems. The yellow-green flowers are borne in dense cones on separate stalks from the leaves.
Habitat/distribution Native to southeast Asia, introduced and widely grown in tropical zones.

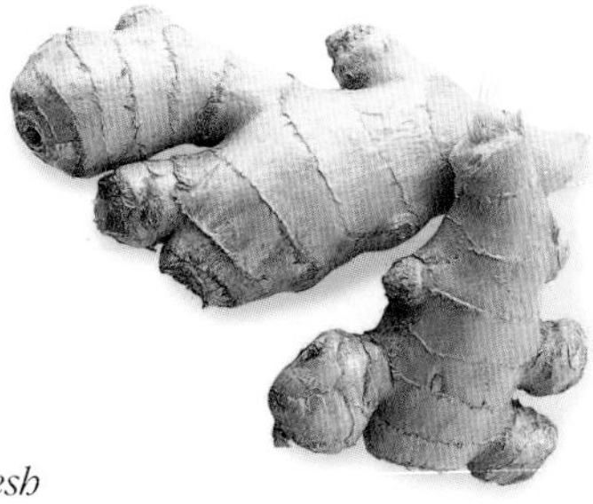

Right *Fresh ginger root and crystallized ginger.*

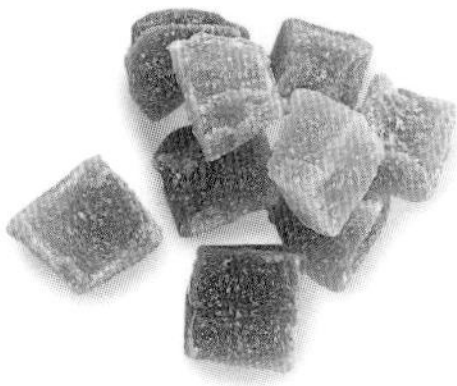

Growth A tender, tropical plant, grown in fertile, humus-rich, well-drained soil with plenty of moisture and humidity. It is usually treated as an annual crop. Propagated by division.
Parts used Rhizomes – fresh, or dried, whole or ground.

USES Medicinal Ginger has antiseptic, expectorant properties, promotes sweating and is taken in decoctions for colds, chills and feverish infections. It is taken in tablet form or as a tincture for nausea, travel sickness, indigestion, stomach upsets and menstrual pain. The essential oil is taken in drops on sugar lumps for fevers, nausea and digestive upsets, and added to massage oil to ease rheumatic pain and aching joints. It reduces wind and enhances peripheral circulation. Clinical trials have shown ginger is as effective as anti-inflammatory pain killers. It is warming and can help ease PMS bloating and menstrual cramps.
Culinary Fresh ginger is grated and added to stir-fry dishes, and widely used, fresh or dried, in Chinese and Thai cuisines. Dried ground ginger is an ingredient of curry powder, pickles and chutneys and used in Western cookery in biscuits, cakes and desserts. Whole fresh ginger is crystallized in sugar syrup and made into chocolates and confectionery.
Aromatic The essential oil is used in perfumery and as a flavouring in the food industry.

CAUTION Not to be taken in pregnancy or if on anti-coagulants without medical supervision. Not to be taken in high doses.

Index

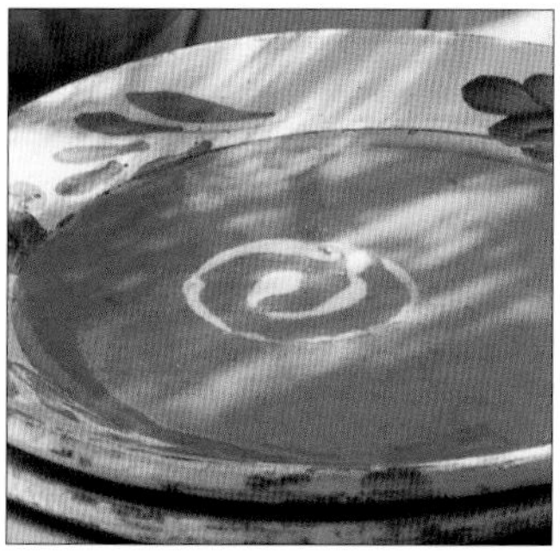

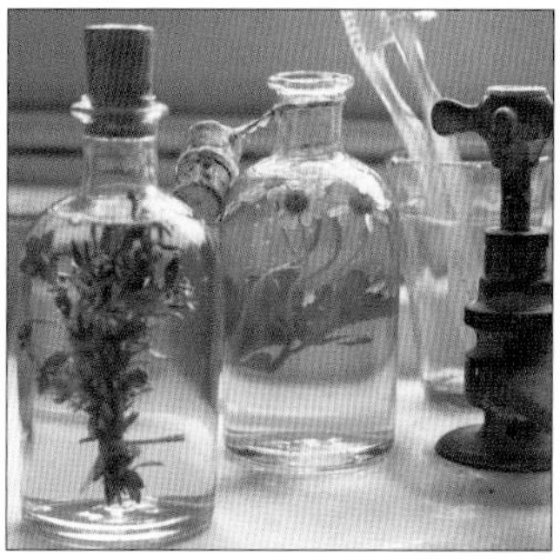

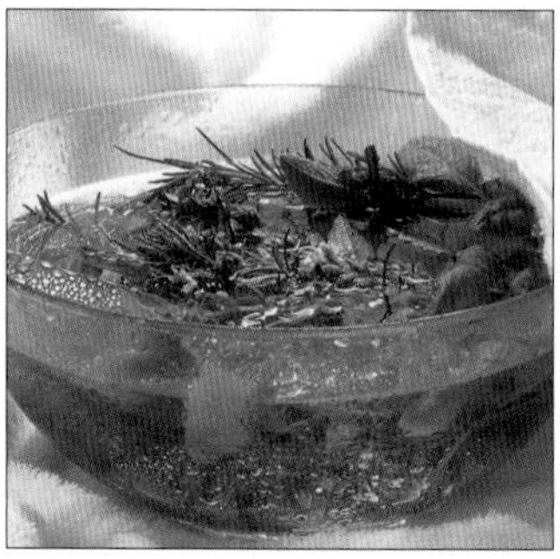

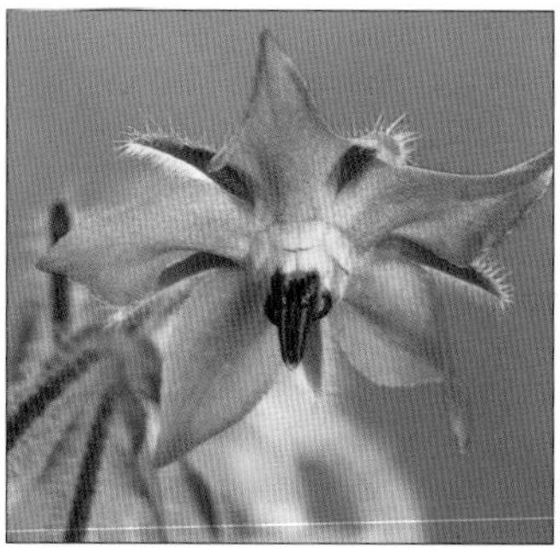

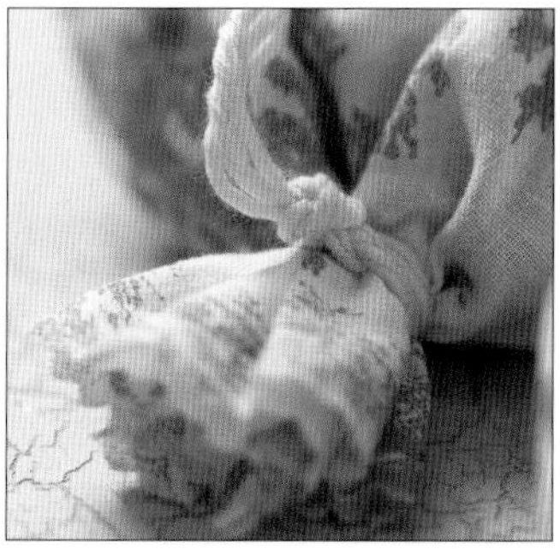

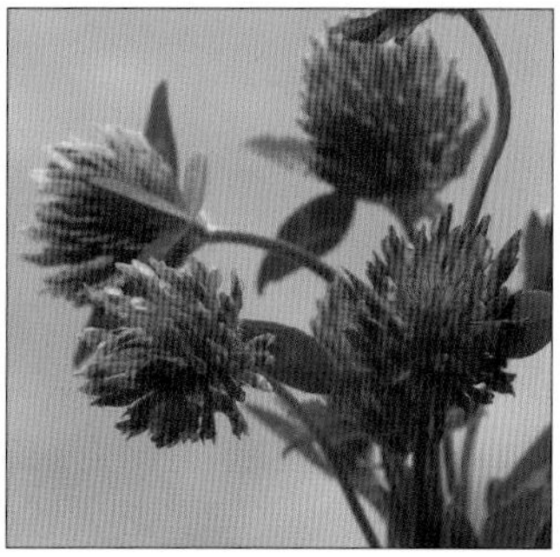

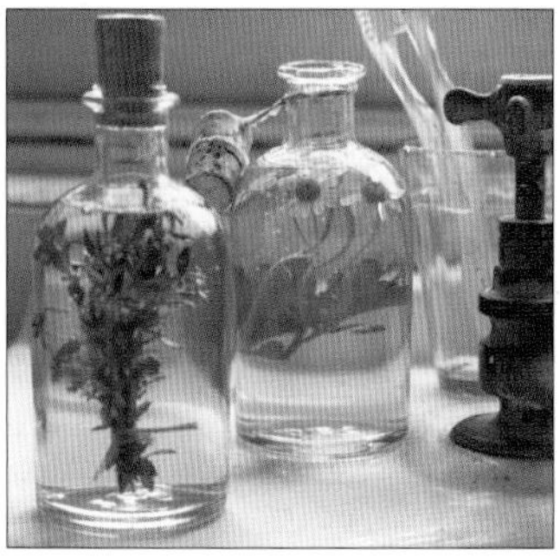

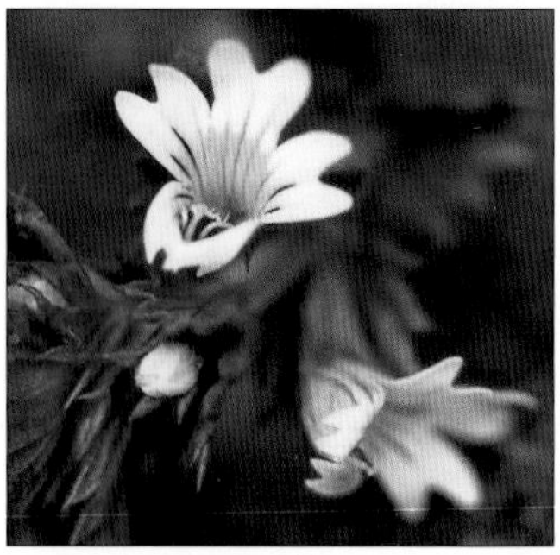

Picture Credits

213tl Alamy; 247tr A–Z Botanical Collection Ltd; 69tc Alamy; 148tr Clive Boursnell; 128tl, 197tl, 204tr Deni Bown; 218cr (Hans Reinhard) Bruce Coleman Ltd; 125br Bob & Clara Calhoun; 150tr Michael R. Chandler; 244tl Anthony Cooper; 161tr Ron Evans; 135tl Vaughn Fleming; 156/7tc Christopher Gallagher; 134cr and br, 161br, 165br, 181br, 183c, 230tr Michelle Garrett; 152tl, 154tr, 168br, 170tl (Dr John Feltwell) Garden & Wildlife Matters; 112tl, 146tr, 157tr John Glover; 135tr Sunniva Harte; 138tl, 146tc, 148tl, 163tr, 206tl, 209bl, 237tl Harry Smith Collection; 109bc, 110tl, 112br, 118tl, 119tl, 120tc, 125bl, 130tl, 131tl, 133tl, 134tl, 137tl, 141tl, 144tl, 155tc, 159bl and tr, 167tc, 168tr, 169tl, 171bc, 176tl, 177tl, 183bc, 193tr, 209tr, 216r, 220tr, 221tl and tr, 225t, 226br, 227tr, 228b, 230tl, 234tl Jessica Houdret; 136tc K. Jayara; 110tr (Brenda Szabo) Kirstenbosch Botanic Garden, South Africa; 156tl Lamontagne; 218tl Harald Lange; 114tr Lucy Mason; 245tr E. Mole; 111tl, 216tl Dr. Eckhart Pott; 206br (Duncan Ross) Poyntzfield Nursery; 139bl Malcolm Richards; 225b (Clive Nichols) The Garden Picture Library; 238tr Adrian Thomas; 135bc, 140tr Brigitte Thomas; 203cl N. Schwihtz; 247tl Bjorn Svensson; 197tc and tr, 203tl Staffen Widstrand

Key: t = top, b = bottom, c = centre, r = right, l = left

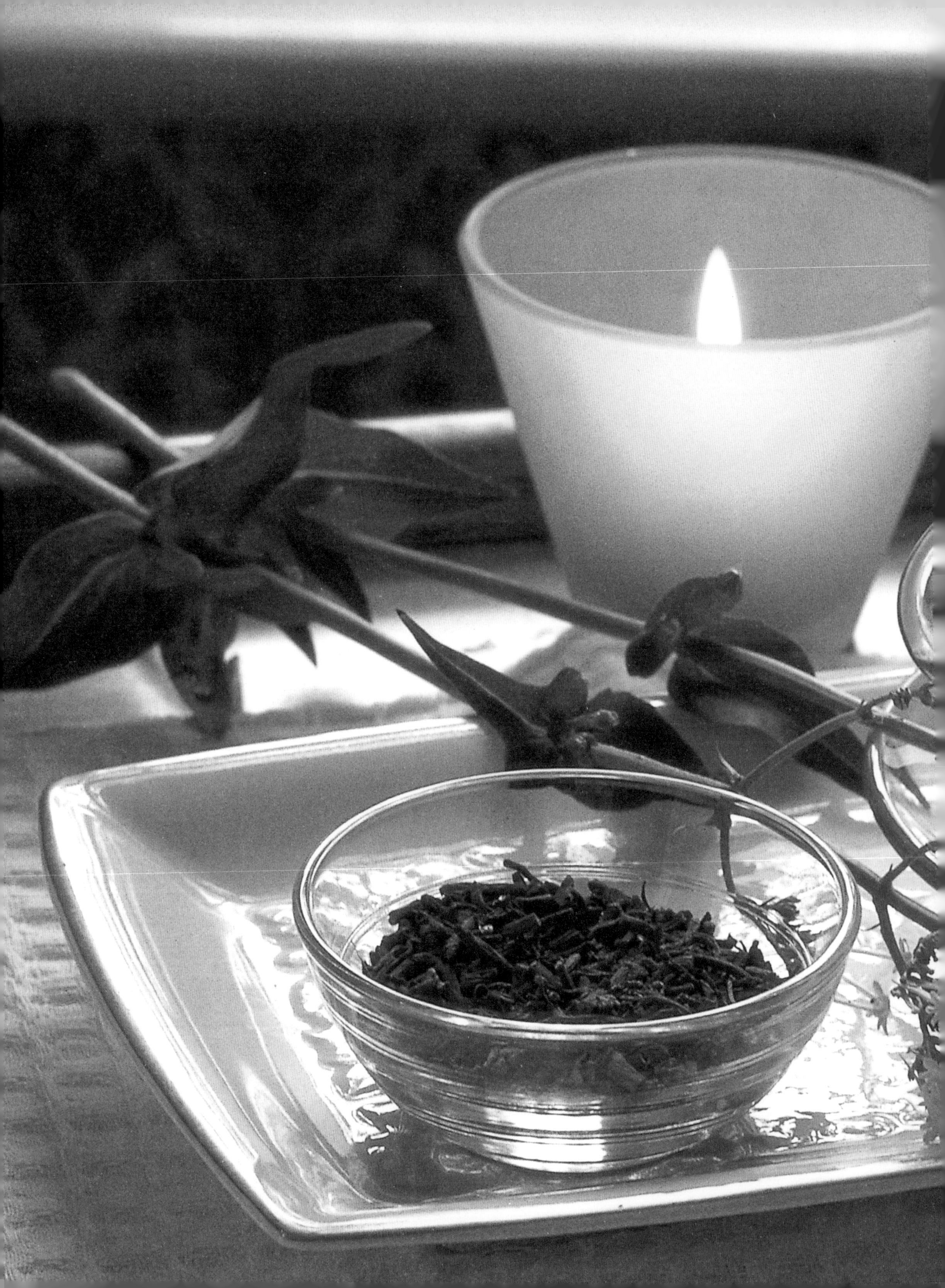